A Clinical Guide to Neurodegeneration

A Clinical Guide to Neurodegeneration

Edited by Antonio Chavez

AMERICAN
MEDICAL PUBLISHERS
www.americanmedicalpublishers.com

American Medical Publishers,
41 Flatbush Avenue,
1st Floor, New York,
NY 11217, USA

Visit us on the World Wide Web at:
www.americanmedicalpublishers.com

ISBN: 978-1-63927-277-8

Cataloging-in-Publication Data

A clinical guide to neurodegeneration / edited by Antonio Chavez.
p. cm.
Includes bibliographical references and index.
ISBN 978-1-63927-277-8
1. Nervous system--Degeneration--Treatment. 2. Nervous system--Degeneration--Treatment--Guidebooks.
3. Nervous system--Diseases--Treatment--Guidebooks. 4. Degeneration (Pathology). I. Chavez, Antonio.
RC394 .D35 C55 2021
616.8--dc23

Table of Contents

Preface VII

Chapter 1 **Cytoplasmic mislocalization of RNA splicing factors and aberrant neuronal gene splicing in TDP-43 transgenic pig brain** 1
Guohao Wang, Huaqiang Yang, Sen Yan, Chuan-En Wang, Xudong Liu, Bentian Zhao, Zhen Ouyang, Peng Yin, Zhaoming Liu, Yu Zhao, Tao Liu, Nana Fan, Lin Guo, Shihua Li, Xiao-Jiang Li and Liangxue Lai

Chapter 2 **The heat shock response in neurons and astroglia and its role in neurodegenerative diseases** 21
Rebecca San Gil, Lezanne Ooi, Justin J. Yerbury and Heath Ecroyd

Chapter 3 **Whole blood gene expression and white matter Hyperintensities** 41
Honghuang Lin, Claudia Satizabal, Zhijun Xie, Qiong Yang, Tianxiao Huan, Roby Joehanes, Chengping Wen, Peter J. Munson, Alexa Beiser, Daniel Levy and Sudha Seshadri

Chapter 4 **Together JUN and DDIT3 (CHOP) control retinal ganglion cell death after axonal injury** 51
Stephanie B. Syc-Mazurek, Kimberly A. Fernandes, Michael P. Wilson, Peter Shrager and Richard T. Libby

Chapter 5 **YKL-40 in the brain and cerebrospinal fluid of neurodegenerative dementias** 64
Franc Llorens, Katrin Thüne, Waqas Tahir, Eirini Kanata, Daniela Diaz-Lucena, Konstantinos Xanthopoulos, Eleni Kovatsi, Catharina Pleschka, Paula Garcia-Esparcia, Matthias Schmitz, Duru Ozbay, Susana Correia, Ângela Correia, Ira Milosevic, Olivier Andréoletti, Natalia Fernández-Borges, Ina M. Vorberg, Markus Glatzel, Theodoros Sklaviadis, Juan Maria Torres, Susanne Krasemann, Raquel Sánchez-Valle, Isidro Ferrer and Inga Zerr

Chapter 6 **Is amyotrophic lateral sclerosis/frontotemporal dementia an autophagy disease?** 85
Zhiqiang Deng, Patricia Sheehan, Shi Chen and Zhenyu Yue

Chapter 7 **Genetic ablation of dynactin p150^{Glued} in postnatal neurons causes preferential degeneration of spinal motor neurons in aged mice** 96
Jia Yu, Chen Lai, Hoon Shim, Chengsong Xie, Lixin Sun, Cai-Xia Long, Jinhui Ding, Yan Li and Huaibin Cai

Chapter 8 **Amyloid-beta modulates microglial responses by binding to the triggering receptor expressed on myeloid cells 2 (TREM2)** 113
Li Zhong, Zongqi Wang, Daxin Wang, Zhe Wang, Yuka A. Martens, Linbei Wu, Ying Xu, Kai Wang, Jianguo Li, Ruizhi Huang, Dan Can, Huaxi Xu, Guojun Bu and Xiao-Fen Chen

Chapter 9 **Apolipoprotein E4 impairs spontaneous blood brain barrier repair following traumatic brain injury**......125
Bevan S. Main, Sonia Villapol, Stephanie S. Sloley, David J. Barton, Maia Parsadanian, Chinyere Agbaegbu, Kathryn Stefos, Mondona S. McCann, Patricia M. Washington, Olga C. Rodriguez and Mark P. Burns

Chapter 10 ***TMEM106B* haplotypes have distinct gene expression patterns in aged brain**......143
Yingxue Ren, Marka van Blitterswijk, Mariet Allen, Minerva M. Carrasquillo, Joseph S. Reddy, Xue Wang, Thomas G. Beach, Dennis W. Dickson, Nilüfer Ertekin-Taner, Yan W. Asmann and Rosa Rademakers

Chapter 11 **Endoplasmic reticulum stress and inflammation in the central nervous system**......153
Neil T. Sprenkle, Savannah G. Sims, Cristina L. Sánchez and Gordon P. Meares

Chapter 12 **Blood cholesterol in late-life and cognitive decline**......170
Chaoran Ma, Zhaoxue Yin, Pengfei Zhu, Jiesi Luo, Xiaoming Shi and Xiang Gao

Chapter 13 **Intrastriatal injection of α-synuclein can lead to widespread synucleinopathy independent of neuroanatomic connectivity**......179
Zachary A. Sorrentino, Mieu M.T. Brooks, Vincent Hudson III, Nicola J. Rutherford, Todd E. Golde, Benoit I. Giasson and Paramita Chakrabarty

Chapter 14 **Glycine-alanine dipeptide repeat protein contributes to toxicity in a zebrafish model of *C9orf72* associated neurodegeneration**......195
Yu Ohki, Andrea Wenninger-Weinzierl, Alexander Hruscha, Kazuhide Asakawa, Koichi Kawakami, Christian Haass, Dieter Edbauer and Bettina Schmid

Permissions

List of Contributors

Index

Preface

Neurodegeneration is a progressive deterioration of the structures and functions of neurons that leads to cognitive disability and dementia. It is an important characteristic of many incurable debilitating diseases such as Alzheimer's disease (AD), Parkinson's disease (PD), Huntington's disease (HD), etc. Neurodegeneration in these conditions manifests in unique ways. In Alzheimer's disease, a loss of neurons and synapses occurs in the cerebral cortex while Parkinson's disease (PD) manifests with cell death in the substantia nigra. Huntington's disease causes loss of medium spiny neurons affecting the striatum, and the frontal and temporal cortices. Aging stands as the major risk factor for such neurodegenerative diseases. This book unravels the recent researches in the field of neurodegeneration. It presents studies performed by experts across the globe. This book attempts to assist those with a goal of delving into the field of neuroscience.

The researches compiled throughout the book are authentic and of high quality, combining several disciplines and from very diverse regions from around the world. Drawing on the contributions of many researchers from diverse countries, the book's objective is to provide the readers with the latest achievements in the area of research. This book will surely be a source of knowledge to all interested and researching the field.

In the end, I would like to express my deep sense of gratitude to all the authors for meeting the set deadlines in completing and submitting their research chapters. I would also like to thank the publisher for the support offered to us throughout the course of the book. Finally, I extend my sincere thanks to my family for being a constant source of inspiration and encouragement.

Editor

1

Cytoplasmic mislocalization of RNA splicing factors and aberrant neuronal gene splicing in TDP-43 transgenic pig brain

Guohao Wang[1,3,4†], Huaqiang Yang[2†], Sen Yan[1,3†], Chuan-En Wang[3], Xudong Liu[1,4], Bentian Zhao[2], Zhen Ouyang[2], Peng Yin[1], Zhaoming Liu[2], Yu Zhao[2], Tao Liu[2], Nana Fan[2], Lin Guo[2], Shihua Li[3], Xiao-Jiang Li[1,3*] and Liangxue Lai[2*]

Abstract

Background: TAR DNA-binding protein 43 (TDP-43) is a nuclear protein, but it is redistributed in the neuronal cytoplasm in both amyotrophic lateral sclerosis (ALS) and frontotemporal lobar degeneration (FTLD). Because small transgenic animal models often lack cytoplasmic TDP-43, how the cytoplasmic accumulation of TDP-43 contributes to these diseases remains unclear. The current study is aimed at studying the mechanism of cytoplasmic pathology of TDP-43.

Results: We established transgenic pigs expressing mutant TDP-43 (M337V). This pig model shows severe phenotypes and early death. We found that transgenic TDP-43 is also distributed in the cytoplasm of neuronal cells in the spinal cord and brain. Transgenic TDP-43 interacts with PSF, an RNA splicing factor that associates with NeuN to regulate neuronal RNA splicing. The interaction of TDP-43, PSF and NeuN causes PSF and NeuN mislocalize into the neuronal cytoplasm in transgenic pigs. Consistently, abnormal PSF-related neuronal RNA splicing is seen in TDP-43 transgenic pigs. The cytoplasmic localization of PSF and NeuN as well as abnormal PSF-related neuronal RNA splicing was also found in ALS patient brains.

Conclusion: Our findings from a large mammalian model suggest that cytoplasmic mutant TDP-43 could reduce the nuclear function of RNA splicing factors, contributing to neuropathology.

Keywords: TDP-43, PSF, NeuN, NMHC II-B, ALS, transgenic Pig

Background

TAR DNA-binding protein 43 (TDP-43) is a multifunctional, nuclear protein that binds RNA to regulate RNA processing, including alternative splicing, miRNA production, and mRNA trafficking and stabilization [1–6]. TDP-43 has two conserved RNA recognition motifs and a C-terminal glycine-rich domain that mediates interactions with other heterogeneous nuclear ribonucleoprotein (hnRNP) family members [7, 8]. Mutations in the C-terminal domain of TDP-43 are associated with both amyotrophic lateral sclerosis (ALS) and frontotemporal lobar degeneration (FTLD) [9–11]. ALS is characterized by progressive degeneration of large motor neurons in the spinal cord and cerebral cortex, and FTLD causes degeneration of neurons in the frontal and temporal cortices. In both diseases, the key pathological change is that pathogenic TDP-43 is accumulated in the cytoplasm and forms cytoplasmic aggregates [12–14]; however, how cytoplasmic mislocalization of TDP-43 contributes to pathogenesis remains to be investigated.

To date, a variety of transgenic TDP-43 animal models have been established and provided us with valuable tools to uncover gene expression alteration and aberrant RNA splicing caused by TDP-43 [5, 7, 15]. Although overexpression of mutant TDP-43 in cultured cells and some rodent models and deletion of the nuclear localization signal in TDP-43 can lead to the cytoplasmic distribution of mutant

* Correspondence: xli2@emory.edu; lai_liangxue@gibh.ac.cn
†Equal contributors
[1]State Key Laboratory of Molecular Developmental Biology, Institute of Genetics and Developmental Biology, Chinese Academy of Sciences, Beijing 100101, China
[2]Key Laboratory of Regenerative Biology, South China Institute for Stem Cell Biology and Regenerative Medicine, Guangzhou Institutes of Biomedicine and Health, Chinese Academy of Sciences, Guangzhou 510530, China
Full list of author information is available at the end of the article

TDP-43, many transgenic TDP-43 mouse models fail to show the cytoplasmic accumulation of mutant TDP-43 [16–24], suggesting that species-dependent differences may account for differential pathology of TDP-43 in small animals and human patients. Given that TDP-43 is a multifunctional nuclear protein whose expression is tightly regulated [25], mutant TDP-43 or altered levels of normal TDP-43 can cause neuropathology. However, because most of current animal models lack the cytoplasmic accumulation of TDP-43, our ability to investigate how the cytoplasmic mislocalization of TDP-43 contributes to the pathogenesis has been limited.

The lack of cytoplasmic mislocalization of TDP-43 in small animals may be due to unknown species differences that regulate the subcellular localization of TDP-43. Because of the greater similarity between pigs and humans, we have used transgenic pigs to investigate the pathology caused by mutant polyglutamine proteins and SOD1 and uncovered unique pathology not seen in small animals [26, 27]. In the current study, we established transgenic miniature pigs expressing mutant TDP-43 and found that transgenic TDP-43 is also distributed in the cytoplasm of neuronal cells and causes severe phenotypes in pigs. Moreover, this new animal model demonstrates that mutant TDP-43 interacts with the RNA splicing factor PSF (Splicing Factor Proline/Glutamine-Rich) and the cytoplasmic localization of PSF as well as reducing nuclear PSF function in RNA splicing. Thus, by establishing a large mammalian model of TDP-43, we provide fresh insight into the role of cytoplasmic mislocalization of mutant TDP-43 in the pathogenesis of ALS and FTLD.

Results

Generation of transgenic pigs expressing mutant TDP-43

There are a number of mutations in human TDP-43, and transgenic expression of wild type human TDP-43 also causes neuropathology in animal models [22, 28]. Considering that generation of transgenic pigs is much more time-consuming and costly than small animal models, we focused on the generation of transgenic pigs expressing human mutant TDP-43 (M337V), but not wild type TDP-43, and compared them with non-transgenic pigs. Using the same somatic cell nuclear transfer (SCNT) approach for generating transgenic pig models of Huntington's disease and ALS [26, 27], we transfected mutant TDP-43 (M337V) in primary pig fetal fibroblasts isolated from 35-day-old Tibetan miniature pig fetus. Mutant TDP-43 is tagged with the flag epitope at its N-terminus and expressed under the control of the human ubiquitin promoter that can drive gene expression ubiquitously, and the transgene also co-expresses EGFP for identifying transfected cells that express TDP-43 (Fig. 1a). The transfected cells expressing TDP-43 were fused to a total of 2270 SCNT embryos, which were transferred into 13 surrogates that exhibited natural estrus. Seven surrogates developed to term and gave birth to 31 healthy Tibetan miniature piglets after 120–130 d of gestation. Of these, 27 piglets were found to be positive for transgenic TDP-43 via PCR (Fig. 1b), as PCR analysis of DNA samples obtained from the ear tissues of piglets showed that the live piglets were positive for the TDP-43 transgene (Fig. 1c).

Newborn transgenic TDP-43 pigs appeared as normal at birth as non-transgenic pigs. However, they started to gain less body weight from 3 months after birth compared to non-transgenic pigs (Fig. 2a and b). The extent of body weight loss appears to be correlated with the expression levels of TDP-43 in pig ear tissues (Fig. 2c). Many transgenic TDP-43 pigs die earlier starting at the age of 4–5 months, and 85 % (21/27) of the TDP-43 transgenic pigs died within one year (Fig. 2d). As a result of gaining considerable less body weight during development, the transgenic TDP-43 pigs often displayed loose skin characterized by wrinkled and sagging skin on their bodies (Fig. 2e). We previously established ALS pigs expressing mutant SOD1, which grew normally without body weight loss but showed an obvious running defect on a treadmill [27]. Like these ALS transgenic pigs, the TDP-43 transgenic pigs also showed progressive weakness and limb movement defects (Fig. 2f). However, following the training for the treadmill test, some TDP-43 pigs died, which did not allow us to use the treadmill to obtain quantified data of the limb movement impairment for TDP-43 pigs. Therefore, we used the surviving TDP-43 pigs, not including those that died right after treadmill test, to assess the growth, life span, and motor deficit of TDP-43 pigs. We found that there was the progressive reduction in the body weight and that transgenic TDP-43 pigs died earlier than non-transgenic pigs. The shorter life span and the more severe motor deficit in TDP-43 pigs than those of our previously reported transgenic SOD1 pigs [27] suggest that mutant TDP-43 elicits more toxicity than mutant SOD1 in transgenic pigs.

Of the dead TDP-43 pigs, we were able to collect brain tissues from some animals for western blotting and immunohistochemical studies. Using anti-TDP-43 (G400, Cell Signaling), which recognizes endogenous pig TDP-43 and flag-tagged transgenic TDP-43 via western blotting, we found that the levels of transgenic TDP-43 in the spinal cord and cerebellar cortex tissues in different transgenic pigs are lower than or equivalent to the endogenous pig TDP-43 (Fig. 3a). Also, transgenic TDP-43 is widely expressed in different brain regions, including the cerebellum, striatum, and brain stem (Fig. 3b). It is known that the expression level of TDP-43 is tightly self-regulated [29]. By measuring the ratios of endogenous pig TDP-43

A

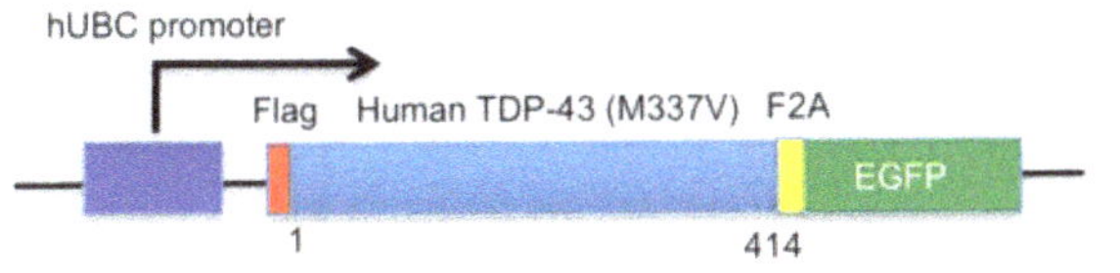

B

Cell lines	Transfer red embryos	No. recipients	No. pregnancies to term	No. born	No. survived	No. transgenic piglets
#2 and #22	1194	7	2	13	13	9
#26 and #27	332	2	2	4	2	2
#15 and #48	372	2	1	4	4	4
#34 and #40	372	2	2	12	12	12

C

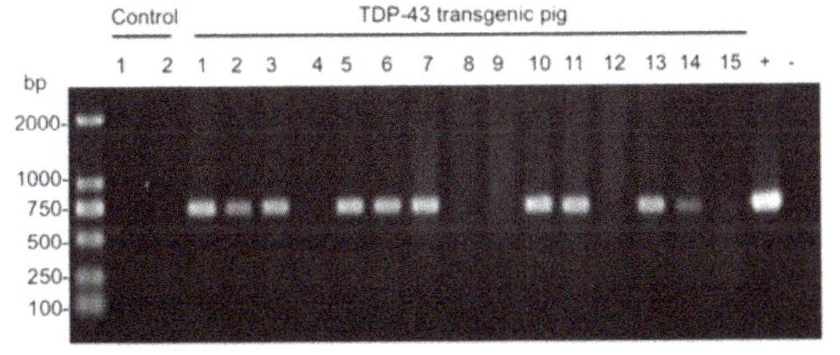

Fig. 1 Generation of transgenic TDP-43 pigs. **a** The plasmid DNA structure for expressing mutant TDP-43 (M337V) under the human ubiquitin promoter in transgenic pigs. F2A is a peptide sequence that can self-cleave to separate TDP-43 from EGFP in cells. **b** The numbers of embryos used and transgenic TDP-43 pigs produced. **c** PCR genotype analysis of ear tissues from 15 transgenic TDP-43 pigs. Two non-transgenic pig (Control) ear tissues served as a control

to actin in non-transgenic pigs and mutant TDP-43 to actin in transgenic TDP-43 pig brains, we found that the expression levels of mutant TDP-43 are not overexpressed (Fig. 3b). Western blotting also revealed small TDP-43 immunoreactive bands (Fig. 3b), which are likely cleaved transgenic TDP-43 fragments as they were not seen in the non-TG control pig brain. In the pig brain cortex, we saw a reduction in the thickness of different layers [(the thickness of layers II-VI (non-TG 1396.9 ± 51.67 μm vs TG 1038.05 ± 36.49 μm (mean ± SE, n = 4)] with a reduced density of NeuN-positive cells in the TDP-43 transgenic pig brain (Fig. 3c), which indicates neurodegeneration in TDP-43 transgenic pig brains.

We know that mutant TDP-43 affects the spinal cord motor neurons to cause ALS [30, 31], so we examined the numbers of motor neurons in the ventral horn of lumbar spinal cords via immunostaining with antibodies to NeuN and CHAT, which is specifically expressed in motor neurons. There were fewer NeuN-positive and CHAT-positive motor neurons (Fig. 4a) in the spinal cord of TDP-43 transgenic pigs. Counting the numbers of these neurons showed that motor neurons were decreased obviously in the ventral horn of lumbar spinal cord of transgenic pigs (Fig. 4b). The degeneration of spinal cord motor neurons causes denervated skeletal muscle in ALS patients. Similarly, we found that size of muscle fibers is markedly reduced in transgenic TDP-43 pigs (Fig. 4c, d). Examination of other peripheral tissues such as heart, liver, stomach, intestines, and kidney did not reveal any significant difference between non-transgenic and transgenic TDP-43 pigs. Although we cannot rule out that the peripheral toxicity of transgenic TDP-43 also contributes to the severe phenotypes of transgenic pigs, the evidence for neurodegeneration in transgenic TDP-43 pigs indicates the important role of neuronal toxicity in transgenic TDP-43 and led us to further explore the mechanism underlying the neurodegeneration.

Interaction of TDP-43 with PSF in the cytoplasm

TDP-43 is involved in gene transcription and RNA splicing via its interactions with other proteins. To identify any pig proteins that could interact with TDP-43 and are involved in TDP-43-mediated toxicity in transgenic pigs, we generated GST-TDP-43 and used it to pull down pig brain cortex proteins. The GST pull-down uncovered a band that is specific to GST-TDP-43 pull-down (Fig. 5a). Via mass spectrometry, this band was identified as the splicing factor proline-glutamine rich (SFPQ/PSF) or PSF, an essential pre-mRNA splicing factor required in spliceosome formation [32–34]. Western blot analysis confirmed the interaction of PSF in pig brain with GST-TDP-43 (Fig. 5b). We also generated His-tagged PSF and purified this recombined protein from bacteria. In vitro binding showed that His-PSF could bind endogenous pig TDP-43 and transgenic hTDP-43 in the pig brain cortex lysates (Fig. 5c). Like TDP-43, PSF contains N-terminal,

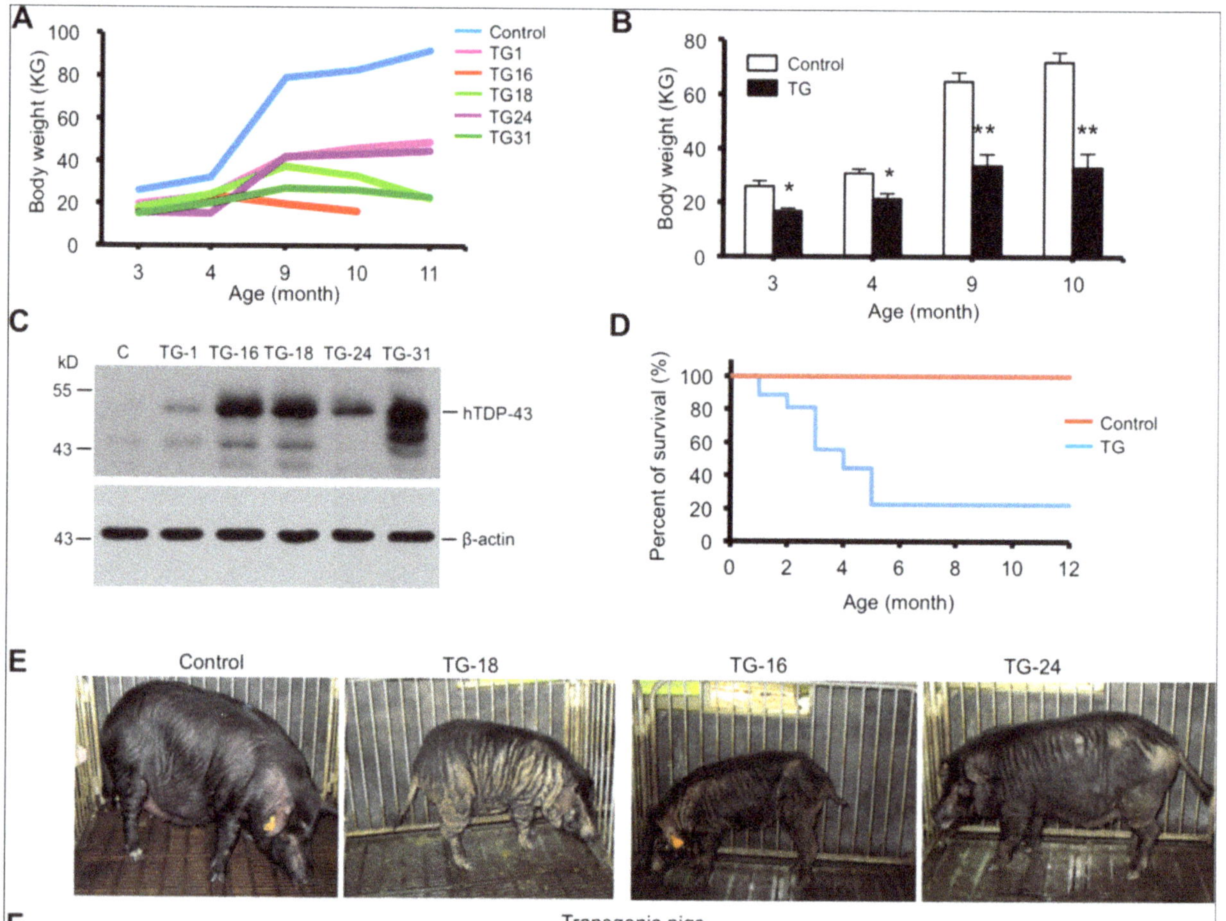

F

	Transgenic pigs																				
	1*	2	3	4	5	6	7	8	9	10	11	12	13	14	15	16*	17	18*	23	24	25	31
Copy number	4	2	3	C	5	6	4	C	C	5	6	C	3	1	1	2	2	2	1	2	3	1
Survival time (m)	11	5	5	alive	2	5	3	alive	alive	4	3	alive	3	1	2	10	alive	11	4	alive	3	alive
Motor deficit	+	ND	ND	–	ND	ND	ND	–	–	ND	ND	–	ND	ND	ND	+	+	+	+	+	ND	+
Body weight loss	+	+	+	–	ND	+	+	–	–	+	ND	–	+	ND	ND	+	+	+	+	+	ND	+

Fig. 2 Progressive phenotypes of transgenic TDP-43 pigs. **a** Body weight reduction in different transgenic TDP-43 pigs at different ages. **b** Body weight (mean ± SE) of non-transgenic and transgenic TDP-43 pigs at 3, 4, 9 and 10 months of age (n = 5 for non-TG (Control) and n = 5 for TDP-43 transgenic pigs (TG)). * $p < 0.05$; ** $p < 0.01$. **c** Western blots analysis of ear tissues showing the expression of transgenic TDP-43 pigs that were monitored for their body weights. **d** Survival plot showing that expression of mutant TDP-43 caused early death of TDP-43 transgenic (TG) pigs (n = 12 for non-TG (Control) and n = 27 for TG). **e** Photographs of representative non-transgenic (Control) and TDP-43 transgenic pig (TG-16, 18, 24) at 9 months of age. **f** Summary of some transgenic pigs for their genotypes and phenotypes. C: Genotype is non-transgenic with the endogenous copies of pig TDP-43

RRM1, RRM2 and C-terminal domains. To define the binding region in TDP-43, we generated GST fusion proteins containing different TDP-43 fragments (1–251, 1–414, and 264–414 amino acids) and used these GST fusion proteins to incubate with His-PSF proteins containing different regions (Fig. 5d). The results revealed that C-terminal PSF (444–707 amino acids) binds GST fusion protein containing C-terminal (264–414 amino acids) TDP-43 (Fig. 5e and f).

PSF is found to interact with NeuN to activate neural cell-specific alternative splicing [35]. We then examined the effect of transfected TDP-43 on the association of PSF

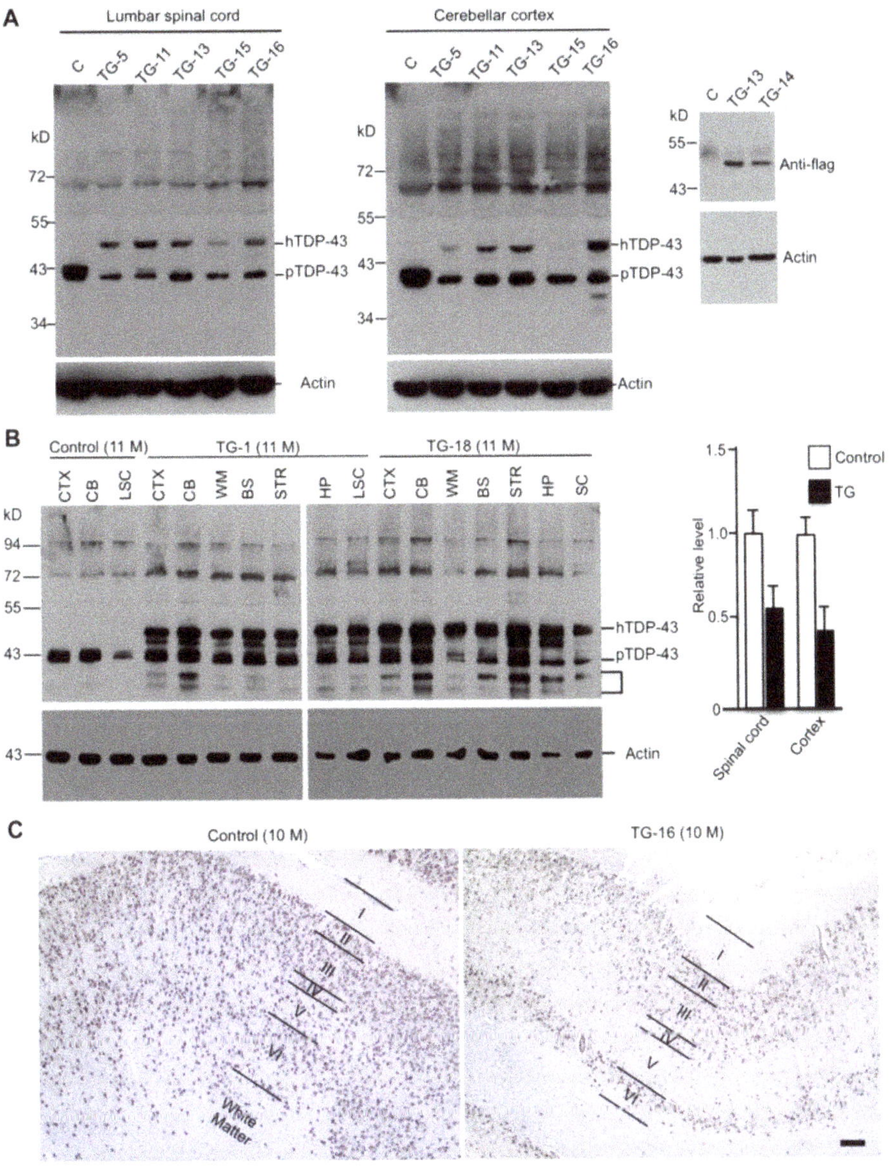

Fig. 3 Expression of transgenic TDP-43 in the pig brain tissues. **a** Western blot analysis the brain cortex and spinal cord tissues of several transgenic TDP-43 pigs using antibodies to TDP-43 and flag. C: non-transgenic. **b** Comparison of the transgenic TDP-43 expression in different brain and peripheral tissues in TG-11 and TG-18 pigs. Bracket indicates degraded fragments of transgenic TDP-43. CTX, cortex; CB, cerebellum; LSC, lumbar spinal cord; WM, white matter; BS, brain stem; STR, striatum; HP, hippocampus; SC, spinal cord. Right panel shows quantification of the ratios of endogenous pig TDP-43 to actin in non-transgenic (Control) pig brains and transgenic TDP-43 to actin on western blots (mean ± SE, n = 5 pigs per group). **c** The brain cortex from non-transgenic (Control) and TDP-43 transgenic pig (TG-16) pigs was stained with anti-NeuN. Layers of the pig brain cortex were indicated, showing a reduced thickness of transgenic TDP-43 pig brain cortex compared to the non-transgenic pig brain cortex. Scale bar: 200 μm

with NeuN. Immunoprecipitation of transfected TDP-43 in mouse N2A cells revealed that mutant TDP-43 (M337V) bound more PSF and NeuN than did wild-type TDP-43 (Fig. 6a). The in vivo interaction of TDP-43 with PSF/NeuN in the pig brain lysates was also verified via immunoprecitation with an antibody to TDP-43 (12892-1-AP from Proteintech) that selectively precipitated and detected human TDP-43 but not endogenous pig TDP-43 (Fig. 6b). We also treated the lysates with RNase to remove RNA before immunopreciptation. Depletion of RNA by this RNase treatment significantly diminished the interactions of TDP-43 with FUS, which is a RNA-binding protein whose interaction with TDP-43 depends on RNA [6, 36, 37]. There was also a slight decrease in the association of TDP-43 with PSF, but not NeuN, compared to those without RNase treatment (Fig. 6b), suggesting that the interactions of TDP-43 with its partners are differentially influenced by RNA in cells.

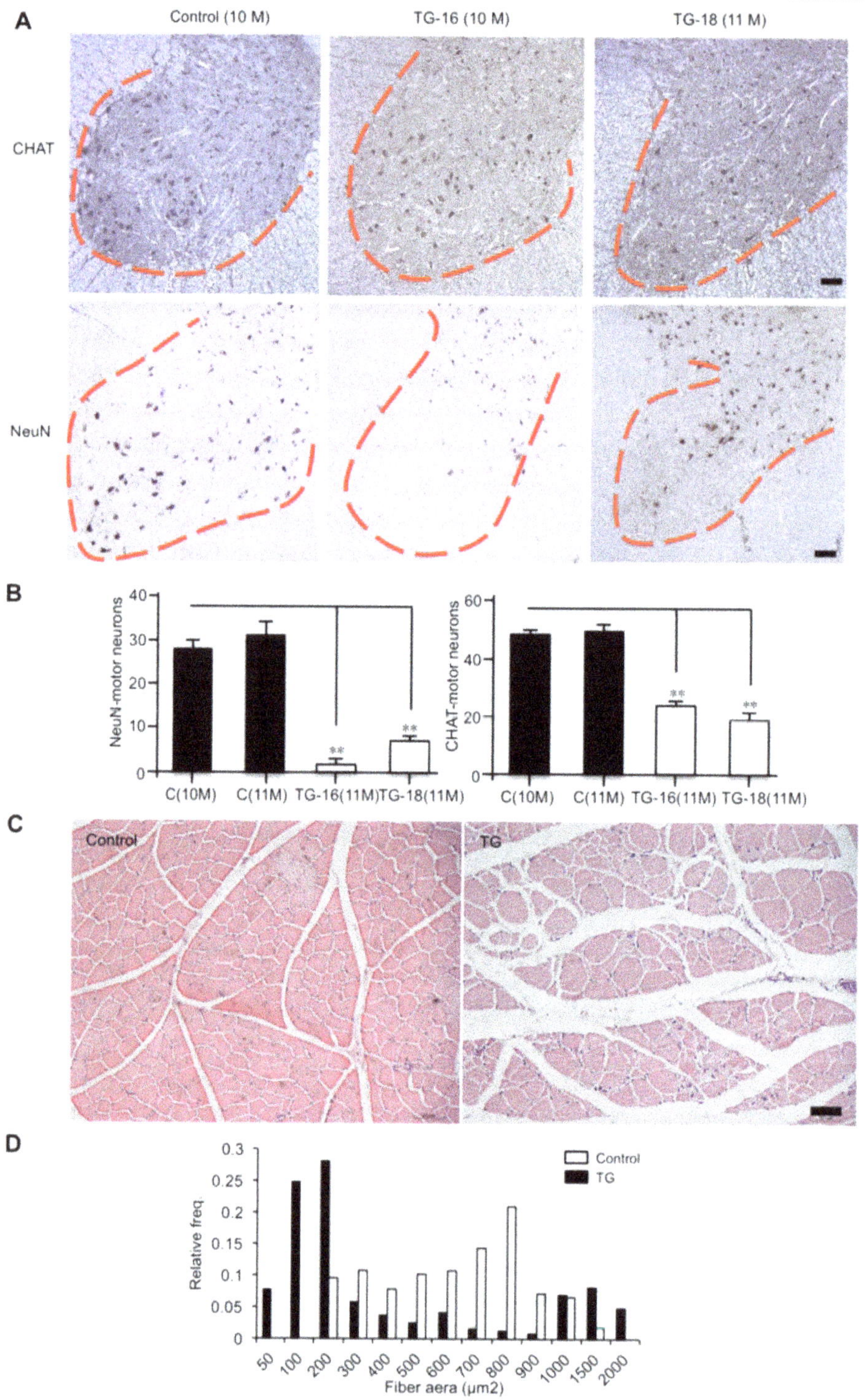

Fig. 4 Expression of mutant TDP-43 in transgenic pigs causes neurodegeneration and muscle atrophy. **a** CHAT- and NeuN-immunostaining of the pig spinal cord showing a reduced number of motor neurons in TDP-43 transgenic pigs (TG-16 and 18) at 10–11 months of age. Control: non-transgenic. Scale bars: 200 μm. **b** Quantitative analysis of the number (mean ± SE) of NeuN- and CHAT-positive neurons per ventral horn in the spinal cord sections. Five-eight images obtained with 20x N.A. 0.8 objective per section and 5 sections per group were analyzed. C: non-transgenic. **c** Skeletal muscle atrophy in TDP-43(M337V) transgenic pigs. Haematoxylin and eosin-stained cross-sections gastrocnemius muscles from 10-month-old non-transgenic (Control) and TDP-43(M337V) transgenic (TG-16) pigs. Scale bar: 50 μm. **d** More than 3 random fields (corresponding to 200–300 cross-sectioned fibers) were examined for quantification of muscle fibers of different sizes

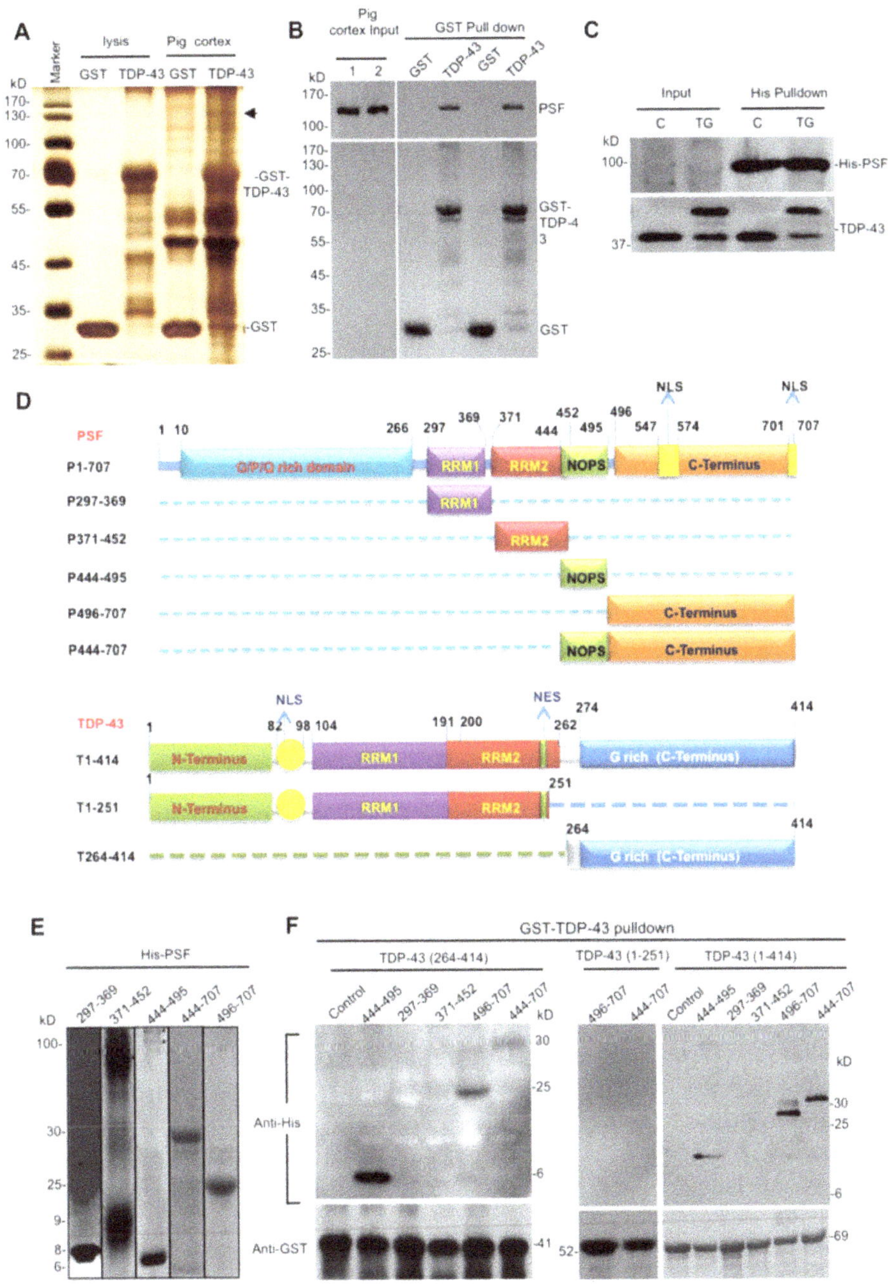

Fig. 5 TDP-43 interacts with PSF and NeuN. **a** Silver-staining of 4-12 % SDS-PAGE gel showing GST-TDP-43 pull-down from pig cortex lysates. GST served as a control. The indicated band was analyzed by mass spectrometry and found to contain PSF. **b** Western blotting with anti-PSF verifying the interaction of GST-TDP-43 and PSF in pig brain cortex lysates. Two GST and GST-TDP-43 pull-down proteins were analyzed. **c** Purified His-PSF was incubated with transgenic pig brain cortex lysates, and the bound proteins were subjected to western blot, which shows the in vitro direct interaction of endogenous pig TDP-43 and transgenic human TDP-43 with His-PSF. Input is 5 % of purified His-PSF, and 40 % of pulldown was loaded into the SDS gel. **d** PSF contains N-terminal, RRM1, RRM2, and C-terminal domains. The N-terminal domain is a glycine/proline/arginine rich domain, the C-terminal and the NOPS regions of PSF were found to bind to TDP-43. TDP-43 contains N-terminal, RRM1, RRM2, and C-terminal (G-rich) domains. **e** Purification of His-PSF containing different domains as indicated with the corresponding amino acid positions. **f** In vitro GST-pull down identifying that the C-terminal regions containing amino acids 444–707 of PSF bind to C-terminal GST-TDP-43 (amino acids 264–414), but not N-terminal TDP-43 (amino acids 1–251)

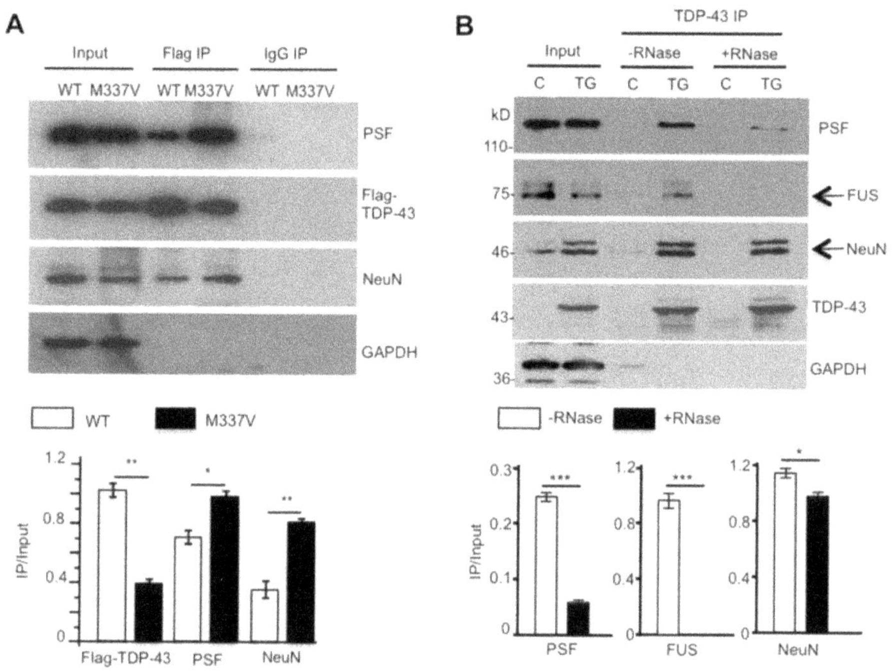

Fig. 6 Interactions of TDP-43 with PSF and NeuN. **a** Representative western blots showing co-immunoprecipitation of transfected flag-TDP-43 (WT or mutant TDP-43 (M337V)) by anti-flag and endogenous PSF, NeuN in mouse N2A cells. IgG immunoprecipitation served as controls. The ratios of precipitated to input were obtained from 3 independent experiments and shown beneath the blots. **b** The *in vivo* interaction of TDP-43 (M337V) with PSF and NeuN in the non-transgenic (C) pig and transgenic TDP-43 (TG) pig brain. The immunoprecipitation was also pre-treated with RNase to remove RNA. An antibody to TDP-43 (12892-1-AP from Proteintech) selectively detected human TDP-43, but not endogenous pig TDP-43. The interaction of FUS with TDP-43, which depends on RNA, served as a control. Quantitative data (ratio of IP/input) are presented beneath the blots. IP bands indicated by arrows were used for quantification. $*p < 0.05$, $**p < 0.01$ and $***p < 0.001$ compared with –RNase treatment

Mutant TDP-43 causes the cytoplasmic mislocalization of PSF and NeuN

After verifying the in vivo association of TDP-43 with PSF and NeuN, we wanted to know whether their subcellular localization is altered in TDP-43 transgenic pig brain. We performed immunocytochemical studies of the spinal cord of transgenic TDP-43 pigs and observed that TDP-43 was concentrated in the nucleus and also distributed in the cytoplasm (Fig. 7a). Immunostaining of PSF in the same tissue showed more cytoplasmic staining of PSF in neuronal cells in the spinal cord of transgenic TDP-43 pigs (Fig. 7a). To validate whether cytoplasmic TDP-43 causes more PSF to mislocalize in the cytoplasm, we performed double immunofluorescent staining. In those neurons that showed cytoplasmic transgenic TDP-43, cytoplasmic transgenic PSF was indeed present (Fig. 7b). Counting neurons in the spinal cord of two non-transgenic (78 neurons) and three TDP-43 pigs (128 neurons) showed that more neurons (32.3 %) in TDP-43 pig spinal cord displayed a strong cytoplasmic distribution of PSF than those in non-transgenic pigs (4.5 %). To provide additional evidence for this cytoplasmic distribution, we performed western blot analysis of TDP-43 immunoprecipitation of cytoplasmic and nuclear fractions of transgenic TDP-43 pig brain cortex tissues. Transgenic mutant TDP-43 was precipitated with anti-flag so its specific precipitation can be verified by comparing with non-transgenic pig tissues. We also saw the distribution of mutant TDP-43, PSF, and NeuN in the cytoplasmic fraction from TDP-43 transgenic pig brain tissue (Fig. 7c and d). Thus, both immunocytochemical and immunoprecipitation results support the idea that transgenic mutant TDP-43 in the cytoplasm caused PSF and NeuN to mislocalize in the cytoplasm via their interactions.

Mutant TDP-43 affects PSF/NeuN-mediated RNA splicing

The interaction of TDP-43 with PSF/NeuN led us to focus on alternative splicing of NMHC II-B (myh 10), nonmuscle myosin heavy chain II-B whose splicing is regulated by PSF and NeuN [35] and is important for neuronal function via regulation of NMDA receptor trafficking [38–40]. NMHC II-B is alternatively spliced via PSF/NeuN to include or exclude a small exon encoding 30 nucleotides, resulting in NMHC II-B +N30 or –N30 isoforms (Fig. 8a). Using RT-PCR analysis, we found that there was more –N30 isoform exclusion in the brain of TDP-43 transgenic pig (Fig. 8b). To examine whether this abnormal splicing affects the expression of NMHC II-B at the protein level, we performed western blotting

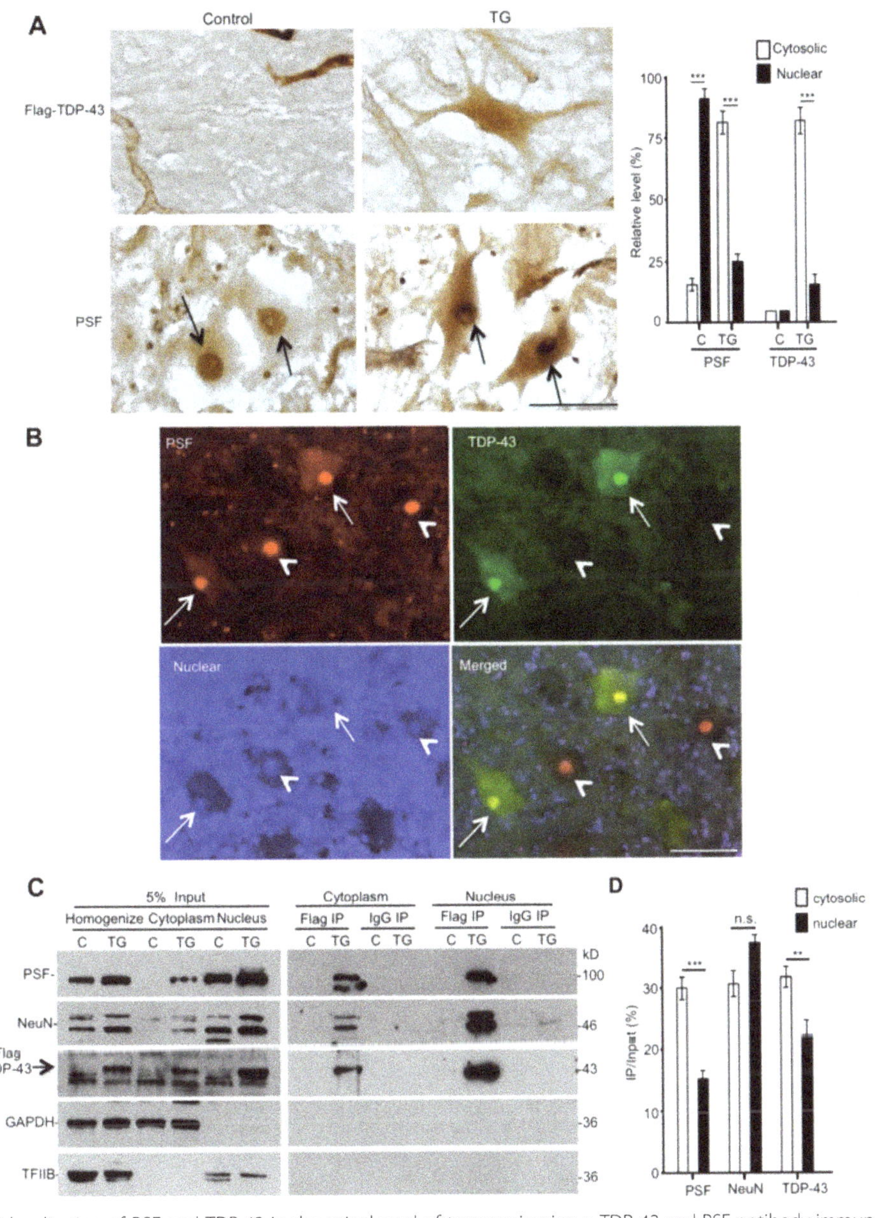

Fig. 7 Cytoplasmic mislocalization of PSF and TDP-43 in the spinal cord of transgenic pigs. **a** TDP-43 and PSF antibody immunocytochemistry of the spinal cord regions of non-transgenic (Control) pig and TDP-43 transgenic (TG-23) pigs. Arrows indicate the nuclei of neurons. Scale bar: 50 μm. **b** Immunofluorescent labeling of the spinal cord sections of the TDP-43 pig (TG-23) showing that in motor neurons (arrows) expressing transgenic TDP-43 (green), cytoplasmic distribution of PSF (red) is also evident. The nuclei were stained with Hoechst. Arrows indicate neurons in which transgenic TDP-43 is localized in both the nucleus and cytoplasm. Note that the nuclei (arrowheads) of large motor neurons were weakly labeled by Hoechst. Scale bar: 50 μm. **c** Flag-TDP-43 immunoprecipitation of the spinal cord sections of the TDP-43 pig revealing that PSF and NeuN were co-precipitated with cytoplasmic TDP-43 from transgenic pig tissues. C: non-transgenic. Rabbit IgG immunoprecipitation and non-transgenic pig brain tissues served as a control. **d** The relative levels (mean ± SE) of proteins (the ratio of IP/Input on the same blot) are presented in the right panel (n.s.: no significant difference; *$p < 0.05$; **$p < 0.01$; ***$p < 0.001$)

analysis of cytosolic and nuclear fractions of the pig brain cortex. We were unable to obtain freshly isolated pig brain tissues for fractionation such that the frozen pig brain tissues may affect the separation of subcellular compartments. However, by comparing non-transgenic and transgenic TDP-43 pig brain fractionation samples, we found that transgenic TDP-43 pig brain showed decreases of NMHC II-B in the total, nuclear, and cytoplasmic fractions, indicating that mutant TDP-43 reduces the level of NMHC II-B (Fig. 8c). To confirm that this decrease also occurred in spinal cord, we performed immunostaining of transgenic TDP-43 pig spinal cord and observed that the NMHC II-B staining of motor neurons is much weaker than that in non-transgenic neurons (Fig. 8d).

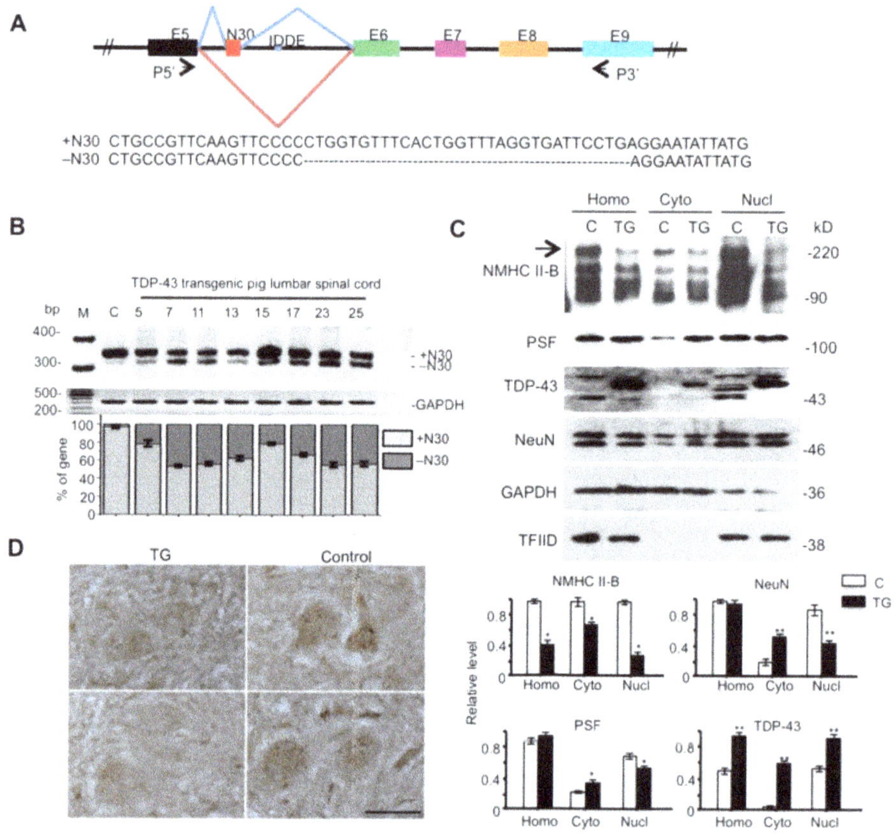

Fig. 8 Mutant TDP-43 causes abnormal splicing of NMHC II-B and promotes NMHC II-B degradation. **a** Diagram of the mouse NMHC II-B gene from exon 5 to exon 9. The exons are shown as boxes and the lines between exons are introns. The IDDE sequence is the NeuN binding region, and the alternative splicing exon N30 is indicated as red box between exon 5 and exon 6. The P5′ and P3′ represent the PCR primers to identify N30 inclusion (+N30) or exclusion (−N30). **b** RT-PCR gel result (upper panel) and quantification (lower panel) of the inclusion (+N30) and exclusion (−N30) of exon N30 in the brain cortex of non-transgenic and transgenic TDP-43 pigs (TG-5, −7, −11, −13, −15, −17, −23, −25). GAPDH served as a control. Relative +N30 and -N30 isoform levels are shown below each lane and are normalized by the total NMHC II-B gene amount. **c** Western blot analysis is unable to distinguish +N30 and −N30 because of their few amino acid differences but shows a decrease of NMHC II-B in homogenates, cytoplasmic, and nuclear fractions from transgenic TDP-43 pig cortex compared with non-transgenic (C) pig. GAPDH and TFIID are cytoplasmic and nuclear marker proteins, respectively. The relative levels of NMHC II-B, NeuN, PSF, and TDP-43 in the homogenates (Hom) (ratios of homogenate proteins to GAPDH) as well as cytosolic (Cyto) (ratios of cytoplasmic proteins to GAPDH) and nuclear (ratios of nuclear proteins to TFIID) fractions are presented beneath the blot. The data are mean ± SE (n = 3 animals per group). *$p < 0.05$; **$p < 0.01$ compared with non-Tg. **d** Reduced NMHC II-B immunostaining in the motor neurons in the spinal cord of transgenic TDP-43 (TG) pig compared with non-Tg (Control) pig. Two representative images are shown. Scale bar: 50 μm

To prove a causal role of TDP-43 in reducing NMHC II-B levels, we transfected mutant TDP-43 in PC12 cells and then examined the half-life of endogenous NMHC II-B using cycloheximide treatment. The transfection of TDP-43 promoted the degradation of endogenous NMHC II-B in PC12 cells (Fig. 9a). Because NMHC II-B consists of +N30 and −N30 isoform and mutant TDP-43 promotes the generation of −N30, we wanted to compare the half-life of +N30 and −N30. Thus, we generated GFP-NMHC II-B (+N30 and-N30) isoforms and expressed them in transfected N2A cells, which allows for high transfection efficiency of this fusion protein. We found that −N30 is degraded faster than +N30 (Fig. 9b). Also, the degradation of −N30 is inhibited by the proteasome inhibitor MG132, but not the autophagy inhibitor BFA (Fig. 9c), suggesting its degradation is mediated by the ubiquitin-proteasome system (UPS). Taken together, our results suggest that TDP-43 affects PSF/NeuN-mediated splicing of NMHC II-B and leads to more −N30 isoform being generated, which is unstable and degraded quickly by the UPS, resulting in a reduced level of NMHC II-B.

Cytoplasmic mislocalization of TDP-43 and NMHC II-B expression in ALS patient brains

We have obtained ALS patient brain tissues that were found to contain TDP-43 aggregates. Because ALS patient brains had undergone extensive neurodegeneration, we had to examine the neurons that were not degenerated and remained clear cell body morphology in order

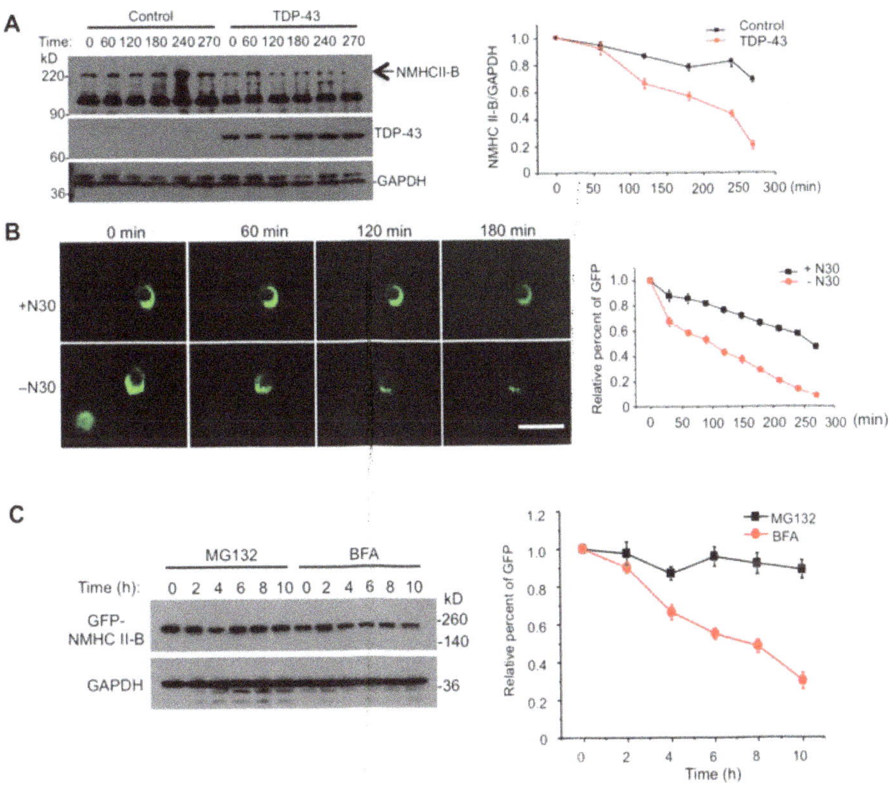

Fig. 9 Mutant TDP-43 increases the degradation of NMHC II-B. **a** The half-life of NMHC II-B after cycloheximide (20 ng/ml) treatment of PC12 cells that were transfected with TDP-43 (M337V). Immunoblots were probed with anti-NMHC II-B for detecting endogenous NMHC II-B, anti-Flag for the transfected TDP-43, and anti-GAPDH for a loading control protein. Arrow indicates NMHC II-B and the band above 90 kDa is a non-specific protein reactive to anti-NMHCII-B. Quantification data of % of 0′ time point are presented in the right panel (n = 3). **b** Fluorescent images of transfected N2A cells expressing GFP-NMHC II-B (+N30) or (−N30) after cycloheximide treatment. The right panel shows quantitative fluorescent signals of transfected proteins over time and demonstrates that (−N30) isoform is degraded faster than (+N30). Scale bar: 20 μm. **c** Western blot (the left panel) and quantification analysis (the right panel) of transfected GFP-NMHC II-B (−N30) degradation in the N2A cells that were treated with cycloheximide (20 ng/ml) and MG132 (5 μM) to inhibit the proteasome or BFA (100 μM) to inhibit autophagy

to assess protein subcellular distribution. We found that those neurons in the ALS brains show more cytoplasmic distribution of PSF and NeuN in the cerebellar cortex and spinal cord than those in the control brains (Fig. 10a). The cytoplasmic colocalization of NeuN and PSF was not seen in the control human brain section and requires the presence of both primary antibodies to NeuN and PSF (Fig. 10b), indicating the specific colocalization in ALS patient brains. Counting the percentage of cells containing cytoplasmic staining of NeuN and PSF also verified that ALS patient brains displayed more cytoplasmic NeuN and PSF (Fig. 10c). Because the postmortem human brain tissues were not well-preserved, there was difficulty in using immuofluorescent staining to analyze these tissues. Despite this, we were also able to find that the ALS patient brain cortex contained more cytoplasmic TDP-43 and PSF than the control individual that was not affected by ALS (Fig. 11a). Immunoprecipitation of TDP-43 from the cytosolic and nuclear fractions of ALS patient and control individual brain cortex tissues revealed that more PSF and NeuN were precipitated by the higher level of cytosolic TDP-43 in the ALS patient sample than the control sample (Fig. 11b and c). All these results from ALS patient samples support the findings from transgenic TDP-43 pig brains for the cytoplasmic distribution of PSF and its interaction with mutant TDP-43.

Next, we wanted to see if NMHC II-B level is also decreased in ALS patient brains. Using RT-PCR to examine alternative splicing of NMHC II-B, we found that tissues from 5 ALS patient cortexes contained more −N30 isoforms than Alzheimer's disease (AD) and control normal individual brains (Fig. 11d). Western blot analysis of the cerebellar cortex tissues from five ALS patients and their controls also validated the decreased levels of NMHC II-B in the ALS patient brains as compared with the control normal individual brains (Fig. 11e). Some AD patient samples show smear by anti-NMHC II-B staining, perhaps because of tissue degeneration in AD brains. However, the increased −N30 band in ALS patient samples (Fig. 11c) and the short half-life of −N30

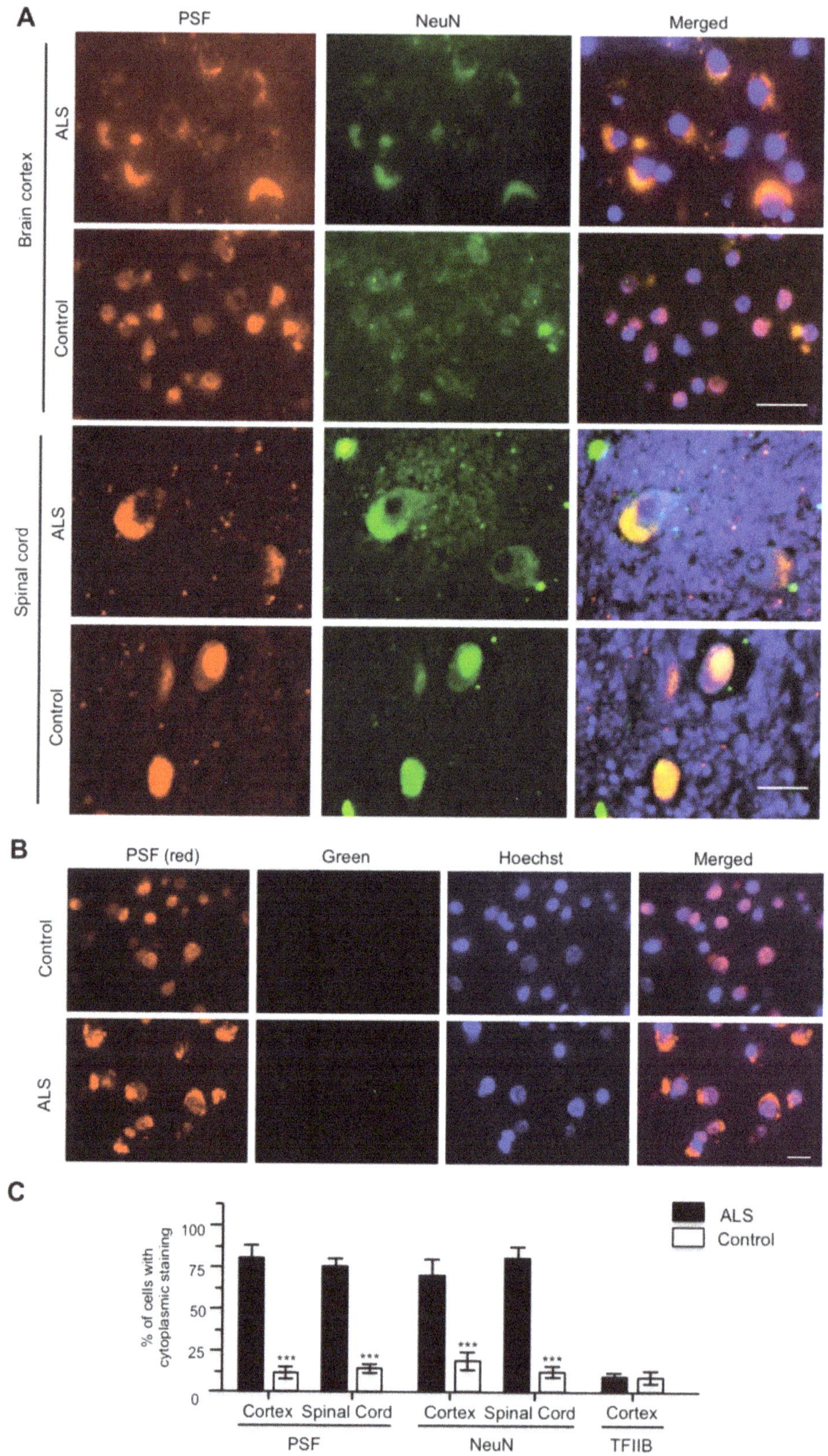

Fig. 10 (See legend on next page.)

(See figure on previous page.)

Fig. 10 Cytoplasmic mislocalization of PSF, reduction of NMHC II-B, and abnormal splicing of NMHC II-B in the brains of ALS patients. **a** Double immunofluorescent staining of the cortex and spinal cord from the ALS patient and non-ALS individual (control) with antibodies to PSF and NeuN. Scale bars: cortex: 10 µm. Spinal cord: 50 µm. Note that ALS patient brain shows cytoplasmic distribution of PSF and NeuN. **b** Immunostaining of the brain cortex in control and ALS patients with single anti-PSF only revealed PSF immunofluorescent staining. **c** Quantitative analysis of the percentage of cells with cytoplasmic PSF and NeuN staining. The staining of the nuclear protein TFIIB served as controls. The data are mean ± SE by counting 60 to 80 cells per sample (n = 3per group). $^{*}p < 0.05$, $^{**}p < 0.01$, $^{***}p < 0.001$

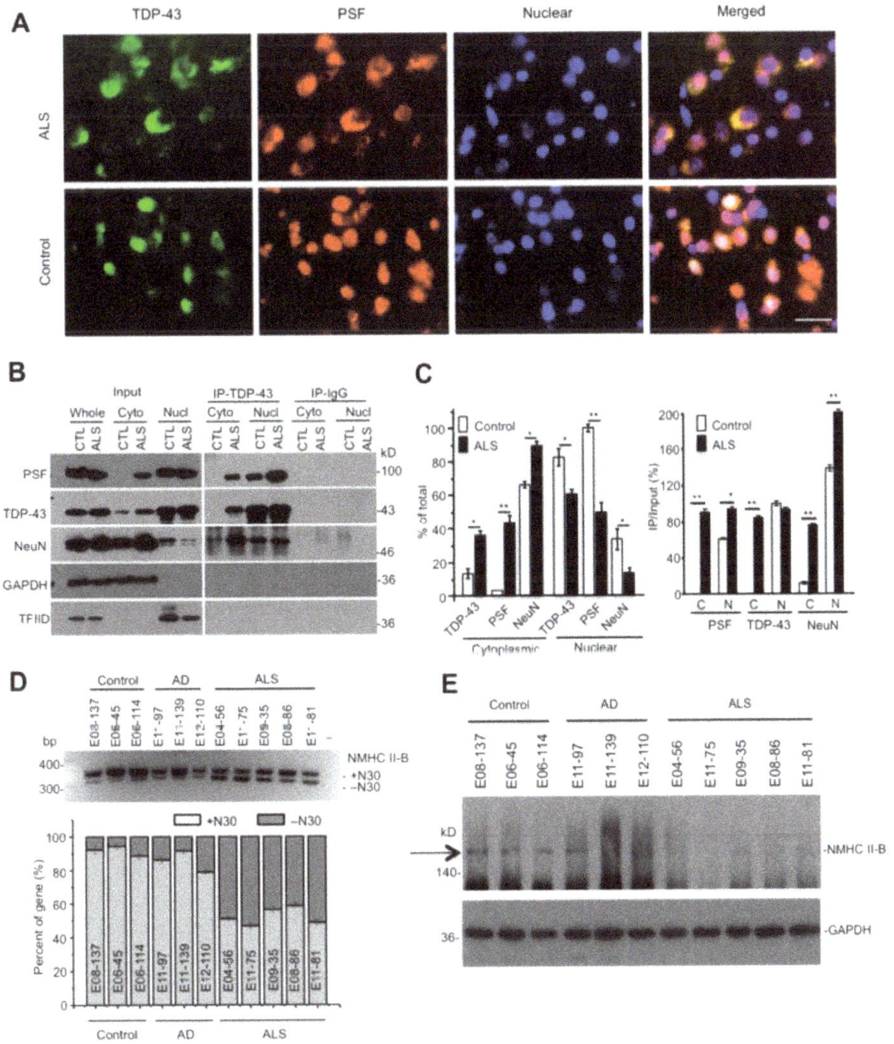

Fig. 11 Interactions of TDP-43 with PSF and reduced NMCH II-B in ALS patient brains. **a** Representative images of cytoplasmic mislocalization of PSF and TDP-43 in the ALS patient brain. Double immunofluorescent staining of the brain cortex from ALS patient and non-ALS individual with antibodies to TDP-43 and PSF. Note that ALS patient brain contains cytoplasmic TDP-43 and PSF. Scale bar: 10 µm. **b** Immunoprecipitation of TDP-43 in the cortex tissue of ALS patient showing the presence of TDP-43, PSF, and NeuN in the cytoplasmic fraction. CTL is the sample from a normal individual. Rabbit IgG served as a control immunoprecipitation. Whole: cortex total lysates; Cyto: cytoplasm of cortex lysates; Nucl: nuclear of cortex lysates; **c** The ratios (mean ± SE, n = 3) of immunoprecipitate (IP) to input and cytoplasmic or nuclear proteins to total lysates on western blots are presented. $^{*}p < 0.05$; $^{**}p < 0.01$ compared with CTL. **d** RT-PCR gel result (the upper panel) and quantification of the relative levels (the lower panel) of +N30 and -N30 isoforms in the brain cortex samples from 3 normal individuals (control), 3 Alzheimer's disease (AD), and 5 ALS patients. **e** NMHC II-B western blot analysis of the brain cortex from normal individuals, Alzheimer's disease (AD) and 5 ALS patients showing decreased expression of NMCH II-B in ALS patient brains

(Fig. 9) support the finding that NMHC II-B is decreased in ALS patient brains.

Since NMHC II-B is important for neuronal intracellular trafficking of receptors like NMDA receptor [38–40] and since the lack of NMHC II-B can affect early development [41] and neurite outgrowth [42], we assumed that overexpression of NMHC II-B should diminish TDP-43-mediated toxicity if TDP-43 reduces NMHC II-B in neuronal cells. To test this idea, we transfected mutant TDP-43 with NMHC II-B (+N30) in cultured primary cortical neurons from mice. Overexpression of mutant TDP-43 could significantly reduce neurite growth of cultured mouse cortical neurons, which is largely dependent on intracellular trafficking of a variety of molecules and receptors. This reduced neurite growth could be alleviated by co-transfection with +N30, but not −N30, NMHC II-B (Fig. 12a). Consistently, by measuring the length of neurites of those mouse cortical neurons expressing M337V with +N30 or −N30 NMHC II-B, we found that +N30 NMHC II-B mitigated TDP-43 toxicity on the neuritis outgrowth (Fig. 12b). However, this protection is partial, indicating that TDP-43 mediates toxicity via multiple pathological pathways. Nevertheless, the protection seen with overexpressed NMHC II-B supports the idea that TDP-43 does affect the expression of NMHC II-B.

Based on the finding that mutant TDP-43 interacts with PSF, we proposed a model for the effects of cytoplasmic mislocalization of mutant TDP-43. In this model, pathogenic TDP-43 is distributed in the cytoplasm. Due to its association with PSF and NeuN, the cytoplasmic mislocalization of TDP-43 may lead to the increased levels of PSF and NeuN in the cytoplasm, thereby reducing the nuclear levels of PSF and NeuN. The reduced PSF/NeuN in the nucleus can impair the nuclear function of these proteins and lead to abnormal RNA splicing, such as greater production of −N30 isoform, which is unstable or becomes toxic. The reduced level of NMHC II-B therefore contributes to the neuropathology caused by mutant TDP-43 (Fig. 12c).

Discussion

TDP-43 contains a bipartite nuclear localization signal sequence and a nuclear export signal that allows nuclear-cytoplasm shuttling [28]. TDP-43 is normally distributed in the neuronal nucleus but pathogenic TDP-43 mislocalizes in the cytoplasm and forms ubiquitinated inclusions in the

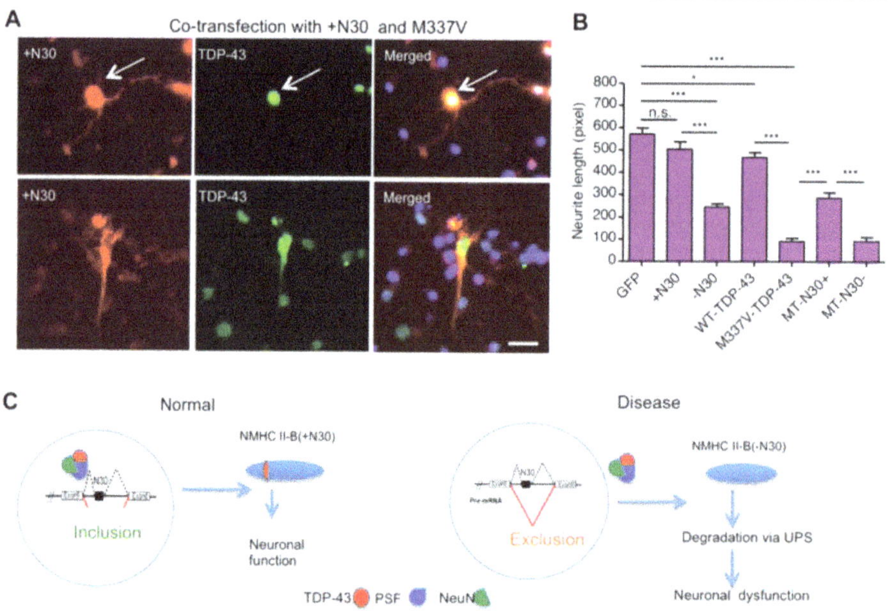

Fig. 12 Overexpression of NMHC II-B reduces TDP-43-mediated neurite toxicity. **a** Representative immunofluorescent images of TDP-43 (green), NMHC II-B (red), and nuclei (blue) in primary neurons from the mouse cortex, which were transfected with mutant TDP-43 (M337V) and NMHC II-B (+N30) or NMHC II-B (−N30). Note that transfected TDP-43 produced much intense immunostaining signals over the background level in non-transfected cells. Scale bars: 10 μm. **b** Quantitative data of neurite length of transfected cells. NMHC II-B (+N30) transfection could promote neurite outgrowth and also partly rescue the neurite outgrowth defect caused by mutant TDP-43. The data were obtained by counting more than 300 transfected cells per group in 3 independent experiments. *$p < 0.05$, **$p < 0.01$ and ***$p < 0.001$ compared with TDP-43 transfection alone. GFP: GFP protein; +N30: NMHC II-B (+N30); −N30: NMHC II-B (−N30); WT-TDP-43: wild type TDP-43; MT-TDP-43: mutant TDP-43 (M337V); MT-N30+: mutant TDP-43 (M337V) and NMHC II-B (+N30); MT-N30-: mutant TDP-43 (M337V) and NMHC II-B (−N30). **c** Proposed model of TDP-43 neuronal toxicity. Because of the interaction of TDP-43 with PSF, the cytoplasmic mislocalization of TDP-43 leads to the cytoplasmic distribution of PSF and NeuN and reduces the nuclear function of PSF and NeuN on the splicing of NMHC II-B, leading to the exclusion of N30, which promotes the degradation of NMHC II-B and affects neuronal function

brains of ALS and FTLD patients [12–14]. The early death, body weight loss, and motor deficit indicate that transgenic mutant TDP-43 affects a variety of brain and body functions, which is consistent with the severe toxicity of mutant TDP-43 in different animals' models. It has been well documented that the levels of TDP-43 are critical for neuropathology, as loss or overexpression of wild type TDP-43 can cause neurotoxicity and phenotypes in animal models [43, 44]. Although western blot analysis of the homogenized pig brain tissues showed that transgenic TDP-43 is not overexpressed as compared to the endogenous pig TDP-43, it remains to be determined whether transgenic TDP-43 is overexpressed in specific types of neurons. In addition, since our study did not include transgenic pigs that express transgenic wild type human TDP-43, we cannot conclude that the phenotypes in our transgenic pigs are definitively caused by the mutation in TDP-43, the expression levels of transgenic TDP-43, or both.

Since transgenic TDP-43 is expressed ubiquitously under the control of the ubiquitin promoter, it is also possible that the toxicity of mutant TDP-43 in peripheral tissues contributes to the severe phenotypes of TDP-43 pigs, which will require further experiments to investigate. An interesting finding in our study is that transgenic mutant TDP-43 is also distributed in the cytoplasm, a phenomenon that is seen in patient brains. Viral vector expression of TDP-43 in cynomolgus monkey spinal cord was found to result in the cytoplasmic distribution of TDP-43 [45]. Thus, large animals that are much closer to humans may share species-specific regulatory mechanisms that underlie the mislocalization of TDP-43 in the neuronal cytoplasm. However, the expression levels of transgenic TDP-43 could also influence its subcellular distribution, which needs to be considered when interpreting this cytoplasmic distribution phenomenon. Although the mechanisms underlying the cytoplasmic distribution of TDP-43 in pathogenic conditions remain to be investigated, this cytoplasmic distribution is likely to occur in the brain with age or under pathological conditions and is certainly associated with genetic mutations in the TDP-43 gene [46–48]. The pathogenic form of TDP-43, which may be phosphorylated or carry specific conformation that can confer interactions with other proteins, is able to mislocalize in the cytoplasm and forms inclusions in the aged brain. Although mutations in TDP-43 could promote the formation of the pathogenic TDP-43, it is possible that protein interactions with pathogenic TDP-43 in neurons may be different or modulated differently in small and large animals, which can explain the cytoplasmic distribution of TDP-43 in transgenic pig brains. Thus, species-related differences underscore the importance of using large animal models to uncover some important pathological changes that may not occur in small animals.

How cytoplasmic distribution of TDP-43 contributes to neuropathology remains unknown. The cytoplasmic mislocalization of TDP-43 is thought to result in the loss of the nuclear TDP-43 and its sequestration of other proteins in the cytoplasm, leading to theories of loss and gain of function caused by TDP-43 [43, 44]. For example, cytoplasmic mutant TDP-43 was found to impair axonal transport of mRNA granules [6]. Using transgenic TDP-43 pigs, we found the evidence that the cytoplasmic mutant TDP-43 can also cause a mislocalization of RNA splicing factors in the cytoplasm, offering a new explanation for the role of cytoplasmic pathogenic TDP-43.

Studies of gene expression in TDP-43 transgenic animal models indicate that mutant TDP-43 affects the splicing and expression of a large number of genes [5, 7, 15, 49]. However, it is likely the effect of mutant TDP-43 on gene expression may not be the same in different cell types and different disease stages. A new finding from our study is that TDP-43 can interact with the splicing factor PSF. The binding region was found in the C-terminal region of TDP-43, consistent with the fact that this C-terminal region associates with many other heterogeneous nuclear ribonucleoproteins (hnRNP) family members. The association of mutations in this C-terminal region with ALS and FTLD [9, 10] also supports the idea that the abnormal interactions of TDP-43 with other hnRNPs or proteins can affect RNA splicing to induce neuropathology. Also, mutations in TDP-43 can alter its subcellular distribution and stability [8, 50, 51], leading to the nuclear and cytoplasmic effects that account for many kinds of abnormal gene expression and RNA splicing.

In TDP-43 transgenic pig brains, we saw diffuse staining of TDP-43 in the cytoplasm without clear aggregates. The formation of cytoplasmic aggregates may be age-dependent or may only occur in old pig brains. The lack of obvious cytoplasmic TDP-43 aggregates supports the idea that soluble TDP-43 is toxic in our TDP-43 transgenic pigs. In fact, this idea has been suggested by the earlier finding that deleting the NLS in mutant TDP-43 could cause the cytoplasmic distribution of mutant TDP-43 and severe phenotypes in transgenic mice without aggregates [52]. Also, aberrant RNA splicing was recently found to occur without aggregation and loss of nuclear TDP-43 [53]. This idea is also supported by the interactions of soluble TDP-43 with PSF/NeuN and abnormal splicing of MNHC II-B in transgenic pig and ALS patient brains. The expression of MNHC II-B is critical for neuronal development [38–40]. Decreased levels of MNHC II-B and its point mutations are found to cause neuronal toxicity and phenotypes in mice and humans [53, 54], making MNHC II-B a good candidate for investigating how TDP-43 mediates neuronal function via affecting NMHC II-B gene slicing and expression.

According to our proposed model, the mislocalization of TDP-43 in the cytoplasm and its interactions with PSF/NeuN may contribute to the cytoplasmic distribution of PSF and NeuN, thereby reducing their effect on RNA splicing in the nucleus. It is possible that the interaction of mutant TDP-43 with PSF/NeuN in the nucleus can impact the function of PSF/NeuN, as the reduced neurite outgrowth of transfected cells showing both cytoplasmic and nuclear distribution of mutant TDP-43 can be alleviated by NMHC II-B. However, TDP-43 is known to interact with a large number of proteins. The contributions of the interactions of TDP-43 with its partners to ALS pathology may depend on cell types, subcellular regions, and species-related factors, which could confer differential posttranslational modifications to modify these interactions.

Conclusions

Using nuclear transfer technology, we established transgenic pigs expressing mutant TDP-43. Like other transgenic TDP-43 animal models, transgenic TDP-43 pigs show severe neurological phenotypes, supporting a toxic gain of function of mutant TDP-43 in large mammalian animals. We also found that mutant TDP-43 is distributed in the cytoplasm in the transgenic pig brain, a phenomenon that is seen in patient brains. By focusing on the TDP-43-PSF interaction and its related RNA splicing function, we provide new evidence for species-dependent cytoplasmic distribution of mutant TDP-43 and a new insight for how the cytoplasmic accumulation of mutant TDP-43 can contribute to abnormal gene expression. These findings should also have implications for identifying other pathological pathways and interacting proteins involved in ALS and FTLD and help uncover therapeutic targets, as well.

Methods

Plasmids and antibodies

pBudCE4.1-PSF was obtained from Dr. V.M. Kalscheuer's lab [55]. pEGFP-NMHC II-B (−N30) was obtained from Addgene, and pEGFP-NMHC II-B (+N30) was constructed by inserting +N30 sequences into pEGFP-NMHC II-B (−N30) using primers and PCR. The shRNA of NMHC II-B (TL711338A, TL711338B, TL711338C and TL711338D) were obtained from Origene. Other constructs of GST-TDP-43(1-414-M337V), GST-TDP-43(1–251), GST-TDP-43(264–414), GST-TDP-43(264-414-M337V), His-PSF(1–707), His-PSF(297–369), His-PSF(444–495), His-PSF (496–707), His-PSF(444–707), pRK-TDP-43(M337V), pRK-C-TDP-43, pRK-C-TDP-43(M337V), pEGFP-TDP-43(M337V) and pEGFP-NMHC II-B (+N30) were generated using the above plasmids or using PCR primers to amplify the first strand cDNAs of human brain tissues and constructed in the pRK5 or pCDNA3 vector. For antibodies, rabbit polyclonal antibody to TDP-43 was raised against GST-TDP-43 at the Institute of Genetics and Developmental Biology in Beijing and was used for immunoprecipitation. Antibodies to PSF (Ab38148), P84 (5E10), Flag (Ab21536) and NMHC II-B [3H2] (ab684) were obtained from Abcam. Other antibodies purchased include: NeuN (mAb377) from Millipore; TDP-43 (12892-1-AP) from Proteintech; TDP-43 (G400) from Cell Signaling; TDP-43 (M01) from Abnova; GFP (GT859) and FUS (GTX63610) from GeneTex; GAPDH (G-9), beta-actin (C-4), Adpatin B (N-19), hnRNPK (D-6), TFIID (N-12), GST (A-6) and His (H-15) from Santa Cruz Biotechnology.

Transgenic pigs

Animal use followed the NIH Guide for the Care and Use of Laboratory Animals. The animal use protocol was approved by the Institutional Animal Care and Use Committees (IACUC) at Guangzhou Institute of Biomedicine and Health (GIBH), Chinese Academy of Sciences. TDP-43 (M337V) cDNA [56] was tagged with the flag epitope at its N-terminal region and fused with EGFP via F2A, a peptide sequence that is self-cleaved to separate TDP-43 from EGFP in cells. EGFP served as a reporter for selecting TDP-43 transfected cells. The cDNA was inserted into the vector (pCAG-Neo) containing the neo-resistant gene and the CAG promoter were replaced with the human ubiquitin (hUPC) promoter. The constructed TDP-43 vector (phUBC-TDP-43(M337V)-F2A-GFP) was then transfected via electroporation (Gene PulserXcell, Bio-Rad, Hercules, CA, USA) into primary pig fetal fibroblasts isolated from a 35-day fetus of a female Tibet miniature pig. The fetal fibroblasts were cultured in Dulbecco's modified Eagle's medium (DMEM, HyClone, Logan, UT, USA) supplemented with 15 % fetal bovine serum (FBS, HyClone, Logan, UT, USA) and 1 % (v:v) penicillin/streptomycin (10,000 U/ml penicillin, 10,000 μg/ml streptomycin; GIBCO-BRL, Grand Island, NY, USA) at 39 °C in an incubator with 5 % CO_2. After 48 h, 500 μg/ml G418 (Merck, Darmstadt, Germany) was added to the medium to select transfected cell colonies, and the plates were incubated in media containing G418 for approximately 10 d. The surviving cell colonies were selected and propagated in a fresh 48-well plate. Colonies that proliferated well were then expanded and screened for the expression of TDP-43.

The ovaries of pigs were collected from long white pigs at a local slaughterhouse. The cumulus-oocyte complexes were isolated and cultured as described previously [26, 27]. After 42–44 h of culture, oocytes were separated from cumulus cells by vigorous vortex for 4 min in TL-Hepes supplemented with 0.1 % polyvinyl alcohol (P8136; Sigma) and 0.1 % hyaluronidase (H3506; Sigma). Denuded mature oocytes were enucleated and injected with a single donor cell into the perivitelline space of the oocyte in contact with the oocyte membrane. Fusion and activation were induced simultaneously with 2 successive

DC pulses of 1.1 kV/cm for 30 ms using an Electro Cell Manipulator 200 (Genetronics, San Diego, CA, USA). Reconstructed embryos (50–100) were transferred to 500 μl of culture medium covered with mineral oil in a four-well multi dish and cultured in 5 % CO_2 for 18–22 h at 39 °C. The embryos were then surgically transferred into the oviduct of a surrogate female on the first day of standing estrus. Pregnancy status was monitored using an ultrasound scanner between days 30–35 post-transplantation. Transgenic piglets were identified by PCR using primers (forward primer: 5'-TTGAACT ATGCGCTCGGGGTTG-3' and reverse primer: 5'-GTTC GGTTGTTTTCCATGGGAGAC-3') and western blot analysis with anti-TDP-43 antibodies.

Animal behavioral studies

The movement capabilities of transgenic pigs were tested by treadmill running as described in our recent study [27]. A suitable cage was placed onto the treadmill to keep the pig and make it run on the conveyer belt. Pigs were trained 3 times for running on treadmill and then were tested from the age of 3 months. The speed of treadmill was kept at 3.0 km/h for 1 min when the pig ran on it. Non-transgenic littermates or age- and body weight-matched non-transgenic pigs were used as controls. Due to their severe phenotypes, TDP-43 transgenic pigs often died in the course of training or formal test of their motor function such that we did not test all TDP-43 transgenic pigs.

Human tissue acquisition

Human cortex and spinal cord tissues were obtained and archived via an institutional review board and Health Insurance Portability and Accountability Act-compliant process at neuropathology/histochemistry core of Emory University. Autopsies were performed following death with post-mortem interval of 6–13 h. The spinal cord and cortex tissues were obtained from the postmortem brains of ALS patients (04–56, E11-75, E09-35, E-86, and E-81) who died at 67–74 years of age and were confirmed to have TDP-43 aggregates via post-mortem histologic analysis. Non-ALS tissues were obtained from neurologically unaffected patients (E08-137, E06-45, and E06-114) and Alzheimer's disease patients (E11-97, E11-139, and E12-110) who died at 53–92 years of age. For immunofluorescence studies, tissues were fixed in formalin and embedded by paraffin, sectioned, and stored at room temperature (16-25 °C). For Co-IP and RT-PCR analysis, tissue segments stored at −80 °C were used.

GST pulldown assays

GST-TDP-43 recombinant fusion proteins were produced in bacteria (BL21) and purified with glutathione-sepharose beads (Sigma). Pig cortex tissues (0.1 g/ml) in NP-40 lysis buffer (50 mM Tris pH7.4, 50 mM NaCl, 0.1 % Triton X-100, 1 % NP40) were homogenized using a Teflon homogenizer for 30 strokes. The lysates were added with protease inhibitor cocktail (Sigma, P8340) plus proteasome inhibitor and kept on ice for 30 min. Lysates were sonicated for 10 s and centrifuged at 1000 × g for 2 min. The supernatants (5 μg/μl protein) were pre-cleaned by incubating with 100 μg GST protein and 30 μL glutathione-sepharose beads for 4 h at 4 °C and then subjected to GST-TDP-43 pull-down assay. Analysis of the GST-TDP-43 pull down bands was performed by AB SCIEX TripleTOF® 5600 system at Institute of Genetics and Developmental Biology in Beijing.

Co-immunoprecipitation and western blot

Cultured cells or brain tissues were homogenized in NP-40,1 × PBS or RIPA buffer with 1× protease inhibitor as previously described [57]. For immunoprecipitation, the lysates were centrifuged at 800 × g for 5 min, and supernatants were incubated with antibody and Protein A beads (Sigma-Aldrich) at 4 °C overnight, followed by washing with lysis buffer 4 times. The samples were subjected to 4-12 % SDS-PAGE (Invitrogen) and detected with SuperSignal West Dura Extended Duration Substrate (Thermo). For RNase treatment, pig cortex lysates were incubated with 200 μg/ml RNase A for 30 min at 25 °C before immunoprecipitation.

Subcellular fractionations

The cytosolic fraction was obtained by centrifuging the brain lysates at a high speed 15000 × g for 15 min, the supernatant was used as cytoplasmic for Western Blot and Co-Immunoprecipitation. For nuclear fractionation, we added 1000 μl of NP-40 buffer to 0.1 g pig brain cortex tissue on ice for 10 min. The tissues were then homogenized with a glass homogenizer for 30 strokes and sonicated of 15 s. The lysates were centrifuged at 4 °C at 800 × g for 10 min. The pellets were re-suspended in 374 μl of buffer (5 mM HEPES, 1.5 mM MgCl2, 0.2 mM EDTA, 0.5 mM DTT, 26 % glycerol (v/v), pH 7.9) with 26 μl of 4.6 M NaCl to give the final concentration at 300 mM NaCl and then homogenized with 20 full strokes in Teflon homogenizer on ice and sonicated for 10 s. The homogenized samples were kept on ice for 20 min and then centrifuged at 24,000 × g for 20 min at 4 °C. The supernatant was used for western blotting or Immunoprecipitation.

Cell cultures

PC12 cells stably expressing flag-TDP-43-EGFP were described in our recent study [56]. HEK293T and SK-N-SH cells were purchased from the ATCC and cultured according to the guidelines recommended by the ATCC. All cells were maintained at 37 °C with 5 % CO_2. PC12 cells were maintained in DMEM/F12 medium with 5 % fetal bovine serum and 10 % horse serum, 100 U/ml penicillin at 37 °C in an atmosphere of 5 % CO_2 and 95 % humidity. NGF was used at 100 ng/ml (N6009, Sigma) to induce neurite extension for the PC12 cells.

Culture of primary neurons from mouse brain cortex was performed as described previously [57]. Briefly, cortical neurons were isolated from the cortex of postnatal day 1 mice. Dissected tissue was treated with 0.0625 mg/ml trypsin and 0.0625 mg/ml DNase (Life Technology) in 1 × HBSS buffer without calcium and magnesium for 10 min at 37 °C, followed by triturating with a 1-ml pipette tip for 20 times. Cells were then washed once with the tissue culture medium and spun down at 1500 g for 3 min. Cells were placed on top of a layer of astrocytes and grown initially in a 50 % glial-conditioned medium [DMEM containing 0.25 % glucose, 2 mM glutamate, 10 % FCS, 500 nm insulin, 1 × vitamin mixture (M6895; Sigma), and 1 % antibiotic–antimycotic (Invitrogen)]. The cells were then cultured in neurobasal/B27 medium.

Immunofluorescence, immunohistochemistry, and quantification

Sections from human or pig brains were fixed in 4 % paraformaldehyde/1 × PBS, embedded in paraffin or Tissue ® Tek O.C.T compound (SAKURA), and sectioned to 10 or 40 μm slices. The paraffin embedded sections were deparaffinized with xylene and sequential ethanol (70 %, 80 %, 100 % X 2 times) and rehydrated with water. Rehydrated slices were heat-treated for antigen retrieval in citrate buffer. The treated slices were then stained by antibodies to TDP-43, NeuN, and PSF and detected using DAB staining. Images of micrographs were taken using a Zeiss microscope (Axiovert 200 MOT).

To quantify neurons expressing transgenic TDP-43 in transgenic pig brains and ALS patient brains, we used 5–8 images obtained with 20 × N.A. 0.8 objective per section and 5 sections per group (n = 3-5 samples per group). To quantify cultured cells, we examined more than total 300 cells per group in at least three independent experiments. To measure the lengths of neurites of cultured neurons, imaged cells were selected at random, and all visible processes of selected neurons were imaged. The transfected neurons whose neurites could be clearly identified were selected to measure the lengths of their neurites using a fluorescent microscope of ZEISS Axiovrert 200 M microscope. The images were analyzed by measuring the longest branch of each neurite and the relative length was quantified as pixel using NeuronJ plugin image software, which is used for quantification of elongated structures.

For analyzing histological changes in the muscle sections, a minimum of 3 random fields (corresponding to 200–300 cross-sectioned fibers) were photo micrographed for gastrocnemius muscle of non-transgenic and TDP-43 transgenic pigs; all type fibers were analyzed for their size using Scion Image software (v. alpha 4.0.3.2, Scion, Frederick, MD).

Statistical analysis

For statistical analysis, data were obtained from three or more independent experiments. Statistical analysis was performed using Microsoft Excel and Student's *t*-test (two tailed) for comparing two different groups. A value of $p < 0.05$ or $p < 0.01$ was indicated with one asterisk (*) or two asterisk (**), which represent statistically significant.

Ethical approval

Animal use followed the NIH Guide for the Care and Use of Laboratory Animals. The animal use protocol was approved by the Institutional Animal Care and Use Committees (IACUC) at Guangzhou Institute of Biomedicine and Health (GIBH), Chinese Academy of Sciences. Human cortex and spinal cord tissues were obtained and archived via an institutional review board and Health Insurance Portability and Accountability Act-compliant process at neuropathology/histochemistry core of Emory University.

Abbreviations

TDP-43: TAR DNA-binding protein 43; PSF: Splicing factor, proline- and glutamine-rich; NeuN: Feminizing Locus on X-3, Fox-3, Rbfox3, or Hexaribonucleotide Binding Protein-3; NMHC II-B: nonmuscle myosin heavy chain II-B; SOD1: Superoxide dismutase [Cu-Zn] also known as superoxide dismutase 1; ALS: Amyotrophic lateral sclerosis; FTLD: Frontotemporal lobar degeneration; hnRNP: heterogeneous nuclear ribonucleoproteins.

Competing interests

The authors declare that they have no competing interests.

Authors' contributions

SL X-JL and LL designed and supervised experiments. G W, SY, C-E W, XL, PY performed molecular and biochemical studies. H Y, BZ, ZO, ZL YZ, TL performed experiments on generation of transgenic pigs. N F and LG provided technical assistance. X-JL wrote the manuscript with help of GW and HY All authors read and approved the final manuscript.

Acknowledgments

This work was supported by grants from the National Basic Research Program of China (973 program) (2011CB944203), the Natural Science Foundation of China (31071293) awarded to L.L.; the National Institutes of Health (NS036232, NS041669, and NS045016) to X.L. and S.L. We would like to thank the staffs of the pig farm for animal husbandry and assistance in the behavioral tasks, the neuropathology/histochemistry core of Emory University for providing human brain tissue samples, and Dr. V.M. Kalscheuer for providing the PSF plasmid. We thank Cheryl Strauss for critically reading this manuscript.

Author details

[1]State Key Laboratory of Molecular Developmental Biology, Institute of Genetics and Developmental Biology, Chinese Academy of Sciences, Beijing 100101, China. [2]Key Laboratory of Regenerative Biology, South China Institute for Stem Cell Biology and Regenerative Medicine, Guangzhou Institutes of Biomedicine and Health, Chinese Academy of Sciences, Guangzhou 510530, China. [3]Department of Human Genetics, Emory University School of Medicine, Atlanta, GA 30322, USA. [4]University of Chinese Academy of Sciences, Beijing 100049, China.

References

1. Krecic AM, Swanson MS. hnRNP complexes: composition, structure, and function. Curr Opin Cell Biol. 1999;11(3):363–71.
2. Polymenidou M, Lagier-Tourenne C, Hutt KR, Huelga SC, Moran J, Liang TY, et al. Long pre-mRNA depletion and RNA missplicing contribute to neuronal vulnerability from loss of TDP-43. Nat Neurosci. 2011;14(4):459–68.
3. Tollervey JR, Curk T, Rogelj B, Briese M, Cereda M, Kayikci M, et al. Characterizing the RNA targets and position-dependent splicing regulation by TDP-43. Nat Neurosci. 2011;14(4):452–58.
4. Kawahara Y, Mieda-Sato A. TDP-43 promotes microRNA biogenesis as a component of the Drosha and Dicer complexes. Proc Natl Acad Sci U S A. 2012;109(9):3347–52.
5. Cohen TJ, Lee VM, Trojanowski JQ. TDP-43 functions and pathogenic mechanisms implicated in TDP-43 proteinopathies. Trends Mol Med. 2011;17(11):659–67.
6. Alami NH, Smith RB, Carrasco MA, Williams LA, Winborn CS, Han SS, et al. Axonal transport of TDP-43 mRNA granules is impaired by ALS-causing mutations. Neuron. 2014;81(3):536–43.
7. Freibaum BD, Chitta RK, High AA, Taylor JP. Global analysis of TDP-43 interacting proteins reveals strong association with RNA splicing and translation machinery. J Proteome Res. 2010;9(2):1104–20.
8. Ling SC, Albuquerque CP, Han JS, Lagier-Tourenne C, Tokunaga S, Zhou H, et al. ALS-associated mutations in TDP-43 increase its stability and promote TDP-43 complexes with FUS/TLS. Proc Natl Acad Sci U S A. 2010;107 (30):13318–23.
9. Lattante S, Rouleau GA, Kabashi E. TARDBP and FUS mutations associated with amyotrophic lateral sclerosis: summary and update. Hum Mutat. 2013;34(6):812–26.
10. Pesiridis GS, Lee VM, Trojanowski JQ. Mutations in TDP-43 link glycine-rich domain functions to amyotrophic lateral sclerosis. Hum Mol Genet. 2009;18 (R2):R156–62.
11. Gendron TF, Rademakers R, Petrucelli L. TARDBP mutation analysis in TDP-43 proteinopathies and deciphering the toxicity of mutant TDP-43. J Alzheimers Dis. 2013;33 Suppl 1:S35–45.
12. Arai T, Hasegawa M, Akiyama H, Ikeda K, Nonaka T, Mori H, et al. TDP-43 is a component of ubiquitin-positive tau-negative inclusions in frontotemporal lobar degeneration and amyotrophic lateral sclerosis. Biochem Biophys Res Commun. 2006;351(3):602–11.
13. Neumann M, Sampathu DM, Kwong LK, Truax AC, Micsenyi MC, Chou TT, et al. Ubiquitinated TDP-43 in frontotemporal lobar degeneration and amyotrophic lateral sclerosis. Science. 2006;314(5796):130–3.
14. Chen-Plotkin AS, Lee VM, Trojanowski JQ. TAR DNA-binding protein 43 in neurodegenerative disease. Nat Rev Neurol. 2010;6(4):211–20.
15. Arnold ES, Ling SC, Huelga SC, Lagier-Tourenne C, Polymenidou M, Ditsworth D, et al. ALS-linked TDP-43 mutations produce aberrant RNA splicing and adult-onset motor neuron disease without aggregation or loss of nuclear TDP-43. Proc Natl Acad Sci U S A. 2013;110(8):E736–45.
16. Ash PE, Zhang YJ, Roberts CM, Saldi T, Hutter H, Buratti E, et al. Neurotoxic effects of TDP-43 overexpression in C. elegans. Hum Mol Genet. 2010;19(16):3206–18.
17. Wegorzewska I, Bell S, Cairns NJ, Miller TM, Baloh RH. TDP-43 mutant transgenic mice develop features of ALS and frontotemporal lobar degeneration. Proc Natl Acad Sci U S A. 2009;106(44):18809–14.
18. Kabashi E, Lin L, Tradewell ML, Dion PA, Bercier V, Bourgouin P, et al. Gain and loss of function of ALS-related mutations of TARDBP (TDP-43) cause motor deficits in vivo. Hum Mol Genet. 2010;19(4):671–83.
19. Li Y, Ray P, Rao EJ, Shi C, Guo W, Chen X, et al. A Drosophila model for TDP-43 proteinopathy. Proc Natl Acad Sci U S A. 2010;107(7):3169–74.
20. Shan X, Chiang PM, Price DL, Wong PC. Altered distributions of Gemini of coiled bodies and mitochondria in motor neurons of TDP-43 transgenic mice. Proc Natl Acad Sci U S A. 2010;107(37):16325–30.
21. Wils H, Kleinberger G, Janssens J, Pereson S, Joris G, Cuijt I, et al. TDP-43 transgenic mice develop spastic paralysis and neuronal inclusions characteristic of ALS and frontotemporal lobar degeneration. Proc Natl Acad Sci U S A. 2010;107(8):3858–63.
22. Xu YF, Gendron TF, Zhang YJ, Lin WL, D'Alton S, Sheng H, et al. Wild-type human TDP-43 expression causes TDP-43 phosphorylation, mitochondrial aggregation, motor deficits, and early mortality in transgenic mice. J Neurosci. 2010;30(32):10851–9.
23. Swarup V, Phaneuf D, Dupre N, Petri S, Strong M, Kriz J, et al. Deregulation of TDP-43 in amyotrophic lateral sclerosis triggers nuclear factor kappaB-mediated pathogenic pathways. J Exp Med. 2011;208(12):2429–47.
24. Huang C, Tong J, Bi F, Zhou H, Xia XG. Mutant TDP-43 in motor neurons promotes the onset and progression of ALS in rats. J Clin Invest. 2012;122 (1):107–18.
25. Avendano-Vazquez SE, Dhir A, Bembich S, Buratti E, Proudfoot N, Baralle FE. Autoregulation of TDP-43 mRNA levels involves interplay between transcription, splicing, and alternative polyA site selection. Genes Dev. 2012;26(15):1679–84.
26. Yang D, Wang CE, Zhao B, Li W, Ouyang Z, Liu Z, et al. Expression of Huntington's disease protein results in apoptotic neurons in the brains of cloned transgenic pigs. Hum Mol Genet. 2010;19(20):3983–94.
27. Yang H, Wang G, Sun H, Shu R, Liu T, Wang CE, et al. Species-dependent neuropathology in transgenic SOD1 pigs. Cell Res. 2014;24(4):464–81.
28. Winton MJ, Igaz LM, Wong MM, Kwong LK, Trojanowski JQ, Lee VM. Disturbance of nuclear and cytoplasmic TAR DNA-binding protein (TDP-43) induces disease-like redistribution, sequestration, and aggregate formation. J Biol Chem. 2008;283(19):13302–9.
29. Ayala YM, De Conti L, Avendano-Vazquez SE, Dhir A, Romano M, D'Ambrogio A, et al. TDP-43 regulates its mRNA levels through a negative feedback loop. EMBO J. 2011;30(2):277–88.
30. Sumi H, Kato S, Mochimaru Y, Fujimura H, Etoh M, Sakoda S. Nuclear TAR DNA binding protein 43 expression in spinal cord neurons correlates with the clinical course in amyotrophic lateral sclerosis. J Neuropathol Exp Neurol. 2009;68(1):37–47.
31. Braak H, Ludolph A, Thal DR, Del Tredici K. Amyotrophic lateral sclerosis: dash-like accumulation of phosphorylated TDP-43 in somatodendritic and axonal compartments of somatomotor neurons of the lower brainstem and spinal cord. Acta Neuropathol. 2010;120(1):67–74.
32. Patton JG, Porro EB, Galceran J, Tempst P, Nadal-Ginard B. Cloning and characterization of PSF, a novel pre-mRNA splicing factor. Genes Dev. 1993;7 (3):393–406.
33. Kaneko S, Rozenblatt-Rosen O, Meyerson M, Manley JL. The multifunctional protein p54nrb/PSF recruits the exonuclease XRN2 to facilitate pre-mRNA 3' processing and transcription termination. Genes Dev. 2007;21(14):1779–89.
34. Tapia-Paez I, Tammimies K, Massinen S, Roy AL, Kere J. The complex of TFII-I, PARP1, and SFPQ proteins regulates the DYX1C1 gene implicated in neuronal migration and dyslexia. FASEB J. 2008;22(8):3001–9.
35. Kim KK, Kim YC, Adelstein RS, Kawamoto S. Fox-3 and PSF interact to activate neural cell-specific alternative splicing. Nucleic Acids Res. 2011;39(8):3064–78.
36. Kim SH, Shanware NP, Bowler MJ, Tibbetts RS. Amyotrophic lateral sclerosis-associated proteins TDP-43 and FUS/TLS function in a common biochemical complex to co-regulate HDAC6 mRNA. J Biol Chem. 2010;285 (44):34097–105.
37. Honda D, Ishigaki S, Iguchi Y, Fujioka Y, Udagawa T, Masuda A, et al. The ALS/FTLD-related RNA-binding proteins TDP-43 and FUS have common downstream RNA targets in cortical neurons. FEBS Open Bio. 2013;4:1–10.
38. Amparan D, Avram D, Thomas CG, Lindahl MG, Yang J, Bajaj G, et al. Direct interaction of myosin regulatory light chain with the NMDA receptor. J Neurochem. 2005;92(2):349–61.
39. Kioussi C, Appu M, Lohr CV, Fischer KA, Bajaj G, Leid M, et al. Co-expression of myosin II regulatory light chain and the NMDAR1 subunit in neonatal and adult mouse brain. Brain Res Bull. 2007;74(6):439–51.
40. Bajaj G, Zhang Y, Schimerlik MI, Hau AM, Yang J, Filtz TM, et al. N-methyl-D-aspartate receptor subunits are non-myosin targets of myosin regulatory light chain. J Biol Chem. 2009;284(2):1252–66.
41. Wang A, Ma X, Conti MA, Liu C, Kawamoto S, Adelstein RS. Nonmuscle myosin II isoform and domain specificity during early mouse development. Proc Natl Acad Sci U S A. 2010;107(33):14645–50.
42. Tullio AN, Bridgman PC, Tresser NJ, Chan CC, Conti MA, Adelstein RS, et al. Structural abnormalities develop in the brain after ablation of the gene encoding nonmuscle myosin II-B heavy chain. J Comp Neurol. 2001;433 (1):62–74.
43. Lee EB, Lee VM, Trojanowski JQ. Gains or losses: molecular mechanisms of TDP43-mediated neurodegeneration. Nat Rev Neurosci. 2012;13(1):38–50.
44. Xu ZS. Does a loss of TDP-43 function cause neurodegeneration? Mol Neurodegener. 2012;7:27.
45. Uchida A, Sasaguri H, Kimura N, Tajiri M, Ohkubo T, Ono F, et al. Non-human primate model of amyotrophic lateral sclerosis with cytoplasmic mislocalization of TDP-43. Brain. 2012;135(Pt 3):833–46.
46. Nishimura AL, Shum C, Scotter EL, Abdelgany A, Sardone V, Wright J, et al. Allele-specific knockdown of ALS-associated mutant TDP-43 in neural stem

cells derived from induced pluripotent stem cells. PLoS One. 2014;9(3): e91269.
47. Serio A, Bilican B, Barmada SJ, Ando DM, Zhao C, Siller R, et al. Astrocyte pathology and the absence of non-cell autonomy in an induced pluripotent stem cell model of TDP-43 proteinopathy. Proc Natl Acad Sci U S A. 2013;110(12):4697–702.
48. Barmada SJ, Skibinski G, Korb E, Rao EJ, Wu JY, Finkbeiner S. Cytoplasmic mislocalization of TDP-43 is toxic to neurons and enhanced by a mutation associated with familial amyotrophic lateral sclerosis. J Neurosci. 2010;30 (2):639–49.
49. Lagier-Tourenne C, Polymenidou M, Hutt KR, Vu AQ, Baughn M, Huelga SC, et al. Divergent roles of ALS-linked proteins FUS/TLS and TDP-43 intersect in processing long pre-mRNAs. Nat Neurosci. 2012;15(11):1488–97.
50. Barmada SJ, Serio A, Arjun A, Bilican B, Daub A, Ando DM, et al. Autophagy induction enhances TDP43 turnover and survival in neuronal ALS models. Nature Chem Biol. 2014;10(8):677–85.
51. Watanabe S, Kaneko K, Yamanaka K. Accelerated disease onset with stabilized familial amyotrophic lateral sclerosis (ALS)-linked mutant TDP-43 proteins. J Biol Chem. 2013;288(5):3641–54.
52. Igaz LM, Kwong LK, Lee EB, Chen-Plotkin A, Swanson E, Unger T, et al. Dysregulation of the ALS-associated gene TDP-43 leads to neuronal death and degeneration in mice. J Clin Invest. 2011;121(2):726–38.
53. Ma X, Kawamoto S, Hara Y, Adelstein RS. A point mutation in the motor domain of nonmuscle myosin II-B impairs migration of distinct groups of neurons. Mol Biol Cell. 2004;15(6):2568–79.
54. Tuzovic L, Yu L, Zeng W, Li X, Lu H, Lu HM, et al. A human de novo mutation in MYH10 phenocopies the loss of function mutation in mice. Rare Dis. 2013;1:e26144.
55. Kunde SA, Musante L, Grimme A, Fischer U, Muller E, Wanker EE, et al. The X-chromosome-linked intellectual disability protein PQBP1 is a component of neuronal RNA granules and regulates the appearance of stress granules. Hum Mol Genet. 2011;20(24):4916–31.
56. Yan S, Wang CE, Wei W, Gaertig MA, Lai L, Li S, et al. TDP-43 causes differential pathology in neuronal versus glial cells in the mouse brain. Hum Mol Genet. 2014;23(10):2678–93.
57. Weng L, Lin YF, Li AL, Wang CE, Yan S, Sun M, et al. Loss of Ahi1 affects early development by impairing BM88/Cend1-mediated neuronal differentiation. J Neurosci. 2013;33(19):8172–84.

2

The heat shock response in neurons and astroglia and its role in neurodegenerative diseases

Rebecca San Gil, Lezanne Ooi, Justin J. Yerbury and Heath Ecroyd*

Abstract

Protein inclusions are a predominant molecular pathology found in numerous neurodegenerative diseases, including amyotrophic lateral sclerosis and Huntington's disease. Protein inclusions form in discrete areas of the brain characteristic to the type of neurodegenerative disease, and coincide with the death of neurons in that region (e.g. spinal cord motor neurons in amyotrophic lateral sclerosis). This suggests that the process of protein misfolding leading to inclusion formation is neurotoxic, and that cell-autonomous and non-cell autonomous mechanisms that maintain protein homeostasis (proteostasis) can, at times, be insufficient to prevent protein inclusion formation in the central nervous system. The heat shock response is a pro-survival pathway induced under conditions of cellular stress that acts to maintain proteostasis through the up-regulation of heat shock proteins, a superfamily of molecular chaperones, other co-chaperones and mitotic regulators. The kinetics and magnitude of the heat shock response varies in a stress- and cell-type dependent manner. It remains to be determined if and/or how the heat shock response is activated in the different cell-types that comprise the central nervous system (e.g. neurons and astroglia) in response to protein misfolding events that precede cellular dysfunctions in neurodegenerative diseases. This is particularly relevant considering emerging evidence demonstrating the non-cell autonomous nature of amyotrophic lateral sclerosis and Huntington's disease (and other neurodegenerative diseases) and the destructive role of astroglia in disease progression. This review highlights the complexity of heat shock response activation and addresses whether neurons and glia sense and respond to protein misfolding and aggregation associated with neurodegenerative diseases, in particular Huntington's disease and amyotrophic lateral sclerosis, by inducing a pro-survival heat shock response.

Keywords: Neurodegeneration, Amyotrophic lateral sclerosis, Huntington's disease, Proteostasis, Heat shock response, Heat shock factor 1, Motor neurons, Striatal neurons, Astroglia

Background

Neurodegenerative diseases (NDs), such as amyotrophic lateral sclerosis (ALS) and Huntington's disease (HD), are thought to manifest through either a loss of function of the wild-type (WT) protein or toxic gain-of-function as a result of its oligomerization and aggregation [1]. The neuron-specific degeneration observed in discrete regions of the brain in NDs suggests that specific neuronal sub-types are particularly vulnerable to protein misfolding and aggregation. This may be the result of: (i) a post-mitotic inability to dilute toxic protein species through cell-division; (ii) an age-related decline in the systems that maintain protein homeostasis (proteostasis); (iii) a failure of the proteostasis network to detect pathogenic protein aggregates; or (iv) a combination of these factors [2–4].

Molecular chaperones are a central component of the proteostasis network as they act to facilitate the correct folding of nascent polypeptides, maintain partially-folded protein intermediates in folding-competent states and re-fold damaged proteins [5–8]. A recent comprehensive analysis of the human "chaperome" identified 332 chaperone genes, 142 of which correspond to the heat shock protein subfamilies (Hsp90, Hsp70, Hsp60, Hsp40 and sHsps) [4]. The Hsps are a family of evolutionarily

* Correspondence: heathe@uow.edu.au
Illawarra Health and Medical Research Institute and School of Biological Sciences, University of Wollongong, Northfields Ave, Wollongong 2522, Australia

conserved chaperones with diverse functions in proteostasis. In addition to their well characterized molecular chaperone functions, Hsps also stabilize the cytoskeleton, regulate stress responses, mitigate apoptotic signalling and shuttle damaged proteins for degradation by the ubiquitin proteasome system or by autophagy [9, 10].

There is a dramatic up-regulation of Hsp expression in cells upon induction of the heat shock response (HSR). The activation of this pathway is a primary defense mechanism that protects cells from stress conditions that promote protein misfolding, aggregation and cell death. It has previously been shown that components of the HSR may be neuroprotective due to their ability to interact with the earliest misfolded proteins that trigger pathogenic aggregation. Indeed, numerous studies have shown that Hsps can prevent the aggregation of various disease-associated proteins in vitro, for example, mutant superoxide dismutase 1 (SOD1) in ALS [11–15]. Heat shock proteins can also interact with pathogenic proteins in vivo and have been found co-localized with plaques and inclusions in transgenic mouse models of NDs and patient post-mortem tissues [16–19]. For example, Hsc70 was co-localized with inclusion bodies in spinal cord sections of $SOD1^{G93A}$, $SOD1^{G85R}$, and $SOD1^{G37R}$ transgenic mice, and human sporadic ALS cases [17]. The co-localization of Hsps with inclusions suggests that Hsps are diverted into inclusions and therefore unavailable to perform normal "housekeeping" functions.

Little is known about how and/or if the HSR is induced in neuronal and glial cells by pathogenic protein aggregation. Elucidating whether the HSR is triggered by protein aggregation and, if so, the mechanism(s) by which this occurs, is important for future work aimed at developing proteostasis-modulating therapeutics to ameliorate ND pathologies. The objectives of this review are to summarize what is currently known about the activation of the HSR in different tissues and cell-types during cellular stress, and explore evidence regarding the involvement of the HSR in rescuing neurons and astroglia from pathological stress associated with NDs. Due to the diversity in how different NDs manifest in the CNS (i.e. dysfunction of different neuronal and non-neuronal cell types across different brain regions), this review seeks to provide a comprehensive summary of the literature surrounding the HSR in cells associated with HD and ALS. We conclude by drawing correlations between our core findings in the HD and ALS literature with NDs in general. In doing so, progress in this field of research is evaluated, gaps in our knowledge are highlighted and possible solutions are discussed.

The HSR

Proteotoxic cellular insults have a common effect of damaging proteins and inducing the accumulation of partially-folded protein intermediates. This in turn can activate transcription factors and induce the HSR. The human genome encodes four heat shock transcription factors (HSF), HSF1 – HSF4, which have unique and overlapping functions [20]. Heat shock transcription factor 1 is the prime integrator of transcriptional responses during stress and is responsible for the induction of the HSR. The role of HSF1 in the activation and attenuation of the HSR in cells under conditions of cellular stress is discussed briefly below.

Heat shock transcription factor 1

Heat shock transcription factor 1 is constitutively expressed in most tissues and cell types and, apart from its role in the HSR, is involved in a wide range of processes including organismal development, insulin signaling and cancer metastasis (for recent comprehensive reviews see [21, 22]). Post-translational modifications are critical in modulating the activity of HSF1 [23]: it can be acetylated [24, 25], SUMOylated [26] and extensively phosphorylated [27] (Fig. 1). The type and site of each post-translational modification have been predominantly identified by proteomic mass spectrometry and site-directed mutagenesis experiments [22, 23, 28]. Whilst the activation of HSF1 is complex and only partially understood, previous studies highlight the importance post-translational modifications play in stabilising, activating and inhibiting the transcriptional activity of HSF1 [28]. For example, conversion of HSF1 into a transcriptionally active trimer occurs concurrently with extensive post-translational modifications including stress-inducible hyperphosphorylation of S230, S326 and T142 [29–31], such that hyperphosphorylated HSF1 is used as a marker of HSF1 activation [32–35]. Aside from (extensive) phosphorylation, acetylation and SUMOylation of HSF1 also play important roles in regulating the strength and duration of the HSR (for comprehensive reviews see [21, 36]).

HSR activation and attenuation

Under conditions of cellular stress, HSF1 monomers form activated homo-trimers and translocate into the nucleus. Trimerization is mediated through the formation of leucine zippers on adjacent HSF1 oligomerization domains (Fig. 2) [37, 38]. Activated HSF1 trimers bind to *cis*-regulatory elements on DNA composed of nGAAn pentamers (where n is any base), collectively called heat shock elements [39–42]. The extent and duration of HSF1-mediated transcription is influenced by the number of heat shock elements, the exact sequence of nGAAn pentamers in the promoter regions of HSF1 target genes, and post-translational modifications on HSF1 itself [21]. In addition to the rapid up-regulation of Hsp expression in response to cellular stress, HSF1 also coordinates the expression of many transcriptional and translational regulators, co-chaperones, ubiquitin, signaling molecules and mitotic regulators [21, 43, 44].

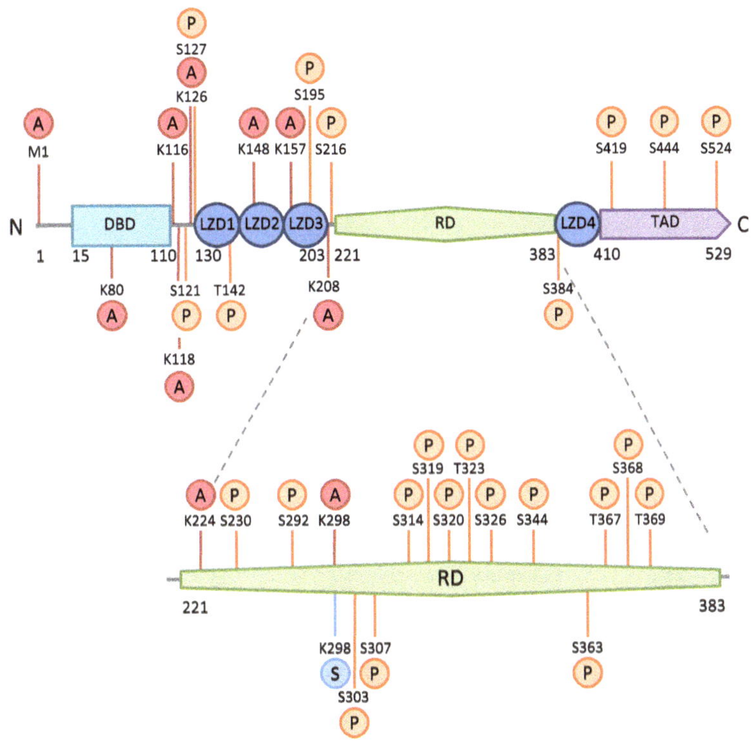

Fig. 1 Post-translational modifications of HSF1 in relation to the functional domains in the protein. The HSF1 protein consists of a DNA-binding domain (DBD), four leucine zipper domains (LZD), a regulatory domain (RD) and a transactivating domain (TAD). The proposed sites of serine/threonine phosphorylation (P), lysine acetylation (A) and phosphorylation-dependent lysine SUMOylation (S) are marked on the HSF1 amino acid chain. These post-translational modifications are mediated by numerous kinases, acetylases and SUMOylases and act to modulate the stabilization and activity of HSF1 and thus the strength and duration of the HSR

Heat shock factor 1-mediated transcription is attenuated by an auto-regulatory mechanism, whereby HSF1-induced Hsps competitively inhibit HSF1 trimer activity [22, 28]. This negative feedback loop provides an important mechanism by which cells can regulate the activation and attenuation of an HSR via the presence and concentration of Hsps in the cell. The trimerisation of HSF1 is suppressed by interaction of the monomer with a multi-chaperone complex composed of Hsp90, co-chaperone p23 and immunophilin FK506-binding protein 5 [45, 46]. In addition, the chaperonin TRiC/CCT can also interact with HSF1 to inhibit its activation [47]. Active HSF1 trimers in the nucleus can be inhibited by the binding of Hsp70 and its co-chaperone Hsp40, possibly through recruitment of the Hsp70-interacting transcriptional co-repressor, CoREST [48, 49]. Further characterization of the mechanisms that modulate HSF1 activity (and therefore, the HSR) may help elucidate additional targets for therapies that could be used to boost the HSR in the context of disease such as NDs.

The HSR in the mammalian CNS

In mammals, the HSR varies both in terms of kinetics (i.e. how fast stress-induced transcripts are generated) and magnitude (i.e. the fold increase in Hsp levels) between tissues and even between cells in the same tissue [50–52]. Analysis of the human "chaperome" shows that the constitutive expression of housekeeping chaperones and co-chaperones varies between tissues [52]. For example, sHsps are overrepresented in skeletal and cardiac muscle compared to the brain [52]. With regard to inducing the HSR, whole organism hyperthermia results in an HSR that varies substantially across tissues types [50]. For example, in heat-stressed rats, the kinetics of the response and magnitude of induction where found to vary between the brain, liver and skin when assessed over time by northern blot of Hsp70 and Hsp27 stress-induced mRNA [50]. Moreover, cells in the same tissue can display different capacities to induce the HSR. For example, cultured astrocytes elicit faster and higher levels of Hsp70 expression after heat shock (45 °C for 30 min) compared to cultured cortical neurons [51]. These studies strongly suggest that the capacity of a cell to sense stress and elicit an HSR differs in a cell-type dependent manner.

An attenuated HSR may be an intrinsic characteristic of neurons [35, 53–55]. Indeed, this hypothesis is supported by several animal studies that have challenged

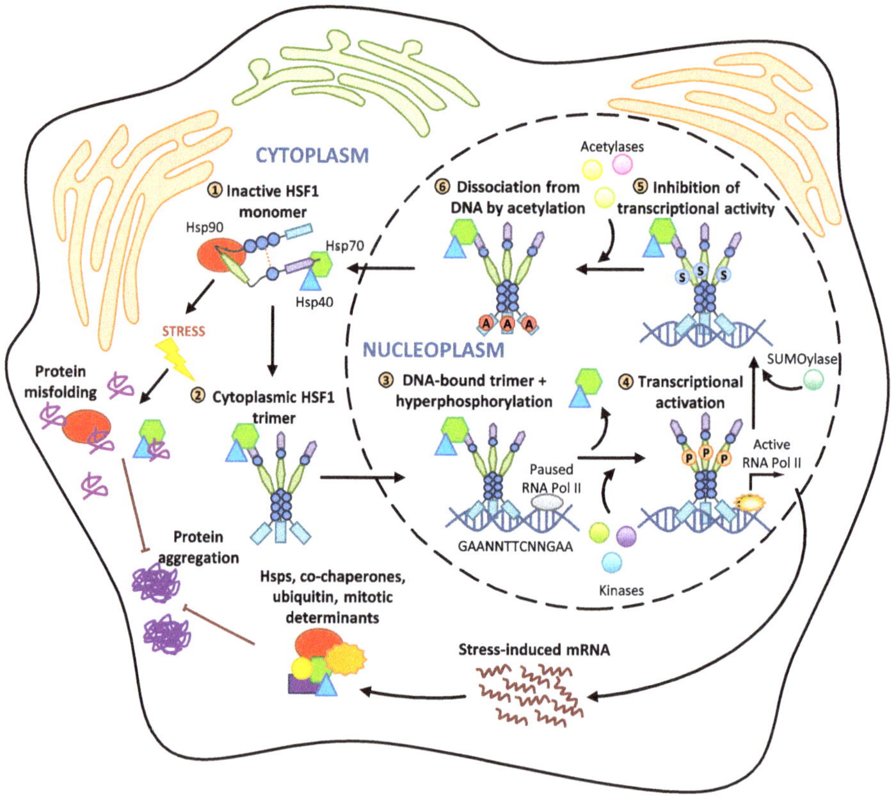

Fig. 2 The activation of HSF1 and its binding to DNA is regulated by a multi-step pathway that involves nuclear accumulation, intramolecular and intermolecular protein interactions, and post-translational modifications. (1) In the absence of stress, HSF1 is maintained in a monomeric state through the regulatory actions of several post-translational modifications, intramolecular contacts, and interactions with Hsps in inhibitory complexes. Cellular stress results in the accumulation of misfolded and damaged proteins, which compete with HSF1 for binding to Hsps. (2) HSF1 monomers are released and undergo a conformational change conducive to trimerization. (3) Concurrent nuclear accumulation, HSE-binding and hyperphosphorylation of trimeric HSF1 occur. (4) This process releases RNA PolII from a paused to an active state to initiate the transcription of stress-induced genes. (5) SUMOylation at K298 and binding of Hsp40/Hsp70 represses the transcriptional activity of HSF1 trimers. (6) Acetylation at K80 disrupts HSF1 binding to DNA and HSF1 trimers dissociate and re-join the monomeric pool in the cytosol. Stress-inducible Hsps participate in a negative-feedback loop to inhibit further HSF1 activation

rodents with hyperthermia or ischemic injury and shown that neurons do not induce Hsp70 expression after exposure to these stressors, whereas surrounding astroglial cells do [35, 51, 54–59]. These seminal studies show that under conditions of acute cellular stress, neurons are inherently poor activators of the HSR, whereas astroglia readily activate the HSR. This prompts the question of whether neuronal and astroglial cells respond to chronic ND-relevant stressors (such as protein aggregation) and, if so, whether there is a difference in the response of neuronal and astroglial cells to this stress. In an attempt to address these questions, the remainder of this review deals with what is known about HSR activation in the context of two NDs, HD and ALS.

Huntington's Disease

Huntington's disease is characterized by the formation of intracellular inclusions composed primarily of the ubiquitous protein huntingtin (Htt) and by the subsequent death of striatal medium spiny neurons and cortical pyramidal neurons [60, 61]. The genetic basis for the pathogenesis of HD is a CAG codon repeat expansion in the Huntingtin (*HTT*) gene, which leads to a mutant protein that contains an expanded poly-glutamine (polyQ) sequence [62]. Expansions of the polyQ tract beyond 36 glutamines result in an aggregation-prone Htt protein; the length of the polyQ-expansion correlates with the age of disease onset and severity (i.e. the longer the polyQ tract, the earlier the onset of disease and the more rapid the disease progression) [63]. Well-characterized cell and transgenic mouse models of HD have been used in investigations into the impact of the HSR on the pathogenicity of polyQ-expansions.

PolyQ-expanded Htt may interact differently with the proteostasis network compared to other disease-associated proteins. Evidence for this comes from studies that have shown that polyQ-expanded Htt^{103Q} (i.e. Htt with a polyQ stretch of 103 glutamines) partitions exclusively into perivacuolar inclusion bodies (IPODs: Insoluble PrOtein Deposits) that store terminally aggregated proteins [64]. Fluorescence recovery after photobleaching experiments showed that Htt^{103Q} proteins sequestered into IPODs are immobile [65] indicating that sequestration into IPODs prevents possible interactions of the aggregated protein with components of the proteostasis network, exacerbating the formation of inclusions in cells [64, 66]. Recent evidence also suggests that Htt inclusion body formation deactivates apoptosis and results in slow necrotic cell death [67]. This contrasts with quality control partitioning of other aggregation-prone disease-associated proteins, such as SOD1, which accumulate in juxtanuclear compartments (JUNQ: JUxtaNuclear Quality control) for presentation to molecular chaperones for re-folding and/or the ubiquitin proteasome system for degradation [64, 66, 68, 69]. Therefore, findings pertaining to the HSR in the context of HD may uniquely apply to this ND due to the propensity of polyQ-expanded Htt to misfold directly into terminal aggregates and become stored in IPODs (as opposed to the JUNQ).

The HSR in striatal neurons

The expression and cellular accumulation of pathogenic polyQ-expanded Htt is not sufficient to induce an HSR in cell and animal models of HD. The expression of Htt^{91Q} does not induce an HSR (as assessed by an Hsp70 promoter driven EGFP expression construct) [70]. Notably, the expression of Htt^{111Q} in striatal cells was not sufficient to up-regulate Hsp expression nor activate HSF1 [32]. Likewise, primary cultures of rat cortical and striatal neurons expressing Htt^{111Q} showed low levels of Hsp70 mRNA transcripts and protein compared to cerebellar granule cells, which have high levels of Hsp70 and are resistant to degeneration [71]. Studies using transgenic mouse models of HD have demonstrated that there is a reduction in Hsp70 (and other molecular chaperones) in the brain as the disease progresses (Table 1) [72]. Taken together, these results show that cells expressing polyQ-expanded Htt do not sense or respond to this aggregation-prone protein by inducing an HSR.

The expression of polyQ-expanded Htt sensitizes neurons to heat stress [32, 73]. Heat shock (42 °C for 6 h) of primary murine striatal neurons expressing pathogenic Htt^{111Q} resulted in a 6-fold increase in caspase activity compared to heat shocked cells expressing non-pathogenic Htt^{7Q} [32]. Furthermore, cells expressing Htt^{111Q} had a reduced capacity to express Hsp70, Hsp25 (the mouse orthologue of Hsp27) and Hsp90 after heat shock compared to those expressing Htt^{7Q} [32]. These findings suggest that expression of polyQ-expanded Htt attenuates the capacity of striatal neurons to up-regulate the expression of Hsps after heat shock, which is normally a very strong activator of the HSR.

Based on these findings, it is pertinent to question whether the observed inability of striatal neurons to induce an HSR in the context of HD is the result of insufficient levels of HSF1, a failure to activate HSF1, a lack of HSF1 binding to DNA, or a combination of these deficiencies (Fig. 3). Quantification of total HSF1 protein by immunoblot demonstrated that primary striatal neurons expressing Htt^{111Q}, and the striata and cerebella of HD mouse models, have lower total HSF1 levels compared to controls [32]. New evidence implicates CK2α'

Table 1 List of Hsps and whether their expression is up-regulated (↑), down-regulated (↓), or not changed (No Δ) across rodent models of HD compared to transgenic WT or non-transgenic mouse controls

Hsps	Transgenic disease models	Tissue or cell type	Reference
HSF1	STHdh(Q111) knock-in mice	IB: 80% ↓striatal and cerebellar tissue homogenates	[32, 74]
αB-c (HSPB5)	R6/2	IB: No Δ whole brain homogenates	[72]
	Htt-N171-82Q	IB: No Δ spinal cord homogenates	[79]
Hsp25 (HSPB1)	R6/2	IB: No Δ whole brain homogenates	[72]
	Htt-N171-82Q	IB: No Δ spinal cord homogenates	[79]
Hsp40	R6/2	IB: 60% ↓Hdj1 whole brain homogenates IB: 25% ↓Hdj2 whole brain homogenates	[72]
Hsp60	R6/2	LC-MS: 4-fold ↓ in protein abundance in the cortex LC-MS: 4-fold ↑ in protein abundance in the striatum	[80]
Hsp70	STHdh(Q111) knock-in mice	IB: 80% ↓striatal and cerebellar tissue homogenates	[32]
	R6/2	IB: ↓ whole brain homogenates IB: No Δ Hsc70 whole brain homogenates	[72]
Hsp90	R6/2	IB: No Δ Hsp90 whole brain homogenates IB: No Δ Hsp84 whole brain homogenates	[72]
Hsp105	–	–	–

These results are from immunoblot (IB), or liquid chromatography coupled with quantitative mass spectrometry (LC-MS) of affected CNS regions

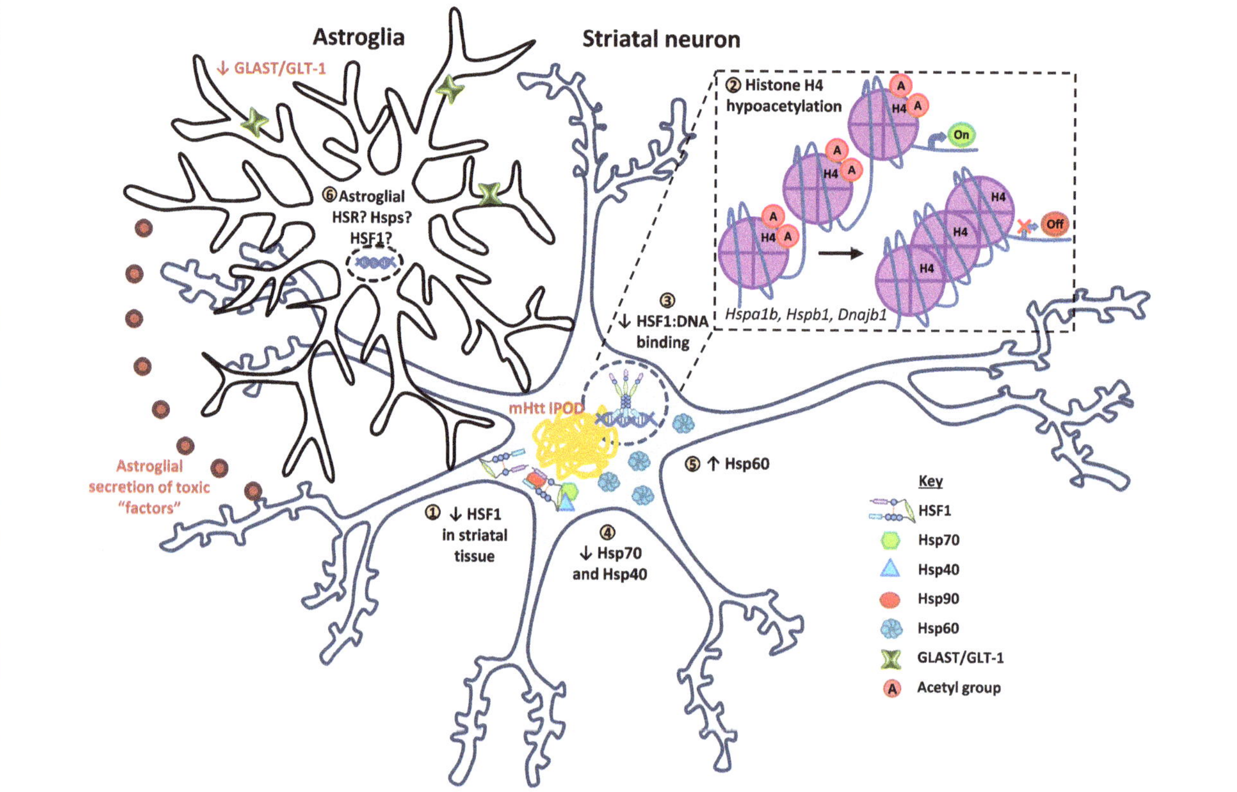

Fig. 3 Proposed summary of changes in the HSR and its components in polyQ-expanded Htt over-expression models of HD. Huntington's disease onset and progression into late stage is dependent on the molecular pathologies developed in striatal neurons (e.g. formation of polyQ-expanded Htt aggregates or IPODs) and astroglia (e.g. decline in GLAST/GLT-1 expression and the secretion of unidentified toxic "factors"). The susceptibility of striatal neurons to degeneration from HD-associated stresses could be the result of a polyQ-expanded Htt-mediated attenuation of the HSR. Over-expression of polyQ-expanded Htt in CNS tissues results in a (1) reduction in HSF1 levels. (2) Histone H4 acetylation has been shown to be a strong promoter of HSF1 binding to DNA of target genes. However, hypoacetylation of histone H4 at HSF1 targets (e.g. *Hspa1b*, *Hspb1*, and *Dnajb1*) with disease progression can explain (3) the decrease in HSF1 binding to DNA observed in polyQ-expanded Htt expressing striatal neurons. (4) HD disease progression is also associated with a decline in Hsp70 and Hsp40 family members and (5) a striatal-specific increase in Hsp60. (6) There have been few investigations regarding HSF1 activation and DNA-binding in astroglia. Therefore, the capacity of polyQ-expanded Htt over-expressing astroglia to activate HSF1 and induce an HSR is currently unknown

kinase and Fbxw7 Fbox protein (an E3 ubiquitin ligase) in the enhanced degradation of HSF1 in cells expressing polyQ-expanded Htt [74]. The proposed model suggests that polyQ-expanded Htt up-regulates CK2α′ kinase expression and increases the phosphorylation of HSF1 at S303 and S307. This in turn recruits Fbxw7, which ubiquitinylates phospho-HSF1 targeting it for degradation by the ubiquitin proteasome system [74]. Enhanced degradation of HSF1 by the proteasome has also been implicated in a mouse model and human post-mortem tissues of α-synucleinopathies, whereby elevated levels of the ubiquitin ligase, NEDD4, ubiquitinates HSF1 for degradation [25]. Whilst expression of Htt^{111Q} is not sufficient to induce HSF1 activation in cerebellar granule cells, heat shock does result in activated (hyperphosphorylated) HSF1 trimers accumulating in the cell nucleus [32, 71]. Similarly, HSF1 dissociation from Hsp90, hyperphosphorylation, and nuclear translocation are not impaired in HD mice upon treatment with the Hsp90 inhibitor NVP-HSP990, which is able to penetrate into the brain [71]. Therefore, there is a reduction in total HSF1 levels in the striatum; however, HSF1 can become hyperphosphorylated and translocate into the nucleus in HD models.

With regard to the DNA binding capacity of HSF1 in HD models, evidence suggests that the expression of polyQ-expanded Htt attenuates HSF1 binding to DNA in striatal cells [73]. Genome-wide chromatin immunoprecipitation (ChIP) experiments demonstrated that in primary striatal neurons expressing Htt^{111Q}, HSF1 is only capable of binding 39% of its target genes after heat shock (1159 bound genes) compared to cells expressing Htt^{7Q} (2943 bound genes) [73]. Microarray data show that the reduced HSF1 binding to DNA in heat shocked cells expressing Htt^{111Q} corresponds with a decline in the transcription of several Hsps (*Dndjb5*, *Dnajb12* and *Hspb6*). Furthermore, mRNA levels of Hsp70, Hsp40 and Hsp25 were reduced in the cerebral cortices of HD mouse models compared to controls following treatment with NVP-HSP990 [75]. Therefore, since HSF1 activation appears to be unimpaired, low levels of HSF1 and its compromised ability to bind DNA could account for the observed inability of cells expressing polyQ-expanded Htt to elicit an HSR. This dysregulation of chaperone gene expression likely plays a key role in the pathology of HD.

Altered chromatin architecture in HD may explain the reduced capacity of HSF1 to bind to target genes in striatal neurons under stress [75–78]. Quantitative PCR coupled with ChIP analysis after NVP-HSP990 (Hsp90 inhibitor) treatment demonstrated significant hypoacetylation of histone H4 at *Hspa1b, Hspb1, Dnajb1* genes in Htt^{111Q} expressing primary striatal neurons compared to Htt^{7Q} [75]. Hypoacetylation of these Hsp genes may change the chromatin landscape sufficiently to interfere with HSF1 binding to DNA (Fig. 3). Stress-inducible binding of HSF1 to DNA is associated with histone acetylation, H3K4 trimethylation, RNA polymerase II and other co-activators [77]. Furthermore, tetra-acetyl histone H4 has previously been suggested to be a strong modulator of HSF1 binding to DNA [77]. Therefore, it follows that histone H4 hypoacetylation in HD models may reduce chromatin accessibility of HSF1 at heat shock genes, consequently impairing the HSR.

At the tissue level, there are several studies that have investigated Hsp expression, and therefore HSR activation, in affected and non-affected tissues in mouse models of HD (Table 1). Immunoblot analysis of whole brain or spinal cord homogenates from HD mice have shown that overall there is no change in the total protein levels of the sHsps Hsp25 or αB-crystallin (αB-c, HSPB5) or Hsp90 family members compared to mice expressing non-pathogenic Htt [72, 79]. Whole tissue homogenates from HD mice showed a reduction in HSF1, Hsp70, and two Hsp40 family members (Hdj1 and Hdj2; Fig. 3) [32, 72]. Conversely, striatal homogenates from HD mice were found to have a 4-fold increase in Hsp60 levels compared to control mice [80]. A lack of immunohistochemistry in these studies makes it impossible to determine (i) where changes occur at the cellular level and (ii), whether small cell populations or specific cell-types induce an HSR, which is undetectable in bulk cell analyses. Employing immunohistochemistry in parallel to this work, or more powerful omics-based single-cell analyses, such as the proteomics approach undertaken by Sharma et al. [81], has the potential to resolve cell-type and brain-region specific differences in the presence or absence of disease. In this way, cell-type specific differences in the ability to induce a pro-survival HSR will be identified.

The role of glial cells in HD

There is evidence that the onset and progression of HD is both cell-autonomous and non-cell autonomous. One study showed that a transgenic mouse with pan-neuronal expression of Htt^{103Q} developed pathologies associated with end-stage disease, including astrogliosis, motor deficits and neurodegeneration [82, 83]. However, when Htt^{103Q} expression was restricted to either striatal neurons or cortical pyramidal neurons, pathologies associated with end-stage disease did not develop despite these cells having nuclear polyQ-expanded Htt aggregates and alterations in NMDA receptor function [82, 83]. These studies showed for the first time that HD pathogenesis and propagation depends on interactions between neuronal subtypes. Neuron-astroglia interactions have also been implicated in the non-cell autonomous progression of HD. A study that investigated transgenic mice that expressed Htt^{98Q} in both neurons and astroglia observed that these mice displayed more severe neurological symptoms and earlier death compared to mice in which Htt^{98Q} expression was restricted to either neurons or astroglia alone [84]. Therefore, it seems likely that both neuron-neuron and neuron-astroglia interactions are responsible for the onset and progression of HD.

The combination of molecular pathologies that develop in neurons and astroglia work in tandem to progress HD (Fig. 3). However, the mechanisms that underlie astroglial-mediated toxicity in HD are only partially understood. Astroglia expressing polyQ-expanded Htt secrete neurotoxic factors and decrease the expression of the glutamate transporters, GLAST and GLT-1 [85–87]. Indeed, polyQ-expanded Htt-expressing astroglia have been shown to increase the vulnerability of striatal and cortical neurons in co-culture to excitotoxic stresses [88]. Conversely, in co-culture experiments, astrocytes expressing non-pathogenic Htt^{23Q} protected 78% of the Htt^{130Q}-expressing cortical neurons from glutamate toxicity [88]. Furthermore, conditioned medium derived from WT astroglial cultures protects Htt^{111Q}-expressing striatal neuronal progenitor cells from neurotoxic insults (e.g. H_2O_2, glutamate, 3-nitropropionic acid) [89].

With respect to neurotoxic factors secreted by astroglia, an elegant study by Liddelow et al. [86], demonstrated that pro-inflammatory microglia can activate a neurotoxic phenotype in astroglia (defined in the work as A1 astroglia). They showed that A1 astrocyte formation is a pathological response of the CNS in mice treated with systemic injections of lipopolysaccharide and acute CNS injury, and in patients with NDs [86]. The proportion of neurotoxic (A1) astroglia in the caudate nucleus of HD patients was significantly greater than in controls (60% in HD tissue compared to 25% in the control) [86]. Furthermore, qPCR of A1 astroglia-associated transcripts showed a 60-fold increase in the caudate nucleus of

HD patients compared to controls [86]. Thus, cell-cell interactions and dysfunctions of striatal or cortical pyramidal neurons and astroglia are likely to work synergistically to progress HD into late-stages. Therefore, it is important to maintain astrocytes in the striatum in a healthy and neurotrophic condition to minimize neurodegeneration in the striatum. The focus of research investigating pro-survival mechanisms and the proteostasis network in HD has thus far been predominantly focused on striatal neurons. However, considering accumulating evidence that implicates astroglia in the pathogenesis of HD, it is relevant to also investigate these pathways in astroglia.

The HSR in striatal astrocytes

Studies investigating HSR-inducing compounds have provided valuable insights into the capacity of different cell populations to induce an HSR in the absence of the expression of polyQ-expanded Htt. Primary striatal astrocytes derived from WT mice showed a stronger induction of the HSR compared to striatal projection neurons after treatment with the Hsp90 inhibitor, NVP-HSP990: treated striatal astroglia showed an 18-fold increase in Hsp70 and 4-fold increase in Hsp25 mRNA levels [90]. In contrast, NVP-HSP990 treated striatal projection neurons only showed an 8-fold increase in Hsp70, 3-fold increase in Hsp40, and no change in Hsp25 mRNA levels [90]. In the vehicle treated mice, there were no significant differences compared to non-treated mice in the synthesis of any of the Hsp mRNAs investigated (Hsp70, Hsp40, Hsp90 or HSF1), with the exception of Hsp25, which showed a 7-fold increase in astroglia compared to striatal projection neurons [90]. Together these findings suggest that, in the absence of polyQ-expanded Htt expression, striatal astroglia are "pre-loaded" with greater levels of Hsp25 mRNA and can induce a stronger HSR compared to striatal projection neurons.

The size and frequency of formation of polyQ-expanded Htt inclusions varies across different cell-types in the CNS. Striatal and frontal cortex glial fibrillary acidic protein (GFAP)-positive astroglia demonstrated a significant reduction in the size and the proportion of cells with Htt^{210Q} inclusions compared to neurons in these CNS regions in a mouse model of HD [91]. This difference was attributed to a possible increase in proteostasis network components (including heat shock proteins) in reactive astroglia. However, there is insufficient evidence from models of HD, with regards to the Hsp content of striatal astroglia, to draw relationships between inclusion size and number and proteostasis capacity of striatal astroglia (Fig. 3).

Determining mechanisms that maintain astroglia in a healthy and neurotrophic state should be a priority in future HD research, given that polyQ-expanded Htt expression decreases the levels of glutamate transporters and induces a neurotoxic phenotype of astroglia. Indeed, a recent study demonstrated that the over-expression of the sHsp, αB-c, in astroglia ameliorates the pathologies associated with HD in transgenic mice that express full-length Htt^{97Q} [92]. Over-expression of αB-c in astroglia significantly reduced the number of large (> 1 μm) Htt^{97Q} inclusions in the striatum and cortex, and resulted in a 14% increase in the number of NeuN-positive neurons in the striatum [92]. This provides an elegant example of how increasing Hsps in astroglia can ameliorate HD neuropathologies in a non-cell autonomous manner and provides support for increased investigation into the HSR in astroglia in the context of HD.

Summary of the HSR in HD

It has been demonstrated using a range of cell and animal models of HD that striatal neurons do not sense or respond to polyQ-expanded Htt expression by up-regulating Hsps. Moreover, striatal neurons expressing polyQ-expanded Htt have an attenuated capacity to induce an HSR after heat shock. This could be due to decreased levels of HSF1 in striatal tissue observed in HD models. In addition, the altered chromatin landscape caused by histone H4 hypoacetylation at Hsp genes observed in a HD mouse model, may also lead to decreased binding of HSF1 to DNA, and down-regulation of Hsp70 and Hsp40. In the absence of polyQ-expanded Htt expression, striatal astroglia, compared to striatal projection neurons, have greater levels of Hsp25 mRNA and can induce a stronger HSR. However, the effect of polyQ-expanded Htt on HSR induction in astroglia remains to be elucidated.

Previous research has demonstrated that a variety of Hsps can inhibit polyQ-expanded Htt protein aggregation. However, the affected neurons in HD appear not to sense the initial stages of pathogenic protein misfolding as a cellular stress and therefore do not activate an HSR. As the neurons and surrounding astroglia in the CNS appear to be incapable of activating an HSR in the context of HD, therapeutics that can induce Hsp expression in early stages of disease may prove beneficial.

Amyotrophic lateral sclerosis

Amyotrophic lateral sclerosis is characterized by a loss of motor neurons in the primary motor cortex, corticospinal tracts, brainstem and spinal cord. Only 5–10% of ALS cases are familial (fALS) and some of these arise from mutations in one of 13 (or more) genes leading to the expression of aberrant aggregation-prone proteins. Mutations in *SOD1* (copper/zinc ion-binding superoxide dismutase), *FUS* (fused in sarcoma), *TDP-43* (TAR DNA binding protein), *CCNF* (cyclin F) [93], *OPTN* (optineurin), *ANG* (angiogenin, ribonuclease, RNase A family,

5), *UBQLN2* (ubiquitin-like ubiquilin2), and others, as well as repeat expansions in *C9ORF72* (chromosome 9 open reading frame 72), are all associated with fALS (recently reviewed by [94, 95]). The remaining 90–95% of ALS cases are idiopathic and sporadic. In ALS, motor neurons are selectively susceptible to degeneration as a consequence of mutant ALS-associated protein expression, despite the ubiquitous presence of these same mutant forms in neuronal and non-neuronal cells [96]. Motor neurons have functional and morphological characteristics that may make them particularly vulnerable to toxic protein misfolding and aggregation, neuroinflammation, excitotoxic insults, oxidative damage and subsequent degeneration in ALS [96]. For example, motor neurons have a high metabolic load, high energy demands, long axons, and rely on rapid signaling of neurotransmitters to other neurons and muscle tissue by axonal transport. Malfunction of each of these characteristics of motor neurons have been associated with ALS pathology (for reviews see [97–99]). In addition, recent findings have shown that multiple housekeeping and stress-response pathways involved in maintaining proteostasis (e.g. the ubiquitin proteasome system and endoplasmic reticulum unfolded protein response) are dysregulated in ALS-affected motor neurons, which would further exacerbate their degeneration [96, 100–105]. However, it remains to be established whether affected cell-types in the CNS can induce an HSR as a result of pathogenic protein aggregation associated with ALS as a protective response to this chronic proteotoxic stress.

The HSR in motor neurons

Motor neurons may have a relatively high threshold for HSR induction compared to surrounding non-neuronal cells. Batulan et al. [53] investigated the endogenous expression of HSF1 in motor neurons and their capacity to activate the HSR. In these studies, immunohistochemistry of motor neurons in spinal cord cultures demonstrated the presence of HSF1, but not Hsp70, in these cells. The capacity of motor neurons to induce an HSR was assessed following heat shock (42 °C for 1 h) by monitoring the stress-inducible expression of an Hsp70 promoter driven EGFP construct. The lack of EGFP fluorescence in motor neurons after heat shock suggested that HSF1 was not activated and thus did not bind to the HSE used in this reporter construct [53]. Other studies have also shown that spinal cord motor neurons in situ fail to transcribe and express Hsp70 following heat shock [58, 106]. However, it is not clear from this work whether HSF1 was (i) not activated and therefore not capable of binding DNA and/or (ii) not present at sufficient levels in these cells to induce an HSR.

To determine which of these possibilities was responsible for these observations, WT HSF1 ($HSF1^{WT}$) and a constitutively active mutant of HSF1 ($HSF1^{+}$) were over-expressed in primary murine motor neurons [53]. Simply increasing the level of $HSF1^{WT}$ in cells was not sufficient to enhance their capacity to express Hsp70 [53]. Conversely, over-expression of $HSF1^{+}$ resulted in an up-regulation of Hsp70, Hsp40, and Hsp25 levels in 96.1 ± 3.4%, 100 ± 0%, and 14.6 ± 7.3% in motor neurons, respectively [53, 107]. Furthermore, expression of $HSF1^{+}$ in motor neurons expressing pathogenic $SOD1^{G93A}$ significantly reduced the formation of inclusions and conferred cytoprotection, compared to $HSF1^{WT}$ [107]. Together, these findings suggest that the attenuated capacity of motor neurons to induce an HSR in the context of heat shock is due to their inability to activate HSF1, not insufficient levels of HSF1 in these cells (Fig. 4).

The over expression and aggregation of mutant SOD1 (mSOD1) in mouse models may not be sufficient to induce an HSR in motor neurons. Primary murine motor neurons expressing mSOD1 demonstrate no change in expression levels of Hsp70, Hsp105, Hsp90, Hsp60, or Hsp40 compared to those expressing $SOD1^{WT}$ and non-transgenic control motor neurons (Table 2). Furthermore, a reduction in Hsp105 levels was observed in spinal cord tissue homogenates of $SOD1^{G93A}$ mice [108]. Hsp105 is a chaperone expressed in neurons and glia- in the CNS and can inhibit the aggregation of mSOD1 in cell-based models [108]. Therefore, the decline in Hsp105 expression, combined with the inability of rodent motor neurons to up-regulate Hsp70, Hsp90, Hsp60, or Hsp40, suggests that the HSR is either unable to be activated or is impaired in these models of ALS (Fig. 4).

In the absence of disease, the endogenous and constitutive expression of Hsp27 in motor neurons of the spinal cord plays an important role in the housekeeping of proteostasis. Hsp27 is a well characterized molecular chaperone that also has potent anti-apoptotic functions [109]. Hsp27 can inhibit the release of mitochondrial cytochrome c and associate with Daxx, thereby inhibiting a motor neuron-specific apoptosis pathway mediated by Fas-Ask1-p38 [109–112]. However, in transgenic mouse models Hsp25 levels become dysregulated and decline in motor neurons during ALS progression (Table 2). Studies have shown that pre-symptomatic mSOD1 mice have Hsp25 levels comparable to age-matched controls [113, 114]. However, immediately prior to the onset of disease symptoms, Hsp25 levels decline in spinal cord motor neurons as demonstrated by immunohistochemistry of spinal cord sections [113, 114]. In contrast, by the late stages of the disease, both Hsp25 and αB-c are up-regulated in spinal cord astroglia, a finding consistent in numerous studies [79, 113–116]. Future research could

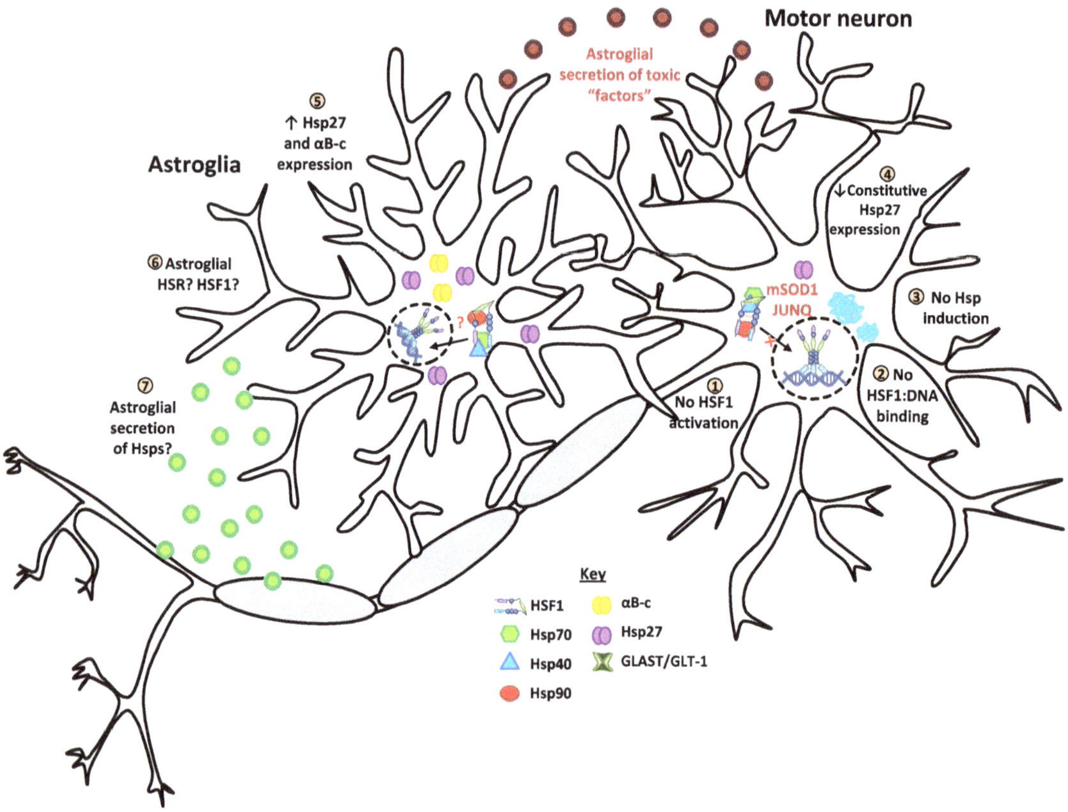

Fig. 4 Proposed mechanism of the HSR and its components in motor neurons and astroglia of mSOD1 over-expressing models of ALS. Motor neuron disease initiation and progression is dependent on the molecular pathologies developed in motor neurons (e.g. formation of mSOD1 aggregates or JUNQ) and astroglia (e.g. secretion of unidentified toxic "factors"). The susceptibility of motor neurons to degeneration is likely due to an inability of motor neurons and astroglia to induce a cytoprotective HSR in response to increasing quantities of misfolded proteins (e.g. mSOD1). (1 and 2) HSF1 in motor neurons has a relatively high threshold for activation and the over-expression of mSOD1 and subsequent molecular pathologies do not activate HSF1 nor induce HSF1 binding to DNA. (3) There is no detectable basal expression or up-regulation of Hsps in mSOD1 over-expressing motor neurons, with the exception of (4) Hsp27, which gradually declines with disease progression. (5) Astroglia in mSOD1 over-expressing mice have increased amounts of Hsp27 and αB-c with disease progression; however, the levels of other Hsps are not changed. (6) There have been few investigations regarding HSF1 activation and DNA-binding in astroglia in the context of ALS. Therefore, the capacity of mSOD1 over-expressing astroglia to activate HSF1 and induce an HSR remains unknown. (7) There is increasing evidence that extracellular vesicles containing Hsps are secreted by astroglia, and these vesicles are endocytosed by motor neurons and facilitate transfer of Hsps

address whether this decline in Hsp25 in mSOD1 expressing motor neurons correlates with an increase in Hsp25 sequestered in insoluble protein deposits. This could be achieved by immunoblot analysis of soluble and insoluble protein fractions and immunohistochemistry. The decrease in Hsp25 in motor neurons during the later stages of ALS in these transgenic mouse models may increase their susceptibility to neurodegeneration as a consequence of toxic protein accumulation and other ALS-related stresses (Fig. 4).

With regards to ALS in humans, immunohistochemistry of human motor neurons in cervical spinal cord sections obtained at autopsy showed no change in Hsp70 or Hsp27 levels compared to age-matched controls [53]. The combined evidence suggests that the toxicity of mSOD1 in spinal cord motor neurons is not sufficient to elicit the stress-inducible expression of Hsps in rodents or humans. In contrast, Hsp70 (but not Hsp27) immunoreactivity was occasionally observed to be higher in neighboring glial cells in fALS or sporadic ALS patients [53]. This suggests that astroglia in humans and rodents are capable of up-regulating certain Hsps in response to stresses associated with ALS. This further supports the hypothesis that motor neurons intrinsically have a high threshold for induction of the HSR and suggests that misfolded mSOD1 can go undetected by this inducible arm of the proteostasis network in these cells.

There is a lack of diversity in the models that have been used in work investigating the HSR in association with ALS. Data regarding neuronal and glial Hsp expression in ALS is derived primarily from mSOD1 rodent models, with the exception of one study that used the TDP-43$^{WT \times Q331K}$ transgenic mouse model of ALS [117]. Therefore, it remains to be determined whether these findings

Table 2 List of Hsps and whether their expression is up-regulated (↑), down-regulated (↓), or not changed (No Δ) in rodent models of motor neuron disease at the late-stage of disease compared to age-matched transgenic WT or non-transgenic mouse controls

Hsps	Transgenic disease models	Tissue or cell type	Reference
HSF1	TDP-43$^{WT×Q331K}$	IB: ↓ spinal cord tissue homogenates	[117]
	SOD1^{G93A}	IB: ↓ spinal cord tissue homogenates	[174]
αB-c (HSPB5)	SOD1^{L126Z}	IHC: ↑ spinal cord astroglia IHC: ↓ spinal cord oligodendrocytes	[115]
	SOD1^{G93A}	IHC: ↑ spinal cord astroglia	[116, 175]
	SOD1^{G37R}	IHC: ↑ spinal cord astroglia	[116]
Hsp22 (HSPB8)	SOD1^{G93A}	IHC: ↑ spinal cord motor neurons	[176, 177]
Hsp25 (HSPB1)	SOD1^{G93A}	IHC: ↑ spinal cord astroglia IHC: ↓ spinal cord oligodendrocytes	[53, 113, 114, 116]
	SOD1^{G37R}	IHC: ↑ astroglia in the inferior colliculus, cerebellar white matter, brain stem, spinal cord	[79]
	SOD1^{L126Z}	IHC: ↓ spinal cord motor neurons	[115]
	SOD1^{G93A}, SOD1^{G85R}, SOD1^{G37R}, SOD1$^{H46R/H48Q}$	IHC: ↑ spinal cord astroglia IHC: ↑ spinal cord undefined neurons	[178]
Hsp40	SOD1^{G93A}	IHC: No Δ spinal cord	[79]
	SOD1^{G93A}, SOD1^{G85R}, SOD1^{G37R}, SOD1$^{H46R/H48Q}$	IB: No Δ spinal cord tissue homogenates	[178]
	TDP-43$^{WT×Q331K}$	IB: No Δ spinal cord tissue homogenates	[117]
Hsp60	SOD1^{G93A}	IHC: No Δ spinal cord	[79]
	SOD1^{G93A}, SOD1^{G85R}, SOD1^{G37R}, SOD1$^{H46R/H48Q}$	IB: No Δ spinal cord tissue homogenates	[178]
Hsp70	SOD1^{G93A}, SOD1^{G85R}, SOD1^{G37R}, SOD1$^{H46R/H48Q}$	IB: No Δ spinal cord tissue homogenates	[53, 79, 115, 178]
	SOD1^{G93A}	IHC: ↑ "sick-appearing" spinal cord motor neurons	[179]
	SOD1^{G85R}	IB: ↑ spinal cord tissue homogenates	[145]
Hsp90	SOD1^{G93A}	IHC: No Δ spinal cord	[79]
	SOD1^{G93A}, SOD1^{G85R}, SOD1^{G37R}, SOD1$^{H46R/H48Q}$	IB: No Δ spinal cord tissue homogenates	[178]
Hsp105	SOD1^{G93A}	IB: ↓ in spinal cord tissue homogenates	[108]

These results are from immunoblot (IB) or immunohistochemical (IHC) staining and microscopy of different CNS regions

also apply to other fALS-associated mutations (e.g. *FUS*). This is of particular relevance if each aggregation-prone protein engages a specific set of Hsps, as has been previously proposed [118]. Therefore, additional research is required in other rodent models of ALS to advance our understanding of the HSR in this disease.

The role of glial cells in ALS

There is strong evidence that ALS can be characterized as a non-cell autonomous disease [99, 119]. As such, ALS initiation and progression depends on both the molecular pathologies developed within motor neurons, and the subsequent reactivity of surrounding non-neuronal cell populations such as astroglia and microglia. For example, transgenic mice expressing SOD1^{G37R} specifically in motor neurons in the ventral horn of spinal cords remained healthy for up to 1.5 years of age compared to mice that ubiquitously express this mSOD1 isoform, which die at 4 months of age [120, 121]. Moreover, knock out of SOD1^{G37R} expression in motor and dorsal root ganglion neuron progenitors of transgenic mice results in an 18 day delay to disease onset and 31 day delay to early disease progression compared to controls [122]. Together, these findings demonstrate that mSOD1 expression in motor neurons plays a role in early disease initiation and mSOD1 expression in other cells is required for disease progression. In support of this, selective deletion of SOD1^{G37R} expression from GFAP-positive spinal cord astroglia or cluster of differentiation molecule 11B (CD11b)-positive microglia did not slow disease onset or early disease progression, but significantly delayed late disease progression resulting in an overall extension of survival by 60 and 99 days, respectively [122, 123]. These two studies demonstrate that mSOD1 expression in astroglia and microglia plays a significant role in late disease progression and overall survival. This work and the work of many others emphasizes the importance of astroglia and microglia in the pathogenic cascade associated with ALS (for in-depth reviews examining the non-cell-autonomous nature of ALS see [99, 119, 124]).

The non-cell-autonomous progression of ALS by glial cells has also recently been demonstrated in a mutant

TDP-43 model of ALS [125]. In a TDP-43^{Q331K} expressing transgenic mouse model of ALS, cre recombinase excision of the TDP-43^{Q331K} transgene from motor neurons completely rescued motor neuron death [125]. However, despite the increase in motor neuron survival, there was no significant difference in the number of degenerating axons and neuromuscular junctions or glial-mediated neuroinflammation in end-stage disease mice when the TDP-43^{Q331K} transgene was excised in motor neurons [125]. These findings are supported by research that showed that astroglial-specific expression of TDP-43^{M337V} in rats results in the death of spinal cord motor neurons and denervation of skeletal muscles [126]. One proposed mechanism for the neurotoxicity of astroglia in mutant TDP-43 expressing models is that neurotrophic genes are suppressed and neurotoxic genes are up-regulated (e.g. *LCN2* and *CHI3L1*) [127]. Combined, these studies suggest that the expression of mutant TDP-43 in astroglia is sufficient to cause non-cell-autonomous death of motor neurons. Furthermore, the non-cell-autonomous progression of ALS is not confined to mSOD1-expressing mouse models, but may represent a generic mode of ALS progression.

The ubiquitous expression of mutant ALS-associated protein in the CNS may not alone facilitate the transition of astroglia from a neurotrophic to neurotoxic phenotype in ALS. Co-culture with A1 astrocytes induces the rapid death of a range of neurons, including spinal cord α-motor neurons [86]. Interestingly, there was a significant increase in the proportion of A1 astroglia in the motor cortex of patients with ALS (40% of ALS astroglia were A1 compared to 15% in controls) [86]. Likewise, there was a 60-fold increase in A1-related transcripts in the motor cortex of ALS patients compared to controls [86]. The mechanism by which these A1 astrocytes induce toxicity was proposed to be through the secretion of a 'toxic factor' [86]. Other studies have also suggested that mSOD1-expressing astrocytes release a soluble 'toxic factor', which significantly reduces the viability of motor neurons in co-culture [128–131]. The identity of this neurotoxic factor is currently unknown and additional research is required to determine its mode of action. In any case, it is important to consider cytoprotective mechanisms that maintain the neurotrophic functions of glia in ALS, such as the HSR leading to Hsp expression.

The HSR in astroglia

It is generally regarded that astroglia are capable of activating an HSR in response to stress, including whole animal hyperthermia [51, 57–59]. In the context of ALS, astroglia have higher levels of the sHsps, αB-c and Hsp25, compared to WT controls at the end-stage of disease, but not Hsp90, Hsp70, Hsp60 or Hsp40 (Table 2, Fig. 4). Interestingly, these findings suggest that the over-expression of unstable and misfolded mSOD1 species in the CNS fails to activate the HSR. Moreover, the expression of sHsps and other Hsp families may not be under the same transcriptional and translational controls.

In astroglia, there is a scarcity of published work investigating HSF1-activation and HSR induction at the molecular level using biochemical techniques (Fig. 4). However, the discord between sHsps being up-regulated and other Hsps not being affected in astroglia in the context of ALS suggests that there are additional layers of regulation of the HSR in these cells that are either HSF1-mediated or post-translational. In recent work, Zheng et al. [28] hypothesized that the phosphorylation of HSF1 at serine and threonine residues serves to fine-tune HSF1 transcription at promoter regions, rather than acting solely as an on/off switch. Thus, HSF1 phosphorylation could serve to regulate the kinetics and magnitude of the HSR in a cell-type dependent manner. Additional unidentified mechanisms of HSF1 regulation, including those that are cell-type specific, could explain the complete absence of HSR induction in motor neurons compared to astroglia in mSOD1-expressing transgenic mice. In fact, the HSF1-mediated HSR in the different cell-types that comprise the CNS is likely to be much more complex than our current models of HSR induction and attenuation (Fig. 2), which are based primarily on findings from *Saccharomyces cerevisiae, Drosophila melanogaster,* cell-lines or studies using recombinant human HSF1 in solution [38, 132–134]. Future research should elucidate mechanisms of HSR induction in astroglia, particularly astroglia that are affected in the spinal cord in ALS.

Knowledge of the precise mechanism by which HSF1 mediates the induction of specific Hsps in astroglia is important as it may uncover new therapeutic targets for the rescue of motor neurons from degeneration associated with ALS progression. This knowledge could be harnessed to up-regulate specific sets of Hsps that have been shown to interact with aggregating proteins associated with ALS [118]. For example, Hsp70 and HspB8 interact with TDP-43 and Hsc70, Hsp70, DNAJB1, DNAJB2a/b, Hsp27, αB-c, and HspB8 interact with SOD1 to prevent protein aggregation and decrease cytotoxicity [118]. It has been proposed that other Hsps are also likely to prevent the aggregation of TDP-43 and SOD1 since there are numerous 'non-canonical' members of the Hsp families that have not been tested for anti-aggregation or anti-apoptotic activities in these assays [118]. Up-regulation of cytoprotective Hsps in astroglia could maintain them in a healthy neurotrophic state to support motor neuronal viability and prevent conversion of astroglia to a neurotoxic (A1) phenotype. However, further research is needed to investigate mechanisms of HSF1-mediated HSR induction across different CNS cell-types in the presence and absence of disease-associated protein aggregation.

One mechanism by which astroglia may provide cytoprotection to motor neurons is through the exchange of extracellular vesicles containing Hsps [135]. Extracellular vesicles derived from chick spinal cord primary astroglial cultures following heat shock contain Hsp70 and Hsc70 [136]. In another study investigating glial-neuronal interactions, T98G glioma cells were shown to secrete Hsp70 into the culture medium and LA-N-5 neuroblastoma cells took up this Hsp70 [137]. The Hsp70 uptake increased the stress tolerance of the LA-N-5 cells to heat shock and staurosporine-induced apoptosis [137]. It would be interesting to extend on this work to investigate whether extracellular vesicles from more physiologically relevant cell-models (e.g. primary murine astroglia and motor neurons) also facilitate the trafficking of Hsps. The mechanisms of astroglial exocytosis and neuronal endocytosis used to traffic Hsps are also yet to be elucidated. This non-cell-autonomous mechanism(s) by which astroglia provide products of the HSR to neurons could be exploited to increase Hsp levels in motor neurons. This strategy could enhance the stress tolerance of motor neurons and decrease degeneration in the spinal cord in ALS (Fig. 4).

Summary of the HSR in ALS

Spinal cord motor neurons from primary cell or animal models of ALS are unable to activate HSF1 and hence lack a stress-induced up-regulation of Hsps. The levels of Hsp27 in motor neurons decline with disease progression. Motor neurons have an inherently high threshold for the activation of the HSR and the expression and accumulation of mSOD1 in the cell is not sufficient to activate the HSR. In contrast, spinal cord astroglia have elevated levels of αB-c and Hsp25 (rodent) or Hsp70 (human) at the end-stage of disease. However, the precise mechanisms by which these Hsps are up-regulated are unknown. Overall, there is a distinct lack of research into the HSR in spinal cord astroglia and its potential role in ALS.

Due to the non-cell-autonomous nature of ALS, future research should focus on maintaining affected spinal cord astroglia in a neurotrophic state to support motor neuron viability. Furthermore, investigation of Hsp70 (and other Hsp) transfer between astroglia and motor neurons could represent an exciting new mechanism for the development of therapeutics that target the proteostasis network in ALS.

Studying the therapeutic effects of increasing HSR components

The plaques and inclusions that are characteristic of ALS, HD and other NDs all share common morphological and biochemical features and this points to the highly related nature of these diseases [138, 139]. In addition, plaques and inclusion bodies are co-localized with various components of the proteostasis network, which may represent an irreversible sequestration and subsequent loss of function of these vital housekeeping components [140]. The sequestration of these chaperones, in conjunction with the possibility that toxic misfolded proteins are not sufficient to induce an HSR in the CNS, are likely to be important molecular mechanisms that lead to neurodegeneration in these diseases. However, there appears to be mechanistic differences in the way that these pathological proteins inhibit or evade detection by the HSR. In the case of Htt, there is evidence to suggest that the misfolded proteins themselves may directly impair mechanisms of the proteostasis network by changing the chromatin landscape (Fig. 3). The absence of a stress-induced up-regulation of Hsps in early disease allows the formation of toxic protein species, which precede a cascade of cellular dysfunctions in NDs. Therefore, in the absence of an HSR in affected neurons and surrounding glia in the CNS, boosting the HSR pharmacologically represents a promising therapeutic intervention for the treatment of these diseases at an early stage.

A significant amount of work has investigated the effects of over-expressing individual Hsps or activating an HSF1-mediated HSR in rodent models of NDs (for comprehensive reviews see [9, 36, 140–144]). Determining which of the HSR components are the most efficacious in preventing protein aggregation and subsequent neurotoxicity is an important step in elucidating targets for the development of therapeutics that ameliorate NDs. Over-expression of individual chaperones in mSOD1 mouse models of ALS has resulted in modest effects with regards to a reduction in the amount of insoluble protein and increased motor neuron survival (Table 3) [145–150]. However, this does not correlate with an increase in overall survival of the double transgenic animals (Table 3) [145–150]. Conversely, up-regulation of the HSR by treatment with withaferin A, celastrol or arimoclomol results in an increase in the number of surviving motor neurons and the lifespan of mSOD1 expressing mice [151–154]. This same trend was observed in mouse models of HD, whereby over-expression of HSJ1a and Hsp70 has no effect on overall survival but over-expression of an active mutant of HSF1 extended survival by 15 days (Table 4) [155]. The exceptions to this are DNAJB1, DNAJB6 and QBP-Hsc70 binding motif which, when over-expressed, were

Table 3 The effect of the over-expression of Hsps and up-regulation of the HSR on the molecular pathologies developed in rodent models of MND

Transgenic model/ Therapeutic compound	MND model	Increase in Hsp in Tg mouse	Extended lifespan	% ↑/↓ in surviving motor neurons	% ↑/↓ in levels of inclusions	References
Hsp27 Tg	SOD1^{G93A}	40-fold ↑spinal cord 25-fold ↑ cortex, cerebellum, hippocampus Expressed in MN + GFAP^{+ve} astroglia	No Δ (prolonged 4.2 days)	–	No Δ	[146]
	SOD1^{G93A}	–	No Δ (died 6 days sooner)	24% ↑	No Δ	[147]
HSJ1a Tg	SOD1^{G93A}	7-fold ↑	No Δ	61% ↑	No Δ	[148]
Hsp70 Tg	SOD1^{G93A}	10-fold ↑	No Δ (prolonged 1.4 days)	–	–	[145]
	SOD1^{G85R}	10-fold ↑ spinal cord	No Δ	–	–	
	SOD1^{G37R}	10-fold ↑	No Δ	–	–	
Hsp70 administered exogenously	SOD1^{G93A}	rhHsp70 injected 3× weekly (20μg)- detected in muscle not CNS	9 days	12.5% ↑	–	[149]
HSF1 Tg	SOD1$^{H46R/H48Q}$	3-fold ↑	No Δ	–	34% ↓	[151]
SIRT1 Tg	SOD1^{G93A}	3-fold ↑	15 days	–	40% ↓	[150]
Withaferin A	SOD1^{G93A}	2.6-fold ↑ Hsp25 2.2-fold ↑ Hsp70 Phosphorylated HSF1	8 days	30% ↑	39% ↓	[152]
	SOD1^{G37R}	–	18 days	–	–	
Celastrol	SOD1^{G93A}	–	16 days	30% ↑		[153]
Arimoclomol	SOD1^{G93A}	3-fold ↑ Hsp70 2.5-fold ↑ Hsp90 Phosphorylated HSF1	28 days	74% ↑	–	[154]
NXD30001	SOD1^{G93A}	No ↑ in Hsps in the CNS ↑ Hsp70 in skeletal muscle	–	–	–	[170]

Double transgenic (Tg) mice were bred for the over-expression of an Hsp and a SOD1 mutant associated with ALS. Alternatively, mice that over-express mSOD1 were treated with a therapeutic compound for the activation of the HSR. The fold increase in Hsp levels (and, if reported, the tissue-type in which this occurs), number of extended days of life, percent increase (↑) or decrease (↓) in spinal cord motor neurons, and percent ↑ or ↓ in the levels of inclusions is reported for each study

capable of reducing insoluble Htt and extending survival by 17, 21 and 32 days, respectively [156–159]. These findings illustrate how specific sets of Hsps may be more efficacious against aggregating proteins associated with HD. Furthermore, molecules that activate HSF1 and up-regulate the HSR (and therefore increase expression of a broad range of stress-related proteins) appear to be more capable of reducing protein aggregate load, preventing neurodegeneration and increasing lifespan of mouse models of NDs compared to up-regulation of individual chaperones.

Investigations into the therapeutic benefit of pharmacological activation of the HSR in the context of NDs are currently in progress. There are two classes of therapeutics under investigation, each target different aspects of the HSR pathway. One class of therapeutics activate HSF1 and/or up-regulate downstream products of the HSR. These include celastrol, arimoclomol, withaferin A, acetyl, L-carnitine and pyrrolidine dithiocarbamate [160–164]. Thus far, arimoclomol is the most promising HSR-mediating therapeutic. Administration of arimoclomol to mouse models of ALS (10 mg/kg/day), spinal and bulbar muscular atrophy (120 mg/kg/day) and inclusion body myositis (120 mg/kg/day) ameliorated neuropathologies associated with each disease, and arimoclomol successfully passed phase I human clinical trials in 2008 [154, 165–167]. However, there is currently limited information regarding that status of phase II/III trials of arimoclomol in ALS patients.

Another class of therapeutics targets the HSF1 inhibitory complex composed of Hsp90, co-chaperone p23 and immunophilin FK506-binding protein 5. Since, Hsp90 activities are ATP-dependent, this complex can be targeted by small molecules that compete with ATP for binding to Hsp90. Radicicol, NVP-HSP990, geldanamycin and geldanamycin-derived 17-allylaminogeldanamycin are Hsp90 inhibitors that act in this way and have been investigated for the treatment of NDs [72, 75, 168, 169]. In HD mouse models, NVP-HSP990-induced induction of the HSR in CNS tissues but this effect declined with increasing age of mice and despite a 20% decline in inclusion load, no extension of life was observed [75]. Furthermore,

Table 4 The effect of the over-expression of Hsps and up-regulation of the HSR on the molecular pathologies developed in rodent models of HD

Transgenic model/Therapeutic compound	HD model	Increase in Hsp in Tg mouse	Extended lifespan	% ↑/↓ in surviving neurons	% ↑/↓ in levels of inclusions	References
αB-c Tg (astroglia only)	BACHD	–	–	12.5% ↑	50% ↓	[92]
Hsp27 Tg	R6/2	12-fold ↑	–	–	No Δ	[180]
Hsp70 Tg	R6/2	Rat Hsp70	–	–	No Δ	[72]
		5–15-fold ↑ human Hsp70	No Δ	No Δ	No Δ	[181]
rAAV-QBP1-Hsc70 binding motif	R6/2	Injected into the striatum	32 days	–	90.8% ↓	[158]
rAAV-DNAJB1	R6/2	Injected into the striatum	17 days	–	39.2% ↓	[159]
DNAJB6 Tg	R6/2	Brain-specific up-regulation (nestin promoter)	21 days	–	33% ↓	[157]
HSJa Tg	R6/2	Brain specific up-regulation	No Δ	No Δ	35% ↓	[182]
Hsp104	N171-82Q HD	"Strongly" expressed in the brain, heart kidneys, testis	–	–	No Δ	[183]
HSF1^{Active} Tg	R6/2	Expressed in skeletal muscle, heart and testes	15 days	No Δ	79% ↓	[155]
NVP-HSP990 treatment	R6/2	2.7-fold ↑ Hsp70 3.8-fold ↑ Hsp25 1.6-fold ↑ Hsp40	No Δ	–	20% ↓	[75]
HSF1 KO	R6/2	–	105 day decrease in lifespan	–	15% ↑	[184]
HSF2 KO	R6/2	–	91 day decrease in lifespan	–	20% ↑	[185]

Double transgenic (Tg) mice were bred for the over-expression of an Hsp and polyQ-expanded Htt associated with HD. Alternatively, HSF1 and HSF2 genes were knocked-out (KO) of HD mouse models. Lentiviral vectors for the expression of QBP1-Hsc70 binding motif and DNAJB1 were injected directly into the striatum of R6/2 mice. In one case, mice that over-express polyQ-expanded Htt were treated with NVP-HSP990, a therapeutic compound for the activation of the HSR. The fold increase in Hsp levels (and, if reported, the tissue-type in which this occurs), number of extended days of life, percent increase (↑) or decrease (↓) in spinal cord motor neurons, and percent ↑ or ↓ in the levels of inclusions is reported for each study

in ALS mouse models, NXD30001 failed to induce the HSR in the CNS, despite the brain permeability of this molecule [170]. In vivo assessments investigating the efficacy of these compounds in the induction of the HSR has led to the conclusion that Hsp90 inhibitors are cytotoxic and not promising candidates to pursue for clinical trials.

A novel molecule identified in a yeast-based high-throughput screen, HSF1A, activates HSF1 by interacting with components of the inhibitory TRiC/CCT complex [171]. Treatment of cells with HSF1A results in HSF1 nuclear accumulation, trimerization, and enhanced binding to DNA [171]. Treatment of PC12 cells expressing polyQ-expanded Htt with HSF1A resulted in the reduction of inclusion bodies formed and protected cells against toxicity [171]. Furthermore, recent evidence shows that treatment of Neuro-2a cells transfected to express TDP-43-ΔNLS-K145Q with HSF1A results in a ~ 60% reduction in the number of aggregates formed compared to the vehicle control [172]. This indicates that the activation of endogenous HSF1 by HSF1A is sufficient to suppress mutant TDP-43 expression in this cell-based model [172]; however, it remains to be established whether HSF1A provides protection in vivo, in transgenic mouse models of NDs.

The therapeutic strategy of activating HSF1 in the CNS in the context of NDs is a promising one. Over 3 decades of research has provided strong in vitro evidence that activating HSF1 can reduce protein inclusion formation and ameliorate other molecular pathologies associated with a range of NDs [155, 172, 173]. However, progress towards the development of therapeutic compounds, that activate the HSR in affected tissues and cell-types in NDs has been slow. This is the likely due to the complexity of HSR induction in vivo, for example, in CNS tissues, Hsps may be provided to neurons in a non-cell autonomous manner that cannot be assessed in initial drug screens that are performed in vitro. Drug screens need to move beyond simple cell-based models and begin to incorporate more advanced tissue culture approaches to consider the responses from the multiple cell types present in tissues.

Conclusions

This review has highlighted the complexity of the HSF1-mediated HSR and demonstrated that the generic model for its induction and attenuation does not take into account additional layers of regulation that are stress- and cell-type specific. This review highlights that regulation in the induction of the HSR differs not only between cell types (e.g. neurons and astroglia) but also between neuronal sub-types in different regions of the brain (e.g. striatal neurons and motor neurons). It is these regulatory aspects of the HSR that are of particular interest with regards to the cells that comprise the CNS, where protein inclusion formation associated with NDs occurs. We propose that the appearance of protein inclusions in discrete neuronal populations in NDs may result from low (or no) basal levels of Hsps and/or a high threshold of HSR induction in these cells. Indeed, two recent findings in an α-synucleinopathy and HD suggest a possible generic underlying pathology in NDs, whereby HSF1 is targeted for degradation by the proteasome through elevated expression or activity of ubiquitinases [25, 74]. Furthermore, evidence from a range of models of NDs indicates that the species formed during protein misfolding and aggregation do not cause sufficient cellular stress to induce an HSR in affected neurons and astroglia. This suggests that cell-autonomous and non-cell-autonomous mechanisms that maintain protein homeostasis are insufficient to prevent protein aggregation associated with NDs in the CNS and highlights that the HSR is a promising pathway to target in the development of novel therapeutics for these diseases.

Future research should investigate basal and stress-inducible HSR proteins in neurons and astroglia, preferably using quantitative, high throughput and single-cell analysis techniques, which circumvent contamination by other cell types. This is particularly important due to the growing body of evidence that implicates neuronal-astroglial interactions in the progression of ALS and HD into late- and end-stage disease (as is also the case for other NDs). In addition, it is important to investigate the mechanisms by which astroglia can be maintained in a neurotrophic (rather than neurotoxic) phenotype in NDs. In compiling this review, it highlighted to us that there is a scarcity of research that has investigated the HSR in astroglia in the context of ALS or HD (and indeed most NDs). Furthermore, the ability of astroglia to provide non-cell-autonomous support to neurons by trafficking Hsps and other neurotrophic factors in exosomes is currently understudied in physiologically relevant models. Future research in this field should investigate the HSR in NDs by adopting a more holistic approach and focus on defining the cell-autonomous and non-cell-autonomous HSR within different cells-types of the CNS.

Abbreviations

ALS: Amyotrophic lateral sclerosis; ANG: Angiogenin; C9ORF72: Chromosome 9 open reading frame 72; CCNF: Cyclin F; CD11b: Cluster of differentiation molecule 11B; ChIP: Chromatin immunoprecipitation; CNS: Central nervous system; DBD: DNA binding domain; DNA: Deoxyribonucleic acid; fALS: Familial amyotrophic lateral sclerosis; FUS: Fused in sarcoma; GFAP: Glial fibrillary acidic protein; GLAST: Glutamate aspartate transporter; GLT-1: Glutamate transporter; HD: Huntington's disease; HSE: Heat shock element; HSF1: Heat shock transcription factor 1; Hsps: Heat shock proteins; HSR: Heat shock response; Htt: Huntingtin; IPOD: Perivacuolar inclusion bodies; JUNQ: Juxtanuclear compartments; KO: Knock-out; LZD: Leucine zipper domain; mRNA: Messenger ribonucleic acid; mSOD1: Mutant superoxide dismutase 1; NDs: Neurodegenerative diseases; NMDA: N-methyl-D-aspartate; OTPN: Optineurin; PCR: Polymerase chain reaction; PolyQ: Polyglutamine; QBP: Polyglutamine binding peptide; qPCR: Quantitative polymerase chain reaction; RD: Regulatory domain; RNA: Ribonucleic acid; sHsps: Small heat shock proteins; SOD1: Superoxide dismutase 1; SUMO: Small ubiquitin like modifier; TAD: Transactivation domain; TDP-43: TAR DNA binding protein; Tg: Transgenic; TRiC/CCT: T-complex protein-1 ring complex/chaperonin containing TCP1; UBQLN2: Ubiquilin 2; WT: Wild-type; αB-c: AlphaB-crystallin

Acknowledgements

We thank the Illawarra Health and Medical Research Institute for their technical and administrative support.

Funding

RSG is supported by an Australian Government Research Training Program Scholarship. JJY is supported by an NHMRC Career Development Fellowship (1084144).

Authors' contributions

RSG, LO, JJY and HE conceived of the review. RSG wrote the initial review and constructed the figures. RSG, LO, JJY and HE contributed to the editing of the manuscript. All authors read and approved the final manuscript.

Authors' information

Not applicable.

Competing interests

The authors declare that they have no competing interests.

References

1. Chiti F, Dobson CM. Protein misfolding, functional amyloid, and human disease. Annu Rev Biochem. 2006;75:333–66.
2. Verbeke P, Fonager J, Clark BF, Rattan SI. Heat shock and aging: mechanisms and implications. Cell Biol Int. 2001;25:845–57.
3. Douglas PM, Dillin A. Protein homeostasis and aging in neurodegeneration. J Cell Biol. 2010;190:719–29.
4. Brehme M, Voisine C, Rolland T, Wachi S, Soper JH, Zhu Y, Orton K, Villella A, Garza D, Vidal M, et al. A chaperome subnetwork safeguards proteostasis in aging and neurodegenerative disease. Cell Rep. 2014;9:1135–50.
5. Hartl FU, Bracher A, Hayer-Hartl M. Molecular chaperones in protein folding and proteostasis. Nature. 2011;475:324–32.
6. Balchin D, Hayer-Hartl M, Hartl FU. In vivo aspects of protein folding and quality control. Science. 2016;353.
7. Kampinga HH, Bergink S. Heat shock proteins as potential targets for protective strategies in neurodegeneration. Lancet Neurol. 2016;15:748–59.
8. Wyatt AR, Yerbury JJ, Ecroyd H, Wilson MR. Extracellular chaperones and proteostasis. Annu Rev Biochem. 2013;82:295–322.
9. Leak RK. Heat shock proteins in neurodegenerative disorders and aging. J Cell Commun Signal. 2014;8:293–310.
10. Treweek TM, Meehan S, Ecroyd H, Carver JA. Small heat-shock proteins: important players in regulating cellular proteostasis. Cell Mol Life Sci. 2015; 72:429–51.

11. Yerbury JJ, Gower D, Vanags L, Roberts K, Lee JA, Ecroyd H. The small heat shock proteins alphaB-crystallin and Hsp27 suppress SOD1 aggregation in vitro. Cell Stress Chaperon. 2013;18:251–7.
12. Robertson AL, Headey SJ, Saunders HM, Ecroyd H, Scanlon MJ, Carver JA, Bottomley SP. Small heat-shock proteins interact with a flanking domain to suppress polyglutamine aggregation. Proc Natl Acad Sci U S A. 2010;107: 10424–9.
13. Evans CG, Wisen S, Gestwicki JE. Heat shock proteins 70 and 90 inhibit early stages of amyloid beta-(1–42) aggregation in vitro. J Biol Chem. 2006;281: 33182–91.
14. Wilhelmus MM, Boelens WC, Otte-Holler I, Kamps B, de Waal RM, Verbeek MM. Small heat shock proteins inhibit amyloid-beta protein aggregation and cerebrovascular amyloid-beta protein toxicity. Brain Res. 2006;1089:67–78.
15. Muchowski PJ, Schaffar G, Sittler A, Wanker EE, Hayer-Hartl MK, Hartl FU. Hsp70 and Hsp40 chaperones can inhibit self-assembly of polyglutamine proteins into amyloid-like fibrils. Proc Natl Acad Sci U S A. 2000;97:7841–6.
16. Howarth JL, Glover CPJ, Uney JB. HSP70 Interacting protein prevents the accumulation of inclusions in polyglutamine disease. J Neurochem. 2009; 108:945–51.
17. Watanabe M, Dykes-Hoberg M, Cizewski Culotta V, Price DL, Wong PC, Rothstein JD. Histological evidence of protein aggregation in mutant SOD1 transgenic mice and in amyotrophic lateral sclerosis neural tissues. Neurobiol Dis. 2001;8:933–41.
18. Wilhelmus MMM, Otte-Höller I, Wesseling P, De Waal RMW, Boelens WC, Verbeek MM. Specific association of small heat shock proteins with the pathological hallmarks of Alzheimer's disease brains. Neuropath Appl Neuro. 2006;32:119–30.
19. Jana NR, Tanaka M, Wang G-H, Nukina N. Polyglutamine length-dependent interaction of Hsp40 and Hsp70 family chaperones with truncated N-terminal huntingtin: their role in suppression of aggregation and cellular toxicity. Hum Mol Genet. 2000;9:2009–18.
20. Åkerfelt M, Morimoto RI, Sistonen L. Heat shock factors: integrators of cell stress, development and lifespan. Nat Rev Mol Cell Biol. 2010;11:545–55.
21. Vihervaara A, Sistonen L. HSF1 At a glance. J Cell Sci. 2014;127:261–6.
22. Anckar J, Sistonen L. Regulation of HSF1 function in the heat stress response: implications in aging and disease. Annu Rev Biochem. 2011;80:1089–115.
23. Xu Y-M, Huang D-Y, Chiu J-F, Lau ATY. Post-translational modification of human heat shock factors and their functions: a recent update by proteomic approach. J Proteome Res. 2012;11:2625–34.
24. Westerheide SD, Anckar J, Stevens SM Jr, Sistonen L, Morimoto RI. Stress-inducible regulation of heat shock factor 1 by the deacetylase SIRT1. Science. 2009;323:1063–6.
25. Kim E, Wang B, Sastry N, Masliah E, Nelson PT, Cai H, Liao F-F. NEDD4-Mediated HSF1 degradation underlies α-synucleinopathy. Hum Mol Genet. 2016;25:211–22.
26. Hietakangas V, Ahlskog JK, Jakobsson AM, Hellesuo M, Sahlberg NM, Holmberg CI, Mikhailov A, Palvimo JJ, Pirkkala L, Sistonen L. Phosphorylation of serine 303 is a prerequisite for the stress-inducible SUMO modification of heat shock factor 1. Mol Cell Biol. 2003;23:2953–68.
27. Velichko A, Markova E, Petrova N, Razin S, Kantidze O. Mechanisms of heat shock response in mammals. Cell Mol Life Sci. 2013;70:4229–41.
28. Zheng X, Krakowiak J, Patel N, Beyzavi A, Ezike J, Khalil AS, Pincus D. Dynamic control of Hsf1 during heat shock by a chaperone switch and phosphorylation. elife. 2016;5:e18638.
29. Guettouche T, Boellmann F, Lane W, Voellmy R. Analysis of phosphorylation of human heat shock factor 1 in cells experiencing a stress. BMC Biochem. 2005;6:4.
30. Holmberg CI, Hietakangas V, Mikhailov A, Rantanen JO, Kallio M, Meinander A, Hellman J, Morrice N, MacKintosh C, Morimoto RI, et al. Phosphorylation of serine 230 promotes inducible transcriptional activity of heat shock factor 1. EMBO J. 2001;20:3800–10.
31. Soncin F, Zhang X, Chu B, Wang X, Asea A, Stevenson M, Sacks D, Calderwood S. Transcriptional activity and DNA binding of heat shock factor-1 involve phosphorylation on threonine 142 by CK2. Biochem Biophys Res Commun. 2003;303:700–6.
32. Chafekar SM, Duennwald ML. Impaired heat shock response in cells expressing full-length polyglutamine-expanded huntingtin. PLoS One. 2012;7:e37929.
33. Mathur SK, Sistonen L, Brown IR, Murphy SP, Sarge KD, Morimoto RI. Deficient induction of human hsp70 heat shock gene transcription in Y79 retinoblastoma cells despite activation of heat shock factor 1. Proc Natl Acad Sci U S A. 1994;91:8695–9.
34. Raychaudhuri S, Loew C, Körner R, Pinkert S, Theis M, Hayer-Hartl M, Buchholz F, Hartl FU. Interplay of acetyltransferase EP300 and the proteasome system in regulating heat shock transcription factor 1. Cell. 2014;156:975–85.
35. Yang J, Oza J, Bridges K, Chen KY, Liu AY. Neural differentiation and the attenuated heat shock response. Brain Res. 2008;1203:39–50.
36. Neef DW, Jaeger AM, Thiele DJ. Heat shock transcription factor 1 as a therapeutic target in neurodegenerative diseases. Nat Rev Drug Discov. 2011;10:930–44.
37. Sandqvist A, Björk JK, Åkerfelt M, Chitikova Z, Grichine A, Vourc'h C, Jolly C, Salminen TA, Nymalm Y, Sistonen L. Heterotrimerization of heat-shock factors 1 and 2 provides a transcriptional switch in response to distinct stimuli. Mol Biol Cell. 2009;20:1340–7.
38. Rabindran SK, Haroun RI, Clos J, Wisniewski J, Wu C. Regulation of heat shock factor trimer formation: role of a conserved leucine zipper. Science. 1993;259:230–4.
39. Pelham HR. A regulatory upstream promoter element in the Drosophila Hsp 70 heat-shock gene. Cell. 1982;30:517–28.
40. Sorger PK, Pelham HR. Yeast heat shock factor is an essential DNA-binding protein that exhibits temperature-dependent phosphorylation. Cell. 1988;54: 855–64.
41. Amin J, Ananthan J, Voellmy R. Key features of heat shock regulatory elements. Mol Cell Biol. 1988;8:3761–9.
42. Xiao H, Lis J. Germline transformation used to define key features of heat-shock response elements. Science. 1988;239:1139–42.
43. Trinklein N, Chen W, Kingston R, Myers R. Transcriptional regulation and binding of heat shock factor 1 and heat shock factor 2 to 32 human heat shock genes during thermal stress and differentiation. Cell Stress Chaperon. 2004;9:21–8.
44. Trinklein N, Murray J, Hartman S, Botstein D, Myers R. The role of heat shock transcription factor 1 in the genome-wide regulation of the mammalian heat shock response. Mol Biol Cell. 2004;15:1254–61.
45. Bharadwaj S, Ali A, Ovsenek N. Multiple components of the HSP90 chaperone complex function in regulation of heat shock factor 1 in vivo. Mol Cell Biol. 1999;19:8033–41.
46. Guo Y, Guettouche T, Fenna M, Boellmann F, Pratt WB, Toft DO, Smith DF, Voellmy R. Evidence for a mechanism of repression of heat shock factor 1 transcriptional activity by a multichaperone complex. J Biol Chem. 2001;276: 45791–9.
47. Neef DW, Jaeger A, Gomez-Pastor R, Willmund F, Frydman J, Thiele DJ. A direct regulatory interaction between chaperonin TRiC and stress responsive transcription factor HSF1. Cell Rep. 2014;9:955–66.
48. Shi Y, Mosser DD, Morimoto RI. Molecular chaperones as HSF1-specific transcriptional repressors. Genes Dev. 1998;12:654–66.
49. Gómez AV, Gallequillos D, Maass JC, Battaglioli E, Kukuljan M, Andrés ME. CoREST represses the heat shock response mediated by HSF1. Mol Cell. 2008;31:222–31.
50. Blake MJ, Gershon D, Fargnoli J, Holbrook NJ. Discordant expression of heat shock protein mRNAs in tissues of heat-stressed rats. J Biol Chem. 1990;265: 15275–9.
51. Nishimura RN, Dwyer BE, Clegg K, Cole R, de Vellis J. Comparison of the heat shock response in cultured cortical neurons and astrocytes. Mol Brain Res. 1991;9:39–45.
52. Sala AJ, Bott LC, Morimoto RI. Shaping proteostasis at the cellular, tissue, and organismal level. J Cell Biol. 2017;216:1231–41.
53. Batulan Z, Shinder GA, Minotti S, He BP, Doroudchi MM, Nalbantoglu J, Strong MJ, Durham HD. High threshold for induction of the stress response in motor neurons is associated with failure to activate HSF1. J Neurosci. 2003;23:5789–98.
54. Oza J, Yang J, Chen K, Liu AC. Changes in the regulation of heat shock gene expression in neuronal cell differentiation. Cell Stress Chaperon. 2008;13:73–84.
55. Pavlik A, Aneja IS. Cerebral neurons and glial cell types inducing heat shock protein Hsp70 following heat stress in the rat. Prog Brain Res. 2007;162:417–31.
56. Nishimura RN, Dwyer BE. Evidence for different mechanisms of induction of HSP70i: a comparison of cultured rat cortical neurons with astrocytes. Brain Res Mol Brain Res. 1996;36:227–39.
57. Manzerra P, Rush SJ, Brown IR. Tissue-specific differences in heat shock protein Hsc70 and Hsp70 in the control and hyperthermic rabbit. J Cell Physiol. 1997;170:130–7.
58. Manzerra P, Brown IR. Expression of heat shock genes (Hsp70) in the rabbit spinal cord: localization of constitutive and hyperthermia-inducible mRNA species. J Neurosci Res. 1992;31:606–15.

59. Krueger AM, Armstrong JN, Plumier J, Robertson HA, Currie RW. Cell specific expression of Hsp70 in neurons and glia of the rat hippocampus after hyperthermia and kainic acid-induced seizure activity. Brain Res Mol Brain Res. 1999;71:265–78.
60. Vonsattel JP, DiFiglia M. Huntington disease. J Neuropathol Exp Neurol. 1998;57:369–84.
61. Han I, You Y, Kordower JH, Brady ST, Morfini GA. Differential vulnerability of neurons in Huntington's disease: the role of cell type-specific features. J Neurochem. 2010;113:1073–91.
62. MacDonald ME, Ambrose CM, Duyao MP, Myers RH, Lin C, Srinidhi L, Barnes G, Taylor SA, James M, Groot N, et al. A novel gene containing a trinucleotide repeat that is expanded and unstable on Huntington's disease chromosomes. Cell. 1993;72:971–83.
63. Zoghbi HY, Orr HT. Glutamine repeats and neurodegeneration. Annu Rev Neurosci. 2000;23:217–47.
64. Kaganovich D, Kopito R, Frydman J. Misfolded proteins partition between two distinct quality control compartments. Nature. 2008;454:1088–95.
65. Kayatekin C, Matlack KE, Hesse WR, Guan Y, Chakrabortee S, Russ J, Wanker EE, Shah JV, Lindquist S. Prion-like proteins sequester and suppress the toxicity of huntingtin exon 1. Proc Natl Acad Sci U S A. 2014;111:12085–90.
66. Polling S, Mok YF, Ramdzan YM, Turner BJ, Yerbury JJ, Hill AF, Hatters DM. Misfolded polyglutamine, polyalanine, and superoxide dismutase 1 aggregate via distinct pathways in the cell. J Biol Chem. 2014;289: 6669–80.
67. Ramdzan YM, Trubetskov MM, Ormsby AR, Newcombe EA, Sui X, Tobin MJ, Bongiovanni MN, Gras SL, Dewson G, Miller JML, et al. Huntingtin inclusions trigger cellular quiescence, deactivate apoptosis, and lead to delayed necrosis. Cell Rep. 2017;19:919–27.
68. Matsumoto G, Kim S, Morimoto RI. Huntingtin and mutant SOD1 form aggregate structures with distinct molecular properties in human cells. J Biol Chem. 2006;281:4477–85.
69. Farrawell NE, Lambert-Smith IA, Warraich ST, Blair IP, Saunders DN, Hatters DM, Yerbury JJ. Distinct partitioning of ALS associated TDP-43, FUS and SOD1 mutants into cellular inclusions. Sci Rep. 2015;5:13416.
70. Bersuker K, Hipp MS, Calamini B, Morimoto RI, Kopito RR. Heat shock response activation exacerbates inclusion body formation in a cellular model of Huntington disease. J Biol Chem. 2013;288:23633–8.
71. Tagawa K, Marubuchi S, Qi ML, Enokido Y, Tamura T, Inagaki R, Murata M, Kanazawa I, Wanker EE, Okazawa H. The induction levels of heat shock protein 70 differentiate the vulnerabilities to mutant huntingtin among neuronal subtypes. J Neurosci. 2007;27:868–80.
72. Hay DG, Sathasivam K, Tobaben S, Stahl B, Marber M, Mestril R, Mahal A, Smith DL, Woodman B, Bates GP. Progressive decrease in chaperone protein levels in a mouse model of Huntington's disease and induction of stress proteins as a therapeutic approach. Hum Mol Genet. 2004;13:1389–405.
73. Riva L, Koeva M, Yildirim F, Pirhaji L, Dinesh D, Mazor T, Duennwald ML, Fraenkel E. Poly-glutamine expanded huntingtin dramatically alters the genome wide binding of HSF1. J Huntingtons Dis. 2012;1:33–45.
74. Gomez-Pastor R, Burchfiel ET, Neef DW, Jaeger AM, Cabiscol E, McKinstry SU, Doss A, Aballay A, Lo DC, Akimov SS, et al. Abnormal degradation of the neuronal stress-protective transcription factor HSF1 in Huntington's disease. Nat Commun. 2017;8:14405.
75. Labbadia J, Cunliffe H, Weiss A, Katsyuba E, Sathasivam K, Seredenina T, Woodman B, Moussaoui S, Frentzel S, Luthi-Carter R, et al. Altered chromatin architecture underlies progressive impairment of the heat shock response in mouse models of Huntington disease. J Clin Invest. 2011;121:3306–19.
76. Jackrel ME, Shorter J. Shock and awe: unleashing the heat shock response to treat Huntington's disease. J Clin Invest. 2011;121:2972–5.
77. Guertin MJ, Lis JT. Chromatin landscape dictates HSF binding to target DNA elements. PLoS Genet. 2010;6:e1001114.
78. Zuccato C, Belyaev N, Conforti P, Ooi L, Tartari M, Papadimou E, MacDonald M, Fossale E, Zeitlin S, Buckley N, Cattaneo E. Widespread disruption of repressor element-1 silencing transcription factor/neuron-restrictive silencer factor occupancy at its target genes in Huntington's disease. J Neurosci. 2007;27:6972–83.
79. Wang J, Martin E, Gonzales V, Borchelt DR, Lee MK. Differential regulation of small heat shock proteins in transgenic mouse models of neurodegenerative diseases. Neurobiol Aging. 2008;29:586–97.
80. Liu X, Miller BR, Rebec GV, Clemmer DE. Protein expression in the striatum and cortex regions of the brain for a mouse model of Huntington's disease. J Proteome Res. 2007;6:3134–42.
81. Sharma K, Schmitt S, Bergner CG, Tyanova S, Kannaiyan N, Manrique-Hoyos N, Kongi K, Cantuti L, Hanisch U-K, Philips M-A, et al. Cell type- and brain region-resolved mouse brain proteome. Nat Neurosci. 2015;18:1819–31.
82. Gu X, Andre VM, Cepeda C, Li SH, Li XJ, Levine MS, Yang XW. Pathological cell-cell interactions are necessary for striatal pathogenesis in a conditional mouse model of Huntington's disease. Mol Neurodegener. 2007;2:8.
83. Gu X, Li C, Wei W, Lo V, Gong S, Li SH, Iwasato T, Itohara S, Li XJ, Mody I, et al. Pathological cell-cell interactions elicited by a neuropathogenic form of mutant Huntingtin contribute to cortical pathogenesis in HD mice. Neuron. 2005;46:433–44.
84. Bradford J, Shin JY, Roberts M, Wang CE, Sheng G, Li S, Li XJ. Mutant huntingtin in glial cells exacerbates neurological symptoms of Huntington disease mice. J Biol Chem. 2010;285:10653–61.
85. Faideau M, Kim J, Cormier K, Gilmore R, Welch M, Auregan G, Dufour N, Guillermier M, Brouillet E, Hantraye P, et al. In vivo expression of polyglutamine-expanded huntingtin by mouse striatal astrocytes impairs glutamate transport: a correlation with Huntington's disease subjects. Hum Mol Genet. 2010;19:3053–67.
86. Liddelow SA, Guttenplan KA, Clarke LE, Bennett FC, Bohlen CJ, Schirmer L, Bennett ML, Münch AE, Chung W-S, Peterson TC, et al. Neurotoxic reactive astrocytes are induced by activated microglia. Nature. 2017;541:481–7.
87. Bradford J, Shin J-Y, Roberts M, Wang C-E, Li X-J, Li S. Expression of mutant huntingtin in mouse brain astrocytes causes age-dependent neurological symptoms. Proc Natl Acad Sci U S A. 2009;106:22480–5.
88. Shin JY, Fang ZH, Yu ZX, Wang CE, Li SH, Li XJ. Expression of mutant huntingtin in glial cells contributes to neuronal excitotoxicity. J Cell Biol. 2005;171:1001–12.
89. Ruiz C, Casarejos MJ, Gomez A, Solano R, de Yebenes JG, Mena MA. Protection by glia-conditioned medium in a cell model of Huntington disease. PLoS Curr. 2012;4:e4fbca54a2028b.
90. Carnemolla A, Lazell H, Moussaoui S, Bates GP. In vivo profiling reveals a competent heat shock response in adult neurons: implications for neurodegenerative disorders. PLoS One. 2015;10:e0131985.
91. Jansen AHP, van Hal M, Op den Kelder IC, Meier RT, de Ruiter AA, Schut MH, Smith DL, Grit C, Brouwer N, Kamphuis W, et al. Frequency of nuclear mutant huntingtin inclusion formation in neurons and glia is cell-type-specific. Glia. 2017;65:50–61.
92. Oliveira AO, Osmand A, Outeiro TF, Muchowski PJ, Finkbeiner S. AlphaB-crystallin overexpression in astrocytes modulates the phenotype of the BACHD mouse model of Huntington's disease. Hum Mol Genet. 2016;25:1677–89.
93. Williams KL, Topp S, Yang S, Smith B, Fifita JA, Warraich ST, Zhang KY, Farrawell N, Vance C, Hu X, et al. CCNF mutations in amyotrophic lateral sclerosis and frontotemporal dementia. Nat Commun. 2016;7:11253.
94. Chen S, Sayana P, Zhang X, Le W. Genetics of amyotrophic lateral sclerosis: an update. Mol Neurodegener. 2013;8:28.
95. Iguchi Y, Katsuno M, Ikenaka K, Ishigaki S, Sobue G. Amyotrophic lateral sclerosis: an update on recent genetic insights. J Neurol. 2013;260:2917–27.
96. Asea AAA, Brown IR. Heat shock proteins and the brain: implications for neurodegenerative diseases and neuroprotection. In: AAA A, Calderwood SK, editors. Heat shock proteins, vol. 3. New York: Springer; 2008.
97. Bruijn LI, Miller TM, Cleveland DW. Unraveling the mechanisms involved in motor neuron degeneration in ALS. Annu Rev Neurosci. 2004;27:723–49.
98. Rothstein JD. Current hypotheses for the underlying biology of amyotrophic lateral sclerosis. Ann Neurol. 2009;65:S3–9.
99. Boillée S, Vande Velde C, Cleveland Don W. ALS: a disease of motor neurons and their nonneuronal neighbours. Neuron. 2006;52:39–59.
100. Tashiro Y, Urushitani M, Inoue H, Koike M, Uchiyama Y, Komatsu M, Tanaka K, Yamazaki M, Abe M, Misawa H, et al. Motor neuron-specific disruption of proteasomes, but not autophagy, replicates amyotrophic lateral sclerosis. J Biol Chem. 2012;287:42984–94.
101. Cheroni C, Marino M, Tortarolo M, Veglianese P, De Biasi S, Fontana E, Zuccarello LV, Maynard CJ, Dantuma NP, Bendotti C. Functional alterations of the ubiquitin-proteasome system in motor neurons of a mouse model of familial amyotrophic lateral sclerosis. Hum Mol Genet. 2009;18:82–96.
102. Prell T, Lautenschlager J, Witte OW, Carri MT, Grosskreutz J. The unfolded protein response in models of human mutant G93A amyotrophic lateral sclerosis. Eur J Neurosci. 2012;35:652–60.
103. Nishitoh H, Kadowaki H, Nagai A, Maruyama T, Yokota T, Fukutomi H, Noguchi T, Matsuzawa A, Takeda K, Ichijo H. ALS-linked mutant SOD1 induces ER stress- and ASK1-dependent motor neuron death by targeting Derlin-1. Genes Dev. 2008;22:1451–64.

104. Ferrucci M, Fulceri F, Toti L, Soldani P, Siciliano G, Paparelli A, Fornai F: Protein clearing pathways in ALS. Arch Ital Biol 2011, 149:121–149.
105. Taylor JP, Brown RH Jr, Cleveland DW. Decoding ALS: from genes to mechanism. Nature. 2016;539:197–206.
106. Brown IR, Rush SJ. Cellular localization of the heat shock transcription factors HSF1 and HSF2 in the rat brain during postnatal development and following hyperthermia. Brain Res. 1999;821:333–40.
107. Batulan Z, Taylor DM, Aarons RJ, Minotti S, Doroudchi MM, Nalbantoglu J, Durham HD. Induction of multiple heat shock proteins and neuroprotection in a primary culture model of familial amyotrophic lateral sclerosis. Neurobiol Dis. 2006;24:213–25.
108. Yamashita H, Kawamata J, Okawa K, Kanki R, Nakamizo T, Hatayama T, Yamanaka K, Takahashi R, Shimohama S. Heat-shock protein 105 interacts with and suppresses aggregation of mutant Cu/Zn superoxide dismutase: clues to a possible strategy for treating ALS. J Neurochem. 2007;102:1497–505.
109. Charette SJ, Lavoie JN, Lambert H, Landry J. Inhibition of Daxx-mediated apoptosis by heat shock protein 27. Mol Cell Biol. 2000;20:7602–12.
110. Raoul C, Henderson CE, Pettmann B. Programmed cell death of embryonic motoneurons triggered through the FAS death receptor. J Cell Biol. 1999; 147:1049–62.
111. Raoul C, Estevez AG, Nishimune H, Cleveland DW, de Lapeyriere O, Henderson CE, Haase G, Pettmann B. Motoneuron death triggered by a specific pathway downstream of Fas. Potentiation by ALS-linked SOD1 mutations. Neuron. 2002;35:1067–83.
112. Raoul C, Barthelemy C, Couzinet A, Hancock D, Pettmann B, Hueber AO. Expression of a dominant negative form of Daxx in vivo rescues motoneurons from Fas (CD95)-induced cell death. J Neurobiol. 2005;62:178–88.
113. Maatkamp A, Vlug A, Haasdijk E, Troost D, French PJ, Jaarsma D. Decrease of Hsp25 protein expression precedes degeneration of motoneurons in ALS-SOD1 mice. Eur J Neurosci. 2004;20:14–28.
114. Strey CW, Spellman D, Stieber A, Gonatas JO, Wang X, Lambris JD, Gonatas NK. Dysregulation of stathmin, a microtubule-destabilizing protein, and up-regulation of Hsp25, Hsp27, and the antioxidant peroxiredoxin 6 in a mouse model of familial amyotrophic lateral sclerosis. Am J Pathol. 2004;165:1701–18.
115. Wang J, Xu G, Li H, Gonzales V, Fromholt D, Karch C, Copeland NG, Jenkins NA, Borchelt DR. Somatodendritic accumulation of misfolded SOD1-L126Z in motor neurons mediates degeneration: αB-crystallin modulates aggregation. Hum Mol Gen. 2005;14:2335–47.
116. Vleminckx V, Van Damme P, Goffin K, Delye H, Van Den Bosch L, Robberecht W. Upregulation of HSP27 in a transgenic model of ALS. J Neuropathol Exp Neurol. 2002;61:968–74.
117. Chen H-J, Mitchell JC, Novoselov S, Miller J, Nishimura AL, Scotter EL, Vance CA, Cheetham ME, Shaw CE. The heat shock response plays an important role in TDP-43 clearance: evidence for dysfunction in amyotrophic lateral sclerosis. Brain. 2016;139(Pt 5):1417–32.
118. Kakkar V, Meister-Broekema M, Minoia M, Carra S, Kampinga HH. Barcoding heat shock proteins to human diseases: looking beyond the heat shock response. Dis Model Mech. 2014;7:421–34.
119. Lee J, Hyeon SJ, Im H, Ryu H, Kim Y, Ryu H. Astrocytes and microglia as non-cell autonomous players in the pathogenesis of ALS. Exp Neurobiol. 2016;25:233–40.
120. Pramatarova A, Laganiere J, Roussel J, Brisebois K, Rouleau GA. Neuron-specific expression of mutant superoxide dismutase 1 in transgenic mice does not lead to motor impairment. J Neurosci. 2001;21:3369–74.
121. Wong PC, Pardo CA, Borchelt DR, Lee MK, Copeland NG, Jenkins NA, Sisodia SS, Cleveland DW, Price DL. An adverse property of a familial ALS-linked SOD1 mutation causes motor neuron disease characterized by vacuolar degeneration of mitochondria. Neuron. 1995;14:1105–16.
122. Boillée S, Yamanaka K, Lobsiger CS, Copeland NG, Jenkins NA, Kassiotis G, Kollias G, Cleveland DW. Onset and progression in inherited ALS determined by motor neurons and microglia. Science. 2006;312:1389–92.
123. Yamanaka K, Chun SJ, Boillee S, Fujimori-Tonou N, Yamashita H, Gutmann DH, Takahashi R, Misawa H, Cleveland DW. Astrocytes as determinants of disease progression in inherited ALS. Nat Neurosci. 2008;11:251–3.
124. Ilieva H, Polymenidou M, Cleveland DW. Non–cell autonomous toxicity in neurodegenerative disorders: ALS and beyond. J Cell Biol. 2009;187:761–72.
125. Ditsworth D, Maldonado M, McAlonis-Downes M, Sun S, Seelman A, Drenner K, Arnold E, Ling S-C, Pizzo D, Ravits J, et al. Mutant TDP-43 within motor neurons drives disease onset but not progression in amyotrophic lateral sclerosis. Acta Neuropathol. 2017;133:907–22.
126. Tong J, Huang C, Bi F, Wu Q, Huang B, Liu X, Li F, Zhou H, Xia XG. Expression of ALS-linked TDP-43 mutant in astrocytes causes non-cell-autonomous motor neuron death in rats. EMBO J. 2013;32:1917–26.
127. Huang C, Huang B, Bi F, Yan LH, Tong J, Huang J, Xia XG, Zhou H. Profiling the genes affected by pathogenic TDP-43 in astrocytes. J Neurochem. 2014; 129:932–9.
128. Nagai M, Re DB, Nagata T, Chalazonitis A, Jessell TM, Wichterle H, Przedborski S. Astrocytes expressing ALS-linked mutated SOD1 release factors selectively toxic to motor neurons. Nat Neurosci. 2007;10:615–22.
129. Bilsland LG, Nirmalananthan N, Yip J, Greensmith L, Duchen MR. Expression of mutant SOD1G93A in astrocytes induces functional deficits in motoneuron mitochondria. J Neurochem. 2008;107:1271–83.
130. Di Giorgio FP, Carrasco MA, Siao MC, Maniatis T, Eggan K. Non-cell autonomous effect of glia on motor neurons in an embryonic stem cell-based ALS model. Nat Neurosci. 2007;10:608–14.
131. Cassina P, Cassina A, Pehar M, Castellanos R, Gandelman M, de Leon A, Robinson KM, Mason RP, Beckman JS, Barbeito L, Radi R. Mitochondrial dysfunction in SOD1G93A-bearing astrocytes promotes motor neuron degeneration: prevention by mitochondrial-targeted antioxidants. J Neurosci. 2008;28:4115–22.
132. Peteranderl R, Nelson HCM. Trimerization of the heat shock transcription factor by a triple-stranded alpha-helical coiled-coil. Biochemistry. 1992;31:12272–6.
133. Westwood JT, Wu C. Activation of Drosophila heat shock factor: conformational change associated with a monomer-to-trimer transition. Mol Cell Biol. 1993;13:3481–6.
134. Neudegger T, Verghese J, Hayer-Hartl M, Hartl FU, Bracher A. Structure of human heat-shock transcription factor 1 in complex with DNA. Nat Struct Mol Biol. 2016;23:140–6.
135. Frühbeis C, Fröhlich D, Kuo WP, Krämer-Albers E-M. Extracellular vesicles as mediators of neuron-glia communication. Front Cell Neurosci. 2013;7:182.
136. Taylor AR, Robinson MB, Gifondorwa DJ, Tytell M, Milligan CE. Regulation of heat shock protein 70 release in astrocytes: role of signaling kinases. Dev Neurobiol. 2007;67:1815–29.
137. Guzhova I, Kislyakova K, Moskaliova O, Fridlanskaya I, Tytell M, Cheetham M, Margulis B. In vitro studies show that Hsp70 can be released by glia and that exogenous Hsp70 can enhance neuronal stress tolerance. Brain Res. 2001;914:66–73.
138. Bucciantini M, Giannoni E, Chiti F, Baroni F, Formigli L, Zurdo J, Taddei N, Ramponi G, Dobson CM, Stefani M. Inherent toxicity of aggregates implies a common mechanism for protein misfolding diseases. Nature. 2002;416:507–11.
139. Kayed R, Head E, Thompson JL, McIntire TM, Milton SC, Cotman CW, Glabe CG. Common structure of soluble amyloid oligomers implies common mechanism of pathogenesis. Science. 2003;300:486–9.
140. Muchowski PJ, Wacker JL. Modulation of neurodegeneration by molecular chaperones. Nat Rev Neurosci. 2005;6:11–22.
141. Duncan EJ, Cheetham ME, Chapple JP, van der Spuy J. The role of Hsp70 and its co-chaperones in protein misfolding, aggregation and disease. In: Blatch GL, Edkins AL, editors. The networking of chaperones by co-chaperones. Volume 78: Springer International Publishing; 2015. p. 243–73. *Subcellular Biochemistry*.
142. Pratt WB, Gestwicki JE, Osawa Y, Lieberman AP. Targeting Hsp90/Hsp70-based protein quality control for treatment of adult onset neurodegenerative diseases. Annu Rev Pharmacol. 2015;55:353–71.
143. Bose S, Cho J. Targeting chaperones, heat shock factor-1, and unfolded protein response: promising therapeutic approaches for neurodegenerative disorders. Ageing Res Rev. 2017;35.155–75.
144. Calderwood SK, Murshid A. Molecular chaperone accumulation in cancer and decrease in Alzheimer's disease: the potential roles of HSF1. Front Neurosci. 2017;11:192.
145. Liu J, Shinobu LA, Ward CM, Young D, Cleveland DW. Elevation of the Hsp70 chaperone does not effect toxicity in mouse models of familial amyotrophic lateral sclerosis. J Neurochem. 2005;93:875–82.
146. Krishnan J, Vannuvel K, Andries M, Waelkens E, Robberecht W, Van Den Bosch L. Over-expression of Hsp27 does not influence disease in the mutant SOD1G93A mouse model of amyotrophic lateral sclerosis. J Neurochem. 2008;106:2170–83.
147. Sharp PS, Akbar MT, Bouri S, Senda A, Joshi K, Chen H-J, Latchman DS, Wells DJ, de Belleroche J. Protective effects of heat shock protein 27 in a model of ALS occur in the early stages of disease progression. Neurobiol Dis. 2008; 30:42–55.

148. Novoselov SS, Mustill WJ, Gray AL, Dick JR, Kanuga N, Kalmar B, Greensmith L, Cheetham ME. Molecular chaperone mediated late-stage Neuroprotection in the SOD1G93A mouse model of amyotrophic lateral sclerosis. PLoS One. 2013;8:e73944.
149. Gifondorwa DJ, Robinson MB, Hayes CD, Taylor AR, Prevette DM, Oppenheim RW, Caress J, Milligan CE. Exogenous delivery of heat shock protein 70 increases lifespan in a mouse model of amyotrophic lateral sclerosis. J Neurosci. 2007;27:13173–80.
150. Watanabe S, Ageta-Ishihara N, Nagatsu S, Takao K, Komine O, Endo F, Miyakawa T, Misawa H, Takahashi R, Kinoshita M, Yamanaka K. SIRT1 overexpression ameliorates a mouse model of SOD1-linked amyotrophic lateral sclerosis via HSF1/HSP70i chaperone system. Mol Brain. 2014;7:62.
151. Lin P-Y, Simon SM, Koh WK, Folorunso O, Umbaugh CS, Pierce A. Heat shock factor 1 over-expression protects against exposure of hydrophobic residues on mutant SOD1 and early mortality in a mouse model of amyotrophic lateral sclerosis. Mol Neurodegener. 2013;8:43.
152. Patel P, Julien JP, Kriz J. Early-stage treatment with withaferin a reduces levels of misfolded superoxide dismutase 1 and extends lifespan in a mouse model of amyotrophic lateral sclerosis. Neurotherapeutics. 2014;
153. Kiaei M, Kipiani K, Petri S, Chen J, Calingasan NY, Beal MF. Celastrol blocks neuronal cell death and extends life in transgenic mouse model of amyotrophic lateral sclerosis. Neurodegener Dis. 2005;2:246–54.
154. Kieran D, Kalmar B, Dick JR, Riddoch-Contreras J, Burnstock G, Greensmith L. Treatment with arimoclomol, a coinducer of heat shock proteins, delays disease progression in ALS mice. Nat Med. 2004;10:402–5.
155. Fujimoto M, Takaki E, Hayashi T, Kitaura Y, Tanaka Y, Inouye S, Nakai A. Active HSF1 significantly suppresses polyglutamine aggregate formation in cellular and mouse models. J Biol Chem. 2005;280:34908–16.
156. Gillis J, Schipper-Krom S, Juenemann K, Gruber A, Coolen S, van den Nieuwendijk R, van Veen H, Overkleeft H, Goedhart J, Kampinga HH, Reits EA. The DNAJB6 and DNAJB8 protein chaperones prevent intracellular aggregation of polyglutamine peptides. J Biol Chem. 2013;288:17225–37.
157. Kakkar V, Månsson C, de Mattos EP, Bergink S, van der Zwaag M, van Waarde Maria AWH, Kloosterhuis Niels J, Melki R, van Cruchten Remco TP, Al-Karadaghi S, et al. The S/T-rich motif in the DNAJB6 chaperone delays polyglutamine aggregation and the onset of disease in a mouse model. Mol Cell. 2016;62:272–83.
158. Bauer PO, Goswami A, Wong HK, Okuno M, Kurosawa M, Yamada M, Miyazaki H, Matsumoto G, Kino Y, Nagai Y, Nukina N. Harnessing chaperone-mediated autophagy for the selective degradation of mutant huntingtin protein. Nat Biotech. 2010;28:256–63.
159. Popiel HA, Takeuchi T, Fujita H, Yamamoto K, Ito C, Yamane H, Muramatsu S-I, Toda T, Wada K, Nagai Y. Hsp40 Gene therapy exerts therapeutic effects on polyglutamine disease mice via a non-cell autonomous mechanism. PLoS One. 2012;7:e51069.
160. Sharma S, Mishra R, Walker B, Deshmukh S, Zampino M, Patel J, Anamalai M, Simpson D, Singh I, Kaushal S, Kaushal S. Celastrol, an oral heat shock activator, ameliorates multiple animal disease models of cell death. Cell Stress Chaperon. 2015;20:185–201.
161. Kalmar B, Lu C-H, Greensmith L. The role of heat shock proteins in amyotrophic lateral sclerosis: the therapeutic potential of arimoclomol. Pharmacol Therapeut. 2014;141:40–54.
162. Khan S, Rammeloo AW, Heikkila JJ. Withaferin a induces proteasome hnhibition, endoplasmic reticulum stress, the heat shock response and acquisition of thermotolerance. PLoS One. 2012;7:e50547.
163. Abdul HM, Calabrese V, Calvani M, Butterfield DA. Acetyl-L-carnitine-induced up-regulation of heat shock proteins protects cortical neurons against amyloid-beta peptide 1-42-mediated oxidative stress and neurotoxicity: implications for Alzheimer's disease. J Neurosci Res. 2006;84:398–408.
164. DeMeester SL, Buchman TG, Qiu Y, Dunnigan K, Hotchkiss RS, Karl IE, Cobb JP. Pyrrolidine dithiocarbamate activates the heat shock response and thereby induces apoptosis in primed endothelial cells. Shock. 1998;10:1–6.
165. Kalmar B, Novoselov S, Gray A, Cheetham ME, Margulis B, Greensmith L. Late stage treatment with arimoclomol delays disease progression and prevents protein aggregation in the SOD1 mouse model of ALS. J Neurochem. 2008;107:339–50.
166. Malik B, Nirmalananthan N, Gray AL, La Spada AR, Hanna MG, Greensmith L. Co-induction of the heat shock response ameliorates disease progression in a mouse model of human spinal and bulbar muscular atrophy: implications for therapy. Brain. 2013;136:926–43.
167. Ahmed M, MacHado PM, Miller A, Spicer C, Herbelin L, He J, Noel J, Wang Y, McVey AL, Pasnoor M, et al. Targeting protein homeostasis in sporadic inclusion body myositis. Sci Transl Med. 2016;8(331):331ra41.
168. Ortega L, Calvillo M, Luna F, Pérez-Severiano F, Rubio-Osornio M, Guevara J, Limón ID. 17-AAG improves cognitive process and increases heat shock protein response in a model lesion with Aβ25–35. Neuropeptides. 2014;48:221–32.
169. Sittler A, Lurz R, Lueder G, Priller J, Lehrach H, Hayer-Hartl MK, Hartl FU, Wanker EE. Geldanamycin activates a heat shock response and inhibits huntingtin aggregation in a cell culture model of Huntington's disease. Hum Mol Genet. 2001;10:1307–15.
170. Cha JRC, St., KJH L, Tradewell ML, Gentil BJ, Minotti S, Jaffer ZM, Chen R, Rubenstein AE, Durham HD. A novel small molecule HSP90 inhibitor, NXD30001, differentially induces heat shock proteins in nervous tissue in culture and in vivo. Cell Stress Chaperon. 2014;19:421–35.
171. Neef DW, Turski ML, Thiele DJ. Modulation of heat shock transcription factor 1 as a therapeutic target for small molecule intervention in neurodegenerative disease. PLoS Biol. 2010;8:e1000291.
172. Wang P, Wander CM, Yuan CX, Bereman MS, Cohen TJ. Acetylation-induced TDP-43 pathology is suppressed by an HSF1-dependent chaperone program. Nat Commun. 2017;8:82.
173. Jiang YQ, Wang XL, Cao XH, Ye ZY, Li L, Cai WQ. Increased heat shock transcription factor 1 in the cerebellum reverses the deficiency of Purkinje cells in Alzheimer's disease. Brain Res. 2013;1519:105–11.
174. Mimoto T, Morimoto N, Miyazaki K, Kurata T, Sato K, Ikeda Y, Abe K. Expression of heat shock transcription factor 1 and its downstream target protein T-cell death associated gene 51 in the spinal cord of a mouse model of amyotrophic lateral sclerosis. Brain Res. 2012;1488:123–31.
175. Zinkie S, Gentil BJ, Minotti S, Durham HD. Expression of the protein chaperone, clusterin, in spinal cord cells constitutively and following cellular stress, and upregulation by treatment with Hsp90 inhibitor. Cell Stress Chaperon. 2013;18:745–58.
176. Crippa V, Sau D, Rusmini P, Boncoraglio A, Onesto E, Bolzoni E, Galbiati M, Fontana E, Marino M, Carra S, et al. The small heat shock protein B8 (HspB8) promotes autophagic removal of misfolded proteins involved in amyotrophic lateral sclerosis (ALS). Hum Mol Genet. 2010;19:3440–56.
177. Marino M, Papa S, Crippa V, Nardo G, Peviani M, Cheroni C, Trolese MC, Lauranzano E, Bonetto V, Poletti A, et al. Differences in protein quality control correlate with phenotype variability in 2 mouse models of familial amyotrophic lateral sclerosis. Neurobiol Aging. 2015;36:492–504.
178. Wang J, Slunt H, Gonzales V, Fromholt D, Coonfield M, Copeland NG, Jenkins NA, Borchelt DR. Copper-binding-site-null SOD1 causes ALS in transgenic mice: aggregates of non-native SOD1 delineate a common feature. Hum Mol Gen. 2003;12:2753–64.
179. Vlug AS, Teuling E, Haasdijk ED, French P, Hoogenraad CC, Jaarsma D. ATF3 expression precedes death of spinal motoneurons in amyotrophic lateral sclerosis-SOD1 transgenic mice and correlates with c-Jun phosphorylation, CHOP expression, somato-dendritic ubiquitination and Golgi fragmentation. Eur J Neurosci. 2005;22:1881–94.
180. Zourlidou A, Gidalevitz T, Kristiansen M, Landles C, Woodman B, Wells DJ, Latchman DS, de Belleroche J, Tabrizi SJ, Morimoto RI, Bates GP. Hsp27 Overexpression in the R6/2 mouse model of Huntington's disease: chronic neurodegeneration does not induce Hsp27 activation. Hum Mol Genet. 2007;16:1078–90.
181. Hansson O, Nylandsted J, Castilho RF, Leist M, Jäättelä M, Brundin P. Overexpression of heat shock protein 70 in R6/2 Huntington's disease mice has only modest effects on disease progression. Brain Res. 2003;970:47–57.
182. Labbadia J, Novoselov SS, Bett JS, Weiss A, Paganetti P, Bates GP, Cheetham ME. Suppression of protein aggregation by chaperone modification of high molecular weight complexes. Brain. 2012;135:1180–96.
183. Vacher C, Garcia-Oroz L, Rubinsztein DC. Overexpression of yeast hsp104 reduces polyglutamine aggregation and prolongs survival of a transgenic mouse model of Huntington's disease. Hum Mol Genet. 2005;14:3425–33.
184. Hayashida N, Fujimoto M, Tan K, Prakasam R, Shinkawa T, Li L, Ichikawa H, Takii R, Nakai A. Heat shock factor 1 ameliorates proteotoxicity in cooperation with the transcription factor NFAT. EMBO J. 2010;29:3459–69.
185. Shinkawa T, Tan K, Fujimoto M, Hayashida N, Yamamoto K, Takaki E, Takii R, Prakasam R, Inouye S, Mezger V, Nakai A. Heat shock factor 2 is required for maintaining proteostasis against febrile-range thermal stress and polyglutamine aggregation. Mol Biol Cell. 2011;22:3571–83.

3

Whole blood gene expression and white matter Hyperintensities

Honghuang Lin[1,2*], Claudia Satizabal[1,3], Zhijun Xie[4], Qiong Yang[5], Tianxiao Huan[1,6], Roby Joehanes[7,8], Chengping Wen[4], Peter J. Munson[7], Alexa Beiser[1,3,5], Daniel Levy[1,6] and Sudha Seshadri[1,3*]

Abstract

Background: White matter hyperintensities (WMH) are an important biomarker of cumulative vascular brain injury and have been associated with cognitive decline and an increased risk of dementia, stroke, depression, and gait impairments. The pathogenesis of white matter lesions however, remains uncertain. The characterization of gene expression profiles associated with WMH might help uncover molecular mechanisms underlying WMH.

Methods: We performed a transcriptome-wide association study of gene expression profiles with WMH in 3248 participants from the Framingham Heart Study using the Affymetrix Human Exon 1.0 ST Array.

Results: We identified 13 genes that were significantly associated with WMH (FDR < 0.05) after adjusting for age, sex and blood cell components. Many of these genes are involved in inflammation-related pathways.

Conclusion: Thirteen genes were significantly associated with WMH. Our study confirms the hypothesis that inflammation might be an important factor contributing to white matter lesions. Future work is needed to explore if these gene products might serve as potential therapeutic targets.

Keywords: White matter hyperintensities, Gene expression, Epidemiology

Background

Magnetic resonance imaging (MRI) has been frequently used to identify abnormalities of white matter, detectable as white matter hyperintensities (WMH) [1, 2]. The prevalence of these white matter lesions increases with aging [3–5], and they typically happen long before the onset of clinically manifest neurological conditions [6]. WMH are observed in both apparently healthy individuals [2, 7, 8] and in individuals with stroke and dementia [9]. They have been associated with the risk of a variety of neurological diseases and other adverse outcomes, such as dementia [10–12], cognitive dysfunction [5, 9, 13–15], cardiovascular diseases [7], stroke [16–19], and mortality [20, 21]. The progression of WMH has also been used as a biomarker for predicting outcomes following stroke [22] and as a surrogate endpoint for clinical trials of cerebral small-vessel disease [23].

The pathophysiology of WMH remains poorly understood. Cardiovascular disease risk factors such as hypertension and diabetes are also risk factors for WMH, and small vessel arteriosclerotic disease is thought to be a key mechanism leading to WMH. In recent years, increasing evidence has suggested that chronic inflammation and glial proliferation might also be involved in the pathogenesis of WMH [24]. Moreover, it has been shown that WMH is highly heritable, with heritability estimates ranging from 55 to 73% [25–27]. Several genetic loci have been identified to be associated with WMH [28–31], however, they explain only a small portion of the observed heritability.

Gene expression has proved to be an important intermediate phenotype that helps to bridge genetic variations with many phenotypic traits [32–34]. Xu et al. [35] examined the association of gene expression in blood with WMH. Twenty participants with extensive WMH and 18 participants with minimum WMH were enrolled in the study. A total of 241 genes were found to be differentially expressed ($P < 0.005$ and at

* Correspondence: hhlin@bu.edu; suseshad@bu.edu
[1]National Heart Lung and Blood Institute's and Boston University's Framingham Heart Study, Framingham, MA, USA
Full list of author information is available at the end of the article

least 1.2 fold difference), many of which are involved in inflammation, oxidative stress, detoxification and hormonal responses. Another study by Simpson et al. [36] examined the association of gene expression in postmortem central nervous system tissue with WMH. Seven participants with WM lesions and 7 participants without lesions were enrolled in the study, and 502 genes were found to be differentially expressed, including genes involved in immunity and ion transport.

These studies have demonstrated that differential gene expression was associated with WMH. However, they examined small samples of highly selected participants, which limits their generalizability. The objective of this study is to assess the association of gene expression with WMH in over 3000 participants from the Framingham Heart Study (FHS).

Methods

Study samples

The FHS is a community-based, prospective study initiated in 1948 that aimed to investigate cardiovascular disease and its risk factors in the community. Three generations of participants have been enrolled, and multiple examinations have been performed with an interval of 2 to 8 years [37–39]. At each clinical examination, participants go through extensive physical examination, lifestyle and medical history interview. This analysis is restricted to the second generation (Offspring) of participants who attended the eighth Offspring examination (2005–2008), and the Third Generation participants who attended the second examination (2008–2011). All participants gave written informed consent, and the study was approved by the institutional review board at the Boston University Medical Center.

WMH measurement

The details for the MRI protocol in FHS have been described previously [9, 40]. In brief, MRI was performed on a 1.5 Tesla Siemens Avanto scanner. Fluid attenuated inversion recovery (FLAIR) sequences were used for the measurement of WMH. The segmentation and quantification of WMH was performed using a semi-automated procedure [41], which has shown high inter-rater reliability [42]. Total intracranial volume (TCV), based on FLAIR, was quantified using the Quanta 2 software package [41].

RNA extraction and gene expression profiling

Total RNA was isolated from frozen PAXgene blood tubes (PreAnalytiX, Hombrechtikon, Switzerland) and amplified using the WT-Ovation Pico RNA Amplification System (NuGEN, San Carlos, CA) according to the manufacturers' standard operating procedures. The obtained cDNA was hybridized to the Affymetrix Human Exon 1.0 ST Array (Affymetrix, Inc., Santa Clara, CA). The raw data were quantile-normalized and log2 transformed, followed by summarization using Robust Multi-array Average [43]. The gene annotations were obtained from Affymetrix NetAffx Analysis Center (version 31). We excluded transcript clusters that were not mapped to RefSeq transcripts, resulting in 17,873 distinct transcripts (17,324 distinct genes) for downstream analysis.

Given that the gene expression was measured from whole blood, the proportion of different cell types might affect gene expression. However, only 2181 participants from the Third Generation cohort had measured cell counts, of which 1225 were included in the current study. For the remaining participants, we used the partial least square method to estimate the cell counts from those with measured cell counts based on the gene expression data [44]. The percentages of each imputed cell type were then normalized, where the negative predicted values were set to 0 and the sum of the percentages for all cell types was set as 100%. Cross-validated estimates of prediction accuracy (R^2) were 0.61, 0.41, 0.25, 0.83, 0.83, 0.81, 0.89, and 0.25, for white blood cell counts, red blood cell counts, platelet counts, neutrophil percent, lymphocyte percent, monocyte percent, eosinophil percent, and basophil percent, respectively.

Statistical analyses

WMH mesures were log transformed to reduce the skewness of its distribution. Linear mixed effects models were used to test the association between gene expression and WMH volumes, treating the expression of each gene as the dependent measure, and the log-transformed WMH measure as the exposure. The analyses were adjusted for age, sex, and TCV. We also adjusted for the differential cell counts using a fixed effect factor, and for familial relatedness by implementing a random variance-covariance matrix.

In our secondary analyses, we additionally adjusted for smoking, body mass index, systolic blood pressure, diastolic blood pressure, hypertension treatment, total cholesterol, HDL cholesterol, and triglyceride.

In order to correct for multiple testing, we used false discovery rate (FDR) [45], which is defined as the number of incorrectly rejected hypotheses divided by the total number of rejected hypotheses. Significant associations were defined as those with FDR < 0.05. All the analyses were performed using the "lmekin" R package (www.r-project.org/).

Overlap with GWAS loci

The summary statistics of GWAS association was obtained from a meta-analysis of participants from multiple ancestries [46]. Four genetic loci were significantly associated with WMH. At each locus, we obtained all SNPs with *P*-value less than 5×10^{-8} (defined as GWAS SNPs). We then examined if any of GWAS SNPs was associated with gene expression in blood using FHS expression quantitative trait loci (eQTL) database [44]. An eGene was defined if its expression was associated with at least one of GWAS SNPs (FDR < 0.05). The association of each of the eGenes with WMH was then examined as described in the previous section.

We also queried the GWAS catalog [47] and extracted variants significantly associated with stroke or dementia ($P < 5 \times 10^{-8}$). For each of these variants, we searched its eGene, and examined the association of eGenes as described in the previous section.

Construction of gene interaction subnetwork associated with WMH

A dense module searching strategy [48] was used to identify modules enriched with WMH-related genes. The experimentally validated interactions between genes were obtained from the PINA database [49]. Before the searching, each gene was assigned a score to represent its association with WMH. The module searching started with a seed gene that was significantly associated with WMH (FDR < 0.05). Neighboring genes were then added sequentially to the module if the addition increased the overall module score [50], which was defined as $Z_m = \frac{\sum g_i}{\sqrt{k}}$, where k is the number of genes in the module, and g_i is the score of the gene i. The searching stopped if no more genes could be added.

Results

The current study includes 1397 eligible participants from the Offspring Cohort (mean age 66.4 ± 9.0 years, 54.2% women) and 1851 participants from the Third Generation Cohort (mean age 48.0 ± 8.5 years, 54.0% women) who had both gene expression and WMH measured. The descriptive characteristics of the participants are provided in Table 1.

Association of Gene Expression with WMH volume

As shown in Table 2, a total of 13 genes were significantly associated with WMH (FDR < 5%). Six of them were upregulated, and the remaining seven genes were down-regulated. Figure 1 is the volcano plot showing the association between each gene with WMH. The most significant gene was *IL4R* ($P = 1.5 \times 10^{-8}$), which encodes the alpha chain of the interleukin 4 receptor. The result was similar after excluding articipants with stroke, dementia and vascular diseases (Additional file 1: Table S1).

Table 1 Baseline characteristics of the study participants

Characteristics	Offspring cohort (*n* = 1397)	Third generation cohort (*n* = 1851)
Women, *n* (%)	757 (54.2%)	1000 (54.0%)
Age, years (mean ± SD)	66.4 ± 9.0	48.0 ± 8.5
WMH, median (25th, 75th percentile)	2.41 (1.25, 4.69)	1.28 (0.92, 1.75)
Ln(WMH + 1), median (25th, 75th percentile)	1.23 (0.81, 1.74)	0.82 (0.65, 1.01)
Total cranial volume, median (25th, 75th percentile)	1222 (1143, 1307)	1254 (1170, 1344)
Current smoker, n (%)	97 (6.9%)	174 (9.4%)
Hypertension, n (%)	828 (59.3%)	135 (7.3%)
Body mass index (BMI), median (25th, 75th percentile)	27.52 (24.52, 30.78)	27.11 (23.98, 30.72)
Total cholesterol, median (25th, 75th percentile)	185 (162, 210)	184 (163, 207)
HDL, median (25th, 75th percentile)	56 (45, 68)	57 (47, 71)

In the secondary analysis, we adjusted the model for additional clinical factors (see Methods). As shown in Table 2, most of top hits were still significant, although the association were slightly attenuated.

In order to assess potential effects of imputed cell counts, we performed a sensitivity analysis by including only individuals with measured cell counts, and compared the association of gene expression with WMH using either imputed or measured cell counts. As shown in Additional file 1: Figure S1, the statistics of associations were highly correlated using either the imputed and measured cell counts (R2=0.98), suggesting only marginal effect of imputed cell counts. We also additionally adjusted for the RNA integrity number in our statistical model, and found the results remained largely unchanged (Additional file 1: Table S2). We then performed another sensitive analysis by separating Offspring and Third Generation participants and assessed the association of gene expression with WMH separately. As shown in Additional file 1: Table S3, all 13 top genes had the same direction of association. In addition, the association in Offspring cohort showed relatively stronger effects than that in the Third Generation cohort, reflecting relatively older participants and more WMH volumes comparing to the Third Generation participants.

We also compared the top genes from the current study with previous studies. Among the 13 WMH-related genes, *SEPT11* was also reported to be associated with WMH in brain [36].

Overlap with GWAS loci

In our recent GWAS that included more than 20,000 participants from diverse ancestries, we identified 4

Table 2 Most significant genes associated with WMH (FDR < 0.05)

Gene	Primary analysis[a]					Secondary analysis[a]			
	Effect size	SE[b]	P-value	FDR[c]	Direction of effect[d]	Effect size	SE[b]	*P*-value	Direction of effect[d]
IL4R	−0.055	0.010	1.5E-08	2.6E-04	↓	−0.050	0.010	3.6E-07	↓
CD79A	−0.069	0.013	2.7E-07	2.5E-03	↓	−0.067	0.014	1.0E-06	↓
FCRL6	0.068	0.013	5.2E-07	3.1E-03	↑	0.064	0.014	2.8E-06	↑
PAX5	−0.052	0.011	3.1E-06	1.4E-02	↓	−0.049	0.011	1.6E-05	↓
FCRL1	−0.066	0.014	4.8E-06	1.7E-02	↓	−0.059	0.015	5.8E-05	↓
BANK1	−0.060	0.014	8.6E-06	2.1E-02	↓	−0.057	0.014	3.4E-05	↓
ARHGAP10	0.029	0.007	9.4E-06	2.1E-02	↑	0.028	0.007	1.9E-05	↑
YY1	0.018	0.004	9.5E-06	2.1E-02	↑	0.019	0.004	3.5E-06	↑
TGFBR3	0.047	0.011	1.8E-05	3.6E-02	↑	0.044	0.011	6.4E-05	↑
IL1RL2	0.021	0.005	2.2E-05	3.7E-02	↑	0.020	0.005	6.1E-05	↑
SEPT11	0.033	0.008	2.3E-05	3.7E-02	↑	0.034	0.008	1.2E-05	↑
TREML2	−0.029	0.007	2.6E-05	3.9E-02	↓	−0.026	0.007	2.2E-04	↓
ARL17A	−0.100	0.024	3.2E-05	4.4E-02	↓	−0.097	0.025	7.8E-05	↓

[a]Primary analysis was adjusted for age, sex, total cranial volume and cohort, whereas secondary analysis was additional adjusted for smoking, body mass index, systolic blood pressure, diastolic blood pressure, hypertension treatment, total cholesterol, HDL cholesterol, and triglycerides
[b]SE: standard error
[c]FDR: false discovery rate
[d]Direction of effect: ↓ indicates decreased gene expression was associated with increased WMH, whereas ↑ indicates increased gene expression was associated with increased WMH

genetic loci that were significantly associated with WMH [46]. As shown in Table 3, GWAS SNPs at these loci were associated with the expression of 17 genes (FDR < 0.05); three of them was nominally associated with WMH (*SEMA4A, UNC13D* and *WBP2*). As an example, the risk allele of rs2984613 was associated with decreased expression of *SEMA4A*, which was associated with increased WMH. We then searched all eQTLs for the 13 WMH-related genes, and found that these eQTLs were significantly enriched with variants associated with WMH [46] ($P < 2.2e\text{-}16$ by Kolmogorov–Smirnov test). Our results suggest that gene expression might serve as an intermediate phenotype that bridges genetic variations and WMH.

We also examined if previously reported genetic loci for stroke and dementia were associated with 13 WMH-related genes in the current study. GWAS catalog was queried, and 142 genome-wide significant variants ($P < 5 \times 10^{-8}$) were found to be associated with dementia or stroke. We then searched these variants in FHS eQTL database [44] and found that they were associated with the expression of 70 eGenes; 7 of them were nominally associated with WMH, including *ARL17A, SYTL2, PTGDR, POLR2E, MS4A6A, GPR141,* and *RIN3*. Among them, *ARL17A* was the most significant one and it was associated with SNP rs2732703, which was recently found to be associated with Alzheimer's disease among individuals without APOE ε4 allele [51].

Pathway analysis

In order to examine the integrative effects of differentially expressed genes on the biological systems, we examined the enrichment of WMH-related genes in biological pathways using WebGestalt [52]. Given that only 13 genes reached the significance cutoff after correction for multiple testing, we expanded the selection and examined the enrichment of top 1% of genes associated with WMH (including 179 genes). Table 4 shows the top enriched biologic pathways (FDR < 0.05). Many of them are involved in the immune responses and apoptosis, such as antigen processing and presentation (FDR = 0.0019) and apoptosis (FDR = 0.0338).

Gene interaction network associated with WMH

We applied a dense module searching strategy [48] to construct a WMH-specific subnetwork and examined the interaction between top genes associated with WMH. Note that during the construction of subnetwork, genes with weak or no association with WMH might be also added to the subnetwork if the genes could interact with other significant genes, thus their inclusion would increase the overall score of the subnetwork (see Methods). As shown in Fig. 2, the subnetwork is consisted of 40 nodes and 57 edges, where each node represents one gene, and each edge represents the interaction between two genes. Many of these genes are involved in B cell receptor

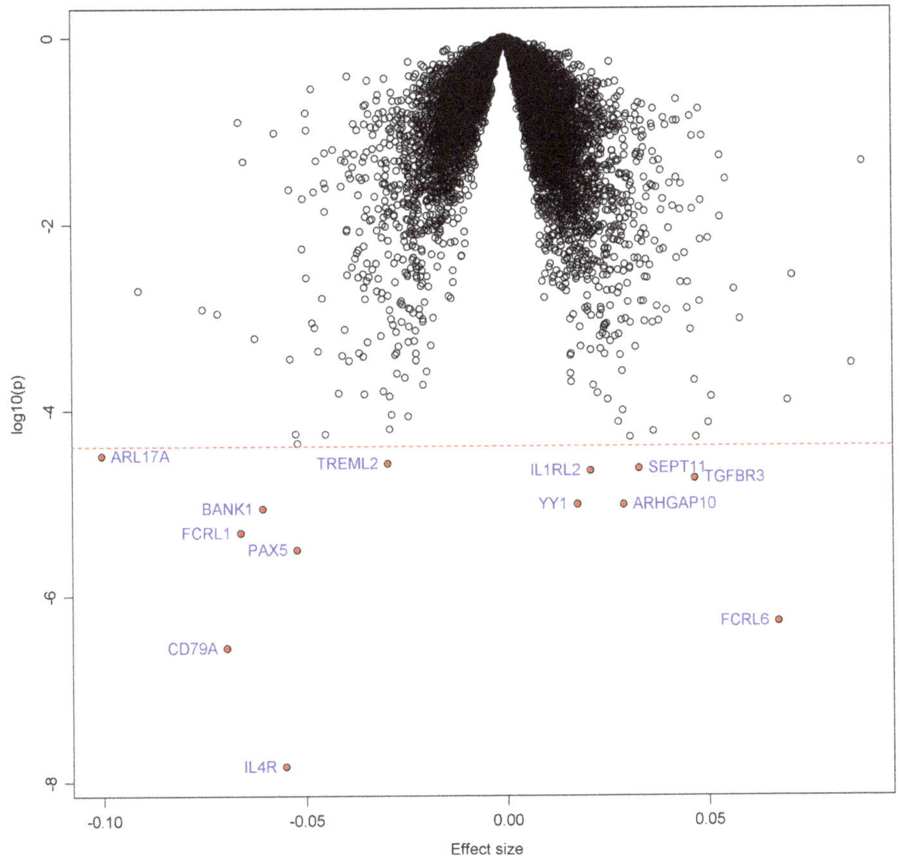

Fig. 1 Volcano plot of gene expression associated with WMH. Each dot represents one gene. The x-axis represents the beta estimation (β) of each gene, whereas the y-axis represents the $\log_{10}(P)$. Positive effects represent that genes were positively associated with WMH, whereas negative effects represent that the genes were negatively associated with WMH. The red dash line indicates FDR < 0.05. The 13 genes that reached significance cutoff were highlighted

signaling pathway and Epstein-Barr virus infection. *CASP3* appears to be one of the pivotal genes in the network that was connected with 9 other genes, although itself was not associated with WMH ($P = 0.79$). Previously studies also have found that the activation of *CASP3* was observed in brain with ischemic lesions [53–55].

Association with neuropsychological performance

The standardized neuropsychological performance testing was described previously [56–58]. Seven matrices were tested, including Hooper Visual Organization Test score, Logical Memories Delayed Recall score, Logical Memories Recognition score, Similarities Test score, Trails Test A score, Trails Test B score, and Trails B–A score. As shown in Additional file 1: Table S4, four genes were significantly associated with at least one cognitive matrix, including *BANK1* for logical memories recognition ($P = 4.5 \times 10^{-4}$), *TGFBR3* for Trails B–A score ($P = 1.8 \times 10^{-3}$) and Trails Test B score ($P = 1.9 \times 10^{-3}$), *FCRL1* for Hooper Visual Organization Test ($P = 2.9 \times 10^{-3}$) and *FCRL6* for Trails B–A score ($P = 3.4 \times 10^{-3}$). Our results suggest potential shared mechanisms between WMH and cognitive function.

Discussion

Increasing evidence has suggested that WMH is an important surrogate of aging and cerebrovascular diseases [26, 28]. However, molecular mechanisms underlying WMH are still poorly understood. In this study, we performed transcriptome profiling on participants who lie across a wide age-range and were ascertained without specific clinical characteristics. We identified 13 genes that were significantly associated with WMH (FDR < 0.05) and examined their integrative effect by the network analysis. *CASP3* appears to be one of pivotal genes that interact with multiple genes associated with WMH.

Table 3 Association of GWAS loci with gene expression. Three genes, *SEMA4A*, *UNC13D*, and *WBP2* were nominally associated with WMH

GWAS SNP	Risk allele[a]	Locus	*P* value (GWAS association with WMH) [46]	Association of SNPs with gene expression by eQTL analysis [44]			Association of eGene expression with WMH (current study)		
				eGene	*P* value	Direction on gene expression[b]	Effect size[a]	SE[c]	*P* value
rs4072479	C	17q25.1	4.6E-14	*WBP2*	1.0E-10	↓	**−0.020**	**0.010**	**4.6E-02**
rs8067275	T	17q25.1	1.9E-13	*MYO15B*	2.3E-05	↑	0.003	0.005	0.52
rs9894244	A	17q25.1	5.2E-10	*GALK1*	2.9E-06	↓	0.001	0.004	0.79
rs9894244	A	17q25.1	5.2E-10	*ITGB4*	2.9E-06	↓	−0.001	0.003	0.79
rs7216615	C	17q25.1	1.1E-09	*H3F3B*	9.2E-29	↓	−0.007	0.008	0.38
rs34143128	C	17q25.1	2.4E-09	*ACOX1*	9.1E-50	↓	0.003	0.009	0.75
rs1135889	A	17q25.1	8.8E-09	*UNC13D*	4.5E-11	↓	**−0.010**	**0.004**	**6.1E-03**
rs1135889	A	17q25.1	8.8E-09	*EXOC7*	9.1E-05	↓	−0.009	0.006	0.86
rs1135889	A	17q25.1	8.8E-09	*ZACN*	9.1E-05	↓	−0.001	0.005	0.86
rs2984613	C	1q22	2.0E-08	*C1orf85*	6.5E-23	↓	−0.003	0.007	0.65
rs2984613	C	1q22	2.0E-08	*TMEM79*	6.5E-23	↓	0.005	0.007	0.65
rs2984613	C	1q22	2.0E-08	*SMG5*	3.3E-20	↓	0.002	0.005	0.72
rs2984613	C	1q22	2.0E-08	*PAQR6*	1.6E-16	↓	0.001	0.006	0.89
rs2984613	C	1q22	2.0E-08	*PMF1*	7.3E-10	↑	−0.001	0.005	0.91
rs2984613	C	1q22	2.0E 08	*SEMA4A*	2.4E-08	↓	**−0.022**	**0.006**	**3.4E-04**
rs10883865	G	10q24.33	4.6E-08	*AS3MT*	7.9E-26	↓	0.011	0.010	0.30
rs10883865	G	10q24.33	4.6E-08	*USMG5*	7.7E-07	↑	0.015	0.011	0.19

[a]Risk allele respresnts the allele that was associated with increased risk of WMH
[b]Direction of effect: ↓indicates the risk allele was associated with decreased gene expression, whereas ↑ indicates the risk allele was associated with increased gene expression
[c]*SE* standard error
Genes with *P*-value less than 0.05 were marked in bold text

Many of the WMH-related genes are involved in the immune response pathway, including the most significant gene, *IL4R* ($P = 1.5 \times 10^{-8}$) and others such as *CD79A*, *TGFBR3* and *IL1RL2*. A variety of studies have suggested a role of inflammatory processes in the development of cerebral large- and small-vessel disease [59, 60]. A high infectious burden is also associated with an increased risk of stroke [61]. Inflammatory markers, such as interleukin-6 and C-reactive protein, have been associated with the presence and progression of white matter lesions across multiple ancestries [24, 62]. Some of top genes are involved in tumorigenesis and Alzheimer type neurodegeneration, which is consistent with prior GWAS.

We found a single gene in the current study overlapping with those reported previously [35, 36]. The lack of overlapping might dues to several reasons. The gene expression in the current study was measured by the Affymetrix Exon 1.0 ST array instead of Affymetrix HU133 Plus 2.0 array, which interrogated different sets of genes with different probesets. In addition, our study focused on whole blood samples but with much larger sample size. Moreover, participants of current study are relatively young and generally healthy, which might represent the WMH burden in the general population. It should be noted that the expression in brain would be more relevant to WMH. However, it is impractical to examine the brain expression in a community-based cohort. We have developed a brain donation program [63], which will be a valuable resource to study brain gene expression profile in future.

We acknowledge several limitations of our study. Gene expression could vary from tissue to tissue over time, but we only measured it in whole blood during a single examination. So we could not study longitudinal changes in gene expression over time, and how this might be related to WMH. Less than half of the studied samples had measured cell counts, and the remaining samples used imputed cell counts, which could introduce some additional variations to our results. In addition, in this cross-sectional study of observational data, we could not infer causal relationships between gene expression and WMH; the observed gene expression changes

Table 4 Most significant pathways enriched with top 1% genes associated with WMH. Two genes, ***IL4R*** and ***CD79A*** were highlighted as they both reached the significance cutoff WMH (FDR < 0.05)

Biological pathway	Total number of genes in the pathway	Ratio of enrichment	*P* value	FDR	Top 1% genes associated with WMH
Hematopoietic cell lineage	97	7.99	6.0E-06	0.0018	*HLA-DOB; HLA-DRA;* **IL4R**; *IL5RA; CD8A; CD19; CD22; CD37*
Antigen processing and presentation	77	8.81	1.3E-05	0.0019	*PSME3; HLA-DOB; HLA-DRA; KLRC3; KLRD1; CIITA; CD8A*
Inflammatory bowel disease (IBD)	65	8.95	5.0E-05	0.0050	*HLA-DOB; HLA-DRA;* **IL4R**; *RORA; STAT4; IL18R1*
Primary immunodeficiency	37	10.48	5.3E-04	0.0338	*CIITA; CD8A; CD19;* **CD79A**
Apoptosis	140	4.85	5.6E-04	0.0338	*BCL2L11; TUBA1B; CTSW; GZMB; BIRC3; TNFRSF10C; MAP3K14*
Graft-versus-host disease	41	9.46	7.9E-04	0.0399	*GZMB; HLA-DOB; HLA-DRA; KLRD1*
Cytokine-cytokine receptor interaction	265	2.93	0.005668	0.231	*CCR7;* **IL4R**; *IL5RA; PDGFRB; CCL4; CXCR5; TNFRSF10C; IL18R1*
B cell receptor signaling pathway	73	5.3	0.006633	0.231	*CD19; CD22; CD72;* **CD79A**
Allograft rejection	38	7.7	0.006858	0.231	*GZMB; HLA-DOB; HLA-DRA*
Type I diabetes mellitus	43	6.8	0.009672	0.285	*GZMB; HLA-DOB; HLA-DRA*

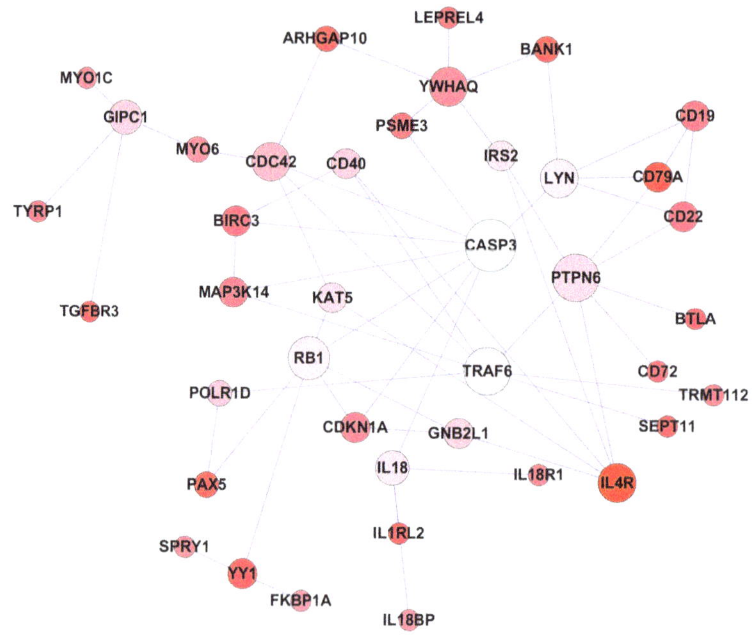

Fig. 2 WMH-related subnetwork derived from protein-protein interaction. Each node represents one gene, wheras each edge represents the interaction between two genes. The nodes were colored to represent their association with WMH: red color represents strong association, and white color represents no association. The node size is proportional to the number of edges that the node connects to

could be a consequence of vascular injury, both systemic and in the brain. Moreover, all participants included in this study were exclusively adults of European descent. Thus it is unclear if our findings could be generalized to other ethnicities/age groups.

Conclusions

In conclusion, we performed a large-scale profiling of gene expression in whole blood in a large community-based cohort, and identified 13 genes whose expression was associated with WMH. Our results are consistent with earlier reports that the immune response might be an important pathway to link gene expression and WMH. We also identified genes in glial proliferation and Alzheimer neurodegeneration pathways as potential links to WMH. Future studies with larger sample sizes and better techniques for measurement of gene expression such as RNA sequencing [64, 65] might uncover additional WMH-related genes and novel preventive and therapeutic targets for white matter lesions.

Additional file

Additional file 1: Table S1. Association of top genes with WMH after excluding samples with stroke, dementia or vascular diseases. **Table S2.** Association of top genes with WMH after additionally adjusted for the RNA integrity number (RIN). **Table S3.** Separated analysis for participants from the Offspring cohort and the Third Generation cohort. **Table S4.** Association of top genes within cognitive performance. **Figure S1.** Correlation between the statistics of WMH associations derived from the imputed cell counts or the measured cell counts using those samples who have measured cell counts. X-axis represents the statistics derived from measured cell counts, while y-axis represents the statistics derived from the imputed cell counts. Strong correlation was observed (R2 = 0.984), suggesting only marginal effect of imputed cell counts.

Abbreviations

eQTL: Expression quantitative trait loci; FDR: False discovery rate; FHS: Framingham Heart Study; GWAS: Genome-wide association study; TCV: Total intracranial volume; WMH: White matter hyperintensities

Acknowledgements

Not applicable

Funding

FHS gene expression profiling was funded through the Division of Intramural Research (Principal Investigator, Daniel Levy), National Heart, Lung, and Blood Institute, National Institutes of Health, Bethesda, MD. The Framingham Heart Study is supported by National Heart, Lung, and Blood Institute contract HHSN268201500001I. Additional support was provided by grants from the National Institute on Aging (R01 AG033193, R01 AG008122, U01 AG049505, R01 AG049607, R01 AG054076) and the National Institute on Neurological Disorders and Stroke (R01 NS017950 and UH2 NS100605). None of the funding agencies had any role in shaping the analyses or presentation of results.

Authors' contributions

HL and SS initiated the study and drafted the manuscript. HL, CS, ZX, QY, CW, AB and SS analyzed and interpreted the result. TH, RJ, PJM and DL generated and processed the gene expression data. All authors critically reviewed and approved the final manuscript.

Competing interests

The authors declare that they have no competing interests.

Author details

[1]National Heart Lung and Blood Institute's and Boston University's Framingham Heart Study, Framingham, MA, USA. [2]Section of Computational Biomedicine, Department of Medicine, Boston University School of Medicine, 72 East Concord Street, B-616, Boston, MA 02118, USA. [3]Department of Neurology, Boston University School of Medicine, 72 East Concord Street, B-602, Boston, MA 02118, USA. [4]College of Basic Medical Science, Zhejiang Chinese Medical University, Hangzhou, Zhejiang Province, China. [5]Department of Biostatistics, Boston University School of Public Health, Boston, MA, USA. [6]Population Sciences Branch, Division of Intramural Research, National Heart, Lung, and Blood Institute, Bethesda, MD, USA. [7]Mathematical and Statistical Computing Laboratory, Center for Information Technology, National Institute of Health, Bethesda, MD, USA. [8]Hebrew Senior Life, 1200 Centre Street Room #609, Boston, MA 02131, USA.

References

1. Debette S, Markus HS. The clinical importance of white matter hyperintensities on brain magnetic resonance imaging: systematic review and meta-analysis. BMJ. 2010;341:c3666.
2. de Leeuw FE, de Groot JC, Bots ML, Witteman JC, Oudkerk M, Hofman A, van Gijn J, Breteler MM. Carotid atherosclerosis and cerebral white matter lesions in a population based magnetic resonance imaging study. Journal of neurology. 2000;247:291–6.
3. de Leeuw FE, de Groot JC, Achten E, Oudkerk M, Ramos LM, Heijboer R, Hofman A, Jolles J, van Gijn J, Breteler MM. Prevalence of cerebral white matter lesions in elderly people: a population based magnetic resonance imaging study. The Rotterdam scan study. J Neurol Neurosurg Psychiatry. 2001;70:9–14.
4. Ylikoski A, Erkinjuntti T, Raininko R, Sarna S, Sulkava R, Tilvis R. White matter hyperintensities on MRI in the neurologically nondiseased elderly. Analysis of cohorts of consecutive subjects aged 55 to 85 years living at home. Stroke. 1995;26:1171–7.
5. Garde E, Mortensen EL, Krabbe K, Rostrup E, Larsson HB. Relation between age-related decline in intelligence and cerebral white-matter hyperintensities in healthy octogenarians: a longitudinal study. Lancet. 2000;356:628–34.
6. Longstreth WT Jr. Brain vascular disease overt and covert. Stroke. 2005;36:2062–3.
7. Launer LJ. Epidemiology of white matter lesions. Top Magn Reson Imaging. 2004;15:365–7.
8. Ylikoski R, Ylikoski A, Erkinjuntti T, Sulkava R, Raininko R, Tilvis R. White matter changes in healthy elderly persons correlate with attention and speed of mental processing. Archives Neurol. 1993;50:818–24.
9. Au R, Massaro JM, Wolf PA, Young ME, Beiser A, Seshadri S, D'Agostino RB, DeCarli C. Association of white matter hyperintensity volume with decreased cognitive functioning: the Framingham heart study. Archives of neurology. 2006;63:246–50.
10. Debette S, Beiser A, DeCarli C, Au R, Himali JJ, Kelly-Hayes M, Romero JR, Kase CS, Wolf PA, Seshadri S. Association of MRI markers of vascular brain injury with incident stroke, mild cognitive impairment, dementia, and mortality: the Framingham offspring study. Stroke. 2010;41:600–6.
11. Kuller LH, Lopez OL, Newman A, Beauchamp NJ, Burke G, Dulberg C, Fitzpatrick A, Fried L, Haan MN. Risk factors for dementia in the cardiovascular health cognition study. Neuroepidemiology. 2003;22:13–22.
12. Meguro K, Ishii H, Kasuya M, Akanuma K, Meguro M, Kasai M, Lee E, Hashimoto R, Yamaguchi S, Asada T. Incidence of dementia and associated risk factors in Japan: the Osaki-Tajiri project. J Neurol Sci. 2007;260:175–82.
13. Bigler ED, Lowry CM, Kerr B, Tate DF, Hessel CD, Earl HD, Miller MJ, Rice SA, Smith KH, Tschanz JT, et al. Role of white matter lesions, cerebral atrophy, and APOE on cognition in older persons with and without dementia: the Cache County, Utah, study of memory and aging. Neuropsychology. 2003; 17:339–52.
14. Burton EJ, Kenny RA, O'Brien J, Stephens S, Bradbury M, Rowan E, Kalaria R, Firbank M, Wesnes K, Ballard C. White matter hyperintensities are associated with impairment of memory, attention, and global cognitive performance in older stroke patients. Stroke. 2004;35:1270–5.
15. Gunning-Dixon FM, Raz N. Neuroanatomical correlates of selected executive functions in middle-aged and older adults: a prospective MRI study. Neuropsychologia. 2003;41:1929–41.
16. Gerdes VE, Kwa VI, ten Cate H, Brandjes DP, Buller HR, Stam J. Amsterdam vascular medicine G: cerebral white matter lesions predict both ischemic strokes and myocardial infarctions in patients with established atherosclerotic disease. Atherosclerosis. 2006;186:166–72.
17. Bokura H, Kobayashi S, Yamaguchi S, Iijima K, Nagai A, Toyoda G, Oguro H, Takahashi K. Silent brain infarction and subcortical white matter lesions increase the risk of stroke and mortality: a prospective cohort study. J Stroke Cerebrovasc Dis. 2006;15:57–63.
18. Wong TY, Klein R, Sharrett AR, Couper DJ, Klein BE, Liao DP, Hubbard LD, Mosley TH. Study AIARiC: cerebral white matter lesions, retinopathy, and incident clinical stroke. JAMA. 2002;288:67–74.
19. Buyck JF, Dufouil C, Mazoyer B, Maillard P, Ducimetiere P, Alperovitch A, Bousser MG, Kurth T, Tzourio C. Cerebral white matter lesions are associated with the risk of stroke but not with other vascular events: the 3-City Dijon study. Stroke. 2009;40:2327–31.
20. Kuller LH, Arnold AM, Longstreth WT Jr, Manolio TA, O'Leary DH, Burke GL, Fried LP, Newman AB. White matter grade and ventricular volume on brain MRI as markers of longevity in the cardiovascular health study. Neurobiol Aging. 2007;28:1307–15.
21. Ikram MA, Vernooij MW, Vrooman HA, Hofman A, Breteler MM. Brain tissue volumes and small vessel disease in relation to the risk of mortality. Neurobiol Aging. 2009;30:450–6.
22. Yamauchi H, Fukuda H, Oyanagi C. Significance of white matter high intensity lesions as a predictor of stroke from arteriolosclerosis. J Neurol Neurosurg Psychiatry. 2002;72:576–82.
23. Schmidt R, Scheltens P, Erkinjuntti T, Pantoni L, Markus HS, Wallin A, Barkhof F, Fazekas F. White matter lesion progression: a surrogate endpoint for trials in cerebral small-vessel disease. Neurology. 2004;63:139–44.
24. Fornage M, Chiang YA, O'Meara ES, Psaty BM, Reiner AP, Siscovick DS, Tracy RP, Longstreth WT Jr. Biomarkers of inflammation and MRI-defined small vessel disease of the brain: the cardiovascular health study. Stroke. 2008;39:1952–9.
25. Carmelli D, DeCarli C, Swan GE, Jack LM, Reed T, Wolf PA, Miller BL. Evidence for genetic variance in white matter hyperintensity volume in normal elderly male twins. Stroke. 1998;29:1177–81.
26. Atwood LD, Wolf PA, Heard-Costa NL, Massaro JM, Beiser A, D'Agostino RB, DeCarli C. Genetic variation in white matter hyperintensity volume in the Framingham study. Stroke; a journal of cerebral circulation. 2004;35:1609–13.
27. Turner ST, Jack CR, Fornage M, Mosley TH, Boerwinkle E, de Andrade M. Heritability of leukoaraiosis in hypertensive sibships. Hypertension. 2004;43:483–7.
28. DeStefano AL, Atwood LD, Massaro JM, Heard-Costa N, Beiser A, Au R, Wolf PA, DeCarli C. Genome-wide scan for white matter hyperintensity: the Framingham heart study. Stroke. 2006;37:77–81.
29. Paternoster L, Chen W, Sudlow CL. Genetic determinants of white matter hyperintensities on brain scans: a systematic assessment of 19 candidate gene polymorphisms in 46 studies in 19,000 subjects. Stroke. 2009;40:2020–6.
30. Turner ST, Fornage M, Jack CR Jr, Mosley TH, Kardia SL, Boerwinkle E, de Andrade M. Genomic susceptibility loci for brain atrophy in hypertensive sibships from the GENOA study. Hypertension. 2005;45:793–8.
31. Fornage M, Debette S, Bis JC, Schmidt H, Ikram MA, Dufouil C, Sigurdsson S, Lumley T, DeStefano AL, Fazekas F, et al. Genome-wide association studies of cerebral white matter lesion burden: the CHARGE consortium. Annals Neurology. 2011;69:928–39.
32. Lin H, Yin X, Lunetta KL, Dupuis J, McManus DD, Lubitz SA, Magnani JW, Joehanes R, Munson PJ, Larson MG, et al. Whole blood gene expression and atrial fibrillation: the framingham heart study. PLoS ONE. 2014;9:e96794.
33. Lin H, Joehanes R, Pilling LC, Dupuis J, Lunetta KL, Ying SX, Benjamin EJ, Hernandez D, Singleton A, Melzer D, et al. Whole blood gene expression and interleukin-6 levels. Genomics. 2014;104:490–5.
34. Joehanes R, Ying S, Huan T, Johnson AD, Raghavachari N, Wang R, Liu P, Woodhouse KA, Sen SK, Tanriverdi K, et al. Gene expression signatures of coronary heart disease. Arterioscler Thromb Vasc Biol. 2013;33:1418–26.
35. Xu H, Stamova B, Jickling G, Tian Y, Zhan X, Ander BP, Liu D, Turner R, Rosand J, Goldstein LB, et al. Distinctive RNA expression profiles in blood associated with white matter hyperintensities in brain. Stroke; a journal of cerebral circulation. 2010;41:2744–9.

36. Simpson JE, Hosny O, Wharton SB, Heath PR, Holden H, Fernando MS, Matthews F, Forster G, O'Brien JT, Barber R, et al. Microarray RNA expression analysis of cerebral white matter lesions reveals changes in multiple functional pathways. Stroke. 2009;40:369–75.
37. Dawber TR, Kannel WB, Lyell LP. An approach to longitudinal studies in a community: the Framingham study. Ann N Y Acad Sci. 1963;107:539–56.
38. Feinleib M, Kannel WB, Garrison RJ, McNamara PM, Castelli WP. The Framingham Offspring Study. Design and preliminary data. Preventive Med. 1975;4:518–25.
39. Kannel WB, Feinleib M, McNamara PM, Garrison RJ, Castelli WP. An investigation of coronary heart disease in families. The Framingham offspring study. Am J Epidemiol. 1979;110:281–90.
40. DeCarli C, Massaro J, Harvey D, Hald J, Tullberg M, Au R, Beiser A, D'Agostino R, Wolf PA. Measures of brain morphology and infarction in the framingham heart study: establishing what is normal. Neurobiology of aging. 2005;26:491–510.
41. DeCarli C, Fletcher E, Ramey V, Harvey D, Jagust WJ. Anatomical mapping of white matter hyperintensities (WMH): exploring the relationships between periventricular WMH, deep WMH, and total WMH burden. Stroke. 2005;36:50–5.
42. Carmichael O, Mungas D, Beckett L, Harvey D, Tomaszewski Farias S, Reed B, Olichney J, Miller J, Decarli C. MRI predictors of cognitive change in a diverse and carefully characterized elderly population. Neurobiol Aging. 2012;33:83–95.
43. Irizarry RA, Hobbs B, Collin F, Beazer-Barclay YD, Antonellis KJ, Scherf U, Speed TP. Exploration, normalization, and summaries of high density oligonucleotide array probe level data. Biostatistics. 2003;4:249–64.
44. Joehanes R, Zhang X, Huan T, Yao C, Ying SX, Nguyen QT, Demirkale CY, Feolo ML, Sharopova NR, Sturcke A, et al. Integrated genome-wide analysis of expression quantitative trait loci aids interpretation of genomic association studies. Genome Biology. 2017;18:16.
45. Benjamini Y, Hochberg Y. Controlling the false discovery rate: a practical and powerful approach to multiple testing. J Royal Stat Soc. 1995;57:289–300.
46. Verhaaren BF, Debette S, Bis JC, Smith JA, Ikram MK, Adams HH, Beecham AH, Rajan KB, Lopez LM, Barral S, et al. Multiethnic genome-wide association study of cerebral white matter hyperintensities on MRI. Circ Cardiovasc Genet. 2015;8:398–409.
47. MacArthur J, Bowler E, Cerezo M, Gil L, Hall P, Hastings E, Junkins H, McMahon A, Milano A, Morales J, et al. The new NHGRI-EBI catalog of published genome-wide association studies (GWAS catalog). Nucleic Acids Res. 2017;45:D896–901.
48. Jia P, Zheng S, Long J, Zheng W. Zhao Z: dmGWAS: dense module searching for genome-wide association studies in protein-protein interaction networks. Bioinformatics. 2011;27:95–102.
49. Cowley MJ, Pinese M, Kassahn KS, Waddell N, Pearson JV, Grimmond SM, Biankin AV, Hautaniemi S, Wu J. PINA v2.0: mining interactome modules. Nucleic Acids Res. 2012;40:D862–5.
50. Ideker T, Ozier O, Schwikowski B, Siegel AF. Discovering regulatory and signalling circuits in molecular interaction networks. Bioinformatics. 2002; 18(Suppl 1):S233–40.
51. Jun G, Ibrahim-Verbaas CA, Vronskaya M, Lambert JC, Chung J, Naj AC, Kunkle BW, Wang LS, Bis JC, Bellenguez C, et al. A novel Alzheimer disease locus located near the gene encoding tau protein. Mol Psychiatry. 2016;21:108–17.
52. Wang J, Duncan D, Shi Z, Zhang B. WEB-based GEne SeT AnaLysis toolkit (WebGestalt): update 2013. Nucleic Acids Res. 2013;41:W77–83.
53. Gorup D, Bohacek I, Milicevic T, Pochet R, Mitrecic D, Kriz J, Gajovic S. Increased expression and colocalization of GAP43 and CASP3 after brain ischemic lesion in mouse. Neuroscience Lett. 2015;597:176–82.
54. Manabat C, Han BH, Wendland M, Derugin N, Fox CK, Choi J, Holtzman DM, Ferriero DM, Vexler ZS. Reperfusion differentially induces caspase-3 activation in ischemic core and penumbra after stroke in immature brain. Stroke. 2003;34:207–13.
55. Didenko VV, Ngo H, Minchew CL, Boudreaux DJ, Widmayer MA, Baskin DS. Caspase-3-dependent and -independent apoptosis in focal brain ischemia. Mol Med. 2002;8:347–52.
56. Au R, Seshadri S, Wolf PA, Elias M, Elias P, Sullivan L, Beiser A, D'Agostino RB. New norms for a new generation: cognitive performance in the framingham offspring cohort. Exp Aging Res. 2004;30:333–58.
57. Therkelsen KE, Preis SR, Beiser A, DeCarli C, Seshadri S, Wolf P, Au R, Fox CS. Neck circumference, brain imaging measures, and neuropsychological testing measures. J Stroke Cerebrovasc Dis. 2016;25:1570–81.
58. Nishtala A, Preis SR, Beiser A, Devine S, Hankee L, Seshadri S, Wolf PA, Au R. Midlife cardiovascular risk impacts executive function: Framingham offspring study. Alzheimer Dis Assoc Disord. 2014;28:16–22.
59. Simpson JE, Ince PG, Higham CE, Gelsthorpe CH, Fernando MS, Matthews F, Forster G, O'Brien JT, Barber R, Kalaria RN, et al. Microglial activation in white matter lesions and nonlesional white matter of ageing brains. Neuropathol Appl Neurobiol. 2007;33:670–83.
60. Fassbender K, Bertsch T, Mielke O, Muhlhauser F, Hennerici M. Adhesion molecules in cerebrovascular diseases. Evidence for an inflammatory endothelial activation in cerebral large- and small-vessel disease. Stroke. 1999;30:1647–50.
61. Palm F, Pussinen PJ, Aigner A, Becher H, Buggle F, Bauer MF, Grond-Ginsbach C, Safer A, Urbanek C, Grau AJ. Association between infectious burden, socioeconomic status, and ischemic stroke. Atherosclerosis. 2016;254:117–23.
62. Nagai K, Kozaki K, Sonohara K, Akishita M, Toba K. Relationship between interleukin-6 and cerebral deep white matter and periventricular hyperintensity in elderly women. Geriatr Gerontol Int. 2011;11:328–32.
63. Au R, Seshadri S, Knox K, Beiser A, Himali JJ, Cabral HJ, Auerbach S, Green RC, Wolf PA, McKee AC. The Framingham brain donation program: neuropathology along the cognitive continuum. Curr Alzheimer Res. 2012;9:673–86.
64. Adam O, Lavall D, Theobald K, Hohl M, Grube M, Ameling S, Sussman MA, Rosenkranz S, Kroemer HK, Schafers HJ, et al. Rac1-induced connective tissue growth factor regulates connexin 43 and N-cadherin expression in atrial fibrillation. J Am Coll Cardiol. 2010;55:469–80.
65. Matkovich SJ, Zhang Y, Van Booven DJ, Dorn GW 2nd. Deep mRNA sequencing for in vivo functional analysis of cardiac transcriptional regulators: application to Galphaq. Circ Res. 2010;106:1459–67.

4

Together JUN and DDIT3 (CHOP) control retinal ganglion cell death after axonal injury

Stephanie B. Syc-Mazurek[1,2], Kimberly A. Fernandes[1], Michael P. Wilson[1], Peter Shrager[3] and Richard T. Libby[1,4,5*]

Abstract

Background: Optic nerve injury is an important pathological component in neurodegenerative diseases such as traumatic optic neuropathies and glaucoma. The molecular signaling pathway(s) critical for retinal ganglion cell (RGC) death after axonal insult, however, is/are not fully defined. RGC death after axonal injury is known to occur by BAX-dependent apoptosis. Two transcription factors JUN (the canonical target of JNK) and DDIT3 (CHOP; a key mediator of the endoplasmic reticulum stress response) are known to be important apoptotic signaling molecules after axonal injury, including in RGCs. However, neither *Jun* nor *Ddit3* deficiency provide complete protection to RGCs after injury. Since *Jun* and *Ddit3* are important apoptotic signaling molecules, we sought to determine if their combined deficiency might provide additive protection to RGCs after axonal injury.

Methods: To determine if DDIT3 regulated the expression of JUN after an axonal insult, mice deficient for *Ddit3* were examined after optic nerve crush (ONC). In order to critically test the importance of these genes in RGC death after axonal injury, RGC survival was assessed at multiple time-points after ONC (14, 35, 60, and 120 days after injury) in *Jun*, *Ddit3,* and combined *Jun/Ddit3* deficient mice. Finally, to directly assess the role of JUN and DDIT3 in axonal degeneration, compound actions potentials were recorded from *Jun*, *Ddit3,* and *Jun/Ddit3* deficient mice after ONC.

Results: Single and combined deficiency of *Jun* and *Ddit3* did not appear to alter gross retinal morphology. *Ddit3* deficiency did not alter expression of JUN after axonal injury. Deletion of both *Jun* and *Ddit3* provided significantly greater long-term protection to RGCs as compared to *Jun* or *Ddit3* deficiency alone. Finally, despite the profound protection to RGC somas provided by the deficiency of *Jun* plus *Ddit3*, their combined loss did not lessen axonal degeneration.

Conclusions: These results suggest JUN and DDIT3 are independently regulated pro-death signaling molecules in RGCs and together account for the vast majority of apoptotic signaling in RGCs after axonal injury. Thus, JUN and DDIT3 may represent key molecular hubs that integrate upstream signaling events triggered by axonal injury with downstream transcriptional events that ultimately culminate in RGC apoptosis.

Keywords: Axonopathy, Neurodegeneration, Retinal ganglion cell, Mitogen-activated protein kinase, Endoplasmic reticulum stress

* Correspondence: richard_libby@urmc.rochester.edu
[1]Department of Ophthalmology, Flaum Eye Institute, University of Rochester Medical Center, Box 314, 601 Elmwood Ave, Rochester, NY 14642, USA
[4]Department of Biomedical Genetics, Rochester, USA
Full list of author information is available at the end of the article

Background

Axonal injury is an important component in neurodegenerative diseases, including traumatic optic neuropathies and glaucoma [1–4]. In glaucomatous neurodegeneration, axonal injury at the lamina of the optic nerve head leads to axonal dysfunction and apoptotic RGC death [2, 4–20]. Several pro-death molecular signaling pathways have been implicated in glaucomatous RGC death including mitogen-activated protein kinase (MAPK) and endoplasmic reticulum (ER) signaling [21–37]. The molecular signaling leading from ocular hypertensive insult to apoptotic RGC death, however, is not well defined. Identifying the molecular events leading to RGC apoptosis after a glaucoma-relevant insult is an important step in identifying the molecules responsible for triggering and signaling axonal and somal degeneration in glaucoma.

MAPK pathway components, including c-Jun N-terminal kinases (JNKs) and their canonical target JUN (also known as cJUN), and ER stress signaling, and its downstream effector DNA damage inducible transcript 3, *Ddit3* (also known as CCAAT/enhancer binding homologous protein (CHOP)/GADD153), are known to be important pro-apoptotic cascades after glaucoma-relevant injuries [21–36]. Activation of either JUN or DDIT3 is known to culminate in BAX activation and *Bax*-dependent apoptosis and BAX is known to be required for RGC death after axonal injury [6, 38, 39]. Importantly, either *Jun* or *Ddit3* deficiency has been shown to protect RGCs after axonal injury. Either *Jun* or *Ddit3* deficiency provided significant, but incomplete protection to RGCs after axonal injury [22, 33]. These data suggest that individually, *Jun* and *Ddit3* are not solely responsible for BAX activation in RGCs after axonal injury. It is possible that JUN and DDIT3 are functioning in the same pathway, and thus protecting RGCs through similar downstream targets. In other systems, ER stress can lead to JNK-JUN activation [40–42]. Furthermore, JUN and DDIT3 may be activated in RGCs by the same upstream kinase, dual leucine kinase (DLK) [35, 36, 43]. Alternatively, JUN and DDIT3 may be independently regulated after axonal injury. Therefore, it must be determined if JUN and DDIT3 act through distinct mechanisms in RGCs and provide additive protection to RGCs after axonal injury.

Here, we sought to evaluate if JUN and DDIT3 independently regulate RGC death after axonal injury or if they might function in the same molecular pathway. Previously we showed that DDIT3 upregulation after axonal injury was not prevented by *Jun* deficiency [23]. We extend these findings and show that similarly, *Ddit3* does not control expression of JUN [23]. Thus, JUN and DDIT3 appear to be independently regulated, suggesting that combined deficiency of both JUN and DDIT3 could provide greater protection than either deficiency alone. To determine if protection afforded by JUN and DDIT3 deficiency is additive, animals deficient in both *Jun* and *Ddit3* were generated and evaluated after mechanical optic nerve injury. Combined deficiency *of Jun* and *Ddit3* was more protective of RGCs after axonal injury than either *Jun* or *Ddit3* deficiency alone, and provided profound long-term protection of RGCs after axonal injury. These results suggest that MAPK and ER stress signaling pathways are together the major regulators of RGCs after axonal injury.

Methods

Mice

Mice were housed on a 12-h light dark cycle and fed chow and water ad libitum. Five different alleles were used to generate four different mice strains: 1) mice deficient in *Jun* (also known as *cJun*), 2) mice deficient in *Ddit3*, 3) mice deficient in both *Jun* and *Ddit3*, and 4) mice deficient in *Dlk*. To generate animals conditionally deficient in *Jun*, a floxed allele of *Jun* [44] and Six3-cre recombinase (a neural retina cre, Jackson Laboratory, Stock# 019755) were crossed to generate 1) animals carrying the recombined floxed alleles, referred to as $Jun^{-/-}$ or *Jun* deficient ($Jun^{fl/fl}$Six3cre$^+$), 2) heterozygote animals referred to as $Jun^{+/-}$($Jun^{+/fl}$Six3cre$^+$), and 3) animals carrying non-recombined floxed alleles or wildtype alleles with or without the cre recombinase referred to as $Jun^{+/+}$ or wildtype (WT, $Jun^{+/+}$Six3cre$^-$, $Jun^{+/+}$Six3cre$^+$, $Jun^{+/fl}$Six3cre$^-$, or $Jun^{fl/fl}$ Six3cre$^-$). Mice carrying the null allele for *Ddit3* were acquired from Jackson Laboratory (Stock# 005530) and intercrossed to generate: 1) animals carrying two copies of the null allele, referred to as $Ddit3^{-/-}$ or *Ddit3* deficient, 2) heterozygote animals carrying one copy of the null allele referred to as $Ddit3^{-/+}$, and 3) animals carrying no copies of the null allele, referred to as $Ddit3^{+/+}$ or WT in the text. Animals deficient in both *Jun* and *Ddit3* were generated by crossing animals carrying the floxed allele of *Jun* and Six3-cre with animals carrying the null allele for *Ddit3* to generate Ddit3$^{-/-}$;$Jun^{fl/fl}$Six3cre$^+$ animals referred to as *Jun/Ddit3* deficient animals in the text. To generate animals conditionally deficient in *Dlk*, a floxed allele of *Dlk* [45] and Six3-cre recombinase (a neural retina cre) were crossed on a C57BL/6 J background to generate 1) animals carrying the recombined floxed alleles, referred to as $Dlk^{-/-}$ or *Dlk* deficient ($Dlk^{f/fl}$Six3cre$^+$) and 2) animals carrying non-recombined floxed alleles or wildtype alleles with or without the cre recombinase referred to as $Dlk^{+/+}$ or WT ($Dlk^{+/+}$Six3cre$^-$, $Dlk^{+/+}$Six3cre$^+$, $Dlk^{+/fl}$Six3cre$^-$, or $Dlk^{fl/fl}$ Six3cre$^-$). The Jun^{fl} and Dlk^{fl} alleles were all backcrossed at least 3 times to the C57BL/6 J genetic background prior to intercrossing with the Six3cre allele that had been backcrossed at least 10 generations into the C57BL/6 J genetic background. The

Ddit3 allele was obtained already backcrossed into C57BL/6 J for 5 generations. All experiments were conducted in adherence with the Association for Research in Vision and Ophthalmology's statement on the use of animals in ophthalmic and vision research and were approved by the University of Rochester's University Committee on Animal Resources.

Optic nerve injury

Mice were anesthetized with 100 mg/kg ketamine and 10 mg/kg xylazine. Optic nerve crush (ONC) was completed as previously described [22, 23, 43, 46]. Briefly, the optic nerve was surgically exposed and crushed immediately behind the eye with a pair of self-closing forceps (Roboz RS-5027) for 5 s. Controls included contralateral eyes that had not been manipulated and eyes in which a sham surgery was performed, where the optic nerve was exposed but not crushed. Animals were harvested at 1, 5, 14, 35, 60, and 120 days following ONC or sham surgery.

Histology and cell counts

Eyes to be processed for retinal morphology were fixed in 2.5% glutaraldehyde, 2% paraformaldehyde (PFA) for 24 h at 4 °C. After dehydration, eyes were embedded in Technovit (Electron Microscopy Services) and sectioned at 2.5 μm. Sections that included the optic nerve were stained with Multiple Stain Solution (Polysciences, Inc). Eyes to be processed for retinal flat mount immunohistochemistry were fixed in 4% PFA for two hours at room temperature. The anterior segment was removed and the posterior segment was processed for retinal flat mount immunohistochemistry as has been previously described [22, 23, 43, 46].

For retinal flat mount immunohistochemistry, retinas were dissected free of the optic cup and were blocked in 10% horse serum in 0.3% TritonX in 1 M PBS (phosphate buffered saline) for 24 h at 4 °C and then incubated in primary antibody for 72 h at 4 °C. Primary antibodies included: rabbit anti-JUN (Abcam, 1:250), rabbit anti-pJUN (Cell Signaling, 1:250) and mouse βIII tubulin (TUJ1; Covance, 1:1000). Whole retinas were washed in PBS and then incubated in secondary antibody, Alexafluor-conjugated secondary antibodies (Invitrogen), for 48 h at 4 °C before being washed in PBS and mounted RGC side up with Fluorogel in TRIS buffer (Electron Microscopy Sciences). Eight 40× fields were obtained for quantification of TUJ1+ and JUN+ cells. Images were taken 220 μm from the edge of the retina and equally spaced around the periphery of the retina (two fields per quadrant) as RGC density is known to vary across different dorso-ventral/medial-lateral retinal quadrants. Quantification was completed using the cell-counter tool in ImageJ.

Western blotting

Mouse retinas were dissected and placed in 100 μl ice cold lysis buffer (1X RIPA buffer (Santa Cruz 24,948) containing 50 μM sodium fluoride, 2 mM PMSF, 2 mM sodium orthovanadate, 1X protease/phosphatase inhibitor cocktail (Cell Signaling 5872S)). Tissue was lysed by sonication (Bransa Digital Sonifier, 10% amplitude for 3 s) prior to spinning down cellular debris in a microcentrifuge (10,000 rotations per minute, 4°C, 5 min). 10 μl of supernatant was combined with 10 μl 2X Laemmli loading buffer (Bio-Rad) and boiled for 10 min. Samples were fractionated by SDS-PAGE on a 12% gel and transferred to a PVDF membrane (transfer buffer: 1X Tris-glycine (Bio-Rad), 20% methanol). Membranes were rinsed with double-distilled H_2O and treated with a Qentix Western Blot Signal Enhancer kit (Thermo Scientific 21,050) according to manufacturer's instructions. Membranes were then blocked at room temperature using 5% milk in TBST buffer for 1 h. Membranes were treated overnight at 4°C with one of the following primary antibodies: rabbit anti-JUN (Cell Signaling 9165S, 1:750) or mouse anti-GAPDH (Calbiochem CB1001, 1:2000). The following day membranes were washed 3X with TBST prior to treatment with secondary antibodies: HRP-conjugated anti-rabbit IgG (Bio-Rad 170–6515, 1:5000) or HRP-conjugated anti-mouse IgG (Bio-Rad 170–6516, 1:5000). Immunoreactive bands were detected using a chemiluminescence kit (Immun-star, Bio-Rad 170–5070) prior to exposure using either film or digital detection equipment (Azure Biosystems c500). Membranes were occasionally stripped following development and treated with another primary antibody (stripping buffer: 0.1 M Tris-Cl pH 6.8, 2% SDS, 0.7% β-mercaptoethanol). Densitometric analysis was conducted using ImageJ software, and pixel densities of experimental bands were normalized to those of GAPDH loading controls.

Electrophysiology

Optic nerve compound action potentials (CAPs) were recorded as described previously [43]. Briefly, animals were euthanized with CO_2, and optic nerves were dissected by transecting close to the eye and to the chiasm. Optic nerves were incubated for a minimum of 60 min in artificial cerebrospinal fluid (ACSF) aerated with 95% oxygen/5% CO_2 at room temperature. ACSF was prepared with (in mM): 125 NaCl, 1.25 NaH_2PO_4, 25 glucose, 25 $NaHCO_3$, 2.5 $CaCl_2$, 1.3 $MgCl_2$, and 2.5 KCl. The recording chamber was temperature controlled and perfused with oxygenated ACSF. The nerve was gently drawn into suction pipette electrodes containing ACSF at both the stimulating (retinal) end and the recording (chiasm) end. Stimuli consisted of supramaximal constant current pulses of 50 microseconds duration. CAP amplitudes were normalized by maintaining the ratio of the recording pipet plus nerve resistance to the recording pipet resistance at 1.7 [43]. All traces were taken at 25 °C. Data were digitized and then analyzed off-line.

Statistical analysis

At least four retinas were analyzed for each genotype for all experimental conditions. The experimenters were masked to genotype and experimental cohort for quantification of cell number. The student's t-test (unpaired) was used to compare differences across two groups. One-way ANOVA followed by the Tukey's post hoc test for multiple comparisons was used for experiments comparing differences at a single time across more than two groups. Statistical significance was considered for P values <0.05.

Results

Jun and *Ddit3* deficiency does not alter retinal morphology

To determine if *Jun* (also known as *cJun*) and/or *Ddit3* (which encodes the protein CHOP) is necessary for retinal development; adult retinas deficient in *Jun, Ddit3,* and combined *Jun/Ddit3* were evaluated. *Jun* was conditionally deleted in the retina using Six3-cre, an established cre recombinase which deletes floxed alleles in the early developing neuroepithelium [47]. Animals carrying the null allele for *Ddit3* were evaluated independently and also crossed with animals carrying the *Jun* floxed allele and Six3-cre to generate animals deficient in both *Jun* and *Ddit3*. Deficiency in either *Jun* or *Ddit3* or the combined deficiency of *Jun* and *Ddit3* did not alter morphology of the retina (Fig. 1A). Furthermore,

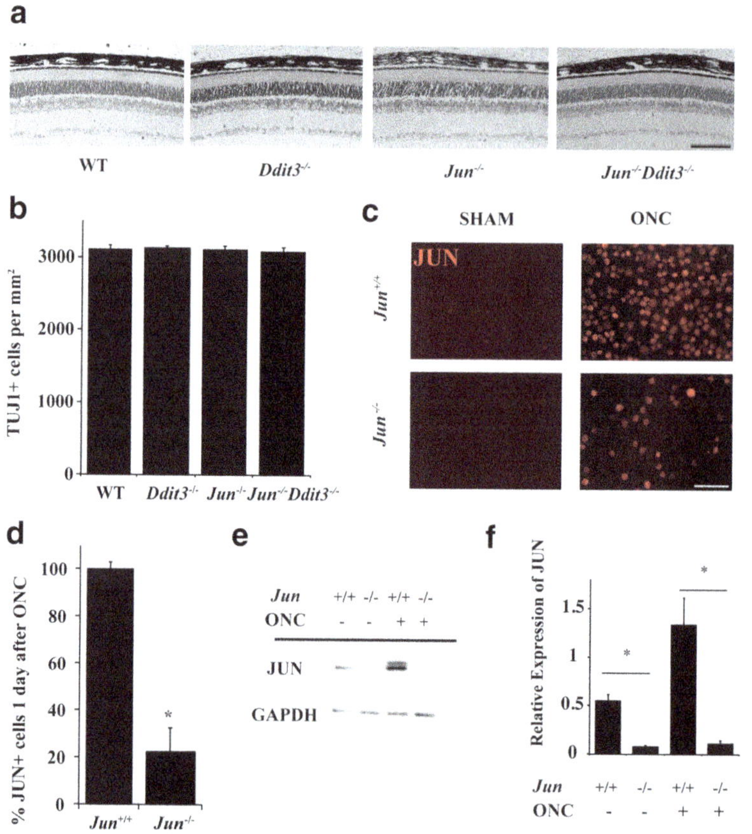

Fig. 1 *Jun* and *Ddit3* deficiency does not alter retinal morphology. **a** Semi-thin retinal cross sections were taken to evaluate the gross structure of the retina in WT, *Jun*, *Ddit3*, and *Jun/Ddit3* deficient animals. *Jun*, *Ddit3*, and combined *Jun/Ddit3* deficiency did not appear to alter gross retinal structure. **b** TUJ1+ cells (a marker of RGCs) were counted in retinal flat mounts in WT, *Jun*, *Ddit3*, *Jun/Ddit3* deficient animals. No difference was observed across genotypes ($P > 0.05$ for each comparison; $n = 8$ per group). **c/d** JUN accumulation was readily detected in the somas of RGCs of wildtype animals after ONC but was not easily detected in sham retinas. To determine the efficiency of *Jun* recombination using Six3-cre, the number of JUN+ cells were counted 1 day after controlled optic nerve ONC, a time when JUN is widely expressed prior to RGC death. JUN+ cells are reduced by 77.7% in *Jun* deficient retinas after ONC (error bars represent standard error of the mean; $n = 6$ per genotype; $P < 0.001$; scale bar 50 μm). **e/f** Western blot analysis was used to determine the level of JUN in wildtype (+/+) and *Jun* deficient (−/−) animals. JUN was significantly reduced in both *Jun* deficient unmanipulated retinas (85%, ONC -) and *Jun* deficient retinas after ONC (92%, ONH +) as compared to wild type animals (* $p < 0.01$)

no differences were observed across subgroups in the number of TUJ1+ RGCs in adult animals (Fig. 1B; $P > 0.05$; $n = 8$ per group). Thus, neither *Jun* nor *Ddit3* deficiency appears to alter the normal development of the retina. To assess the recombination efficiency of Six3-cre, the number of RGCs expressing JUN was evaluated one day after ONC. Consistent with previous studies, JUN accumulation was readily detected in the somas of RGCs of wildtype animals after axonal injury but was not easily detected in sham retinas (Fig. 1C), [22, 23, 48]. In retinas with conditional deletion of *Jun,* JUN accumulation after ONC was detected in approximately 22% of RGCs after ONC compared to wildtype retinas (Fig. 1D, $P<0.001$). Western blot analysis was completed to assess the level of JUN in wildtype and *Jun* deficient animals (Fig. E and F). In unmanipulated eyes, JUN was reduced 85% ($p < 0.001$) in *Jun* deficient retinas as compared to wildtype retinas. After ONC, JUN was reduced 92% ($p = 0.004$) in *Jun* deficient eyes as compared to wildtype animals. Thus, while recombination was not complete, *Jun*-mediated changes should be greatly reduced in *Jun* deficient conditional mutants.

Jun and *Ddit3* are independently regulated after optic nerve injury

Previously, JUN has been shown to be an important pro-apoptotic signaling pathway after glaucoma-relevant axon injury [21–26, 28–30, 35, 36]. DDIT3 has also been shown to be expressed after axonal insult [23, 31, 33, 34]. Furthermore, there is evidence to suggest that DDIT3 and JUN may act in the same signaling pathway. Accumulation of the DDIT3-dependent micro-RNA, miR-216b, has been found to directly target JUN [49]. Previously, *Jun* deficiency was found to not prevent the upregulation of DDIT3 protein after crush [23]. To determine if JUN is regulated by *Ddit3,* immunohistochemistry was performed on wildtype and *Ddit3* deficient retinas. JUN accumulated in RGC somas after optic nerve injury (ONC) in both WT and *Ddit3* deficient retinas (Fig. 2A). Quantification of JUN positive RGCs demonstrated no significant difference between JUN positive RGCs in wildtype and *Ddit3* deficient retinas. Likewise, quantification of phosphorylated JUN positive RGCs demonstrated no significance difference between wildtype and *Ddit3* deficient retinas after ONC (Fig. 2B). Western blot analysis was then completed both in unmanipulated eyes and after ONC to quantify the levels of JUN protein in wildtype and *Ddit3* deficient retinas. No significant difference in JUN levels was observed between wildtype and *Ddit3* deficient retinas in either condition. Together these results suggest that JUN expression is not dependent on *Ddit3* and that *Jun* and *Ddit3* may be independently regulated after optic nerve injury.

Combined deficiency of *Jun* and *Ddit3* is more protective after axonal injury than either *Jun* or *Ddit3* deficiency alone

Since our results suggest that *Jun* and *Ddit3* are independently upregulated after optic nerve injury, animals deficient in both *Jun* and *Ddit3* were generated to determine if the protection afforded by the individual deficiencies is additive. RGC survival was assessed 14, 35, 60, and 120 days after ONC with immunohistochemistry in retinal flat mounts using the RGC specific marker, TUJ1. Consistent with previous reports, deficiency of either *Jun* or *Ddit3* significantly increased RGC survival 14 and 35 days after ONC compared to WT animals [Fig. 3, Tables 1, 22, 33]. *Jun/Ddit3* deficient animals also had increased survival 14 and 35 days after ONC compared to WT animals (14 days after ONC- WT: 29% survival, *Ddit3*: 51%, *Jun*: 93%, *Jun/Ddit3*: 100%; 35 days after ONC- WT: 22%, *Ddit3*: 48%, *Jun*: 75%, *Jun/Ddit3*: 89%; $P < 0.001$ for all comparisons against WT animals) Furthermore, combined *Jun/Ddit3* deficient animals demonstrated increased survival compared to animals deficient in either *Jun* or *Ddit3* alone at 35 days ($p < 0.001$). To determine if the protection afforded to RGCs by *Jun/Ddit3* deficiency was sustained, as in in *Bax* deficient mice [7, 50], a cohort of animals was examined 60 and 120 days after ONC. At both of these time points, RGC survival in *Jun, Ddit3,* and *Jun/Ddit3* deficient retinas was increased compared to WT retinas. RGC survival in combined *Jun/Ddit3* deficient mice was also significantly increased compared to single deletion of *Jun* or *Ddit3* in animals at both 60 days and 120 days after ONC (60 days after ONC- WT: 14 survival, *Ddit3*: 33%, *Jun*: 54%, *Jun/Ddit3*: 83%; 120 days after ONC- WT: 7%, *Ddit3*: 25%, *Jun*: 48%, *Jun/Ddit3*: 75%; $P < 0.001$ for all comparisons). The RGC protection conferred by single *Jun* deficiency and combined *Jun* and *Ddit3* deficiency may be even higher since ~22% of RGCs in *Jun* and *Jun/Ddit3* deficient retinas still express JUN due to incomplete recombination of the *Jun* floxed allele. Thus, the RGC protection afforded by combined *Jun*/*Ddit3* deficiency is sustained after axonal injury. These results demonstrate that JUN and DDIT3 act as the two principal signaling nodes through which all pro-apoptotic signaling converges resulting in RGC death after axonal injury.

Dlk is not the sole shared upstream regulator of *Jun* and *Ddit3* activity

Dual leucine kinase (DLK) is a mitogen-activated protein kinase kinase kinase (MAP3K) and a critical regulator of RGC death after optic nerve injury [35, 36, 43]. Pharmacologic inhibition of DLK has been shown to be protective in rodent models of ocular hypertension suggesting the importance of this molecule in the pathogenesis of

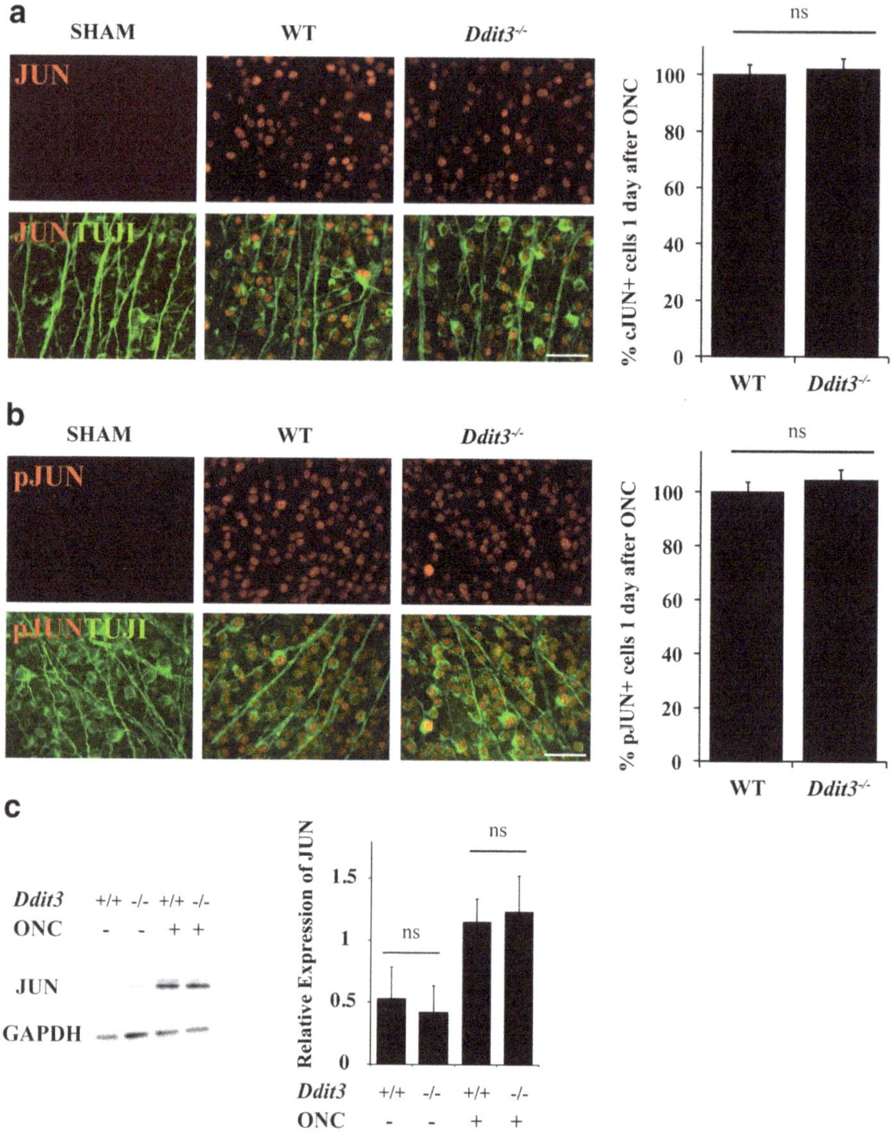

Fig. 2 *Jun* and *Ddit3* are independently regulated after optic nerve injury. To determine if *Ddit3* regulates JUN and pJUN expression, retinal flat mounts (RGC side up) were examined from WT and *Ddit3* deficient retinas one day after ONC. **a** JUN (red) accumulates in RGCs (labeled with TUJ1, a marker of RGCs, green) in WT and *Ddit3* deficient retinas one day after ONC, but not in sham retinas ($n = 4$ per genotype and experimental condition). There was no significance difference (ns) in the number of JUN positive RGCs between wildtype and *Ddit3* deficient retinas. **b** Similarly, pJUN (red) accumulates in RGCs (green) in WT and *Ddit3* deficient retinas one day after ONC. There was no significance difference (ns) in the number of pJUN positive RGCs between wildtype and *Ddit3* deficient retinas. **c** Western blot analysis was used to determine the level of JUN in wildtype (+/+) and *Ddit3* deficient (−/−) animals. There was no significant difference in JUN levels between *Ddit3* deficient and wildtype unmanipulated eyes (ONC -) or between *Ddit3* deficient and wildtype eyes after ONC (ONC +). Previously, DDIT3 has been shown to be expressed in *Jun* deficient retinas after ONC [23]. Scale bar: 50 μm

glaucoma [36]. After axonal injury, DLK is a major activator of JNK signaling and regulates both apoptosis and Wallerian degeneration. After optic nerve injury, *Dlk* deficiency decreases the somal pool of JNK, attenuates somal JUN accumulation, and ultimately increases survival of RGCs as compared to WT animals [35, 36, 43]. Though protective of RGC somas, *Dlk* deficiency does not prevent activation of axonal JNK [43]. *Dlk* has also been proposed to regulate *Ddit3* expression after axonal injury. Unbiased gene expression profiling after mechanical axonal injury demonstrated that *Dlk* deficiency significantly reduced the expression of DDIT3 [35]. Together these results raise the possibility that DLK could be upstream of both *Jun* and *Ddit3,* thus making *Dlk* an important common upstream regulator of RGC death after axonal injury. To test this hypothesis, RGC survival was directly compared in WT, *Dlk,* and *Jun/Ddit3* deficient retinas 35 days after ONC. This time point was chosen because there was significant

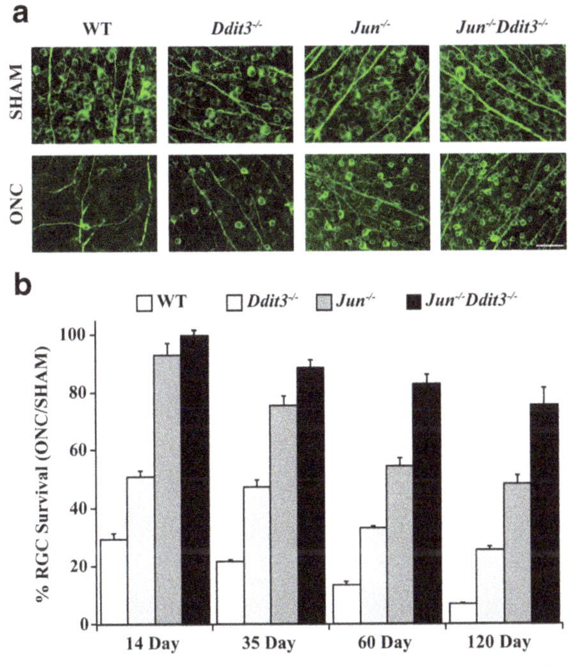

Fig. 3 Combined *Jun/Ddit3* deficiency is more protective after axonal injury than either *Jun* or *Ddit3* deficiency alone. **a** Example of TUJ1 staining in control and experimental eyes at 120 days after ONC (scale bar = 50 μm). **b** *Ddit3, Jun,* and combined *Jun* and *Ddit3* deficient animals had significantly greater RGC survival than WT animals at all time points assessed ($p < 0.001$). Furthermore, there were significant differences ($P < 0.001$) found between the *Ddit3, Jun,* and combined *Jun* and *Ddit3* groups at all time points evaluated expect for between the *Jun,* and combined *Jun* and *Ddit3* 14 days after ONC. Data are plotted as the percentage survival relative to sham animals ($n = 8$ per condition per genotype for 14, 35, and 60 days after ONC, except *Jun* deficient ONC $n = 7$ at 35 days after ONC and $n \geq 6$ per condition per genotype for 120 days after ONC; error bars represent SEM). Raw data in RGCs per mm^2 and *P* values for all comparisons are presented in Table 1

difference in RGC loss between WT, *Jun, Ddit3* and *Jun/Ddit3* deficiency mice after ONC. TUJ1+ cell counts confirmed that both *Dlk* and *Jun/Ddit3* deficiency provide significant protection to RGCs as compared to WT animals (Fig. 4; $P < 0.001$ $n \geq 7$ per group; WT: 20.4% survival, *Dlk*: 64.3%, *Jun/Ddit3*: 88.5%). Furthermore, there was greater protection in *Jun/Ddit3* deficient retinas compared to *Dlk* deficient retinas ($p < 0.001$) suggesting *Dlk* may not be the sole upstream regulator of JUN and DDIT3 activation.

Neither *Jun, Ddit3*, nor combined *Jun* and *Ddit3* deficiency alters axonal degeneration after mechanical optic nerve injury

RGC injury and axonal degeneration are important components of glaucomatous neurodegeneration [2, 8, 9]. After axonal injury, there are differential responses within the RGC somal and axonal compartments [51, 52]. There is spatial compartmentalization of molecular mechanisms that control RGC somal (cell body) and RGC axonal degeneration. Thus, it is necessary to test the role of JUN and DDIT3 in both somal death and axonal degeneration. DDIT3 deficiency promotes optic nerve survival in models of glaucoma, including mechanical optic nerve injury and increased intraocular pressure [33, 34, 37]. *Jun* deficiency has also been shown to protect axons from degeneration in sensory neuron culture [53]. In the DBA/2 J ocular hypertensive mouse model of glaucoma, *Jun* deficiency protected RGC somas but not axons from glaucomatous injury [54]. Thus, JUN does not appear to be required for axonal degeneration in adult RGCs after a glaucomatous injury. To test the hypothesis that single and/or combined deficiency of *Jun* and *Ddit3* may protect against axonal degeneration, optic nerve function was tested after mechanical optic nerve injury. Compound action potentials (CAP) were measured in WT, *Jun, Ddit3,* and *Jun/Ddit3* deficient mice five days after ONC, a time when WT animals demonstrate significant reduction in CAP amplitudes [43]. No differences in amplitudes were observed across the four groups, suggesting that deficiency of *Jun* and *Ddit3,* either singly or together, does not prevent for axonal degeneration after mechanical optic nerve injury (Fig. 5; $P > 0.05$ for all comparisons; $n = 4$ for all groups).

Discussion

Axonal injury is a critical component in many neurodegenerative diseases including glaucomatous neurodegeneration [2, 8, 9, 13, 14, 55, 56]. After axonal injury, RGCs undergo apoptosis in a BAX-dependent manner [5–7]. The molecular pathway that leads from axonal disruption to BAX activation is only partly defined. In fact, no molecule other than BAX is known to be required for BAX dependent RGC death after axonal injury. The transcription factors JUN and DDIT3 are expressed in RGCs after axonal injury [22–26, 31–34, 57, 58]. Both JUN and DDIT3 are known to have pro-death functions in neurons [42, 59, 60]. In RGCs, individual deficiency of *Jun* and *Ddit3* provides significant, but incomplete protection of RGCs after axonal injury [22, 23, 33]. Here, we sought to determine if these pathways are independent of each other and if so, whether combined deficiency of JUN and DDIT3 provides complete protection to RGCs after ONC. JUN and DDIT3 appear to control RGC death independently. Single deficiency of *Jun* or *Ddit3* significantly protected RGCs somas at all time points tested. Combined deficiency of *Jun* and *Ddit3* provided robust protection of RGCs after axonal injury, e.g., 89% survival 35 days after ONC. Furthermore, accounting for the incomplete deletion of *Jun* in RGCs, *Jun/Ddit3* deficiency may protect over 95% of RGCs 120 days after ONC. Thus, combined deficiency of *Jun* and *Ddit3* appears to provide nearly complete protection when accounting for incomplete recombination of the *Jun* allele. Together, JUN and DDIT3

Table 1 Combined *Jun/Ddit3* deficiency is more protective after axonal injury than *Jun* or *Ddit3* deficiency alone. (A) RGC per mm^2 and (B) Percent survival was calculated for WT, *Ddit3* deficient, *Jun* deficient, and combined *Jun/Ddit3* deficient retinas at 14, 35, 60, and 120 days after ONC. Percent survival was defined as the mean number of RGCs after ONC divided by the mean number of RGCs after SHAM. Values are displayed plus/minus SEM. (C) One-way ANOVA followed by the Tukey's post hoc test for multiple comparisons was used to analyze RGC cell counts at 14, 35, 60, and 120 days after ONC

A. RGC per mm^2

	WT	$Ddit3^{-/-}$	$Jun^{-/-}$	$Jun^{-/-}Ddit3^{-/-}$
14 Day ONC	976.4 ± 59.1	1625.4 ± 62.8	2954.5 ± 128.5	3053.9 ± 48.6
14 Day SHAM	3306.8 ± 47.3	3191 ± 25.0	3178.5 ± 73.9	3060.6 ± 42.5
35 Day ONC	681.4 ± 92.5	1484.8 ± 68.7	2340.5 ± 98.8	2729.8 ± 83.9
35 Day SHAM	3149.4 ± 51.7	3125.8 ± 30.6	3103.5 ± 51.7	3085.4 ± 48.0
60 Day ONC	427.2 ± 79.7	1041.4 ± 14.0	1635.9 ± 79.7	2577.4 ± 100.4
60 Day SHAM	3166.7 ± 42.4	3122.9 ± 61.1	3006.3 ± 42.4	3108.2 ± 19.9
120 Day ONC	219.0 ± 8.3	797.0 ± 40.1	1498.0 ± 88.3	2328.0 ± 179.4
120 Day SHAM	3178.0 ± 30.1	3116.0 ± 52.4	3101.1 ± 38.9	3086.0 ± 61.1

B. % Survival (ONC/SHAM)

	WT	$Ddit3^{-/-}$	$Jun^{-/-}$	$Jun^{-/-}Ddit3^{-/-}$
14 Day	29.5 ± 1.8	50.9 ± 0.6	93.0 ± 1.0	99.8 ± 0.3
35 Day	21.6 ± 2.0	47.5 ± 2.2	75.4 ± 0.4	88.5 ± 1.3
60 Day	13.5 ± 4.0	33.3 ± 3.2	54.4 ± 2.6	82.9 ± 2.8
120 Day	6.9 ± 1.6	25.3 ± 2.7	48.3 ± 3.2	75.4 ± 5.8

C. One-way ANOVA followed by the Tukey's post hoc test

	WT	$Ddit3^{-/-}$	$Jun^{-/-}$
14 Days after ONC			
$Ddit3^{-/-}$	<0.0001	–	–
$Jun^{-/-}$	<0.0001	<0.0001	–
$Jun^{-/-}Ddit3^{-/-}$	<0.0001	<0.0001	0.2107
35 Days after ONC			
$Ddit3^{-/-}$	<0.0001	–	–
$Jun^{-/-}$	<0.0001	<0.0001	–
$Jun^{-/-}Ddit3^{-/-}$	<0.0001	<0.0001	0.0024
60 Days after ONC			
$Ddit3^{-/-}$	<0.0001	–	–
$Jun^{-/-}$	<0.0001	<0.0001	–
$Jun^{-/-}Ddit3^{-/-}$	<0.0001	<0.0001	<0.0001
120 Days after ONC			
$Ddit3^{-/-}$	<0.0001	–	–
$Jun^{-/-}$	<0.0001	<0.0001	–
$Jun^{-/-}Ddit3^{-/-}$	<0.0001	<0.0001	<0.0001

activity accounts for the vast majority of apoptotic signaling in RGCs after axonal injury. Furthermore, because JUN and DDIT3 canonically function as transcription factors, it appears that after axonal injury RGC death requires transcriptional events.

JUN and DDIT3 activation may function as key molecular hubs that integrate upstream signaling events triggered by glaucomatous axonal injury. Given that the canonical function of JUN and DDIT3 is to regulate transcription, their activation likely leads to the transcription of pro-

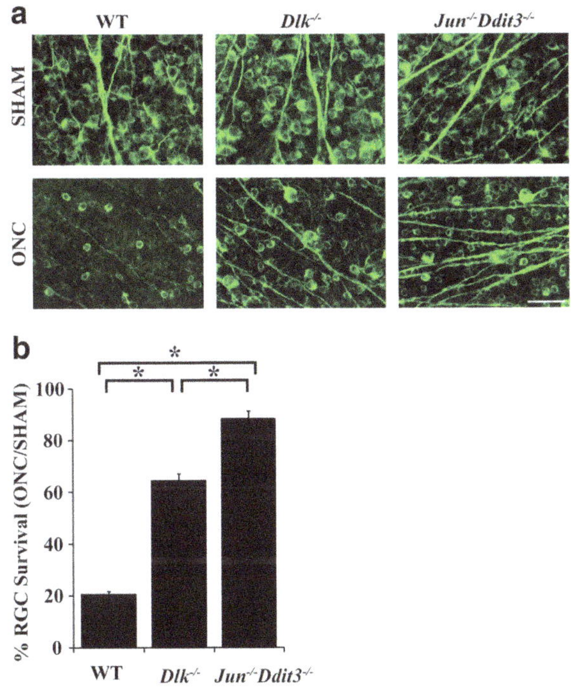

Fig. 4 Combined *Jun/Ddit3* deficiency is more protective after axonal injury than *Dlk* deficiency. **a** Example images of TUJ1 staining in control and experimental eyes 35 days after ONC (scale bar = 50 μm). **b** TUJ1+ cell counts showed that *Dlk* deficient and combined *Jun/Ddit3* deficient animals had significantly greater RGC survival than WT mice 35 days after ONC (% given compared to control eyes of same genotype, WT: 20.4% survival, *Dlk*: 64.3% *Jun/Ddit3:* 88.5%; *, P < 0.001, n = 8 per condition per genotype except n = 7 for *Dlk* deficient animals; error bars represent SEM). Importantly, the protection provided by *Jun/Ddit3* deficiency was significantly greater than the protection provided by *Dlk* deficiency alone (P < 0.001)

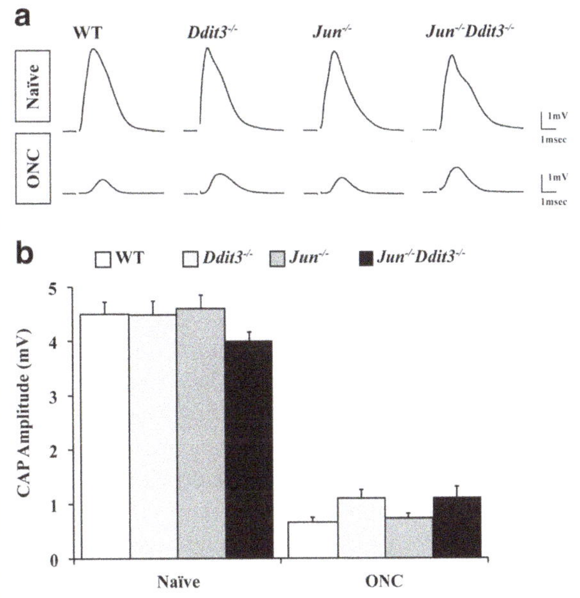

Fig. 5 Neither *Jun*, *Ddit3*, or combined *Jun/Ddit3* deficiency alters axonal degeneration after mechanical optic nerve injury. To assess the role of JUN and DDIT3 in axonal degeneration, compound action potentials (CAPs) were recorded from WT, *Jun*, *Ddit3*, and combined *Jun/Ddit3* animals 5 days after ONC, a time point when there is significant loss of CAP amplitudes in WT mice [43]. **a** Representative traces show that sham eyes from all genotypes had normal action potentials, while amplitudes were reduced about 80% in all cases after ONC. **b** Quantification of CAPs from WT, *Jun*, *Ddit3*, and combined *Jun/Ddit3* animals showed that there were no differences among the CAP amplitudes of naïve, uninjured eyes of all genotypes ($P > 0.05$). All genotypes had significantly reduced amplitudes after ONC as compared to naïve animals (P < 0.001 for all comparisons). CAP amplitudes of *Jun*, *Ddit3*, and combined *Jun/Ddit3* animals were not significantly different after ONC from those of control animals (P > 0.05, $n = 4$ for each genotype and condition)

death genes that ultimately trigger RGC apoptosis. The MAPK and ER stress pathways have both been suggested as pharmacologic targets for glaucomatous injury and there is also some evidence for physiologic overlap [35, 40, 49, 61]. Both systems are known to control pro-death genes in neurons. In RGCs, JUN directly controls the pro-death targets BIM, ATF3, and HRK [23, 46]. In other cell types, DDIT3 has been shown to control pro-death components including DR5 (death receptor-5 or TNFRSF10B), BIM, and GSN [39, 62, 63]. JUN, in RGCs, and DDIT3, in other cell types, have also been shown to inhibit pro-survival targets, such as BCL-2 [23, 64].

Interestingly, JUN and DDIT3 may have overlapping functions. DDIT3 can form protein-protein complexes with JUN and other members of the activator protein-1 (AP-1) transcription factor family [61, 62]. Given these interactions and the fact that activation of both *Jun* and *Ddit3* signaling cascades may culminate in BAX-dependent apoptosis, it is possible that together JUN and DDIT3 may co-regulate downstream effector targets in RGCs after axonal injury. Further work using transcriptomics will be needed to define the downstream effector molecules differentially and mutually controlled by *Jun* and *Ddit3*. In addition to glaucoma-relevant injuries, JUN and DDIT3 have been implicated in other neurodegenerative diseases [42, 60]. Thus, investigation into the downstream molecular targets of JUN and DDIT3 may determine molecular events broadly important for neurodegeneration.

Identification of the upstream regulator(s) of *Jun* and *Ddit3* will be an important step towards defining the critical pathway that leads from axonal injury to RGC degeneration. Potential molecules that have been suggested to activate both MAPK and endoplasmic reticulum stress signaling in other systems include mTOR, TLR4, and ETN1 [65–70]. Further study, however, should be done to identify molecules that activate both JUN and DDIT3 signaling in RGCs. Identified molecules should then be carefully tested in a model of optic nerve injury or preferably, a model of ocular hypertension to determine 1) if these molecules are expressed at a time point consistent with glaucomatous injury 2) if manipulation of these molecules decreases JUN and DDIT3 expression and 3) if deficiency of these molecules protects RGC somas and their axons. These experiments might also reveal early molecular signaling events that occur in axons after a glaucomatous injury. *Dlk* is a MAP3K known to activate JNK-JUN signaling in RGCs and has also been proposed to regulate DDIT3 activation in RGCs [35, 43]. *Dlk* deficiency provided significant protection to RGCs after axonal injury. The level of protection afforded by *Dlk* deficiency was similar to that provided by *Jun* deficiency and about 50% more protection then provided by *Ddit3* deficiency. Like *Jun* deficiency, protection provided by *Dlk* deficiency was not complete. Combined *Jun/Ddit3* deficiency provided greater protection to RGCs than *Dlk* deficiency. Thus, *Dlk* is likely not the sole or only upstream regulator of JUN and DDIT3 in RGCs after axonal injury. While signaling upstream of JUN and DDIT3 may converge, it is also possible that there is not a sole common upstream molecular regulator of all JUN and DDIT3 signaling. The inciting injury in glaucomatous neurodegeneration itself or early sequelae of this perturbation may activate both *Jun* and *Ddit3* through separate mechanisms. Evidence has implicated several distinct cellular events induced by ocular hypertension-induced axonal injury, including: loss of trophic support, noxious glial signaling, neurovascular unit dysfunction, and disruption of the axonal cytoskeleton [16, 20, 71, 72]. Future work to determine a shared upstream regulator of *Jun* and *Ddit3* activation will be important for further defining the major molecular signaling cascades driving RGC degeneration. Regardless of whether the inciting injury in glaucomatous neurodegeneration is extrinsic or intrinsic to RGCs, sequentially stepping upstream of JUN and DDIT3 activation may define the earliest events in glaucoma.

Determining the events leading to MAPK and ER stress activation may be challenging because the MAPK and ER stress signaling pathways are complex. Both routes have multiple parallel pathways with both divergent and convergent elements [59, 73–75]. ER stress is the disruption of normal ER function and activation of the unfolded protein response (UPR) due to the accumulation of unfolded proteins and interruption of normal calcium regulation [76]. The three ER stress response proteins are inositol-requiring transmembrane kinase (IRE1), activating transcription factor-6 (ATF6), and protein kinase RNA-like endoplasmic reticulum kinase (PERK). DDIT3 may be a target of all three protein pathways, but is predominately activated by PERK signaling [77]. Previous work has demonstrated that IRE and ATF6 signaling (the largely pro-survival signals of ER stress) are diminished with persistent ER stress signals, while PERK signaling (largely pro-apoptotic) is maintained [78]. In the same study, overexpression of IRE1, led to enhanced cellular viability after axonal injury. XBP1, a component of the IRE arm, was also activated in RGCs after axonal injury [33, 37], while XBP1 and DDIT3 were differentially expressed [33, 37]. While DDIT3 expression was robust and sustained after axotomy, XBP1 was transiently expressed at modest levels early after injury [33]. Unlike deficiency of *Ddit3*, deficiency of *Xbp1* did not prevent RGC loss after axonal injury suggesting that *Ddit3* dependent signaling was the critical part of the ER stress response for RGC death.

Glaucoma is a chronic, age-related disease which may play out over years and potentially decades [3]. Given the extended time period of glaucomatous injury, chronic ER stress may lead to prolonged activation of PERK-DDIT3 signaling which may override the protective components of ER stress signaling. Furthermore, the unfolded protein response, primarily through the IRE1 arm, has also been shown to initiate phosphorylation of c-Jun N-terminal kinase (JNK) that in turn activates JUN [40–42]. Therefore, in addition to prolonged pro-apoptotic ER stress signaling, activation of ER stress signaling in glaucoma may lead to sustained pro-apoptotic JNK-JUN signaling.

Deficiency in *Jun*, *Ddit3*, or combined *Jun*/*Ddit3* did not prevent loss of axonal function as measured by compound action potential after mechanical axonal injury. It is possible that deficiency in these molecules could lessen morphological degeneration, which was not measured here. *Dlk* deficiency, an upstream regulator of JUN in RGCs, and *Ddit3* deficiency both provided some protection to RGC somas and axons in an acute intraocular pressure elevation mouse model of glaucoma [34, 36] Recently, we showed deficiency in *Jun* does not prevent axonal degeneration in a chronic ocular hypertensive mouse model of glaucoma, though it does provide some protection to RGC somas [54]. It is possible, however, that deficiency in both *Jun* and *Ddit3* will protect RGCs in a chronic, ocular hypertensive model of glaucoma. Interestingly, if combined deficiency of *Jun* and *Ddit3* protects both RGC axons and somas in a glaucoma model it will point to new transcriptional pathways underlying RGC degeneration in glaucoma. This protection would suggest that the transcription events that occur during IOP elevation are critical for axonal degeneration. Such events may not be identified after an acute mechanical axonal injury because of axonal severing. Therefore, it will be important to test the role of *Jun* and *Ddit3* in a chronic, age-related model of ocular hypertension, the DBA/2 J mouse, to determine if *Jun* and *Ddit3* are critical for glaucomatous ocular hypertensive injury.

Conclusions

Jun and *Ddit3* are independently controlled transcription factors that together provide robust, near complete protection of RGCs after axonal injury. *Jun* and *Ddit3* are ideally positioned to integrate cell-signaling cascades after axonal injury with transcriptional regulation of RGC death. *Jun* and *Ddit3* signaling have been shown to be involved in other injuries to RGCs including ischemic injury, diabetic retinopathy, and traumatic optic neuropathy (and traumatic brain injury) [23, 27, 33, 58, 79–82]. Given the robust protection shown here after RGC injury, it will be interesting to determine if dual activation of *Jun* and *Ddit* may define a canonical signaling pathway (culminating in BAX activation) for RGC death. Furthermore, it will be important to test the effectiveness of inhibiting both JNK-JUN and DDIT3-dependent ER stress signaling in other injury paradigms that result in RGC death. As axonal injury is a critical event in many different diseases, it is possible that JUN and DDIT3 may control neural degeneration after axonal injury in other neuron types. Thus, the finding that together JUN and DDIT3 control RGC death after axonal injury may be broadly applicable to understanding the molecular signaling pathways that control neurodegeneration.

Abbreviations

ACSF: artificial cerebrospinal fluid; AP-1: activator protein 1; ATF6: activating transcription factor 6; CAP: compound action potential; CHOP: CCAAT/enhancer binding homologous protein; DDIT3: DNA damage inducible transcript 3; DLK: dual leucine kinase; DR5: death receptor 5; ER: endoplasmic reticulum; IRE1: inositol-requiring transmembrane kinase 1; JNK: c-Jun N-terminal kinase; MAP3K: mitogen-activated protein kinase kinase kinase; MAPK: mitogen-activated protein kinase; ONC: optic nerve crush; PERK: protein kinase RNA-like endoplasmic reticulum kinase; PFA: paraformaldehyde; RGC: retinal ganglion cell; TUJ1: βIII tubulin; UPR: unfolded protein response; WT: wildtype

Acknowledgements

The authors would like to thank Drs. Furuta (Six3-cre) and Wagner (*Jun*[f]) for generously providing mice.

Funding

This work was supported by EY018606 (RTL) and Research to Prevent Blindness, an unrestricted grant to the Department of Ophthalmology at the University of Rochester Medical Center. The funding agencies had no role in the design of the study and collection, analysis, and interpretation of data and in writing the manuscript.

Author's contributions

All authors designed and interpreted the experiments. SBS performed the experiments except for the western blot analysis performed by MW and the compound action potentials that were performed by KAF. SBS and RTL drafted the manuscript. All authors edited the manuscript and read and approved the final manuscript.

Competing interests

The authors declare that they have no competing interests.

Author details

[1]Department of Ophthalmology, Flaum Eye Institute, University of Rochester Medical Center, Box 314, 601 Elmwood Ave, Rochester, NY 14642, USA. [2]Neuroscience Graduate Program, Rochester, USA. [3]Department of Neuroscience, Rochester, USA. [4]Department of Biomedical Genetics, Rochester, USA. [5]The Center for Visual Sciences, University of Rochester Medical Center, Rochester, NY 14642, USA.

References

1. Quigley HA, Addicks EM, Green WR, Maumenee AE. Optic nerve damage in human glaucoma. II. The site of injury and susceptibility to damage. Arch Ophthalmol. 1981;99:635–49.
2. Howell GR, Libby RT, Jakobs TC, Smith RS, Phalan FC, Barter JW, Barbay JM, Marchant JK, Mahesh N, Porciatti V, et al. Axons of retinal ganglion cells are insulted in the optic nerve early in DBA/2J glaucoma. J Cell Biol. 2007;179: 1523–37.
3. Weinreb RN, Aung T, Medeiros FA. The pathophysiology and treatment of glaucoma: a review. JAMA. 2014;311:1901–11.
4. Jakobs TC, Libby RT, Ben Y, John SW, Masland RH. Retinal ganglion cell degeneration is topological but not cell type specific in DBA/2J mice. J Cell Biol. 2005;171:313–25.
5. Li Y, Schlamp CL, Poulsen KP, Nickells RW. Bax-dependent and independent pathways of retinal ganglion cell death induced by different damaging stimuli. Exp Eye Res. 2000;71:209–13.
6. Libby RT, Li Y, Savinova OV, Barter J, Smith RS, Nickells RW, John SW. Susceptibility to neurodegeneration in a glaucoma is modified by Bax gene dosage. PLoS Genet. 2005;1:17–26.
7. Semaan SJ, Li Y, Nickells RW. A single nucleotide polymorphism in the Bax gene promoter affects transcription and influences retinal ganglion cell death. ASN Neuro. 2010;2:e00032.
8. Anderson DR, Hendrickson A. Effect of intraocular pressure on rapid axoplasmic transport in monkey optic nerve. Investig Ophthalmol. 1974; 13:771–83.
9. Quigley HA, Hohman RM, Addicks EM, Massof RW, Green WR. Morphologic changes in the lamina cribrosa correlated with neural loss in open-angle glaucoma. Am J Ophthalmol. 1983;95:673–91.
10. Maes ME, Schlamp CL, Nickells RW. BAX to basics: How the BCL2 gene family controls the death of retinal ganglion cells. Prog Retin Eye Res. 2017;
11. Sun D, Lye-Barthel M, Masland RH, Jakobs TC. The morphology and spatial arrangement of astrocytes in the optic nerve head of the mouse. J Comp Neurol. 2009;516:1–19.
12. Minckler DS, Bunt AH, Johanson GW. Orthograde and retrograde axoplasmic transport during acute ocular hypertension in the monkey. Invest Ophthalmol Vis Sci. 1977;16:426–41.
13. Quigley HA, Anderson DR. Distribution of axonal transport blockade by acute intraocular pressure elevation in the primate optic nerve head. Invest Ophthalmol Vis Sci. 1977;16:640–4.
14. Quigley HA, Addicks EM. Chronic experimental glaucoma in primates. II. Effect of extended intraocular pressure elevation on optic nerve head and axonal transport. Invest Ophthalmol Vis Sci. 1980;19:137–52.
15. Quigley HA, Addicks EM. Regional differences in the structure of the lamina cribrosa and their relation to glaucomatous optic nerve damage. Arch Ophthalmol. 1981;99:137–43.
16. Howell GR, Soto I, Libby RT, John SW. Intrinsic axonal degeneration pathways are critical for glaucomatous damage. Exp Neurol. 2013;246:54–61.
17. Radius RL, Anderson DR. Rapid axonal transport in primate optic nerve. Distribution of pressure-induced interruption. Arch Ophthalmol. 1981;99:650_4.
18. Calkins DJ: Age-related changes in the visual pathways: blame it on the axon. *Invest Ophthalmol Vis Sci* 2013, 54:ORSF37–41.
19. Calkins DJ. Critical pathogenic events underlying progression of neurodegeneration in glaucoma. Prog Retin Eye Res. 2012;31:702–19.
20. Nickells RW, Howell GR, Soto I, John SW. Under pressure: cellular and molecular responses during glaucoma, a common neurodegeneration with axonopathy. Annu Rev Neurosci. 2012;35:153–79.
21. Tezel G, Chauhan BC, LeBlanc RP, Wax MB. Immunohistochemical assessment of the glial mitogen-activated protein kinase activation in glaucoma. Invest Ophthalmol Vis Sci. 2003;44:3025–33.
22. Fernandes KA, Harder JM, Fornarola LB, Freeman RS, Clark AF, Pang IH, John SW, Libby RT. JNK2 and JNK3 are major regulators of axonal injury-induced retinal ganglion cell death. Neurobiol Dis. 2012;46:393–401.

23. Fernandes KA, Harder JM, Kim J, Libby RT. JUN regulates early transcriptional responses to axonal injury in retinal ganglion cells. Exp Eye Res. 2013;112:106–17.
24. Levkovitch-Verbin H, Quigley HA, Martin KR, Harizman N, Valenta DF, Pease ME, Melamed S. The transcription factor c-jun is activated in retinal ganglion cells in experimental rat glaucoma. Exp Eye Res. 2005;80:663–70.
25. Isenmann S, Bahr M. Expression of c-Jun protein in degenerating retinal ganglion cells after optic nerve lesion in the rat. Exp Neurol. 1997;147:28–36.
26. Munemasa Y, Ohtani-Kaneko R, Kitaoka Y, Kumai T, Kitaoka Y, Hayashi Y, Watanabe M, Takeda H, Hirata K, Ueno S. Pro-apoptotic role of c-Jun in NMDA-induced neurotoxicity in the rat retina. J Neurosci Res. 2006;83:907–18.
27. Roth S, Shaikh AR, Hennelly MM, Li Q, Bindokas V, Graham CE. Mitogen-activated protein kinases and retinal ischemia. Invest Ophthalmol Vis Sci. 2003;44:5383–95.
28. Gesslein B, Hakansson G, Carpio R, Gustafsson L, Perez MT, Malmsjo M. Mitogen-activated protein kinases in the porcine retinal arteries and neuroretina following retinal ischemia-reperfusion. Mol Vis. 2010;16:392–407.
29. Kwong JM, Caprioli J. Expression of phosphorylated c-Jun N-terminal protein kinase (JNK) in experimental glaucoma in rats. Exp Eye Res. 2006;82:576–82.
30. Lukas TJ, Wang AL, Yuan M, Neufeld AH. Early cellular signaling responses to axonal injury. Cell Commun Signal. 2009;7:5.
31. Doh SH, Kim JH, Lee KM, Park HY, Park CK. Retinal ganglion cell death induced by endoplasmic reticulum stress in a chronic glaucoma model. Brain Res. 2010;1308:158–66.
32. Ghosh AS, Wang B, Pozniak CD, Chen M, Watts RJ, Lewcock JW. DLK induces developmental neuronal degeneration via selective regulation of proapoptotic JNK activity. J Cell Biol. 2011;194:751–64.
33. Hu Y, Park KK, Yang L, Wei X, Yang Q, Cho KS, Thielen P, Lee AH, Cartoni R, Glimcher LH, et al. Differential effects of unfolded protein response pathways on axon injury-induced death of retinal ganglion cells. Neuron. 2012;73:445–52.
34. Yang L, Li S, Miao L, Huang H, Liang F, Teng X, Xu L, Wang Q, Xiao W, Ridder WH 3rd, et al. Rescue of Glaucomatous Neurodegeneration by Differentially Modulating Neuronal Endoplasmic Reticulum Stress Molecules. J Neurosci. 2016;36:5891–903.
35. Watkins TA, Wang B, Huntwork-Rodriguez S, Yang J, Jiang Z, Eastham-Anderson J, Modrusan Z, Kaminker JS, Tessier-Lavigne M, Lewcock JW. DLK initiates a transcriptional program that couples apoptotic and regenerative responses to axonal injury. Proc Natl Acad Sci U S A. 2013;110:4039–44.
36. Welsbie DS, Yang Z, Ge Y, Mitchell KL, Zhou X, Martin SE, Berlinicke CA, Hackler L Jr, Fuller J, Fu J, et al. Functional genomic screening identifies dual leucine zipper kinase as a key mediator of retinal ganglion cell death. Proc Natl Acad Sci U S A. 2013;110:4045–50.
37. Hu Y. Axon injury induced endoplasmic reticulum stress and neurodegeneration. Neural Regen Res. 2016;11:1557–9.
38. Papadakis ES, Finegan KG, Wang X, Robinson AC, Guo C, Kayahara M, Tournier C. The regulation of Bax by c-Jun N-terminal protein kinase (JNK) is a prerequisite to the mitochondrial-induced apoptotic pathway. FEBS Lett. 2006;580:1320–6.
39. Puthalakath H, O'Reilly LA, Gunn P, Lee L, Kelly PN, Huntington ND, Hughes PD, Michalak EM, McKimm-Breschkin J, Motoyama N, et al. ER stress triggers apoptosis by activating BH3-only protein Bim. Cell. 2007;129:1337–49.
40. Urano F, Wang X, Bertolotti A, Zhang Y, Chung P, Harding HP, Ron D. Coupling of stress in the ER to activation of JNK protein kinases by transmembrane protein kinase IRE1. Science. 2000;287:664–6.
41. Sano R, Reed JC. ER stress-induced cell death mechanisms. Biochim Biophys Acta. 1833;2013:3460–70.
42. Lindholm D, Wootz H, Korhonen L. ER stress and neurodegenerative diseases. Cell Death Differ. 2006;13:385–92.
43. Fernandes KA, Harder JM, John SW, Shrager P, Libby RT. DLK-dependent signaling is important for somal but not axonal degeneration of retinal ganglion cells following axonal injury. Neurobiol Dis. 2014;69:108–16.
44. Behrens A, Sibilia M, David JP, Mohle-Steinlein U, Tronche F, Schutz G, Wagner EF. Impaired postnatal hepatocyte proliferation and liver regeneration in mice lacking c-jun in the liver. EMBO J. 2002;21:1782–90.
45. Miller BR, Press C, Daniels RW, Sasaki Y, Milbrandt J, DiAntonio A. A dual leucine kinase-dependent axon self-destruction program promotes Wallerian degeneration. Nat Neurosci. 2009;12:387–9.
46. Harder JM, Fernandes KA, Libby RT. The Bcl-2 family member BIM has multiple glaucoma-relevant functions in DBA/2J mice. Sci Rep. 2012;2:530.
47. Furuta Y, Lagutin O, Hogan BL, Oliver GC. Retina- and ventral forebrain-specific Cre recombinase activity in transgenic mice. Genesis. 2000;26:130–2.
48. Koistinaho J, Hicks KJ, Sagar SM. Long-term induction of c-jun mRNA and Jun protein in rabbit retinal ganglion cells following axotomy or colchicine treatment. J Neurosci Res. 1993;34:250–5.
49. Xu Z, Bu Y, Chitnis N, Koumenis C, Fuchs SY, Diehl JA. miR-216b regulation of c-Jun mediates GADD153/CHOP-dependent apoptosis. Nat Commun. 2016;7:11422.
50. Harder JM, Libby RT. BBC3 (PUMA) regulates developmental apoptosis but not axonal injury induced death in the retina. Mol Neurodegener. 2011;6:50.
51. Whitmore AV, Libby RT, John SW. Glaucoma: thinking in new ways-a role for autonomous axonal self-destruction and other compartmentalised processes. Prog Retin Eye Res. 2005;24:639–62.
52. Raff MC, Whitmore AV, Finn JT. Axonal self-destruction and neurodegeneration. Science. 2002;296:868–71.
53. Simon DJ, Pitts J, Hertz NT, Yang J, Yamagishi Y, Olsen O, Tesic Mark M, Molina H, Tessier-Lavigne M. Axon Degeneration Gated by Retrograde Activation of Somatic Pro-apoptotic Signaling. Cell. 2016;164:1031–45.
54. Syc-Mazurek SB, Fernandes KA, Libby RT. JUN is important for ocular hypertension-induced retinal ganglion cell degeneration. Cell Death Dis. 2017;8:e2945.
55. Schlamp CL, Li Y, Dietz JA, Janssen KT, Nickells RW. Progressive ganglion cell loss and optic nerve degeneration in DBA/2J mice is variable and asymmetric. BMC Neurosci. 2006;7:66.
56. Anderson DR, Hendrickson AE. Failure of increased intracranial pressure to affect rapid axonal transport at the optic nerve head. Invest Ophthalmol Vis Sci. 1977;16:423–6.
57. Yang L, Wu L, Wang D, Li Y, Dou H, Tso MO, Ma Z. Role of endoplasmic reticulum stress in the loss of retinal ganglion cells in diabetic retinopathy. Neural Regen Res. 2013;8:3148–58.
58. Nashine S, Liu Y, Kim BJ, Clark AF, Pang IH. Role of C/EBP homologous protein in retinal ganglion cell death after ischemia/reperfusion injury. Invest Ophthalmol Vis Sci. 2015;56:221–31.
59. Wang M, Kaufman RJ. Protein misfolding in the endoplasmic reticulum as a conduit to human disease. Nature. 2016;529:326–35.
60. Kim EK, Choi EJ. Pathological roles of MAPK signaling pathways in human diseases. Biochim Biophys Acta. 1802;2010:396–405.
61. Ubeda M, Vallejo M, Habener JF. CHOP enhancement of gene transcription by interactions with Jun/Fos AP-1 complex proteins. Mol Cell Biol. 1999;19: 7589–99.
62. Li T, Su L, Lei Y, Liu X, Zhang Y, Liu X. DDIT3 and KAT2A Proteins Regulate TNFRSF10A and TNFRSF10B Expression in Endoplasmic Reticulum Stress-mediated Apoptosis in Hum0an Lung Cancer Cells. J Biol Chem. 2015;290: 11108–18.
63. Wang XZ, Kuroda M, Sok J, Batchvarova N, Kimmel R, Chung P, Zinszner H, Ron D. Identification of novel stress-induced genes downstream of chop. EMBO J. 1998;17:3619–30.
64. McCullough KD, Martindale JL, Klotz LO, Aw TY, Holbrook NJ. Gadd153 sensitizes cells to endoplasmic reticulum stress by down-regulating Bcl2 and perturbing the cellular redox state. Mol Cell Biol. 2001;21:1249–59.
65. Shanware NP, Bray K, Eng CH, Wang F, Follettie M, Myers J, Fantin VR, Abraham RT. Glutamine deprivation stimulates mTOR-JNK-dependent chemokine secretion. Nat Commun. 2014;5:4900.
66. Babcock JT, Nguyen HB, He Y, Hendricks JW, Wek RC, Quilliam LA. Mammalian target of rapamycin complex 1 (mTORC1) enhances bortezomib-induced death in tuberous sclerosis complex (TSC)-null cells by a c-MYC-dependent induction of the unfolded protein response. J Biol Chem. 2013;288:15687–98.
67. Kuper C, Beck FX, Neuhofer W. Toll-like receptor 4 activates NF-kappaB and MAP kinase pathways to regulate expression of proinflammatory COX-2 in renal medullary collecting duct cells. Am J Physiol Renal Physiol. 2012;302:F38–46.
68. Gadea A, Schinelli S, Gallo V. Endothelin-1 regulates astrocyte proliferation and reactive gliosis via a JNK/c-Jun signaling pathway. J Neurosci. 2008;28: 2394–408.
69. Jain A. Endothelin-1-induced endoplasmic reticulum stress in disease. J Pharmacol Exp Ther. 2013;346:163–72.
70. Afrazi A, Branca MF, Sodhi CP, Good M, Yamaguchi Y, Egan CE, Lu P, Jia H, Shaffiey S, Lin J, et al. Toll-like receptor 4-mediated endoplasmic reticulum stress in intestinal crypts induces necrotizing enterocolitis. J Biol Chem. 2014;289:9584–99.

71. Almasieh M, Wilson AM, Morquette B, Cueva Vargas JL, Di Polo A. The molecular basis of retinal ganglion cell death in glaucoma. Prog Retin Eye Res. 2012;31:152–81.
72. Libby RT, Gould DB, Anderson MG, John SW. Complex genetics of glaucoma susceptibility. Annu Rev Genomics Hum Genet. 2005;6:15–44.
73. Plotnikov A, Zehorai E, Procaccia S, Seger R. The MAPK cascades: signaling components, nuclear roles and mechanisms of nuclear translocation. Biochim Biophys Acta. 1813;2011:1619–33.
74. Chang L, Karin M. Mammalian MAP kinase signalling cascades. Nature. 2001; 410:37–40.
75. Cao SS, Kaufman RJ. Unfolded protein response. Curr Biol. 2012;22:R622–6.
76. Ron D, Walter P. Signal integration in the endoplasmic reticulum unfolded protein response. Nat Rev Mol Cell Biol. 2007;8:519–29.
77. Kim I, Xu W, Reed JC. Cell death and endoplasmic reticulum stress: disease relevance and therapeutic opportunities. Nat Rev Drug Discov. 2008;7:1013–30.
78. Lin JH, Li H, Yasumura D, Cohen HR, Zhang C, Panning B, Shokat KM, Lavail MM, Walter P. IRE1 signaling affects cell fate during the unfolded protein response. Science. 2007;318:944–9.
79. Shimazawa M, Inokuchi Y, Ito Y, Murata H, Aihara M, Miura M, Araie M, Hara H. Involvement of ER stress in retinal cell death. Mol Vis. 2007;13:578–87.
80. Ho FM, Lin WW, Chen BC, Chao CM, Yang CR, Lin LY, Lai CC, Liu SH, Liau CS. High glucose-induced apoptosis in human vascular endothelial cells is mediated through NF-kappaB and c-Jun NH2-terminal kinase pathway and prevented by PI3K/Akt/eNOS pathway. Cell Signal. 2006;18:391–9.
81. Ortolano F, Colombo A, Zanier ER, Sclip A, Longhi L, Perego C, Stocchetti N, Borsello T, De Simoni MG. c-Jun N-terminal kinase pathway activation in human and experimental cerebral contusion. J Neuropathol Exp Neurol. 2009;68:964–71.
82. Begum G, Yan HQ, Li L, Singh A, Dixon CE, Sun D. Docosahexaenoic acid reduces ER stress and abnormal protein accumulation and improves neuronal function following traumatic brain injury. J Neurosci. 2014;34: 3743–55.

5

YKL-40 in the brain and cerebrospinal fluid of neurodegenerative dementias

Franc Llorens[1,2*], Katrin Thüne[1,3], Waqas Tahir[2], Eirini Kanata[4], Daniela Diaz-Lucena[1], Konstantinos Xanthopoulos[4,12], Eleni Kovatsi[4], Catharina Pleschka[5], Paula Garcia-Esparcia[1,6], Matthias Schmitz[2,3], Duru Ozbay[2], Susana Correia[2], Ângela Correia[2], Ira Milosevic[7], Olivier Andréoletti[8], Natalia Fernández-Borges[9], Ina M. Vorberg[5], Markus Glatzel[10], Theodoros Sklaviadis[4], Juan Maria Torres[9], Susanne Krasemann[10], Raquel Sánchez-Valle[11], Isidro Ferrer[1,6†] and Inga Zerr[2,3†]

Abstract

Background: YKL-40 (also known as Chitinase 3-like 1) is a glycoprotein produced by inflammatory, cancer and stem cells. Its physiological role is not completely understood but YKL-40 is elevated in the brain and cerebrospinal fluid (CSF) in several neurological and neurodegenerative diseases associated with inflammatory processes. Yet the precise characterization of YKL-40 in dementia cases is missing.

Methods: In the present study, we comparatively analysed YKL-40 levels in the brain and CSF samples from neurodegenerative dementias of different aetiologies characterized by the presence of cortical pathology and disease-specific neuroinflammatory signatures.

Results: YKL-40 was normally expressed in fibrillar astrocytes in the white matter. Additionally YKL-40 was highly and widely expressed in reactive protoplasmic cortical and perivascular astrocytes, and fibrillar astrocytes in sporadic Creutzfeldt-Jakob disease (sCJD). Elevated YKL-40 levels were also detected in Alzheimer's disease (AD) but not in dementia with Lewy bodies (DLB). In AD, YKL-40-positive astrocytes were commonly found in clusters, often around β-amyloid plaques, and surrounding vessels with β-amyloid angiopathy; they were also distributed randomly in the cerebral cortex and white matter. YKL-40 overexpression appeared as a pre-clinical event as demonstrated in experimental models of prion diseases and AD pathology.

CSF YKL-40 levels were measured in a cohort of 288 individuals, including neurological controls (NC) and patients diagnosed with different types of dementia. Compared to NC, increased YKL-40 levels were detected in sCJD ($p < 0.001$, AUC = 0.92) and AD ($p < 0.001$, AUC = 0.77) but not in vascular dementia (VaD) ($p > 0.05$, AUC = 0.71) or in DLB/Parkinson's disease dementia (PDD) ($p > 0.05$, AUC = 0.70). Further, two independent patient cohorts were used to validate the increased CSF YKL-40 levels in sCJD. Additionally, increased YKL-40 levels were found in genetic prion diseases associated with the *PRNP*-D178N (Fatal Familial Insomnia) and *PRNP*-E200K mutations.

Conclusions: Our results unequivocally demonstrate that in neurodegenerative dementias, YKL-40 is a disease-specific marker of neuroinflammation showing its highest levels in prion diseases. Therefore, YKL-40 quantification might have a potential for application in the evaluation of therapeutic intervention in dementias with a neuroinflammatory component.

Keywords: Chitinase 3-like 1, YKL-40, Neuroinflammation, Cerebrospinal fluid, Neurodegenerative dementias, Brain

* Correspondence: franc.llorens@gmail.com
[†]Equal contributors
[1]Network Center for Biomedical Research in Neurodegenerative Diseases (CIBERNED), Institute Carlos III, Ministry of Health, Feixa Llarga s/n, 08907 L'Hospitalet de Llobregat, Barcelona, Spain
[2]Department of Neurology, University Medical School, Göttingen, Germany
Full list of author information is available at the end of the article

Background

YKL-40 is a glycoprotein secreted by various cell-types including macrophages, chondrocytes, vascular smooth muscle cells and some types of cancer cells [1–4]. In normal adult human tissue higher YKL-40 expression is observed in cells with high cellular activity [5]. Although its precise function is not well understood, it is hypothesized to be involved in tissue remodelling during inflammation and in angiogenic processes mediating infiltration, differentiation and maturation of macrophages, and it is therefore considered a marker of inflammation and endothelial dysfunction [6–9]. Elevated YKL-40 is reported in many pathological conditions such as cancer, diabetes mellitus, cardiovascular disorders and inflammatory diseases of different aetiologies including, among others: bacterial infections, osteoarthritis, hepatic fibrosis, ulcerative colitis, Crohn's disease, rheumatoid arthritis, asthma, chronic obstructive pulmonary disease and liver cirrhosis [4, 10–14].

In the brain, YKL-40 is upregulated in several neurological disorders such as stroke, lentiviral encephalitis, traumatic brain injury, amyotrophic lateral sclerosis, multiple sclerosis and Alzheimer's disease (AD) [15–18]. Although YKL-40 was initially associated with the macrophage lineage [19–21], evidence suggests that during neuroinflammatory processes, its expression is abundant in reactive astrocytes and residual in microglial cells [16, 22]. Indeed, astrocytic YKL-40 expression has been reported in both acute and chronic neurological conditions [16] and in close vicinity to amyloid plaques and neurofibrillary tangles in AD [23]. In CSF, YKL-40 is elevated in several acute and chronic neuroinflammatory conditions [16] and in preclinical and prodromal AD/mild cognitive impairment (MCI) [23–26], which is in agreement with the potential role of astrocytosis in early AD pathogenesis [27]. Interestingly, YKL-40 is associated with cerebral morphometric patterns different from those linked to phospho-tau (p-tau)-related neurodegeneration [28], indicating a dissociation between astrocytic activation and p-tau pathology in early AD. Increased CSF YKL-40 levels have been reported in multiple AD cohorts [29–34], and in frontotemporal dementia (FTD) cases [34–36] but not in vascular dementia (VaD) and in DLB/PDD [32, 35], indicating that its deregulation is associated with disease-specific alterations and further suggesting that elevated CSF YKL-40 levels is not a specific signature for AD pathogenesis. However, conflicting data regarding non-AD dementias has been reported [35, 37]. Moreover, absence of studies reporting YKL-40 levels in prion diseases, which present the highest neuroinflammatory component among all dementia conditions [38], impedes establishment of the precise accuracy of YKL-40 quantification in the differential diagnostic context of neurodegenerative dementias. Further, brain YKL-40 expression patterns in different dementia types, and the potential correlation between brain and CSF levels is largely unknown, indicating that more research regarding YKL-40 expression patterns is required. Based on the data presented before, YKL-40 is in the spot light of biomarker research.

In this study, we investigated the sources of YKL-40 in the brain and evaluated its levels in the CSF in different types of neurodegenerative dementias, allowing us to determine the accuracy of YKL-40 quantification in the differential diagnostic context. Our data revealed that YKL-40 expression, while residual in the white matter of control cases, was highly increased in reactive protoplasmic and perivascular astrocytes in sCJD and AD cases. Among the different disease groups studied, highest YKL-40 levels in brain and CSF were observed in sCJD cases, followed by AD and DLB.

Methods

Reagents and antibodies

Detection of human YKL-40 by western blot was performed using the Human Chitinase 3-like 1 Antibody AF2599 (R&D Biosystems). Detection of murine YKL-40 by western blot, and human and murine YKL.40 by immunohistochemistry and immunofluorescence was performed using the Chitinase 3-like 1 antibody PA5–43746 (Thermo Fisher).

Anti-GAPDH 9484, anti-β-actin 8226 and anti-vimentin 92547 antibodies were from Abcam. Mouse anti-GFAP MAB360 was from Millipore. Rabbit Anti-GFAP Z0334 and anti-amyloid beta (β-amyloid) M0872 were from Dako. Anti-PrP(12F10) A03221 was from SPI Bio. Thioflavin was from Sigma. Chimeric recombinant prion protein (PrP), composed of the Syrian hamster residues 23–137 followed by sheep residues 141–234 (of the R154 Q171 polymorphism), was from Thermo Fisher.

Demographics and human cases

Brain tissue was obtained from the Institute of Neuropathology Brain Bank (HUB-ICO-IDIBELL Biobank) and the Biobank of Hospital Clinic-IDIBAPS following relevant guidelines of both Spanish legislation and the local ethics committee. Neuropathological examination and characterization were carried out on paraffin-embedded samples in every case. Detailed information on neuropathology and inflammatory profiling of the sCJD and AD cohorts has been previously reported [39–42]. sCJD MM1 and VV2 cases were selected due to their higher prevalence, but different clinical phenotypes [43]. The presence of infectious, metabolic and neoplastic diseases was ruled out in control samples. No correlation between post-mortem delay or sample storage time and levels of proteins and mRNA analysed was observed. A full summary of the cases is available in Additional file 1.

In order to establish the potential diagnostic utility of CSF YKL-40 measurement in the context of differential diagnosis of neurodegenerative dementias, we utilized samples from three independent cohorts: i) cases recruited at the Clinical Dementia Center at the University Medical Center Göttingen (Germany) (cohort 1), ii) cases recruited at the Hospital Clinic de Barcelona (Spain) (cohort 2) and iii) cases recruited at hospitals of northern Greece that were further processed at the Laboratory of Pharmacology (School of Pharmacy, Aristotle University of Thessaloniki), as part of additional molecular analysis to enhance disease diagnosis (cohort 3). Lumbar puncture was performed for diagnostic purposes followed by analysis of CSF standard parameters. YKL-40, tau, 14–3-3 and Aβ42 were analysed at the point of the first diagnostic work-up. In cohort 1, the neurological control group was composed of patients with either clinically or pathologically defined alternative diagnoses [44, 45]. This group included cases of psychiatric disorders, ischemic stroke, epilepsy, autoimmune diseases, alcohol abuse, headache, vertigo, pain syndromes, acute hypoxia and non-related neurological conditions. Control cases did not present biomarker profiles indicating the presence of a neurodegenerative disease. Diagnosis of AD was based on the International Classification of Diseases, Tenth Revision (ICD-10) definition for AD (F.00-G.30). Rapidly progressive Alzheimer's disease (rpAD) was defined by a velocity of cognitive decline >6pts/yr. on the Mini Mental Status Examination scale [46]. Velocity of decline was calculated using linear regression (least square method) in accordance with Villemagne et al. [47]. The diagnosis of DLB was based on the criteria of McKeith [17] and PDD as dementia in patients with PD. VaD diagnosis was based on ICD 10 definition (F01) and NINDS-AIREN criteria [48]. In cohort 2, controls were neurologically healthy individuals with no neurological clinical diagnosis and normal neuropsychological assessment. AD patients were diagnosed with probable AD using the National Institute of Neurological and Communicative Disorders and Stroke/Alzheimer's Disease and Related Disorders Association criteria [49] and displayed the typical CSF biomarker profile, characteristic of AD (low levels of amyloid beta 1–42 (Aβ42) and elevated t-tau and p-tau levels). In cohort 3, controls were composed of subjects with cognitive impairment/dementia (of unknown kind) with excluded prion diagnosis. sCJD cases were classified as definite cases by neuropathological examinations or as probable cases according to diagnostic consensus criteria [50, 51]. Genetic prion cases were confirmed by genetic testing (*PRNP* D178N and E200K mutations). Additional file 2 provides information on demographics and CSF biomarkers results.

Experimental mouse models

As a sCJD MM1 mouse model, the tg340 mouse line expressing about 4-fold level of human PrP M129 on a mouse PrP null background [52] was used. Control or sCJD MM1 brain tissues were inoculated as 10% (*w*/*v*) homogenates in 6–10 week-old mice in the right parietal lobe using a 25-gauge disposable hypodermic needle. Mice were observed daily and the neurological status was assessed weekly. The animals were sacrificed at pre-symptomatic (pre-clinical: 120 day post inoculation (dpi) and symptomatic (early clinical: 160 dpi and late clinical: 183 dpi) stages. Additionally, sCJD MM1 inoculum dilutions were performed to study prolonged disease times; animals were sacrificed at 210 dpi (10–1 dilution). Part of the brain was fixed by immersion in 10% buffered formalin to quantify spongiform degeneration and perform immunohistological analyses. The remaining brain was snap frozen and stored at −80 °C for protein and RNA studies. The 5xFAD mouse line harbouring the APP KM670/671NL (Swedish), APP I716V (Florida), APP V717I (London), PSEN1 M146 L (A>C), PSEN1 L286 V mutations was used as a model of AD pathogenesis. This widely-used model recapitulates several AD-related phenotypes displaying severe amyloid pathology and gliosis at about 2–3 months, cognitive alterations at 4–5 months and synaptic and neuronal loss at 9 of age [53, 54]. For scrapie infections with prion strains RML (immunohistochemical data) and 22 L (qPCR data), all animal experiments were in strict accordance with the principles of laboratory animal care (NIH publication No. 86–23, revised 1985) and the recommendations in the Guide for the Care and Use of Laboratory Animals of the German Animal Welfare Act on protection of animals. Animals were maintained under specific pathogen-free conditions. Mice were anesthetized with Ketamine/ Xylazin hydrochloride prior to inoculation. Eight weeks old mice were inoculated intracerebrally (i.c.) with RML 5.0-prions (immunohistochemical data) and 22 L prions (qPCR data). Animals were checked daily and were taken at indicated time points or were allowed to progress to clinical prion disease (presenting with slowness, ataxia, weight loss, trembling and ungroomed fur). For scrapie infections with RML strain (qPCR data), all experiments were performed in the animal facility of the Neurological Department, AHEPA University Hospital. Approximately 8–12 weeks old mice were inoculated. Infectious material corresponding to 100 μl of 1% brain homogenate from terminally ill RML-infected C57Bl/6 mice (104.5 × LD50) was intraperitoneally administered in fourteen animals; ten age-matched unchallenged mice were used as controls. RML-infected C57Bl/6 mice developed the first clinical symptoms, corresponding to abnormal gait, at approximately 130 days post inoculation. More severe symptoms, including loss of muscle tone, hind limb weakness, ataxia, weight loss and ruffled coat, appeared at approximately 160 days post inoculation. Whole brain was harvested from three animals per group at pre-clinical (120 dpi) and end-point clinical (180 dpi) disease stages.

Organotypic slice cultures

Organotypic cerebellar slice preparations from postnatal day 9–13 (P9–13) pups of C57BL/6JRj mice, further infection with 22 L scrapie strain, sample collection and detection of PK-resistant Prion Protein (PrPres) were performed as described previously [55].

CSF analysis

Total tau was measured using INNOTEST™ hTAU Ag; (Fujirebio). Levels of amyloid β1–42 (Aβ42) were measured with an ELISA kit (INNOTEST™ AMYLOID (1–42); Fujirebio). YKL-40 was measured using the MicroVue YKL-40 EIA ELISA kit from Quidel following the manufacturer's instructions. Protein 14–3-3 was detected with western blot as previously described [56].

RNA purification and RT-qPCR

RNA from different human and mouse brain regions was purified using the miRVANA RNA isolation kit following the manufacturer's protocol. For human samples, regions utilized for RNA extraction and corresponding age and gender information is summarized in Additional file 1. RNA was extracted from the following murine brain regions: tg340MM1-CJDMM1: cerebral cortex, RML scrapie: whole brain, 22 L scrapie: cerebral cortex and cerebellum. RNAs were treated with DNase Set (Qiagen) to eliminate genomic DNA contamination. Sample concentration was measured using a NanoDrop 2000 spectrophotometer (Thermo Scientific) and RNA integrity was assessed based on the RNA Integrity Number (RIN value) measured by an Agilent 2100 Bioanalyzer (Agilent). RNA samples were retrotranscribed using the High Capacity cDNA Archive kit (Applied Biosystems). Quantitative PCR assays were performed in duplicates on cDNA samples, in a LightCycler® 480 System (Roche). The reactions were set using 20xTaqMan Gene Expression Assays and 2xTaqMan Universal PCR Master Mix (Applied Biosystems) and conducted under the following conditions: 50 °C for 2 min, 95 °C for 10 min, 40 cycles at 95 °C for 15 s and 60 °C for 1 min. Fold changes were estimated using the 2-ΔΔCT equation. Fold changes in mRNA expression were determined relative to the control cases after normalization with housekeeping genes; statistical significances were calculated using GraphPad Prism 6.01. As housekeeping genes, *GAPDH* and *GUSB* as well as *Gusb* and *Hprt* were used as in human and mouse samples respectively. The Taqman probes used were: CHI3L1 (YKL-40) human: Hs01072228_m1, GFAP human: Hs00909240_m1, AIF1 (IBA-1) human: Hs00741549_g1, GAPDH human: Hs03929097_g1, GUSB human: Hs00939627_m1, Chi3l1 (YKL-40) mouse: Mm00801477_m1, Hprt mouse: Mm03024075_m1, GusB mouse: Mm00446958_g1.

Western blotting

Human and mouse tissues were lysed in lysis buffer containing: 100 mM Tris pH 7, 100 mM NaCl, 10 mM EDTA, 0.5% NP-40 and 0.5% sodium deoxycolate plus protease and phosphatase inhibitors (Sigma). Samples were centrifuged (14,000×g for 20 min at 4 °C) and supernatants were quantified for protein concentration using the Bradford method (Biorad). Samples were mixed with SDS-PAGE sample buffer, heated to 95 °C for 10 min, and resolved by SDS-PAGE analysis. Gels were transferred onto PVDF membranes, blocked and incubated with anti-YKL-40 antibodies (1:1000 dilution) as indicated above. Following incubation with HRP-conjugates, species-specific secondary antibody, the membranes were processed for specific immunodetection using the ECL reagent. GAPDH and β-actin antibodies at 1:5000 dilutions were used as loading controls. Fold changes (in arbitrary units) were determined from densitometric analysis relative to the control cases.

Immunohistochemistry and immunofluorescence

The immunohistochemical study was performed on 4-μm thick dewaxed brain sections. Endogenous peroxidases were blocked with peroxidase (Dako, Glostrup) followed by 10% normal goat serum. Following incubation with the anti-YKL-40 antibody (diluted 1:200) at room temperature overnight, the sections were incubated with EnVision1 system peroxidase (Dako) for 15 min at room temperature. The peroxidase reaction was visualized with diaminobenzidine (DAB) and H_2O_2. Primary antibody was omitted in some sections as immunostaining control and no signal was detected after incubation with the secondary antibody. Sections were counterstained with haematoxylin. For immunofluorescence, 4 μm thick dewaxed sections were stained with a saturated solution of Sudan black B (Merck, Germany) for 15 min to block the autofluorescence of lipofuscin granules present in cell bodies, and then rinsed in 70% ethanol and washed in distilled water. The sections were boiled in citrate buffer to enhance antigenicity, blocked for 30 min at room temperature with 10% fetal bovine serum diluted in phosphate buffered saline, and incubated at 4 °C overnight with primary antibodies. Double-labelling immunofluorescence was performed using a combination of YKL-40 (1:100) and GFAP (1:200 or 1:400) antibodies or PrP (12F10) (1:200) and either Aβ (1:50), YKL40 (1:100) or GFAP (1:400) antibodies. After washing, the sections were incubated with Alexa (Molecular Probes) fluorescence secondary antibodies (Alexa-Fluor 488 and 555 conjugated secondary antibodies). Nuclei were stained with DRAQ5™ (Biostatus Ltd., Shepshed, UK). After washing, the sections were mounted in Immuno-Fluore mounting medium (ICN Biomedicals, Irvine, CA), sealed and dried overnight. Confocal images were acquired using a microscope Leica DMIRE2 and Leica confocal software. Z-Stack image interval was 0.5 μm. Single plane images for quantification were obtained by Nikon Eclipse E800 microscope with ProgRes® CapturePro 2.7.7 software (JENOPTIK). Quantification of YKL-40 and/or GFAP positive cells was performed manually using Fiji ImageJ software in 13–15 areas per section in 3 different patients.

Immunofluorescence of frozen brain sections in 5xFAD mice was carried out as described [57]. For the analysis of human samples, two to four cases per diagnostic group were used and three to four sections from every case were analysed. For immunohistochemical analysis upon prion infection, tissues were fixed with 4% buffered formalin, prion infected samples were inactivated by immersion in 98% formic acid for one hour, post fixed in 4% buffered formalin overnight and processed for paraffin embedding. Sections (2 μm) were subjected to staining with the CHI3L1 antibody (YKL-40, 1:100) using a Ventana Benchmark XT (Ventana, Tuscon, Arizona, USA). Sections were incubated with primary antibody for 1 h, anti-rabbit Histofine Simple Stain MAX PO Universal immunoperoxidase polymer (Nichirei Biosciences, Wedel, Germany) was used as secondary antibody. Detection of secondary antibodies and counter staining was performed with an ultraview universal DAB detection kit from Ventana (Ventana, Tuscon, Arizona, USA). Representative images were taken with a Leica DMD108 digital microscope.

Elisa

Detection of murine YKL-40 in tissue homogenates was performed using the Mouse Chitinase 3-like 1/YKL-40 PicoKine™ ELISA Kit (Bosterbio) following the manufacturer's instructions. Inter- and intra assay coefficients of variation were below 15%. Dilution linearity tested from neat CSF to 1:8 dilution factor. Percent linearity was 85–112%. For the assays, CSF was diluted 1:3.

Real-time quaking induced conversion (RT-QuIC)

RT-QuIC was performed as described previously [58, 59] with minor modifications. Briefly, 85 μl of reaction buffer containing recombinant PrP (10 μg) was mixed with 15 μl of a 1:100 dilution of 10%*w*/*v* brain homogenates. Tissues for RT-QuIC analysis were lysed in PBS 0.1% SDS and clarified by centrifugation for 10 min at 10000×g. Reactions were set at a final volume of 100 μl and placed in 96-well black optical bottom plates (Fisher Scientific). Each sample was run in triplicate. Plates were sealed and incubated in a FLUO Star OPTIMA plate reader (BMG Labtech Ortenberg, GE) at 42 °C for 80 h with intermittent shaking cycles, consisting of 1 min double orbital shaking at the highest speed (600 rpm) followed by a 1 min break.

Statistical analysis

For two-group comparisons the *Mann–Whitney* test (non-parametric distribution) and unpaired t-test (parametric distribution) were used. In multiple comparisons, the *Kruskal–Wallis* test was used. Dunn's multiple comparison test was used for post-hoc analysis. Values of $p < 0.05$ were considered significant. *Pearson* (parametric distribution) and *Spearman* (non-parametric distribution) tests were used to detect correlations between biomarkers, demographic data and mRNA expression levels. Two-way ANOVA followed by Bonferroni's post-hoc was used in the quantification YKL-40 and GFAP positive cells. Receiver operating characteristic (ROC) curves and derived area under the curve (AUC; AUC = 0.5 no discrimination and AUC = 1 perfect discrimination) were calculated. The best cut-off value, sensitivity and specificity were estimated based on the *Youden* index [60] (point on an ROC curve providing the best balance of both sensitivity and specificity). ROC curves and statistical analyses were performed using the Graph Pad Prism 6.01 software.

Genetic testing

For detection of a prion disease-associated mutation, genetic testing was performed on genomic DNA isolated from blood or brain tissue [61]. Informed consent for the prion protein gene (*PRNP*) analysis was obtained from each patient or legal guardian.

Results

YKL-40 expression in sCJD patients

Expression of YKL-40 was initially analysed in sCJD as this neurodegenerative dementia presents the highest neuroinflammatory profile, including massive gliosis [39] and regulation of inflammatory mediators [38] compared to other neurodegenerative dementias [38, 40]. mRNA analysis showed that YKL-40 was highly increased in the frontal cortex (FC) and cerebellum (CB) of sCJD subtypes MM1 and VV2 ($p < 0.001$). No statistically significant differences were observed between sCJD subtypes in the two regions studied. Mean fold change values for controls versus sCJD comparisons were 6.1 in the FC and 11.5 in the CB (Fig. 1a). YKL-40 levels were normalized with GAPDH, and similar results were obtained for GUSB normalization (Additional file 3A). In agreement with mRNA data, YKL-40 protein levels were increased in the FC and CB of sCJD subtypes MM1 and VV2 ($p < 0.001$). Mean fold change values for controls versus

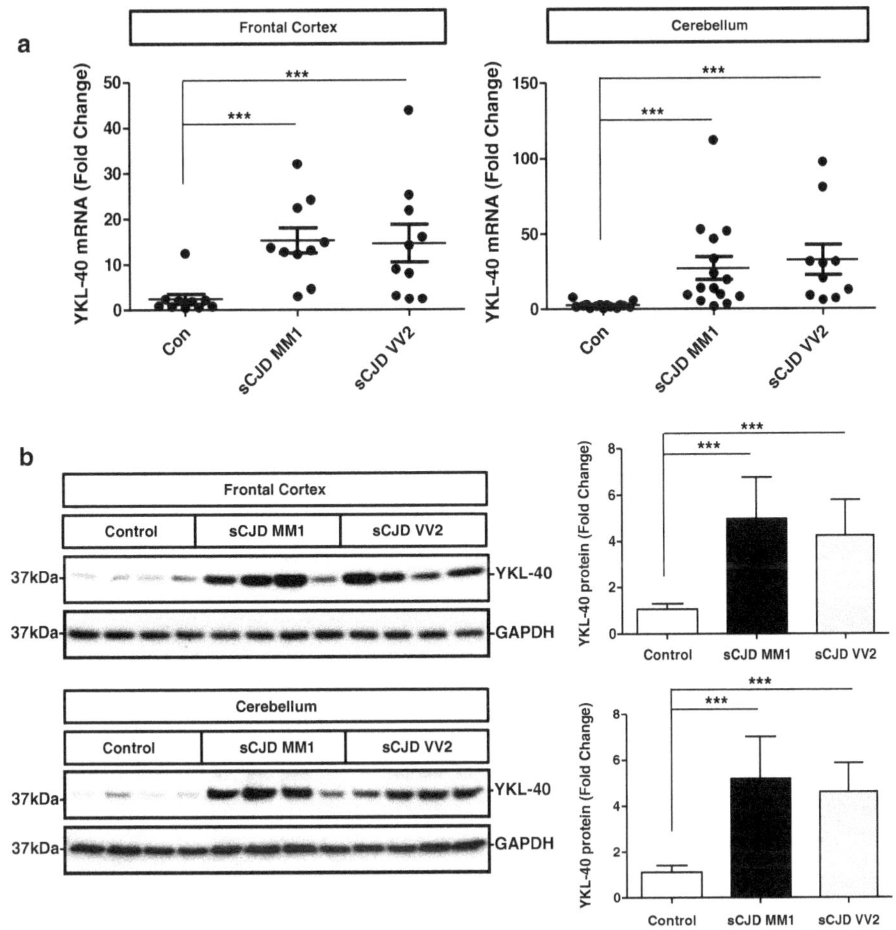

Fig. 1 YKL-40 expression in the brain tissue of sCJD and related mouse model. **a** RT-qPCR analysis of YKL-40 in the frontal cortex (left panel) and cerebellum (right panel) of control, sCJD MM1 and sCJD VV2 samples. GAPDH was used for normalization. **b** Western blot analysis of YKL-40 in the frontal cortex (upper panel) and cerebellum (bottom panel) of control, sCJD MM1 and sCJD VV2 samples. For normalization GAPDH was used. Graphical representation of Western Blot data acquired from the analysis of eight samples per group. Fold changes in the expression of mRNA and protein were determined relative to the control cases. Kruskal-Wallis and Dunn's post-hoc tests were used to determine statistical differences. $^{***}p < 0.001$

sCJD comparisons were 4.5 in the FC and 4.6 in the CB (Fig. 1b).

Further, immunohistochemistry was used for the study of YKL-40 expression and distribution in control and sCJD brains. YKL-40 immunoreactivity in normal brain was restricted to fibrillar astrocytes (stellate astrocytes with long processes) in the white matter and was increased in both the cerebral cortex and white matter of sCJD brain tissue sections compared to controls (Fig. 2a). YKL-40 was localized predominately in reactive protoplasmic and perivascular astrocytes, in addition to increased signal in fibrillar astrocytes of the white matter. Increased YKL-40 immunoreactivity was also detected in the Bergmann glia in the CB of sCJD cases (Fig. 2b). No apparent correlation was observed between PrPSc amorphous deposits in the CB in VV2 and YKL-40-positive astrocytes (data not shown). Specific expression of YKL-40 in astrocytes was confirmed by a positive co-localization between YKL-40 and GFAP in FC (Fig. 2c). Interestingly, double PrP-GFAP and PrP-YKL-40 immunostaining in the FC of sCJD revealed the presence of astrocytic processes within the PrP plaque-like deposits (Additional file 4A and 4B).

Additionally, we found a positive correlation between mRNA levels of YKL-40 and the astrocytic marker GFAP ($p < 0.01$) in the FC of sCJD cases, while no correlation was observed with the microglial marker AIF1 ($p > 0.05$) (Fig. 2d). As positive but moderate correlation between GFAP and YKL-40 expression levels were observed, the association between YKL-40+ and GFAP+ astrocytes was further explored. Quantification of double-labelled GFAP and YKL-40 immunoreactive cells showed co-localization in a majority of cells (GFAP+/YKL-40+ = 251 ± 8 cells/mm2) whereas the number of cells showing only GFAP staining or only YKL-40 staining was significantly smaller (44 ± 15

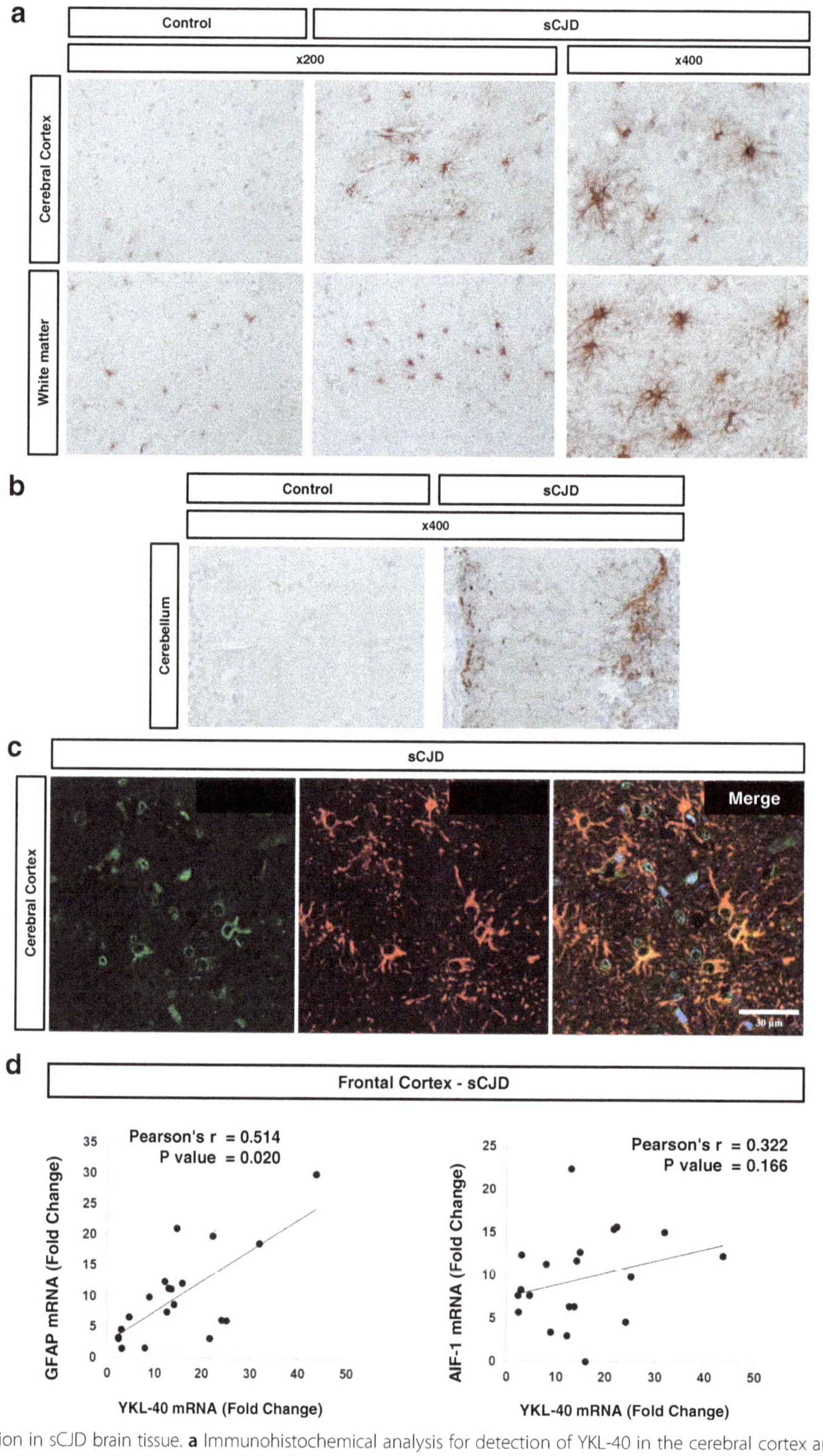

Fig. 2 YKL-40 expression in sCJD brain tissue. **a** Immunohistochemical analysis for detection of YKL-40 in the cerebral cortex and white matter of control and sCJD cases. **b** Immunohistochemical analysis of YKL-40 in the cerebellum of control and sCJD cases. Brown staining corresponds to YKL-40 staining and light blue to haematoxylin counterstaining. **c** Immunofluorescence analysis of YKL-40 (green) and GFAP (red) in cerebral cortex region of sCJD. Nuclei were stained with DAPI (blue). **d** Correlation between the expression levels of YKL-40 and GFAP mRNA (left panel) or AIF-1 mRNA (right panel) in the frontal cortex of sCJD cases. Normalization was performed using GAPDH. Pearson test was used to determine the correlations between mRNA expression levels

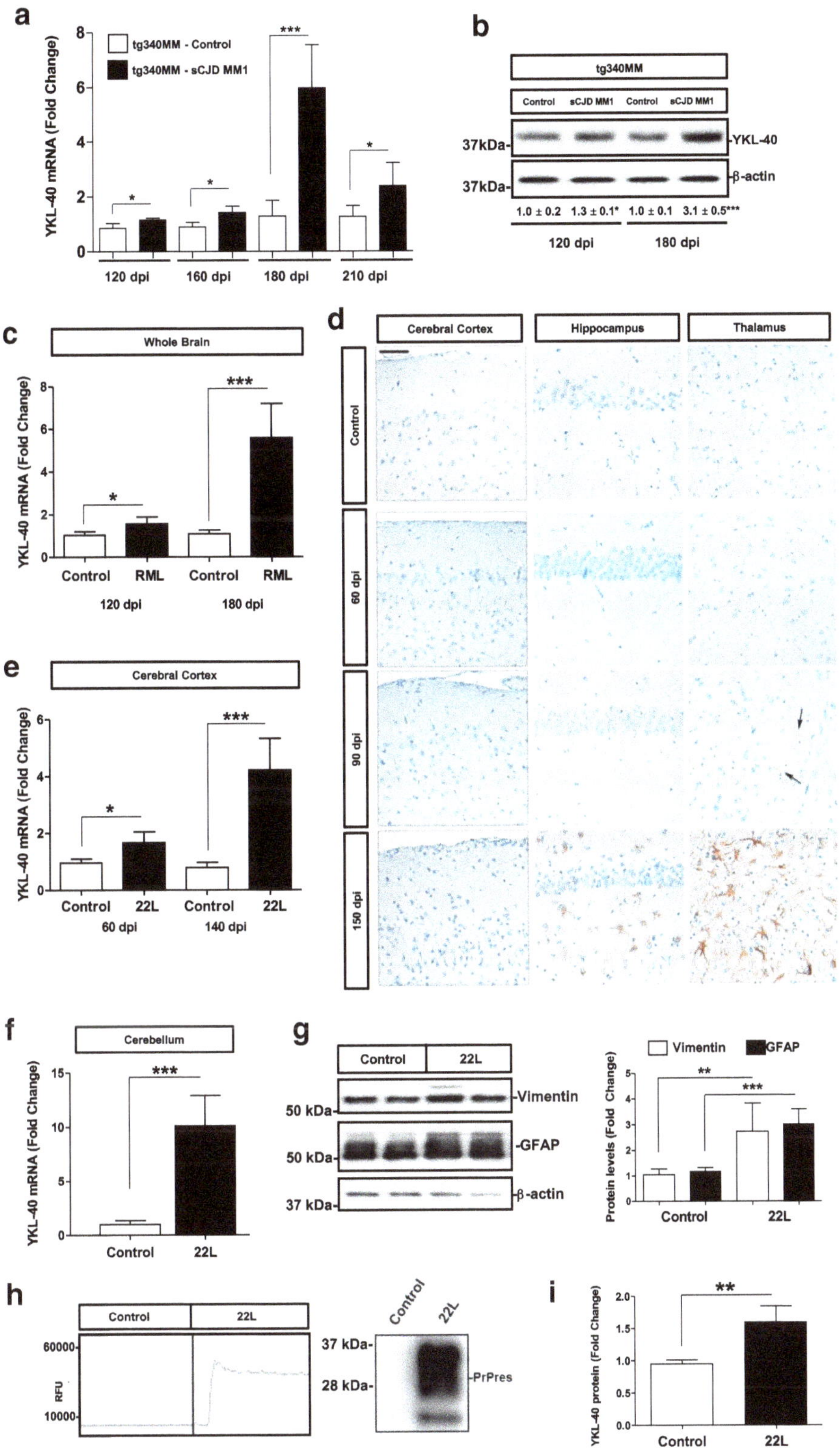

Fig. 3 (See legend on next page.)

(See figure on previous page.)
Fig. 3 YKL-40 expression in experimental models of prion diseases. **a** RT-qPCR analysis of YKL-40 in the cortex of control and sCJD MM1 inoculated tg340*PRNP*129MM mice at 120 dpi (pre-clinical), 160 dpi (early clinical), 180 dpi (clinical) and 210 dpi (clinical with 10–1 diluted inoculum). Four animals per group were analyzed. Normalization was performed using Hprt. **b** Representative Western-blot analyses for YKL-40 immunodetection in the cortex of control and sCJD MM1-inoculated tg340*PRNP*129MM mice at 120 dpi (pre-clinical) and 180 dpi (clinical). Three animals per group were analyzed. Normalization was based on β-actin levels. Numbers indicate densitometry results from three animals per group. Unpaired t-tests were performed to determine statistical differences. **c** RT-qPCR analysis of YKL-40 in the whole brain of control and RML scrapie-infected mice at pre-clinical (120 dpi) and clinical disease (180 dpi) stages. GAPDH was used for normalization. Similar results were acquired when normalization was based on Hprt expression levels (not shown). Unpaired t-tests were used for estimation of statistical differences. **d** Immunohistochemical analysis of YKL-40 expression in the cerebral cortex, hippocampus and thalamus of control and RML scrapie-infected mice at pre-clinical (60 and 90 dpi) and clinical (150 dpi) disease stages. Scale bar = 50 μm. Arrows indicate YKL-40 positive reactive astrocytes. Three animals per time point were used. Two sections were stained per animal (sagittal and coronal sections were used). Brown staining corresponds to YKL-40 staining and light blue to haematoxylin counterstaining. **e** RT-qPCR analysis of YKL-40 in the cerebral cortex of control and 22 L scrapie-infected mice at pre-clinical (60 dpi) and clinical (140 dpi) disease stages. **f** RT-qPCR analysis of YKL-40 in the cerebellum of control and 22 L scrapie-infected mice at clinical (140 dpi) disease stages. In all cases GAPDH was used for normalization. Similar results were obtained when Hprt was used for normalization (not shown). Unpaired t-tests were used to determine statistical differences. **g** Western blot analysis of Vimentin and GFAP in control and 22 L-scrapie infected COCS. β-actin was used for normalization. Graphic representation of densitometry analysis of five cerebellar tissues per condition is shown. Statistical differences were determined with unpaired t-tests. **h** RT-QuIC analysis of control and 22 L-scrapie infected COCS. A representative graph of three cerebellar tissues per condition is shown. All control tissues were tested negative, while all 22 L-infected tissues were tested positive (left panel); western-blot showing the presence of PrPres in 22 L-infected cells (right panel). **i** ELISA analysis of YKL-40 levels in control and 22 L-scrapie infected COCS. Statistical differences were determined with unpaired t-tests. Fold changes in the expression of mRNA and protein were determined relative to the control cases. $^{*}p < 0.05$, $^{**}p < 0.01$, $^{***}p < 0.001$

cells/mm2 and 3 ± 2 cells/mm2, respectively ($p < 0.001$) (Additional file 5A and B).

YKL-40 expression in in vivo experimental models of prion disease

To gain insight into the expression levels of YKL-40 in pre-clinical and early clinical sCJD stages, we took advantage of the tg340-*PRNP*-129MM mouse line inoculated with sCJD MM1 brain homogenate, which fully recapitulates the neuroinflammatory profile of human patients [40]. Analysis of the mRNA levels indicated that YKL-40 was increased at pre-clinical (120 dpi) and early-clinical (160 dpi) disease stages ($p < 0.05$). Differences between control and sCJD MM1-inoculated animals were more significant at clinical stages (180 dpi, $p < 0.001$ and 210 dpi, $p < 0.01$), resembling observations in sCJD post-mortem brains (Fig. 3a). Western blots from the same set of inoculated animals validated the presence of elevated YKL-40 at pre-clinical ($p < 0.05$) and clinical ($p < 0.001$) disease stages at the protein level as well (Fig. 3b).

To ascertain whether increased YKL-40 expression was also present in non-human prion diseases, wild-type mice inoculated with 22 L and RML scrapie strains were utilized. Increased YKL-40 mRNA levels were detected in the whole brain of RML-infected animals at late pre-clinical (120 dpi, $p < 0.05$) and clinical (180 dpi, $p < 0.001$) stages of the disease (Fig. 3c). Immunohistochemical analysis of RML-infected mice revealed the presence of YKL-40 positive astrocytes in the hippocampus and thalamus at clinical stages. In contrast to sCJD infected mice no staining was detected in cortical regions (Fig. 3d). At pre-clinical stages sparse positive YKL-40 positive cells were detected in the thalamic nuclei (Fig. 3d). In contrast, mice inoculated with the 22 L strain, which led to a faster clinical onset and a distinct neuropathology including more cortical PrPSc deposition pattern, presented increased YKL-40 mRNA levels in the cerebral cortex at pre-clinical ($p < 0.05$) and clinical ($p < 0.001$) disease stages (Fig. 3e). Additionally, YKL-40 mRNA levels were highly increased in the cerebellum of 22 L infected mice (Fig. 3f) ($p < 0.001$).

YKL-40 expression in ex vivo experimental models of prion disease

The observation of increased YKL-40 in the cerebellum of 22 L infected mice allowed to speculate that (22 L)-infected cultured organotypic cerebellar slices (COCS), which recapitulate most of the morphological and neuropathological hallmarks associated with prion infection and serve as an excellent ex vivo tool for the study of prion pathogenesis [55, 62], could recapitulate the alterations in YKL-40 expression observed in in vivo scrapie models. Ten weeks post-22 L infection, we detected astrogliosis by means of vimentin and GFAP expression (Fig. 3g). This was accompanied by positive seeding ability of pathogenic PrP by means of RT-QuIC analysis and presence of PrPres demonstrating the presence of prion infection on the COCS (Fig. 3h). At this time point, increased YKL-40 protein was detected in scrapie-infected COCS compared to mock treated cells ($p < 0.01$) (Fig. 3i).

YKL-40 expression in AD patients and in AD experimental model

Compared to controls, YKL-40 mRNA levels were increased in the FC of AD cases at early (AD I-III,

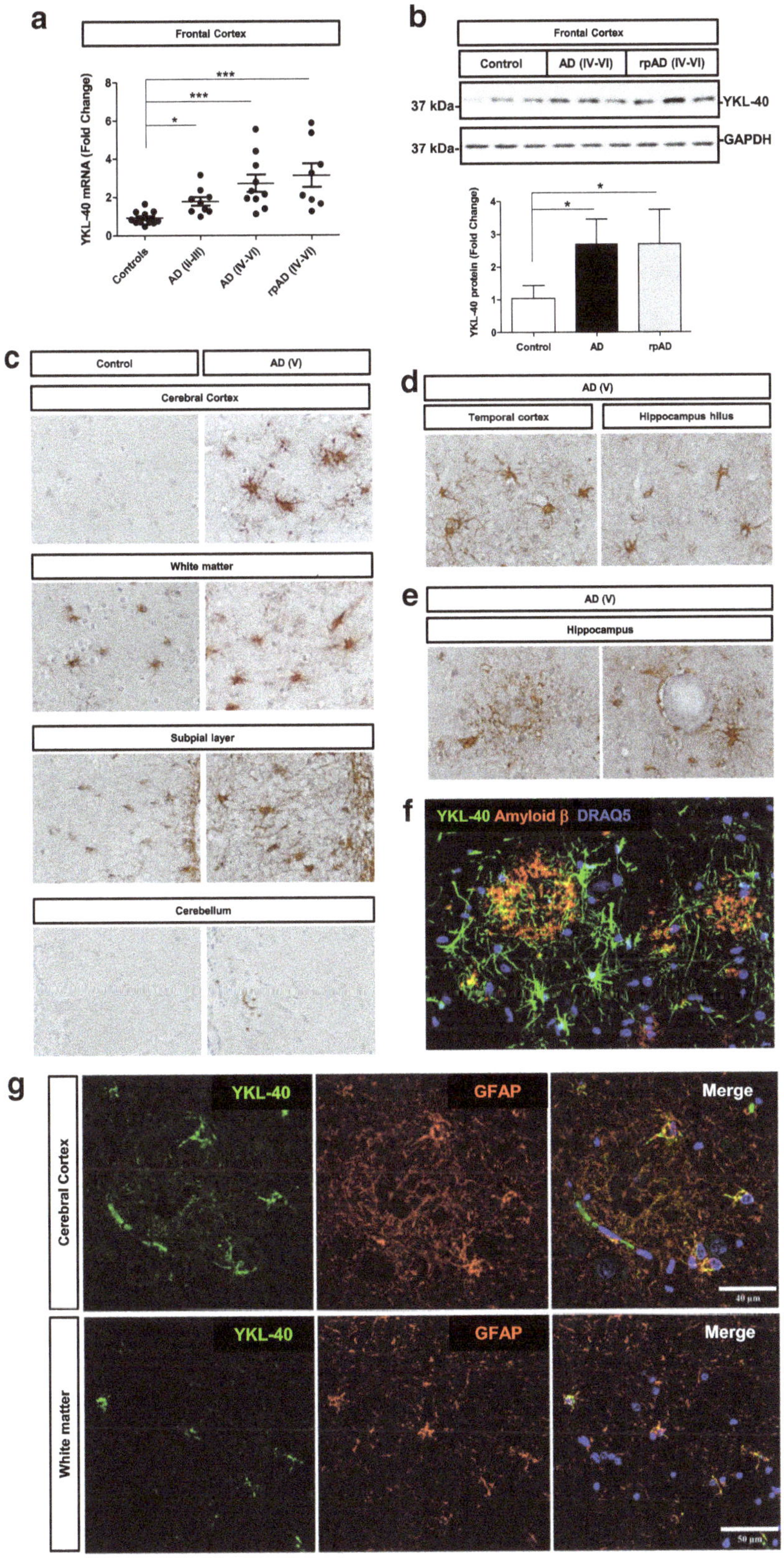

Fig. 4 (See legend on next page.)

(See figure on previous page.)
Fig. 4 YKL-40 expression in AD brain tissue (**a**) RT-qPCR analysis of YKL-40 in the frontal cortex of control, AD (I-III), AD (IV-VI) and rpAD (IV-VI) samples. GAPDH was used for normalization. Kruskal-Wallis and Dunn's post-hoc tests were used to estimate statistical differences. **b** Western blot analysis of YKL-40 in the frontal cortex of control, AD (IV-VI) and rpAD (IV-VI) samples. Normalization was based on GAPDH levels. Graphic summary of densitometry analyses performed on western blot results acquired from 8 control, 8 AD and 6 rpAD samples. **c** Immunohistochemical analysis of YKL-40 in the cerebral cortex, white matter, subpial layer and cerebellum in control and AD cases. **d** Immunohistochemical analysis of YKL-40 in the temporal cortex and hippocampus in AD cases. **e** Immunohistochemical analysis of YKL-40+ astrocytes surrounding β-amyloid plaques (left) and in blood vessels with amyloid angiopathy (right) in the hippocampal region of AD cases Brown staining corresponds to YKL-40 staining and light blue to haematoxylin counterstaining. **f** Double-labeling immunofluorescence of YKL-40 (green) and amyloid β (red) in the hippocampus of AD. **g** Double-labeling immunofluorescence of YKL-40 (green) and GFAP (red) in cerebral cortex and white matter in AD tissues. Fold changes in expression of mRNA and protein were determined relative to the control cases. $^{*}p < 0.05$, $^{***}p < 0.001$

$p < 0.05$) and late (AD IV-VI and rpAD IV-VI, $p < 0.001$) neurofibrillary tangle Braak stages (Fig. 4a). Mean fold change values for controls versus AD comparisons were 1.8 for AD II-III and, 2.9 for AD IV-VI and 3.2 for rpAD IV-VI. No differences were detected between AD and rpAD cases ($p < 0.05$). YKL-40 mRNA levels were normalized with GAPDH, and similar results were obtained for GUSB normalization (Additional file 3B). In agreement with mRNA data, YKL-40 expression at protein level was increased in the FC of AD IV-VI (fold change 2.58) and rpAD IV-VI (fold change 2.59) cases ($p < 0.05$) (Fig. 4b).

Moreover, YKL-40 expression was analysed by immunohistochemical staining in several AD brain regions. Increased YKL-40 expression was detected in the cerebral cortex, white matter and subpial layer of AD sections compared to controls, while it remained unchanged in the cerebellum of AD cases (Fig. 4c). Increased expression was also detected in the temporal cortex and throughout the hippocampus region of AD brain sections (Fig. 4d, and Additional file 6A). YKL-40 staining was mainly detected in astrocytes, similarly to the patterns observed in sCJD cases. In contrast with the diffuse distribution of YKL-40-immunoreactive astrocytes in sCJD, YKL-40-positive astrocytes in the cerebral cortex in AD predominated in clusters often surrounding a core of fibrillar β-amyloid (Fig. 4e). YKL-40-positive astrocytes were also present around blood vessels with β-amyloid (Fig. 4e and Additional file 6B). Double-labelling with YKL-40 and β-amyloid antibodies was used to demonstrate the presence of YKL-40 positive astrocytes surrounding senile and diffuse β-amyloid plaques in the hippocampus of AD cases (Fig. 4f and Additional file 7).

Fibrillar astrocytes in the subcortical white matter and deep white matter were also strongly YKL-40 immunoreactive. Specific expression of YKL-40 in GFAP-immunoreactive astrocytes in the cerebral cortex and white matter regions (Fig. 4g) in AD brains was confirmed by double-labelling immunofluorescence and confocal microscopy. Quantitative assessment of double-labelled GFAP and YKL-40 cells indicated a significant superior number of astrocytes showing co-localization of GFAP and YKL-40 (238 ± 23 cells/mm2), compared to those showing only GFAP or only YKL-40 staining (28 ± 6 cells/mm2 and 17 ± 3 cells/mm2, respectively) ($p < 0.001$) (Additional file 5C and D).

As an in vivo model of AD pathogenesis we used the 5xFAD mouse model. At 3 months of age, 5xFAD animals presented glial changes and amyloid plaques but do not show clinical signs or behavioural alterations [53, 54]. At this time point, we found increased YKL-40 and GFAP protein levels ($p < 0.05$) (Additional file 8A). At immunohistochemical level, widespread astrocytic YKL-40 expression was detected in 10-month-old 5xFAD animals, especially in the cerebral cortex and hippocampus (Additional file 8B) as well as in the thalamus, caudate putamen and midbrain, while sparse YKL-40 positive astrocytes could be detected in the molecular layer of cerebellum. At this stage, animals showed clear clinical and behavioural signs.

YKL-40 in DLB

YKL-40 mRNA expression was further analysed in the FC of DLB cases. Despite increased mean values of YKL.40 detected in DLB and rapid forms of DLB (rpDLB) compared to controls, no statistically significant alterations were found between these groups (Fig. 5a). Similarly, no differences at the protein level were detected between control and DLB cases (Fig. 5b). Sparse YKL-40-positive astrocytes were observed in the cortical regions, white matter and subpial layer in DLB cases; sparse clusters of YKL-40-positive astrocytes were not uncommon due to the fact of the associated low burden of AD-related pathology in DLB (Fig. 5c).

CSF YKL-40 in the differential diagnosis of neurodegenerative dementias

When CSF YKL-40 was analysed in the differential diagnostic context of neurodegenerative dementias (cohort 1, Additional file 2), significantly higher YKL-40 levels were detected in sCJD cases (480 ± 178 pg/mL) compared to neurological controls (NC) (250 ± 77 pg/mL) and to the other dementia groups ($p < 0.001$) (Fig. 6a, Additional file 2). Compared to NC, YKL-40 was also increased in AD patients (386 ± 221 pg/mL, $p < 0.001$) but not in VaD (323 ± 96 pg/mL, $p > 0.05$) and DLB/

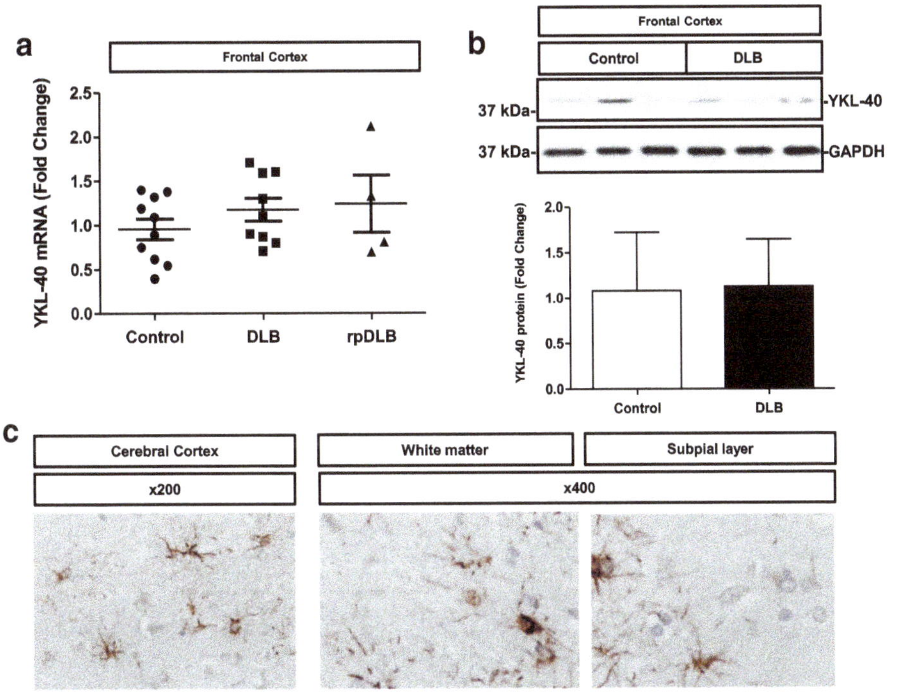

Fig. 5 YKL-40 expression in DLB brain tissue. **a** RT-qPCR analysis of YKL-40 in the frontal cortex of control, DLB and rpDLB samples. Normalization was based on GAPDH levels. **b** Western blot analysis of YKL-40 in the frontal cortex of control, DLB and rpDLB samples. Normalization was carried out with GAPDH. Kruskal-Wallis and Dunn's post-hoc tests were used for determination of statistical differences. **c** Immunohistochemical analysis of YKL-40 in the cerebral cortex, white matter and subpial layer in DLB cases. Brown staining corresponds to YKL-40 staining and light blue to haematoxylin counterstaining. Fold changes in expression (mRNA and protein) were determined relative to the control cases

PDD cases (314 ± 103 pg/mL, $p > 0.05$). To calculate the clinical accuracy of YKL-40 in discriminating between dementia and NC groups, we estimated the AUC values. As expected, the highest values were detected when comparing NC and sCJD cases (AUC: 0.92, 95% CI: 0.87–0.96) (Fig. 6b). Using an optimal cut-off at 315 pg/mL defined by the *Youden* index, an overall sensitivity of 85% and specificity of 84% could be achieved. For the rest of the dementias AUC values were far below those detected for sCJD cases: NC vs AD; AUC: 0.77, 95% CI: 0.68–0.84, NC vs VaD; AUC: 0.71, 95% CI: 0.60–0.84 and NC vs DLB: AUC: 0.70, 95% CI: 0.60–0.80 (Fig. 6b). Next we explored the ability of CSF YKL-40 to discriminate sCJD from the rest of dementia groups. While YKL-40 could not discriminate sCJD from AD with high accuracy (AUC: 0.70, 95% CI: 0.62–0.78), values were higher for sCJD vs DLB/PDD (AUC: 0.81, 95% CI: 0.72–0.89) and sCJD vs VaD (AUC: 0.77, 95% CI: 0.67–0.88) comparisons.

Further we analysed whether YKL-40 levels could be influenced by the rate of cognitive decline and/or disease duration. For this reason, we stratified AD cases into slow and fast progressive AD (AD versus rpAD) and sCJD samples according to codon 129*PRNP* polymorphism, which plays a role in the clinico-pathological phenotype of the disease and, as a consequence, in disease duration [43, 63, 64]. No differences in CSF YKL-40 levels were observed between AD (387 ± 244 pg/mL) and rpAD (384 ± 128 pg/mL) cases or between sCJD cases according to their codon 129 polymorphism: sCJD MM (462 ± 195 pg/mL), MV (519 ± 203 pg/mL) and VV (456 ± 79 pg/mL) (Fig. 6c, d).

Next we sought to investigate the potential correlation between YKL-40 and tau, disease duration and age in sCJD cases. A significant positive correlation of YKL-40 with CSF tau was found ($p < 0.05$) (Fig. 7a), but no correlation of YKL-40 levels with CSF Aβ42, disease duration and age at disease onset was detected ($p > 0.05$) (Fig. 7b and c).

Validation of increased YKL-40 levels in the CSF of prion diseases

In order to validate the presence of increased YKL-40 levels in sCJD, two independent cohorts were used. The first validation cohort (cohort 2, Additional file 2) included healthy controls (HC), AD and sCJD cases. Compared to HC (226 ± 82 pg/mL), YKL-40 levels were significantly increased in sCJD (411 ± 157 pg/mL, $p < 0.001$) and AD (311 ± 113 pg/mL, $p < 0.01$) (Fig. 8a, cohort 2 Additional file 2). Similar results were obtained for the second validation cohort (cohort 3, Additional file 2), where YKL-40 levels in sCJD were significantly higher (603 ± 198 pg/mL) than those detected in cognitive impairment/dementia cases (358 ± 129 pg/mL,

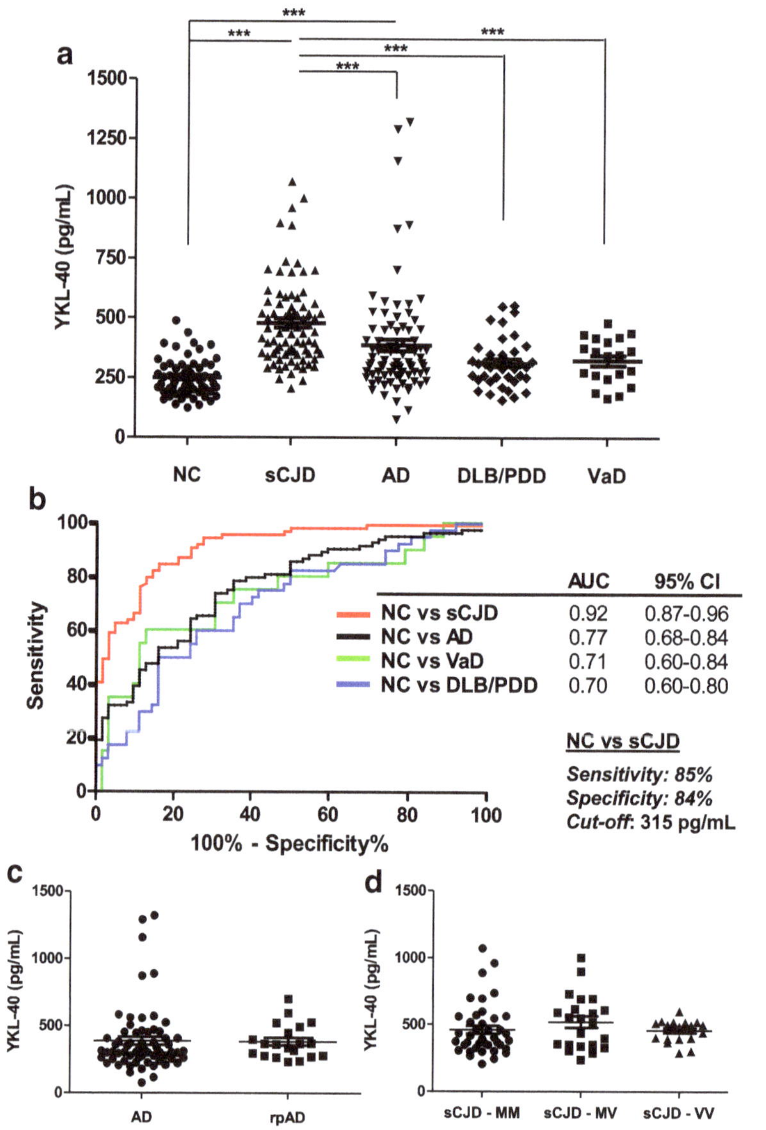

Fig. 6 CSF YKL-40 in the differential diagnosis of neurodegenerative dementia. **a** CSF YKL-40 in NC (n = 62), sCJD (n = 84), AD (n = 84), DLB/PDD (n = 40) and VaD (n = 20) cases (cohort 1). Number of cases analyzed and statistical significance of differences between groups is indicated. Kruskal-Wallis and Dunn's post-hoc tests were used for estimation of statistical differences. **b** ROC curves for YKL-40 quantification in the differential diagnosis of dementia groups compared to NC. In the legend, AUC values, corresponding to the area under ROC curves, and 95% confidence intervals are reported. Diagnostic parameters (cut-off, sensitivity and specificity) are indicated for NC versus sCJD comparison. **c** Stratification of AD cases in slow progressive (AD) (n = 64) and rapid progressive (rpAD) (n = 20) cases. Statistical differences were tested with Mann–Whitney test. **d** Stratification of sCJD cases according to *PRNP* codon 129 polymorphism (MM, n = 40, MV, n = 22 and VV, n = 20). Kruskal-Wallis and Dunn's post-hoc tests were used for statistical differences estimation. ***$p < 0.001$

$p < 0.01$) (Fig. 8b, cohort 3 Additional file 2). Finally, we aimed to determine the usefulness of CSF YKL-40 levels in the discrimination of prion disease from genetic etiology. For this purpose, we analysed genetic cases from two cohorts and compared them with their respective controls and sCJD groups. The study included Controls, sCJD, gCJD *PRNP*-E200K and Fatal Familial Insomnia (FFI) (*PRNP*-D178N mutation) cases (cohort 1 and cohort 2, Additional file 2). In both cohorts gCJD cases harbouring the E200K mutation showed similar YKL-40 levels compared to sCJD cases and were statistically different from controls ($p < 0.001$). In contrast, YKL-40 levels in FFI cases were lower than in sCJD cases, but significantly higher compared to control subjects ($p < 0.05$) (Fig. 9a and b and cohort 1 and cohort 2, Additional file 2).

Discussion

Neuroinflammation in dementia has been identified as a major contributor to disease pathogenesis and as a

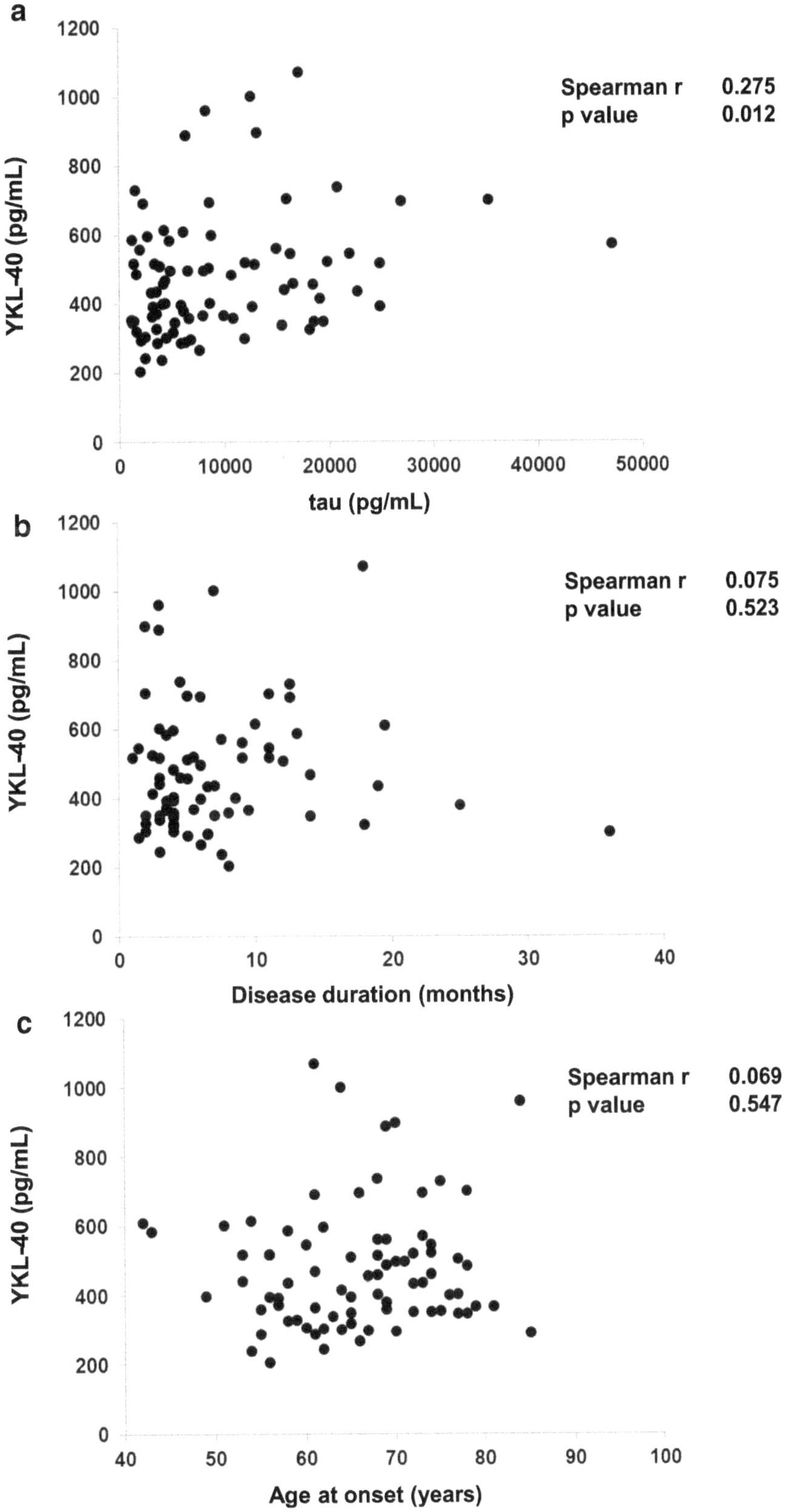

Fig. 7 (See legend on next page.)

(See figure on previous page.)

Fig. 7 Correlation of CSF YKL-40 levels with CSF tau levels, disease duration and age at onset. Correlation analysis between CSF YKL-40 and (**a**) CSF tau levels, (**b**) disease duration (as time in months from disease onset to death) and (**c**) age at onset. The association between CSF YKL-40 and either biomarkers or demographics parameters was investigated with the Spearman correlation. Positive correlation was detected only for CSF YKL-40 versus CSF tau comparison

potentially causative effect of neurodegeneration in chronic profiles [65–67]. However, the precise regional and temporal contribution of glial activation to the pathogenic process is far from understood. Similar to microglial activation, sustained astrocytic activation may lead to a switch from a neuroprotective and neurotrophic to a neurodegenerative phenotype, increasing neuronal vulnerability to chemokines, pro-inflammatory cytokines and reactive oxygen species [68–70]. This is exemplified by proteins such as S100B, which is released from astrocytes with neurotrophic or neurotoxic effects on neurons depending on their concentration and on the astrocytic activation state [71, 72]. In turn, increased expression and secretion of S100B from astrocytes may be reflected in the CSF patterns as reported in traumatic brain injury [73], AD [74, 75] and sCJD [76]. Consequently, astrocytes are turning into a potential target for therapeutic intervention in neurodegenerative diseases associated with an inflammatory component [77], indicating that astrocyte-associated metabolites may be potential biomarkers in biological fluids. Thus, studies on expression patterns and function of secreted, astrocytic-

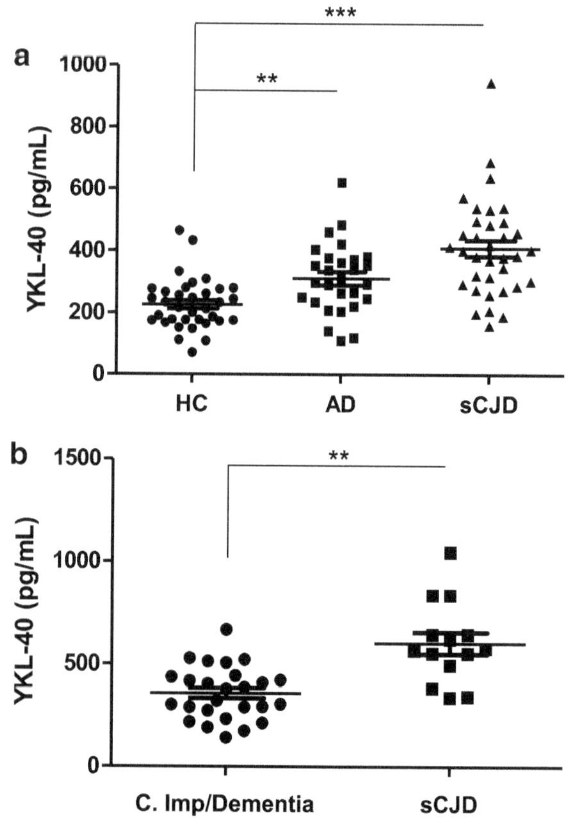

Fig. 8 Independent validation of increased CSF YKL-40 level in sCJD patients. **a** CSF YKL-40 levels in HC (n = 35), AD (n = 28) and sCJD (n = 35) cases (cohort 2). Kruskal-Wallis and Dunn's post-hoc tests were used for statistical differences estimation. **b** CSF YKL-40 levels in Cognitive Impairment/Dementia (n = 26) and sCJD cases (n = 14) (cohort 3). Statistical differences were estimated with the Mann–Whitney test.$^{**}p < 0.01$, $^{***}p < 0.001$

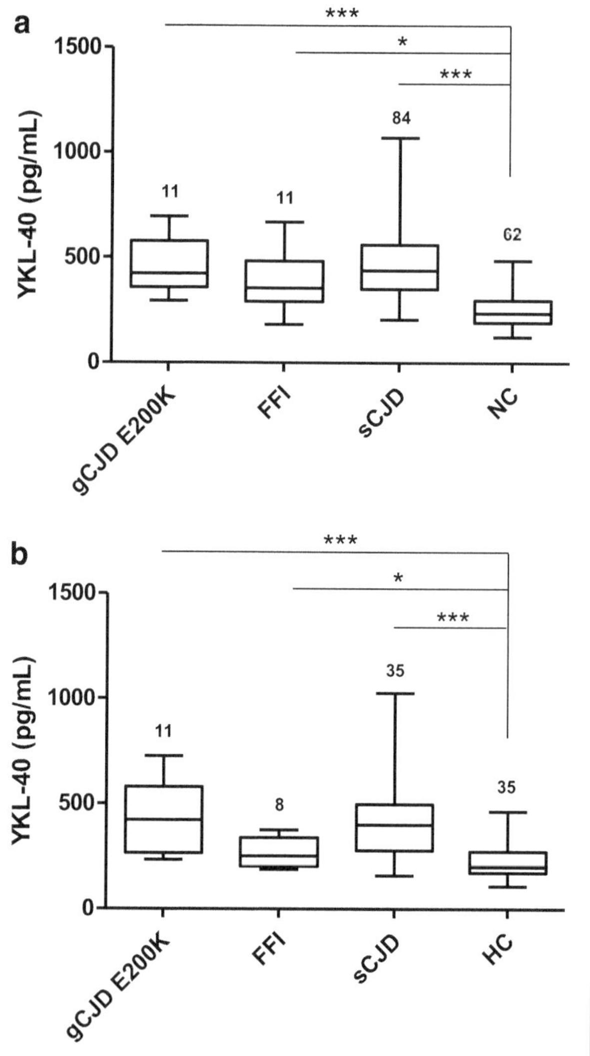

Fig. 9 Detection of CSF YKL-40 levels in gCJD E200K and Fatal Familial Insomnia. **a** CSF YKL-40 levels in gCJD E200K, Fatal Familial Insomnia (FFI) and NC (cohort 1). **b** CSF YKL-40 levels in gCJD E200K, Fatal Familial Insomnia (FFI) and HC (cohort 2). Statistical differences were determined with Kruskal-Wallis and Dunn's post-hoc tests. $^{*}p < 0.05$, $^{***}p < 0.001$

related molecules under pathological or stress conditions are gaining experimental momentum.

The functional role of YKL-40 during neuroinflammation is unclear. However, a neuroprotective effect has been assigned to YKL-40 by an in vivo study, according to which YKL-40 knock-out mice presented more severe neuropathology and more prominent gliosis than their wild-type littermates in a model of controlled cortical impact [78]. These results indicated that YKL-40 modulates the neuroinflammatory response associated with traumatic brain impact (TBI). In agreement with this, YKL-40 knock-out mice present exacerbated experimental autoimmune encephalomyelitis clinical scores accompanied by increased lymphocytic and macrophage infiltrates and gliosis compared to wild-type animals [79], suggesting that YKL-40 is necessary for the proper resolution of inflammation. Importantly, astrocytic YKL-40 expression is under the control of microglial stimuli since YKL-40 transcription, accompanied by morphological changes and increased migratory capacity characteristic of reactive gliosis, is induced by the macrophage-released pro-inflammatory mediators Interleukin-1β (IL-1β) and tumor necrosis factor-α [22]. Interestingly, both cytokines are highly expressed in the microglia of TBI, sCJD, AD and related mouse models [40, 41, 80], suggesting a cross-talk between microglial and astrocytic activation in the regulation of YKL-40-mediated functions in chronic inflammatory profiles associated with neurodegeneration. These data are supported by the finding that YKL-40 expression correlates with the expression of IL-1β and Interleukin-6 and that both cytokines are able to synergistically up-regulate YKL-40 expression in primary astrocytes in vitro in a STAT3 dependent-manner [81], which in turn, has been seen to be activated in the FC of sCJD brains [40]. In this regard, it has been recently shown that a subtype of reactive astrocytes present in neurodegenerative diseases is induced by secreted cytokines from activated microglia [82], reinforcing the suggested role of astrocyte-microglia cross-talk during neurodegeneration [83, 84].

Aiming at a better characterization of YKL-40's role in neurodegenerative disorders, we studied its mRNA and protein levels and its expression in different brain regions in several neurodegenerative conditions. Astrocytic YKL-40 overexpression was prominent in both sCJD and AD, in agreement with the well-known chronic inflammatory profile of both diseases [38]. Most of the YKL-40+ astrocytes were stained with GFAP antibodies, both in sCJD and AD. However, a small population of astrocytes with single labelling for one of the two markers was also detected, in agreement with the positive but moderate correlation between GFAP and YKL-40 expression levels detected in sCJD.

Further, the absence of YKL-40 overexpression in DLB was in line with the corresponding low inflammatory profile in DLB [42, 85]. Disease-specific differences were not restricted to expression levels, but also included regional-dependent regulation. Indeed, we demonstrated that YKL-40 overexpression in the cerebellum is restricted to sCJD and absent in AD.

Data obtained from prion models suggest a role of YKL-40 at pre-clinical and early stages of the disease. In RML infected mice, early prion pathology including microglia activation, astrogliosis and PrPSc deposition could be first detected in the thalamus, whereas hippocampus and cortex still remain unchanged at the microscopic level. At clinical disease stages, hippocampus and cerebellum show widespread signs of prion pathology. This is in line with our detection of YKL-40 immunoreactivity in RML infected mice, which was abundant in the thalamus only at preclinical time points, but was more widespread, including hippocampus, at clinical prion disease stages. This is supported by the elevated levels of YKL-40 in cortical region of the sCJD model at pre-clinical disease stage.

Incorporation of new CSF biomarkers in clinical practice not only improves current diagnostic approaches across the disease continuum, but also provides new tools for prognosis and evaluation of therapeutic efficacy once disease-modifying treatments become available [86–88]. Therefore, peripheral biomarkers mirroring specific disease hallmarks such as neuronal/synaptic damage, neuroinflammation and the presence of misfolded proteins will become useful to evaluate therapeutic approaches. In this regard, we demonstrated that CSF YKL-40 patterns resemble expression levels in brain tissue in a disease-specific manner. Additionally, we detected elevated YKL-40 in the brain of early AD (Braak stages I-III). Although data regarding elevated CSF YKL-40 in early stages of AD are contradictory [24, 25, 89, 90], our results support the presence of increased astrocytic YKL-40 expression, together with a role of astrocytosis, in early AD pathogenesis [91]. Similarly, we detected increased YKL-40 in the brain of an AD mouse model and in experimental models of prion diseases at pre-clinical stages, supporting the presence of astrocytic alterations before clinical onset and the usefulness of YKL-40 quantification in the detection of early pathological changes associated with neuroinflammation. Interestingly increase in YKL-40 at pre-clinical stages (120 dpi) of the sCJD mice model occurs when PrPres, but not synaptic damage, is already detectable [92] [Llorens et al. 2017, submitted], supporting the hypothesis that neuroinflammation may precede neuronal dysfunction.

Additionally, it has recently been shown that in MCI and pre-AD stages, APOE ε4 carriers display higher CSF levels of YKL-40 but not of a marker of microglial activation, sTREM2 (soluble triggering receptor expressed on myeloid cells 2), supporting a role of APOE ε4 in the regulation of astroglial response in AD pathology [93]. However, CSF from pre-sCJD stages is not available to rule out a potential role of CSF YKL-40 as pre-clinical marker of prion diseases. In this regard, use of in vivo prion models not only validates regional alterations observed in human tissue, but also supports utilization of humanized sCJD mouse models in the understanding of human pathogenesis at pre-clinical disease stages, since scrapie infected animals present strain-specific regional alterations that differ from those detected in human and mouse sCJD samples.

An interesting finding of our study is the detection of increased CSF YKL-40 levels in FFI, supporting the idea that astrogliosis is a common hallmark in FFI brain tissue even in regions with no major pathological involvement [94, 95]. In contrast, CSF surrogate markers of neuronal damage are less sensitive in detecting FFI cases [44, 96] as neuronal damage is restricted to thalamic nuclei. Elevated YKL-40 levels in gCJD-E200K patients were in line with the similar diagnostic parameters between sCJD and gCJD-E200K for other prion biomarkers [44, 96], due to the common clinico-pathological spectrum of gCJD-E200K and sCJD cases [97, 98]. Despite high CSF YKL-40 levels were found in sCJD and AD, increased YKL-40 levels have also been detected in other neurological and psychiatric conditions such as brain concussions [99], acute ischemic stroke [100], suicidal ideation [101] and bipolar disorder [102], underlining that astrocytic activation is not restricted to neurodegenerative conditions and that neuroinflammation may play a more prominent and common role in the etiology of neurological diseases.

Conflicting data have been reported on the correlation of YKL-40 with markers of neurodegeneration [23, 25, 31, 32, 89] as well as with cognitive decline [28, 31, 36, 89]. The distinct correlations between different surrogate disease markers and cognitive decline suggest that dementia hallmarks may reflect different aspects of neurodegeneration processes which, although potentially associated, may provide independent information about the pathological state of the brain tissue. In this regard, it has been proven that, in early AD, CSF YKL-40 is associated with a cerebral structural signature distinct from that related to p-tau neurodegeneration [28], even when a positive correlation between the levels of the two biomarkers in the CSF is reported [23–25, 34].

For sCJD, the positive correlation between CSF tau and YKL-40 suggests an association between axonal damage and neuroinflammation. Indeed, it is well known that inflammatory patterns in sCJD correlate with the severity of the neuropathological lesions [103]. In contrast, no correlation was detected between age and disease duration, most likely due to the very short disease duration of sCJD cases (mean disease duration = 7.0 ± 5.9 months).

Conclusions

Here we report, for the first time, that higher YKL-40 levels are detectable in the brain and CSF in prion diseases. Further we show that CSF YKL-40 presents a good diagnostic accuracy in the discrimination of sCJD from NC. While YKL-40 is also elevated in AD, it failed discriminating AD, VaD and DLB/PDD cases (AUC < 0.8). In this regard, caution should be taken when interpreting elevated CSF YKL-40 levels in the diagnostic context of neurodegenerative dementias. However, since CSF YKL-40 resembles astrocytic activation in brain tissue we speculate that YKL-40 quantification may be useful for the assessment of neuroinflammatory profiles during therapeutic intervention.

Additional files

Additional file 1: Summary of human brain cases and regions analyzed with qPCR, western blot and immunohistochemical analysis. Number of cases, age (mean ± SD) and gender (number of females and males) are indicated.

Additional file 2: Summary of CSF samples from the three independent cohorts used in this study. Sample group, number of cases, age (mean ± SD), tau levels (pg/mL), Aβ42 levels (pg/mL), 14-3-3 positive cases and YKL-40 levels (pg/mL) are indicated.

Additional file 3: YKL-40 mRNA expression in sCJD and AD using GUSB as housekeeping gene. Validation of alterations in YKL-40 mRNA in sCJD (A) and AD (B) cases using GUSB as qPCR housekeeping gene. (TIFF 59 kb)

Additional file 4: YKL-40-positive astrocytes associated to PrP amyloid plaques. Immunofluorescence images obtained from double-labeling staining with GFAP (A) and YKL-40 (B) (green) and PrP (red) antibodies in the cortex of sCJD. Individual channels as well as merge images are shown for two different cortical areas.

Additional file 5: Quantification of YKL-40 and GFAP overlap in sCJD and AD cases. Immunofluorescence images obtained from double-labelling staining with GFAP (red) and YKL-40 (green) antibodies in the hippocampus of sCJD (n = 3) (A) and AD V (n = 3) (C) cases. Individual channels as well as merge images are shown for two different cortical areas (one cortical image per CJD or AD patient) of two different patients. Quantifications of GFAP +/YKL-40+ (YKL-40-GFAP), GFAP+/YKL-40- (GFAP) and GFAP−/YKL-40+ (YKL-40) astrocytes are shown. Statistical significance differences were detected between YKL-40-GFAP and YKL-40, GFAP groups; ###p < 0.001 and ***p < 0.001, respectively.

Additional file 6: YKL-40 expression in AD. (A) YKL-40 expression in astrocytes in the dentate gyrus of AD. (B) Immunohistochemical analysis of YKL-40+ astrocytes surrounding β-amyloid plaques in AD cases. (TIFF 989 kb)

Additional file 7: YKL-40 positive astrocytes associated to β-amyloid plaques. Confocal Z-stack images obtained from double-labelling staining with YKL-40 (green) and β-amyloid (red) antibodies in the hippocampus of AD tissue. Z-stacks from representative senile β-amyloid plaque (A) and diffuse amyloid plaque (B) is shown. DRAQ5 staining is shown in blue. Individual channels as well as merge images are shown. Distance between-Z Stacks sections = 0.5 μm.

Additional file 8: YKL-40 expression in 5xFAD mice. (A) Western blot analysis of YKL-40 and GFAP in the cortex of 3-month-old control and 5xFAD animals. Four animals per group were analyzed. GAPDH was used for normalization. Numbers represent the summary of densitometric analysis. Unpaired t-test was used for statistical differences estimation. (B) Immunofluorescence analysis of YKL-40 (green) in the cerebellar cortex and hippocampus of 10-month-old 5xFAD mice. Nuclei were stained with DAPI (blue). Three animals per group and three sections per animal were analyzed.

Acknowledgements

The authors thank Kristin Hartmann (Core facility mouse pathology/UKE) and Dr. Thomas Meyer (Department of Psychosomatic Medicine/UMG) for assistance on animal experimentation and Silja Koechy and Nadine Gotzmann (UMG/DZNE) for technical assistance. We also thank Benjamín Torrejón Escribano (CCiT-UB) for the technical support. We are indebted to the Neurological Tissue Bank of the Biobanc-Hospital Clinic-IDIBAPS for sample procurement.

Funding

This study was funded by Robert Koch Institute through funds from the Federal Ministry of Health of Germany (grant no. 1369–341) to IZ, by CIBERNED (Network Center for Biomedical Research of Neurodegenerative Diseases) project BESAD-P to IF, by the Spanish Ministry of Health - Instituto Carlos III/ Fondo Social Europeo (CP16/00041) to FL, by the Red Nacional de Priones (AGL2015–71764-REDT- MINECO) to FL, IZ, JMT, RSV and IF and by the IKYDA project (ID 57260006) to FL, IZ and TS.

Author's contributions

Study conception and design: FL, IF, IZ. Project supervision: FL. Data collection: FL, KT, WT, KX, EK, EKo, CP, DD-L, MS, DO, SC, AC, PG-E, IM, OA, NFB, IMV, MG, TS, JMT, SK, RSV, IF, IZ. Data analysis and interpretation: FL, KT, WT, MG, SK, IF, IZ. Drafting the article: FL, IF. Final approval of the version to be published: All authors.

Ethics approval and consent to participate

The present study was conducted according to the revised Declaration of Helsinki and Good Clinical Practice guidelines and was approved by the local ethics committees. Informed consent was given by all study participants or their legal representative. For animal investigation, principles of laboratory animal care (NIH publication No. 86–23, revised 1985) were followed. All animal experiments were performed in compliance with the French, German and Greek national guidelines, in accordance with the European Community Council Directive 86/609/EEC and approved by local ethics committees. The experimental protocols were approved by the INRA Toulouse/ENVT ethics committee, the Ethical Committee of the Freie und Hansestadt Hamburg, Amt für Gesundheit und Verbraucherschutz (Permit number: G 21307/591–00.33) and the AHEPA University Hospital local veterinary authorities (21/12/2015).

Competing interests

The authors declare that they have no competing interests.

Author details

[1]Network Center for Biomedical Research in Neurodegenerative Diseases (CIBERNED), Institute Carlos III, Ministry of Health, Feixa Llarga s/n, 08907 L'Hospitalet de Llobregat, Barcelona, Spain. [2]Department of Neurology, University Medical School, Göttingen, Germany. [3]German Center for Neurodegenerative Diseases (DZNE), Göttingen, Germany. [4]Laboratory of Pharmacology, School of Health Sciences, Department of Pharmacy, Aristotle University of Thessaloniki, Thessaloniki, Greece. [5]German Center for Neurodegenerative Diseases (DZNE), Bonn, Germany. [6]Bellvitge University Hospital-IDIBELL, Department of Pathology and Experimental Therapeutics, University of Barcelona, Hospitalet de Llobregat, Spain. [7]European Neuroscience Institute, Göttingen, Germany. [8]Institut National de la Recherche Agronomique/Ecole Nationale Vétérinaire, Toulouse, France. [9]Centro de Investigación en Sanidad Animal (CISA-INIA), Madrid, Spain. [10]Institute of Neuropathology, University Medical Center Hamburg-Eppendorf, Hamburg, Germany. [11]Alzheimer's Disease and Other Cognitive Disorders Unit, Neurology Department, Hospital Clínic, Institut d'Investigacions Biomediques August Pi i Sunyer (IDIBAPS), Barcelona, Spain. [12]Present address: Unit of Lymphoid Malignancies, Division of Experimental Oncology, San Raffaele Scientific Institute, Milan, Italy.

References

1. Kazakova MH, Sarafian VS. YKL-40–a novel biomarker in clinical practice? Folia Med. 2009;51:5–14.
2. Renkema GH, Boot RG, Au FL, Donker-Koopman WE, Strijland A, Muijsers AO, et al. Chitotriosidase a chitinase, and the 39-kDa human cartilage glycoprotein, a chitin-binding lectin, are homologues of family 18 glycosyl hydrolases secreted by human macrophages. Eur J Biochem. 1998;251:504–9.
3. Schultz NA, Johansen JS. YKL-40-a protein in the field of translational medicine: A role as a biomarker in cancer patients? Cancers (Basel). 2010;2:1453–91.
4. Shao R. YKL-40 acts as an angiogenic factor to promote tumor angiogenesis. Front. Physiol. 2013;4:122.
5. Ringsholt M, Høgdall EVS, Johansen JS, Price PA, Christensen LH. YKL-40 protein expression in normal adult human tissues – an immunohistochemical study. J Mol Histol [Internet] 2007;38:33–43. Available from: https://www.ncbi.nlm.nih.gov/pubmed/17242979, http://link.springer.com/10.1007/s10735-006-9075-0
6. Shao R, Hamel K, Petersen L, Cao QJ, Arenas RB, Bigelow C, et al. YKL-40, a secreted glycoprotein, promotes tumor angiogenesis. Oncogene. 2009;28: 4456–68. Available from: http://www.pubmedcentral.nih.gov/articlerender.fcgi?artid=2795793&tool=pmcentrez&rendertype=abstract
7. Rathcke CN, Vestergaard H. YKL-40-an emerging biomarker in cardiovascular disease and diabetes. Cardiovasc Diabetol. 2009;8:7.
8. Rehli M, Niller HH, Ammon C, Langmann S, Schwarzfischer L, Andreesen R, et al. Transcriptional regulation of CHI3L1, a marker gene for late stages of macrophage differentiation. J Biol Chem. 2003;278:44058–67.
9. Rehli M, Krause SW, Andreesen R. Molecular characterization of the gene for human cartilage gp-39 (CHI3L1), a member of the chitinase protein family and marker for late stages of macrophage differentiation. Genomics. 1997;43:221–5.
10. Qin G, Li X, Chen Z, Liao G, Su Y, Chen Y, et al. Prognostic value of YKL-40 in patients with Glioblastoma: a systematic review and meta-analysis. Mol Neurobiol. 2017;54:3264-70.
11. Francescone RA, Scully S, Faibish M, Taylor SL, Oh D, Moral L, et al. Role of YKL-40 in the angiogenesis, radioresistance, and progression of glioblastoma. J Biol Chem. 2011;286:15332–43.
12. Xiang W, Menges S, Schlachetzki JC, Meixner H, Hoffmann A-C, Schlötzer-Schrehardt U, et al. Posttranslational modification and mutation of histidine 50 trigger alpha synuclein aggregation and toxicity. Mol. Neurodegener. 2015;10:8.[cited 2015 Aug 18]; Available from: http://www.molecularneurodegeneration.com/content/10/1/8
13. Johansen JS. Studies on serum YKL-40 as a biomarker in diseases with inflammation, tissue remodelling, fibroses and cancer. Dan Med Bull. 2006; 53:172–209.
14. Michelsen AE, Rathcke CN, Skjelland M, Holm S, Ranheim T, Krohg-Sorensen K, et al. Increased YKL-40 expression in patients with carotid atherosclerosis. Atherosclerosis. 2010;211:589–95. Available from: http://ac.els-cdn.com/S0021915010001760/1-s2.0-S0021915010001760-main.pdf?_tid=8d09dab4-77fd-11e5-a89a-00000aab0f01&acdnat=1445436838_1a64d9b28138f5981ecf641d6062a3d0
15. Bonneh-Barkay D, Bissel SJ, Wang G, Fish KN, Nicholl GCB, Darko SW, et al. YKL-40, a marker of simian immunodeficiency virus encephalitis, modulates the biological activity of basic fibroblast growth factor. Am J Pathol 2008; 173:130–43. Available from: http://www.pubmedcentral.nih.gov/articlerender.fcgi?artid=2438291&tool=pmcentrez&rendertype=abstract.
16. Bonneh-Barkay D, Wang G, Starkey A, Hamilton RL, Wiley CA. In vivo CHI3L1 (YKL-40) expression in astrocytes in acute and chronic neurological diseases.J. Neuroinflammation. 2010;7:34. Available from: http://www.pubmedcentral.nih.gov/articlerender.fcgi?artid=2892443&tool=pmcentrez&rendertype=abstract.
17. Bonneh-Barkay D, Zagadailov P, Zou H, Niyonkuru C, Figley M, Starkey A, et al. YKL-40 expression in traumatic brain injury: an initial analysis. J Neurotrauma [Internet]. 2010;27:1215–23. Available from: http://www.pubmedcentral.nih.gov/articlerender.fcgi?artid=2942903&tool=pmcentrez&rendertype=abstract.

18. Comabella M, Fernández M, Martin R, Rivera-Vallvé S, Borrás E, Chiva C, et al. Cerebrospinal fluid chitinase 3-like 1 levels are associated with conversion to multiple sclerosis. Brain. 2010;133:1082–93.
19. Johansen JS, Baslund B, Garbarsch C, Hansen M, Stoltenberg M, Lorenzen I, et al. YKL-40 in giant cells and macrophages from patients with giant cell arteritis. Arthritis Rheum [Internet]. 1999;42:2624–30. Available from: https://www.ncbi.nlm.nih.gov/pubmed/10616010.
20. Junker N, Johansen JS, Andersen CB, Kristjansen PE. Expression of YKL-40 by peritumoral macrophages in human small cell lung cancer. Lung Cancer [Internet]. 2005;48:223–31. Available from: http://www.ncbi.nlm.nih.gov/entrez/query.fcgi?cmd=Retrieve&db=PubMed&dopt=Citation&list_uids=15829322.
21. Létuvé S, Kozhich A, Arouche N, Grandsaigne M, Reed J, Dombret M, et al. YKL-40 is elevated in patients with chronic obstructive pulmonary disease and activates alveolar macrophages. J Immunol. 2008;181:5167–73.
22. Bonneh-Barkay D, Bissel SJ, Kofler J, Starkey A, Wang G, Wiley CA. Astrocyte and macrophage regulation of YKL-40 expression and cellular response in neuroinflammation. Brain Pathol. 2012;22:530–46.
23. Craig-Schapiro R, Perrin RJ, Roe CM, Xiong C, Carter D, Cairns NJ, et al. YKL-40: a novel prognostic fluid biomarker for preclinical Alzheimer's disease. Biol Psychiatry. 2010;68:903–12.
24. Olsson B, Hertze J, Lautner R, Zetterberg H, Nägga K, Höglund K, et al. Microglial markers are elevated in the prodromal phase of Alzheimer's disease and vascular dementia. J Alzheimers Dis. 2013;33:45–53.
25. Antonell A, Mansilla A, Rami L, Lladó A, Iranzo A, Olives J, et al. Cerebrospinal fluid level of YKL-40 protein in preclinical and prodromal Alzheimer's disease. J Alzheimers Dis. 2014;42:901–8.
26. Kester MI, Teunissen CE, Sutphen C, Herries EM, Ladenson JH, Xiong CJ, et al. Cerebrospinal fluid VILIP-1 and YKL-40, candidate biomarkers to diagnose, predict and monitor Alzheimer's disease in a memory clinic cohort. Alzheimers Res Ther. 2015;7:9.
27. Verkhratsky A, Olabarria M, Noristani HN, Yeh CY, Rodriguez JJ. Astrocytes in Alzheimer's disease. Neurotherapeutics. 2010;7:399–412.
28. Gispert JD, Monté GC, Falcon C, Tucholka A, Rojas S, Sánchez-Valle R, et al. CSF YKL-40 and pTau181 are related to different cerebral morphometric patterns in early AD. Neurobiol Aging. 2016;38:47–55.
29. Perrin RJ, Craig-Schapiro R, Malone JP, Shah AR, Gilmore P, Davis AE, et al. Identification and validation of novel cerebrospinal fluid biomarkers for staging early Alzheimer's disease. PLoS One. 2011;6:e16032.
30. Wildsmith KR, Schauer SP, Smith AM, Arnott D, Zhu Y, Haznedar J, et al. Identification of longitudinally dynamic biomarkers in Alzheimer's disease cerebrospinal fluid by targeted proteomics. Mol. Neurodegener. 2014;9:22. Available from: http://www.ncbi.nlm.nih.gov/pubmed/24902845%5Cn, http://www.pubmedcentral.nih.gov/articlerender.fcgi?artid=PMC4061120.
31. Rosen C, Andersson CH, Andreasson U, Molinuevo JL, Bjerke M, Rami L, et al. Increased Levels of Chitotriosidase and YKL-40 in Cerebrospinal Fluid from Patients with Alzheimer's Disease. Dement Geriatr Cogn Dis Extra. 2014;4:297–304. Available from: http://www.ncbi.nlm.nih.gov/pmc/articles/PMC4164083/pdf/dee-0004-0297.pdf.
32. Wennström M, Surova Y, Hall S, Nilsson C, Minthon L, Hansson O, et al. The inflammatory marker YKL-40 is elevated in cerebrospinal fluid from patients with Alzheimer's but not Parkinson's disease or dementia with Lewy bodies. PLoS One. 2015;10:e0135458.
33. Paterson RW, Heywood WE, Heslegrave AJ, Magdalinou NK, Andreasson U, Sirka E, et al. A targeted proteomic multiplex CSF assay identifies increased malate dehydrogenase and other neurodegenerative biomarkers in individuals with Alzheimer's disease pathology. Transl. Psychiatry. 2016;6:e952. Available from: http://www.nature.com/doifinder/10.1038/tp.2016.194.
34. Alcolea D, Carmona-Iragui M, Suarez-Calvet M, Sanchez-Saudinos MB, Sala I, Anton-Aguirre S, et al. Relationship between beta-Secretase, inflammation and core cerebrospinal fluid biomarkers for Alzheimer's disease. J Alzheimers Dis. 2014;42:157–67. Available from: http://content.iospress.com/articles/journal-of-alzheimers-disease/jad140240.
35. Janelidze S, Hertze J, Zetterberg H, Landqvist Waldo M, Santillo A, Blennow K, et al. Cerebrospinal fluid neurogranin and YKL-40 as biomarkers of Alzheimer's disease. Ann. Clin. Transl. Neurol. 2015;3 Available from: http://doi.wiley.com/10.1002/acn3.266.
36. Teunissen CE, Elias N, Koel-Simmelink MJA, Durieux-Lu S, Malekzadeh A, Pham TV, et al. Novel diagnostic cerebrospinal fluid biomarkers for pathologic subtypes of frontotemporal dementia identified by proteomics. Alzheimer's Dement. 2016;2:86–94.
37. Baldacci F, Toschi N, Lista S, Zetterberg H, Blennow K, Kilimann I, et al. Two-level diagnostic classification using cerebrospinal fluid YKL-40 in Alzheimer's disease. Alzheimers. Dement. 2017:1–11. Available from: http://www.alzheimersanddementia.com/article/S1552-5260(17)30047-X/abstract. http://www.ncbi.nlm.nih.gov/pubmed/28263742.
38. López González I, Garcia-Esparcia P, Llorens F, Ferrer I. Genetic and transcriptomic profiles of inflammation in neurodegenerative diseases: Alzheimer, Parkinson, Creutzfeldt-Jakob and Tauopathies. Int J Mol Sci. 2016;17:1–23.
39. Llorens F, Ansoleaga B, Garcia-Esparcia P, Zafar S, Grau-Rivera O, López-González I, et al. PrP mRNA and protein expression in brain and PrP(c) in CSF in Creutzfeldt-Jakob disease MM1 and VV2. Prion. 2013;7:383–93. Available from: http://www.tandfonline.com/doi/abs/10.4161/pri.26416.
40. Llorens F, Lopez-Gonzalez I, Thune K, Carmona M, Zafar S, Andeoletti O, et al. Subtype and regional-specific neuroinflammation in sporadic creutzfeldt-jakob disease. Front Aging Neurosci. 2014;6:198.
41. Lopez-Gonzalez I, Schluter A, Aso E, Garcia-Esparcia P, Ansoleaga B, LL F, et al. Neuroinflammatory signals in Alzheimer disease and APP/PS1 transgenic mice: correlations with plaques, tangles, and Oligomeric species. J Neuropathol Exp Neurol. 2015;74:319–44. Available from: http://www.ncbi.nlm.nih.gov/pubmed/25756590.
42. Garcia-Esparcia P, López-González I, Grau-Rivera O, García-Garrido MF, Konetti A, Llorens F, et al. Dementia with Lewy Bodies: Molecular Pathology in the Frontal Cortex in Typical and Rapidly Progressive Forms. Front. Neurol. 2017;8 Available from: http://journal.frontiersin.org/article/10.3389/fneur.2017.00089/full.
43. Puoti G, Bizzi A, Forloni G, Safar JG, Tagliavini F, Gambetti P. Sporadic human prion diseases: molecular insights and diagnosis. Lancet Neurol. 2012;11:618–28.
44. Llorens F, Schmitz M, Karch A, Cramm M, Lange P, Gherib K, et al. Comparative analysis of cerebrospinal fluid biomarkers in the differential diagnosis of neurodegenerative dementia. Alzheimers Dement. 2015:1–13.
45. Llorens F, Kruse N, Schmitz M, Gotzmann N, Golanska E, Thüne K, et al. Evaluation of α-synuclein as a novel cerebrospinal fluid biomarker in different forms of prion diseases. Alzheimer's Dement. 2016:1–10. Available from: http://linkinghub.elsevier.com/retrieve/pii/S1552526016330552.
46. Schmidt C, Wolff M, Weitz M, Bartlau T, Korth C, Zerr I. Rapidly progressive Alzheimer disease. Arch Neurol. 2011;68:1124–30.
47. Villemagne VL, Burnham S, Bourgeat P, Brown B, Ellis KA, Salvado O, et al. Amyloid beta deposition, neurodegeneration, and cognitive decline in sporadic Alzheimer's disease: a prospective cohort study. Lancet Neurol. 2013;12:357–67.
48. Roman G, Tatemichi T, Erkinjuntti T, Cummings J, Masdeu J, Garcia J, et al. Vascular dementia: diagnostic criteria for research studies: report of the NINDS-AIREN international workshop. Neurology. 1993;43:250–60.
49. McKhann G, Drachman D, Folstein M, Katzman R, Price D, Stadlan EM. Clinical diagnosis of Alzheimer's disease: report of the NINCDS-ADRDA work group* under the auspices of Department of Health and Human Services Task Force on Alzheimer's disease. Neurol Int. 1984;34:939. Available from: http://www.neurology.org/content/34/7/939.
50. Zerr I, Kallenberg K, Summers DM, Romero C, Taratuto A, Heinemann U, et al. Updated clinical diagnostic criteria for sporadic Creutzfeldt-Jakob disease. Brain. 2009;132:2659–68.
51. Zerr I, Pocchiari M, Collins S, Brandel JP, de Pedro Cuesta J, Knight RS, et al. Analysis of EEG and CSF 14-3-3 proteins as aids to the diagnosis of Creutzfeldt-Jakob disease. Neurology. 2000;55:811–5. Available from: https://www.ncbi.nlm.nih.gov/pubmed/10994001.
52. Padilla D, Béringue V, Espinosa JC, Andreoletti O, Jaumain E, Reine F, et al. Sheep and goat BSE propagate more efficiently than cattle BSE in human PrP transgenic mice. PLoS Pathog. 2011,7(3).e1001319.
53. Oakley H, Cole SL, Logan S, Maus E, Shao P, Craft J, et al. Intraneuronal β-amyloid aggregates, Neurodegeneration, and neuron loss in transgenic mice with five familial Alzheimer's disease mutations: potential factors in amyloid plaque formation. J Neurosci [Internet]. 2006;26:10129–40. Available from: http://www.jneurosci.org/content/26/40/10129.abstract.
54. Eimer WA, Vassar R. Neuron loss in the 5XFAD mouse model of Alzheimer's disease correlates with intraneuronal Aβ42 accumulation and Caspase-3 activation. Mol. Neurodegener. 2013;8:2. Available from: http://www.ncbi.nlm.nih.gov/pubmed/23316765%5Cn, http://www.pubmedcentral.nih.gov/articlerender.fcgi?artid=PMC3552866.
55. Wolf H, Hossinger A, Fehlinger A, Büttner S, Sim V, McKenzie D, et al. Deposition pattern and subcellular distribution of disease-associated prion protein in cerebellar organotypic slice cultures infected with scrapie. Front Neurosci. 2015;9:410.

56. Zerr I, Bodemer M, Gefeller O, Otto M, Poser S, Wiltfang J, et al. Detection of 14-3-3 protein in the cerebrospinal fluid supports the diagnosis of Creutzfeldt-Jakob disease. Ann Neurol. 1998;43:32–40.
57. Milosevic I, Giovedi S, Lou X, Raimondi A, Collesi C, Shen H, et al. Recruitment of endophilin to clathrin-coated pit necks is required for efficient vesicle uncoating after fission. Neuron. 2011;72:587–601.
58. Schmitz M, Cramm M, Llorens F, Collins S, Atarashi R, Satoh K, et al. The real-time quaking-induced conversion assay for detection of human prion disease and study of other protein misfolding diseases. Nat Protoc. 2016;11:2233–42.
59. Cramm M, Schmitz M, Karch A, Mitrova E, Kuhn F, Schroeder B, et al. Stability and reproducibility underscore utility of RT-QuIC for diagnosis of Creutzfeldt-Jakob disease. Mol Neurobiol. 2016;53:1896–904.
60. Youden WJ. Index for rating diagnostic tests. Cancer. 1950;3:32–5.
61. Windl O, Giese A, Schulz-Schaeffer W, Zerr I, Skworc K, Arendt S, et al. Molecular genetics of human prion diseases in Germany. Hum Genet. 1999;105:244–52.
62. Falsig J, Sonati T, Herrmann US, Saban D, Li B, Arroyo K, et al. Prion pathogenesis is faithfully reproduced in cerebellar Organotypic slice cultures. PLoS Pathog. 2012;8(11):e1002985.
63. Hill AF. Molecular classification of sporadic Creutzfeldt-Jakob disease. Brain. 2003;126:1333–46. Available from: http://brain.oxfordjournals.org/cgi/content/abstract/126/6/1333.
64. Heinemann U, Krasnianski A, Meissner B, Varges D, Kallenberg K, Schulz-Schaeffer WJ, et al. Creutzfeldt-Jakob disease in Germany: a prospective 12-year surveillance. Brain. 2007;130:1350–9.
65. Heneka MT, Carson MJ, El KJ, Landreth GE, Brosseron F, Feinstein DL, et al. Neuroinflammation in Alzheimer's disease. Lancet Neurol. 2015; 14(4):388–405.
66. Minter MR, Taylor JM, Crack PJ. The contribution of neuroinflammation to amyloid toxicity in Alzheimer's disease. J. Neurochem. 2016;136(3):457–74.
67. Radford RA, Morsch M, Rayner SL, Cole NJ, Pountney DL, Chung RS. The established and emerging roles of astrocytes and microglia in amyotrophic lateral sclerosis and frontotemporal dementia. Front. Cell. Neurosci. 2015;9: 414. Available from: http://www.pubmedcentral.nih.gov/articlerender.fcgi?artid=4621294&tool=pmcentrez&rendertype=abstract.
68. Ugbode C, Hu Y, Whalley B, Peers C, Rattray M, Dallas ML. Astrocytic transporters in Alzheimer's disease. Biochem J [Internet]. 2017;474:333–55. Available from: http://biochemj.org/lookup/doi/10.1042/BCJ20160505.
69. Simpson JE, Ince PG, Lace G, Forster G, Shaw PJ, Matthews F, et al. Astrocyte phenotype in relation to Alzheimer-type pathology in the ageing brain. Neurobiol Aging. 2010;31:578–90.
70. Fuller S, Steele M, Münch G. Activated astroglia during chronic inflammation in Alzheimer's disease-Do they neglect their neurosupportive roles? Mutat. Res. 2010;690(1-2):40–9.
71. Donato R, Sorci G, Riuzzi F, Arcuri C, Bianchi R, Brozzi F, et al. S100B's double life: Intracellular regulator and extracellular signal. Biochim. Biophys. Acta. 2009;1793(6):1008–22.
72. Van Eldik LJ, Wainwright MS. The Janus face of glial-derived S100B: beneficial and detrimental functions in the brain. Restor. Neurol. Neurosci. 2003;21:97–108. Available from: http://www.ncbi.nlm.nih.gov/pubmed/14530573.
73. Böhmer AE, Oses JP, Schmidt AP, Perón CS, Krebs CL, Oppitz PP, et al. Neuron-specific enolase, S100B, and glial fibrillary acidic protein levels as outcome predictors in patients with severe traumatic brain injury. Neurosurgery. 2011;68:1624–30.
74. Petzold A, Jenkins R, Watt HC, Green AJE, Thompson EJ, Keir G, et al. Cerebrospinal fluid S100B correlates with brain atrophy in Alzheimer's disease. Neurosci Lett. 2003;336:167–70.
75. Llorens F, Schmitz M, Knipper T, Schmidt C, Lange P, Fischer A, et al. Cerebrospinal Fluid Biomarkers of Alzheimer's Disease Show Different but Partially Overlapping Profile Compared to Vascular Dementia. Front. Aging Neurosci. 2017;9:1–9. Available from: http://journal.frontiersin.org/article/10.3389/fnagi.2017.00289/full.
76. Sanchez-Juan P, Green A, Ladogana A, Cuadrado-Corrales N, Sáanchez-Valle R, Mitrováa E, et al. CSF tests in the differential diagnosis of Creutzfeldt-Jakob disease. Neurology. 2006;67:637–43.
77. Fuller S, Munch G, Steele M. Activated astrocytes: a therapeutic target in Alzheimer's disease? Expert rev Neurother. 2009;9:1585–94. Available from: http://www.ncbi.nlm.nih.gov/pubmed/19903019.
78. Wiley CA, Bonneh-Barkay D, Dixon CE, Lesniak A, Wang G, Bissel SJ, et al. Role for mammalian chitinase 3-like protein 1 in traumatic brain injury. Neuropathology. 2015;35:95–106.
79. Bonneh-Barkay D, Wang GJ, LaFramboise WA, Wiley CA, Bissel SJ. Exacerbation of experimental autoimmune encephalomyelitis in the absence of breast regression protein 39/Chitinase 3-like 1. J Neuropathol Exp Neurol. 2012;71:948–58.
80. Dalgard CL, Cole JT, Kean WS, Lucky JJ, Sukumar G, McMullen DC, et al. The cytokine temporal profile in rat cortex after controlled cortical impact. Front Mol Neurosci. 2012;5:6.
81. Bhardwaj R, Yester JW, Singh SK, Biswas DD, Surace MJ, Waters MR, et al. RelB/p50 complexes regulate cytokine-induced YKL-40 expression. J Immunol. 2015;194:2862–70.
82. Liddelow SA, Guttenplan KA, Clarke LE, Bennett FC, Bohlen CJ, Schirmer L, et al. Neurotoxic reactive astrocytes are induced by activated microglia. Nature. 2017; Available from: http://www.nature.com/doifinder/10.1038/nature21029.
83. Lian H, Litvinchuk A, Chiang AC-A, Aithmitti N, Jankowsky JL, Zheng H. Astrocyte-microglia cross talk through complement activation modulates amyloid pathology in mouse models of Alzheimer's disease. J. Neurosci, Available from. 2016;36:577–89. http://www.ncbi.nlm.nih.gov/pubmed/26758846.
84. Schwab C, McGeer PL. Inflammatory aspects of Alzheimer disease and other neurodegenerative disorders. J Alzheimers Dis. 2008;13:359–69.
85. Shepherd CE, Thiel E, McCann H, Harding AJ, Halliday GM. Cortical inflammation in Alzheimer disease but not dementia with Lewy bodies. Arch. Neurol. 2000;57: 817–22.
86. Llorens F, Kruse N, Karch A, Schmitz M, Zafar S, Gotzmann N, et al. Validation of α-Synuclein as a CSF biomarker for sporadic Creutzfeldt-Jakob disease. Mol. Neurobiol. 2017:1–9. Available from: http://link.springer.com/10.1007/s12035-017-0479-5.
87. Stoeck K, Schmitz M, Ebert E, Schmidt C, Zerr I. Immune responses in rapidly progressive dementia: a comparative study of neuroinflammatory markers in Creutzfeldt-Jakob disease, Alzheimer¿s disease and multiple sclerosis. J. Neuroinflammation, Available from. 2014;11:170. http://www.ncbi.nlm.nih.gov/pubmed/25315814.
88. Llorens F, Karch A, Golanska E, Schmitz M, Lange P, Sikorska B, et al. Cerebrospinal Fluid Biomarker-Based Diagnosis of Sporadic Creutzfeldt-Jakob Disease: A Validation Study for Previously Established Cutoffs. Dement. Geriatr. Cogn. Disord. 2017;43:71–80. Available from: https://www.karger.com/?doi=10.1159/000454802.
89. Hellwig K, Kvartsberg H, Portelius E, Andreasson U, Oberstein TJ, Lewczuk P, et al. Neurogranin and YKL-40: independent markers of synaptic degeneration and neuroinflammation in Alzheimer's disease. Alzheimers. Res. Ther. 2015;7:74. Available from: http://www.pubmedcentral.nih.gov/articlerender.fcgi?artid=4690296&tool=pmcentrez&rendertype=abstract.
90. Mattsson N, Tabatabaei S, Johansson P, Hansson O, Andreasson U, Månsson JE, et al. Cerebrospinal fluid microglial markers in Alzheimer's disease: elevated chitotriosidase activity but lack of diagnostic utility. NeuroMolecular Med. 2011; 13:151–9.
91. Carter SF, Scholl M, Almkvist O, Wall A, Engler H, Langstrom B, et al. Evidence for Astrocytosis in Prodromal Alzheimer Disease Provided by 11C–Deuterium-L-Deprenyl: A Multitracer PET Paradigm Combining 11C–Pittsburgh Compound B and 18F–FDG. J. Nucl. Med. 2012;53:37–46.
92. Llorens F, Thüne K, Sikorska B, Schmitz M, Tahir W, Fernández-borges N. Altered Ca 2 + homeostasis induces Calpain- Cathepsin axis activation in sporadic Creutzfeldt-Jakob disease. Acta Neuropathol Commun. 2017;5(1):35.
93. Gispert JD, Monté GC, Suárez-Calvet M, Falcon C, Tucholka A, Rojas S, et al. The {APOE} ε4 genotype modulates {CSF} YKL-40 levels and their structural brain correlates in the continuum of Alzheimer disease but not those of sTREM2. Alzheimer's Dement. Diagnosis, Assess. Dis. Monit. 2016;6 Available from: http://www.sciencedirect.com/science/article/pii/S2352872916300653.
94. Llorens F, Thune K, Schmitz M, Ansoleaga B, Frau-Mendez MA, Cramm M, et al. Identification of new molecular alterations in fatal familial insomnia. Hum Mol Genet. 2016;0:1–20.
95. Parchi P, Castellani R, Cortelli P, Montagna P, Chen SG, Petersen RB, et al. Regional distribution of protease-resistant prion protein in fatal familial insomnia. Ann Neurol. 1995;38:21–9.
96. Ladogana A, Sanchez-Juan P, Mitrova E, Green A, Cuadrado-Corrales N, Sanchez-Valle R, et al. Cerebrospinal fluid biomarkers in human genetic transmissible spongiform encephalopathies. J Neurol, Available from. 2009;256:1620–8. http://www.ncbi.nlm.nih.gov/pubmed/19444528.
97. Kovács GG, Puopolo M, Ladogana A, Pocchiari M, Budka H, van Duijn C, et al. Genetic prion disease: the EUROCJD experience. Hum Genet. 2005;118:166–74.
98. Gambetti P, Kong Q, Zou W, Parchi P, Chen SG. Sporadic and familial CJD: Classification and characterisation. Br. Med. Bull. 2003;66:213–39.

99. Shahim P, Portelius E, Brody DL. Astroglial activation and altered amyloid metabolism in human repetitive concussion. 2017;
100. Hjalmarsson C, Bjerke M, Andersson B, Blennow K, Zetterberg H, Aberg ND, et al. Neuronal and glia-related biomarkers in cerebrospinal fluid of patients with acute ischemic stroke. J. Cent. Nerv. Syst. Dis. 2014;6:51–8. Available from: http://www.pubmedcentral.nih.gov/articlerender.fcgi?artid=4039292&tool=pmcentrez&rendertype=abstract.
101. Rymo I, Kern S, Bjerke M, Zetterberg H, Marlow T, Blennow K, et al. CSF YKL-40 and GAP-43 are related to suicidal ideation in older women. Acta Psychiatr. Scand. 2017:351–7. Available from: http://doi.wiley.com/10.1111/acps.12701.
102. Jakobsson J, Bjerke M, Sahebi S, Isgren A, Ekman CJ, Sellgren C, et al. Monocyte and microglial activation in patients with mood-stabilized bipolar disorder. J Psychiatry Neurosci. 2015;40:250–8.
103. Van Everbroeck B, Dewulf E, Pals P, Lübke U, Martin JJ, Cras P. The role of cytokines, astrocytes, microglia and apoptosis in Creutzfeldt-Jakob disease. Neurobiol Aging. 2002;23:59–64.

6

Is amyotrophic lateral sclerosis/frontotemporal dementia an autophagy disease?

Zhiqiang Deng[1,2,3], Patricia Sheehan[3], Shi Chen[1,2*] and Zhenyu Yue[3*]

Abstract

Amyotrophic lateral sclerosis (ALS) and frontotemporal dementia (FTD) are neurodegenerative disorders that share genetic risk factors and pathological hallmarks. Intriguingly, these shared factors result in a high rate of comorbidity of these diseases in patients. Intracellular protein aggregates are a common pathological hallmark of both diseases. Emerging evidence suggests that impaired RNA processing and disrupted protein homeostasis are two major pathogenic pathways for these diseases. Indeed, recent evidence from genetic and cellular studies of the etiology and pathogenesis of ALS-FTD has suggested that defects in autophagy may underlie various aspects of these diseases. In this review, we discuss the link between genetic mutations, autophagy dysfunction, and the pathogenesis of ALS-FTD. Although dysfunction in a variety of cellular pathways can lead to these diseases, we provide evidence that ALS-FTD is, in many cases, an autophagy disease.

Keywords: Amyotrophic lateral sclerosis, Frontotemporal dementia, Autophagy, Disease-associated genes, Autophagy-related genes

Background

Though various cellular defects are noted in Amyotrophic Lateral Sclerosis (ALS) and Frontotemporal dementia (FTD) including dysregulation of RNA processing, protein aggregation, and oxidative stress, the detailed disease mechanisms remain poorly understood [1, 2]. Emerging evidence from genetic cases points to a role of autophagy in ALS-FTD. Here, we review how specific disease-linked mutations affect proper autophagic function and protein degradation leading to the speculation that ALS-FTD is, at least in part, an autophagy disease.

ALS and FTD

ALS is an adult-onset devastating neurodegenerative disorder characterized by progressive degeneration and deterioration of upper and lower motor neurons of the primary motor cortex, spinal cord and brain stem [3]. FTD is a form of dementia characterized by focal atrophy of the frontal and anterior temporal lobes of the brain, called frontaltemporal lobar degeneration (FTLD) [4]. The comorbidity of these diseases in patients and the shared genetic risk factors suggest ALS and FTD represent a continuum of neurodegenerative disorders [5]. A common pathological hallmark of both ALS and FTD is the presence of cytoplasmic protein aggregates and inclusions in affected neurons and glia cells [6–8], suggesting that an impairment in protein degradation may contribute to the disease process. In eukaryotic cells, the clearance of toxic-aggregated proteins is critical for cell survival, which relies mainly on two protein degradation systems: the ubiquitin-proteasome system (UPS) and autophagy [9, 10]. The UPS is mainly used for the degradation of short-lived proteins, while autophagy is preferentially used for the selective degradation of long-lived proteins and damaged organelles [11]. While the dysfunction of either the UPS or autophagy has been implicated in the formation of ALS-FTD-linked protein aggregates, accumulating evidence suggests that proper functioning of autophagy is the major determinant of motor neuron survival in ALS [12–15].

* Correspondence: shichen@whu.edu.cn; zhenyu.yue@mssm.edu
[1]Brain center, Zhongnan Hospital, Wuhan University, Wuhan, Hubei 430071, China
[3]Department of Neurology, The Friedman Brain Institute, Icahn School of Medicine at Mount Sinai, New York 10029, USA
Full list of author information is available at the end of the article

Autophagic processing

Autophagy is a highly conserved catabolic cellular pathway used to degrade proteins and organelles at a basal level as well as pathogens and protein aggregates under pathological conditions. The endpoint of all autophagic pathways is the lysosome though, the three major autophagic pathways (i.e., microautophagy, chaperone-mediated autophagy, and macroautophagy) utilize different signaling molecules and protein machinery to prompt lysosomal degradation. This review will focus on the role of macroautophagy (hereafter referred to as autophagy) in ALS-FTD.

Canonical autophagy is under the control of mechanistic target of rapamycin complex 1 (mTORC1), a master regulator of diverse signaling pathways, which is regulated by cellular nutrient levels. Under nutrient-rich conditions, mTORC1 is active, suppressing the induction of autophagy by phosphorylating Unc51-like kinase 1 (ULK1) and Transcription Factor EB (TFEB). Starvation conditions inhibit the activity of mTORC1 and allow the induction of autophagy through the dephosphorylation of ULK1 and TFEB. Upon dephosphorylation, TFEB translocates to the nucleus where it functions to upregulate autophagy and lysosome-associated genes thus promoting autophagic degradation [16]. Once ULK1 is dephosphorylated, it forms a complex that can then phosphorylate Beclin1 [17] and Atg14L [18], two protein subunits in the class III phosphoinositol-3-phosphate kinase VPS34 complex. ULK1-mediated Atg14L phosphorylation activates VPS34 kinase activity, which is required for the nucleation of the phagophore membrane. The phagophore then expands to form the isolation membrane and engulf cytoplasmic contents. This elongation of the isolation membrane is dependent on two ubiquitin-like conjugation systems. The first involves the covalent conjugation of Atg12 to Atg5, a process carried out by Atg7 and Atg10. Atg5-Atg12 complex then binds Atg16. The second requires Atg7 and Atg3, assisted by Atg5-Atg12-Atg16, leading to the conjugation of phosphoethanolamine to LC3 [19]. This lipidation of LC3 allows it to associate with the autophagosome membrane and aid in cargo sequestration by associating with various autophagy receptors. Eventually, the membrane closes and forms a double membrane structure referred to as an autophagosome [19]. Following cargo sequestration, autophagosomes are trafficked along microtubule tracks. During this transport, autophagosomes can then fuse with compartments of the endocytic pathway to form an intermediate structure called an amphisome, which will then fuse with lysosomes for cargo degradation [20]. Additional studies investigating the cellular machinery for these fusion events have identified endosomal or lysosomal proteins (i.e., Rab7, LAMP1, HOPS complex proteins) and various SNARE proteins (i.e., Syntaxin17, SNAP29, VAMP7/8) as key mediators of autophagosome-lysosome fusion [21].

Autophagy was initially characterized as a non-selective degradation process. However, accumulating evidence shows that cargo such as damaged mitochondria and aggregated proteins can be selectively degraded by autophagy to maintain intracellular homeostasis [22–24]. This process of selective autophagy is carried out by autophagy receptors, which recognize specific cargo (including disease-related proteins) through protein modifications of receptors in response to proteotoxic stress [25].

Although growing evidence points to an association of autophagic function and the development of ALS and FTD [8, 26], the precise role of autophagy in the pathogenesis of these diseases remains elusive. Here, we review recent evidence for the role of ALS-FTD-associated genes in autophagic processing.

ALS-FTD-associated genes and autophagy

C9ORF72

The GGGGCC (G_4C_2) hexanucleotide repeat expansion in C9ORF72 is the most common genetic cause of ALS-FTD [27]. Multiple pathogenic mechanisms are thought to underlie the pathology associated with the G_4C_2 expansion. This alteration of C9ORF72 may lead to epigenetic changes [28] that result in decreased mRNA levels and the loss-of-function of C9ORF72 [27]. Alternatively, G_4C_2 expansion containing transcripts may be subject to repeat-associated non-ATG (RAN) translation that could result in a toxic gain-of-function of dipeptide-repeat proteins [29–31]. Multiple groups have initiated studies to develop therapeutic interventions aimed at reducing the toxicity of dipeptide-repeat proteins using gene depletion, peptide, or small molecule strategies to decrease RAN translation [32]. Pathologically, post-mortem analysis of patients carrying the G_4C_2 expansion in C9ORF72 reveals the presence of RNA foci and ubiquitin/p62 positive inclusions [33–35]. Given these findings, much interest has arisen in understanding the potential link between C9ORF72 and autophagic regulation. Accumulating evidence demonstrates the relevance of C9ORF72 to autophagy, though its precise role in regulating autophagy is still unknown. Evidence suggests C9ORF72 acts in a multi-protein complex with SMCR8 and WDR41 to regulate the expression and activity of ULK1 [36]. Further, knockdown of C9ORF72 in MEF cells and mice impairs ULK1-mediated autophagy nduction, suggesting that C9ORF72 promotes autophagy [36, 37]. Acting in the same complex, C9ORF72 functions as a guanine nucleotide exchange factor (GEF) to activate Rab8a and Rab39b, two Rab GTPases with known functions in autophagy [38]. In the same study, depletion of C9ORF72 partly impaired autophagy and enhanced aggregation of TDP-43 and accumulation of p62 aggregates in neurons [38]. Additional studies indicate that C9ORF72 controls the Rab1a-dependent recruitment of the ULK1 complex to the phagophore in order to regulate the initiation of autophagy [39]. Again, the reduction of C9ORF72 protein levels was shown to attenuate autophagy and enhance the formation of p62-positive puncta in cells and primary neurons [39]. Together, these results indicate that C9ORF72 acts as a positive regulator of autophagy with its depletion leading to autophagic dysfunction and protein aggregation. However, in addition to regulating autophagy through direct association with the ULK1 autophagy initiation complex, C9ORF72 is indirectly involved in autophagy through regulation of mTORC1. Active mTORC1 inhibits autophagy by negatively regulating ULK1 activity and TFEB-mediated transcription of autophagy genes [40–42]. In the context of ALS-FTD, depletion of C9ORF72 was shown to impair mTORC1 activity by decreasing the response of mTORC1 to amino acid availability [43], reducing the phosphorylation of S6 K, a substrate of mTORC1, and enhancing autophagic flux [44]. In contrast to the findings discussed earlier, these results suggest that depletion of C9ORF72 enhances autophagy through negative regulation of mTORC1. As it is still unclear what the precise role of C9ORF72 is in autophagy, further study is required to determine whether C9ORF72 depletion results in enhanced or impaired autophagy regulation.

TBK1

TANK-binding kinase 1 (TBK1) was recently identified as an ALS FTD causal gene [45, 46]. ALS-FTD-linked TBK1 mutations are proposed to be loss-of-function mutations as patients show decreased mRNA and protein expression [45, 46]. TBK1 has been implicated in various autophagy-related pathways including antibacterial autophagy (xenophagy), mitophagy, and macroautophagy [47–51]. TBK1 phosphorylates autophagy receptors including p62 and OPTN enhancing the elimination of intracellular pathogens such as Mycobacteria and Salmonella, as well as damaged mitochondria [48–51]. Recent studies have shown that ALS-related mutations of TBK1 inhibit mitophagy by blocking autophagosome formation, disrupting the OPTN-TBK1 interaction [46, 52, 53], and failing to translocate to damaged mitochondria [54]. TBK1 is necessary for the maturation of the autophagosome, which is required for the degradation of p62 and its affiliated cargo [50]. Overexpression of wild-type TBK1, but not the kinase dead variant, facilitates clearance of mutant SOD1, another ALS associated protein [55, 56]. These results indicate that ALS-FTD-associated mutations of TBK1 disrupt autophagy through loss of TBK1-regulated clearance of autophagic cargo, including damaged mitochondria and disease-prone proteins.

Recently, a link between TBK1 and C9ORF72 has been reported. TBK1 phosphorylates SMCR8 at S402 and S796, which forms a complex with C9ORF72 and WDR41 to control autophagy flux [38]. Depletion of SMCR8 impairs autophagy, which can be rescued by expression of phosphomimetic variants of SMCR8 but not non-phosphorylatable variants of SMCR8, suggesting a critical role of TBK1 kinase activity in regulating autophagy through SMCR8. Moreover, knockdown of TBK1 enhances the accumulation of p62 puncta in neuronal cells, which can be rescued by phosphomimetic SMCR8 but not non-phosphorylatable SMCR8. These results imply that TBK1 and C9ORF72 may share a common pathway in regulation of autophagy through SMCR8 [38]. Together, ALS-FTD-causal mutations in TBK1 appear to cause the dysregulation of multiple aspects of autophagic function including mitophagy, toxic protein clearance, and C9ORF72/SMCR8 cellular pathways.

Optineurin (OPTN)

OPTN is involved in a variety of cellular functions, including signal transduction, vesicle trafficking, and axon homeostasis [57]. OPTN is a known autophagy receptor, which promotes the clearance of protein aggregates, infected pathogens, and mitochondria [48, 49, 55]. Several studies report that genetic mutations in OPTN enhance the risk of ALS [58–63]. Multiple lines of evidence suggest that ALS related OPTN mutations impair autophagy. For example, ALS patients with OPTN mutation (E478G) show TDP-43 positive neuronal intracytoplasmic inclusions in medullary and spinal motor neurons [58, 59]. In addition, Wild et al. have shown that ALS-linked OPTN mutations (E478G and F178A) are unable to rescue antibacterial autophagy to the level of wild-type OPTN [48]. More recent studies have shown that ALS-linked mutations of OPTN (Q398X, E478G) disrupt its association with myosin VI, an association that is required for autophagosome maturation. This disruption leads to disturbances in the activation of ER stress, dysfunction in protein secretion, Golgi fragmentation, and autophagosome-lysosome fusion [64].

Post-translation modifications, including phosphorylation and ubiquitination, of OPTN enhance its function in autophagy. OPTN can be phosphorylated at various serine residues by TBK1. In antibacterial autophagy, TBK1 phosphorylates OPTN at S177, which enhances its binding affinity with LC3 and promotes autophagic clearance of cytosolic Salmonella [48]. While in mitophagy, TBK1 phosphorylates OPTN at S473 in the UBA domain, which enhances its binding affinity to ubiquitin chains [49]. In addition, phosphorylation of OPTN at Ser473, which is close to ALS-linked mutant site E478G, enhances its binding to ubiquitin chains and its clearance of damaged mitochondria [49]. However, interactome analysis in another study shows this mutation reduces OPTN interactions with binding partners, including proteins which functions in ubiquitin-dependent protein degradation and ER transport [65]. OPTN can also be ubiquitinated at multiple lysine residues by the tumor-suppressor HACE1, which promotes its interaction with p62 to form an autophagy receptor complex and accelerate autophagic flux [66]. Recently, Shen et al. have shown that compared with wild type OPTN, ubiquitin-binding domain mutants including the ALS-linked E478G and D474N mutations, are defective in clearing inclusion bodies formed by truncated TDP-43 [67]. The same group has also shown that the mutants act as dominant-negative traps to compromise the maturation of autophagosomes, which leads to defects in OPTN-mediated selective autophagy [67]. Future experiments are required to determine whether the phosphorylation or ubiquitination of OPTN is impacted in ALS linked mutations.

As discussed above here, post-translational modifications play a crucial role in modifying the function of OPTN in autophagy. Either phosphorylation or ubiquitination of OPTN increases autophagy and lead to the clearance of autophagy substrates. Therefore, it is conceivable that enhancing phosphorylation or ubiquitination of OPTN could be a novel therapeutic target for ALS patients carrying OPTN mutations.

p62 (SQSTM1)

p62 is an autophagy receptor that plays a major role in the clearance of protein aggregates [68]. Moreover, p62 itself is degraded by autophagy and thus can be used as a general marker for autophagic flux [68, 69]. p62 functions in diverse signaling pathways including proteasomal signaling, amino acid sensing, DNA damage response, and oxidative stress [63, 70, 71]. Pathological analyses of postmortem brains reveal that p62 associates with various disease-relevant protein aggregates [72–74]. Due to the numerous roles of p62 in the clearance of pathogens, protein aggregates, and various client proteins, it has become the most well-characterized autophagy receptor [68, 69]. The UBA domain of p62 can be phosphorylated by Casein kinase 2 (CK2), TBK1, and ULK1. These phosphorylation events increase the affinity of p62 for ubiquitinated cargo and enhance the clearance of ubiquitinated proteins in selective autophagy [50, 68, 75]. Additionally, p62 can be ubiquitinated by TRIM21 and Keap1 to regulate the sequestration required for clearance of ubiquitinated proteins in selective autophagy [76, 77]. More recently, it has been reported that upon ubiquitin stress (e.g., proteasome inhibition), p62 undergoes ubiquitination which disrupts the dimerization at its UBA domain allowing p62 to recognize and bind polyubiquitinated cargoes [78].

Mutations in p62 have also been found in ALS-FTD patients [63, 79–81]. A recent report indicates that some rare variants of p62 in the UBA domain increase FTLD risk [80]. While various mutations in p62 have been identified in ALS-FTD, the relevance of these mutations to disease risk is currently unknown [82]. Limited evidence suggests that disease-associated mutations may confer loss-of-function of p62 in selective autophagy [83, 84]. Knockdown of p62 in zebrafish causes a locomotor phenotype that is improved under mTOR inhibition or re-expression of wild-type p62, but not ALS-FTD-associated UBA domain mutant (P392L) p62 [83]. Further, the ALS-FTD-associated p62 LIR mutant, L341 V, is defective in recognition of LC3B [84]. This recognition is required for p62-mediated delivery of ubiquitinated cargo to the autophagosome suggesting this ALS-FTD related mutation results in failed selective autophagy. Finally, recent evidence suggests that p62 regulates the levels and/or functions of other ALS-FTD disease proteins (e.g., SOD1 and TDP-43) [85, 86], which is consistent with a prominent role of the misregulation of p62 in the disruption of protein homeostasis in ALS-FTD.

Ubiquilin 2 (Ubqln2)

Ubqln2 is ubiquitin-like receptor protein that shuttles polyubiquitinated cargo to the proteasome for degradation via its UBA domain [87]. While the role of Ubqln2 in the UPS has been well established, emerging evidence of an interaction between Ubqln2 and LC3 suggests this protein also has a role in autophagy [88, 89]. Multiple mutations in the PXX repeat region are linked to ALS-FTD [63, 90, 91]. In transgenic rats, neuronal expression of a disease-linked Ubqln2 mutation (P497H) induces the formation of protein aggregates positive for p62 and LC3, however, deletion of Ubqln2 has no effect [92]. As the effects of this mutation do not mimic loss-of-function, this finding suggests that the ALS-FTD-linked Ubqln2 mutation (P497H) confers a gain of toxic function [92]. Furthermore, expression of Ubqln2 mutants results in the accumulation of polyubiquitinated proteins (e.g., TDP-43) in a UBA domain-dependent manner [93]. However, a more recent study has shown that Ubqln2 clears aggregates via the proteasome by interacting with the chaperone protein HSP70 [94]. Disease mutations in Ubqln2 are defective in HSP70 binding leading to the accumulation of aggregated proteins, which suggests loss-of-function mutations in Ubqln2 may underlie ALS-FTD [94].

TDP-43

TDP-43 is an RNA- and DNA-binding protein, which harbors RNA recognition motifs (RRM) and a C-terminal glycine-rich domain (GRD) that are required for its functions in nucleic acid binding and protein-protein interactions, respectively [95]. TDP-43 was detected as a major component of the ubiquitin-positive inclusions in ALS-FTD [96]. During the past several years, the identification of different mutations in ALS-FTD has shown that TDP-43 is a causative gene to these diseases [97]. It is reported that TDP-43, especially aggregated TDP-43, is cleared by autophagy [85, 98, 99] and autophagy activators reduced the formation of TDP-43 positive inclusion in TDP-43 overexpression mouse models [100]. High levels of truncated TDP-43, called TDP-25, are a prominent feature of ALS-FTD and are associated with reduced induction of autophagy [101]. Others have reported that depletion of TDP-43 reduces the mRNA level of Atg7, by destabilizing Atg7 mRNA, which causes an impairment in autophagy and the accumulation of polyubiquitinated proteins and p62 in neuroblastoma cells [102]. However, a recent report showed that loss of TDP-43 increased the biogenesis of autophagosomes and lysosomes by inhibiting mTORC1 activity and enhancing TFEB activity while also disrupting the fusion of autophagosomes and lysosomes [103]. Although these studies show seemingly opposite effects of the loss of TDP-43 on autophagy induction, they each suggest an essential role of full-length TDP-43 in proper autophagy regulation and indicate the dysfunction of multiple steps of autophagy is linked to TDP-43-mediated ALS-FTD.

Stress granules are aggregations of RNA and RNA-binding proteins that are dynamically assembled and disassembled when cells are insulted by stress [104]. These stress granules are essential to the maintenance of RNA homeostasis, the dysregulation of which is highly implicated in ALS pathogenesis [104, 105]. TDP-43 is a major component of stress granules in ALS while another ALS-related protein, FUS, is found in these granules in a subset of cases [106, 107]. FUS is also an RNA binding protein and mutations in FUS account for around 5% of familial ALS cases and result in the loss-of-function of FUS [108, 109]. ALS-associated FUS mutation (R521C) accumulates FUS positive stress granules upon stress conditions and disrupts the release of FUS from stress granules in cultured neurons [110]. Moreover, ALS-linked mutant FUS affects the assembly and morphology of stress granules [111]. As stress granules are degraded by autophagy, it is conceivable that mutant FUS decreases the dynamics of stress granules and leads to their accumulation by disrupting autophagic clearance of

Table 1 ALS-FTD genes and their disease mutations linked to autophagy

Gene symbol	Protein	Cellular functions	The effect of the genetic variants	Autophagy involvement
C9ORF72	C9orf72	Proteostasis and vesicle dynamics	Loss/gain of function	Regulates initiation of autophagy. [36, 37]
TBK1	TBK1 (TANK-binding kinase 1)	Proteostasis and immunity	Loss of function	Phosphorylates autophagy receptors (p62 and OPTN); regulates selective autophagy. [48–51]
OPTN	Optineurin	Proteostasis, vesicle trafficking and axon homeostasis	Loss of function	A substrate of TBK1 and autophagy receptor protein; selective autophagy. [25, 48, 49]
SQSTM1	p62	Pproteostasis, amino acid sensing, DNA damage response, and oxidative stress	Loss of function	A substrate of TBK1 and ULK1; autophagy receptor; selective autophagy. [25, 50, 68]
UBQLN2	Ubiquilin-2 (UBQLN2)	Proteasome, proteostasis, and vesicle trafficking	Gain/loss of function	A potential autophagy receptor. [88, 89]
TARDBP	TDP-43	RNA regulation	Loss/gain of function	Regulates autophagy initiation and autophagosome-lysosome fusion. [103]
FUS	FUS (fused in sarcoma)	RNA regulation, and DNA damage repair	Loss of function	ALS-linked mutations, P525L and R522G, impair autophagy. [165]
VCP	Valosin-containing protein	ER-associated degradation, DNA damage, and membrane dynamics	Loss of function	Regulates the clearance of lysosomes. [128]
SOD1	Superoxide dismutase 1	Dismutation reaction	Gain of function	Mutant SOD1 disrupts autophagy. [139–143]
ALS2	Alsin	Proteostasis and endosome biogenesis	Loss of function	Pathogenic mutations in ALS2 disrupt the formation of amphisomes. [150]
VAPB	Vesicle-associated membrane protein-associated protein B/C	Proteostasis, calcium homeostasis, and proteins trafficking	Loss of function	Regulates ER-mitochondrial contact. [155]
SigR1	Sigma receptor-1	Proteostasis, Ca^{2+} signaling, ion channel activity, synaptic plasticity.	Loss of function	Regulates autophagosome-lysosome fusion. [162, 163]

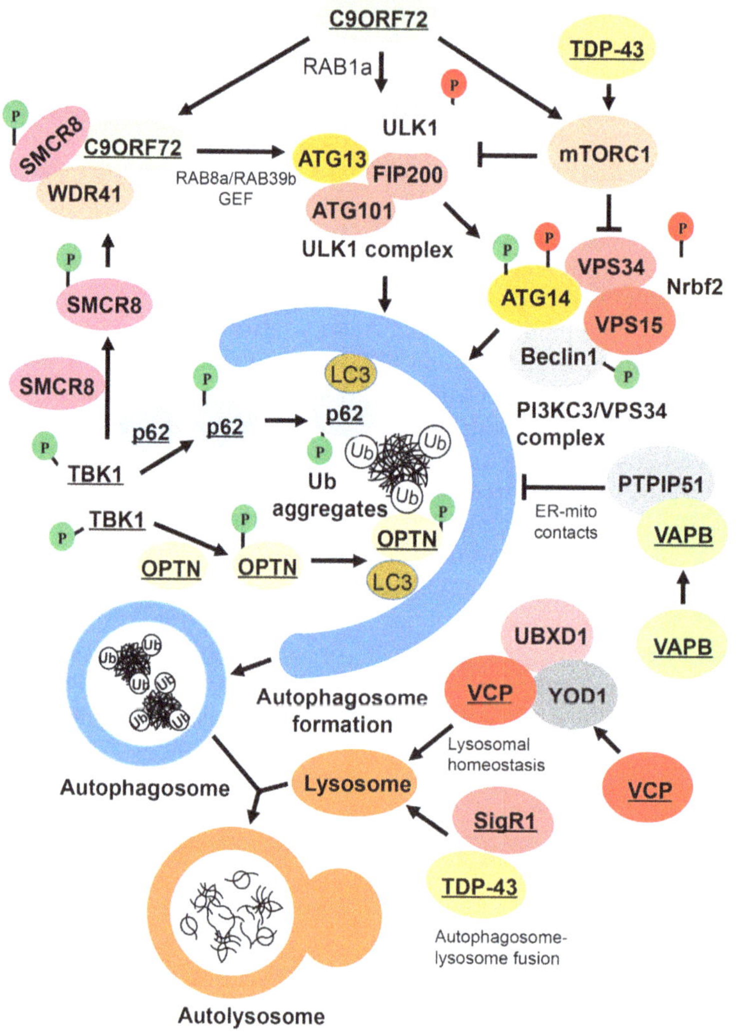

Fig. 1 Interactions of ALS/FTD associated genes with autophagy pathway. Several ALS/FTD genes take part in the selective autophagy pathway, which controls the clearance of ubiquitinated proteins and damaged organelles. Autophagy kinase TBK1 phosphorylates two known autophagy receptors p62 and OPTN to facilitate the clearance of ubiquitinated proteins. TBK1 also phosphorylates SMCR8 to regulate the formation of SMCR8, WDR41 and C9ORF72 complex, which acts as a GEF (GDP/GTP exchange factor) for RAB8a/13b, which is associated with the dynamics of autophagosomes. The C9ORF72 complex potentially regulates the ULK1 kinase activity. C9ORF72 can interact with Rab1a and ULK1 complex to regulate autophagy initiation. Moreover, C9ORF72 can negatively regulate autophagy by increasing mTORC1 activity. TDP-43 regulates mTORC1 activity; however, it can enhance autophagosome–lysosome fusion in an mTORC1 independent manner. VAPB, together with PTPIP51, deregulates autophagy flux by controlling the ER-mitochondria contacts. VCP, which cooperates with UBXD1 and YOD1, maintains lysosomal homeostasis. Underlined genes are linked to ALS/FTD. Abbreviations: ALS: Amyotrophic lateral sclerosis; FTD: Frontal-temporal dementia; TDP-43: Transactive response DNA-binding protein 43; SMCR8; Smith-Magenis Chromosome Region gene 8; WDR41: WD repeat domain 41; ULK1: Unc-51 Like Autophagy Activating Kinase 1; C9ORF72: Chromosome 9 open reading frame 72; GEF: Guanine nucleotide exchange factor; mTORC1: mechanistic target of rapamycin complex 1; TBK1: TANK-binding kinase 1; OPTN: Optineurin; LC3: microtubule-associated protein1 light chain 3; VAPB: Vesicle associated membrane protein associated protein B; VCP: Valosin containing protein; SigR1: Sigma receptor-1; UBXD1: ubiquitin regulatory X (UBX) domain-containing protein 1; YOD1: yeast OTU deubiquinating enzyme 1; ER: endoplasmic reticulum; mito: mitochondria; PTPIP51: protein tyrosine phosphatase interacting protein 51.

these structures [105, 112]. One study suggested that prolonged stress granule formation might contribute to the pathogenesis of ALS. Interestingly, treatment of small molecule inhibitors of eIFα, which is directly correlated with stress granule formation, caused reduction of TDP-43 toxicity [113]. Decrease of TDP-43 toxicity by the same inhibitors has been also shown in other model systems [114], providing the support to the idea of targeting TDP-43 and stress granule in therapeutic development.

VCP

Valosin-contain protein (VCP), also called AAA-ATPase p97, functions in diverse signaling pathways, including endoplasmic reticulum (ER)-associated degradation, transcriptional regulation, DNA damage, and membrane dynamics [115–118]. Loss-of-function mutations in VCP are linked to several human degenerative diseases, including inclusion body myopathy (IBM), ALS-FTD [119, 120]. Histopathological analysis of VCP-associated neurodegenerative diseases show that affected tissues contain prominent inclusions containing ubiquitin and TDP-43 [121–123], and an accumulation of LC3 and p62 [124]. These findings, along with results from recent publications, suggest that VCP is involved in autophagy and specifically functions in the delivery of cargo to lysosomes for degradation [125]. Evidence from yeast has shown an essential role of the VCP orthologue, Cdc48, in the formation of autophagosomes [126] and multiple groups have reported the loss of VCP expression or activity leads to an accumulation of autophagosomes which fail to degrade aggregated proteins due to impaired autophagosome-lysosome fusion [104, 106]. Additional studies have found that mTORC is disrupted in VCP-related diseases, which leads to increased autophagosome biogenesis [127]. This finding, along with recent studies showing a critical role of VCP in the elimination of damaged lysosomes by autophagy, suggests the loss of VCP results in the overproduction of autophagosomes, a disruption in autolysosome formation, and the dysfunction of lysosomes [128]. Other studies have also shown a role for VCP in mitophagy and stress granule degradation [129], suggesting that VCP mutations result in ALS-FTD by disrupting multiple autophagic pathways.

SOD1

The Cu/Zn superoxide dismutase (SOD1) is an ALS causative gene in which mutations account for about 1% of sporadic and 10% of familial cases [130]. Mice expressing mutant SOD1 show an accumulation of aggregated proteins (including mutant SOD1) in the spinal cord, which is comparable with findings in human ALS [131]. Accumulating evidence demonstrates that genetic mutations of SOD1 induce ALS through a dominant toxic gain-of-function rather than the loss of enzymatic function [132, 133]. Previous reports have shown that autophagy can degrade mutant SOD1, preventing its toxicity [134] and antagonizing its cytoplasmic accumulation [135]. Recently, p62 and another ALS-associated gene, ALS2, have been shown to have additive protective roles in antagonizing the toxicity induced by mutant SOD1 [136]. In addition, it has been reported that inhibition of motor neuron autophagy in SOD1-G93A mice induces neuromuscular denervation in the early stages of the disease [137]. Another recent article has shown that bosutinib, which boosts autophagy, can improve the survival of ALS iPSC-derived motor neurons from patients with familial ALS caused by mutations in SOD1 [138]. It is likely that the autophagy-lysosome pathway is disrupted at asymptomatic stages in familial ALS-associated human SOD1-G93A as suggested in a transgenic model [139]. Additionally, the expression of TFEB and Beclin 1, two autophagy-related proteins, is altered in NSC-34 cells and in transgenic mice expressing SOD1-G93A mutation [140, 141]. In other studies, hyperactivity of the autophagy/lysosome pathway was detected in motor neurons of SOD1-linked ALS mice [142], which may account for the accumulation of autophagosomes in transgenic mice expressing mutant SOD1-G93A [143]. Taken together, these studies suggest that mutant SOD1 leads to a misregulation in autophagy. It is intriguing to propose that the disturbance of autophagy-lysosome pathway contributes to the toxicity induced by mutant SOD1, and modulation of autophagy may be a potential strategy for SOD1-mediated ALS treatment.

ALS2 (Alsin)

Mutations in ALS2 were identified in juvenile cases of motor neuron diseases, including ALS [144–146]. Previous reports showed that ALS2 activates Rab5 to regulate the trafficking, fusion, and maturation of endosomes [147–149]. The pathogenic mutations in ALS2 fail to activate Rab5 and disrupt the formation of amphisomes, a hybrid organelle formed through the fusion of autophagosomes and endosomes [150]. Loss of ALS2 in SOD1-H46H transgenic mice results in the accumulation of insoluble high molecular weight SOD1 but also ubiquitinated proteins and p62, while overexpression of ALS2 reduces the toxicity of mutant SOD1 in cultured motor neuronal cells [151]. More recently, ALS2, together with p62, was shown to play an additive protective role in antagonizing the toxicity of mutant SOD1 by promoting the clearance of insoluble mutant SOD1 [136]. These results suggest that the loss-of-function of ALS2, associated with impaired autophagy-induced protein clearance, leads to motor neuron disease associated pathogenesis.

VAPB

Vesicle-associated membrane protein-associated protein B (VAPB, also known as ALS8) is a member of highly conserved VAP family of ER transmembrane proteins [152]. VAPB plays a role in diverse functions including regulating calcium homeostasis in mitochondria and membrane trafficking in dendrites [153, 154]. More recently, Gomez-Suaga et al. have shown that VAPB and PTPIP51, a mitochondrial associated protein, regulate autophagy by modulating calcium delivery at ER-mitochondria contact sites [155]. Following the initial identification of a dominant missense mutation of VAPB in patients with a slowly progressive form of ALS [156], other mutations of VAPB have also been found to cause

ALS [157, 158]. Knock-in mice expressing mutant VAPB-P56S show accumulation of cytoplasmic inclusion containing mutant VAPB and ubiquitinated proteins in motor neurons selectively, implicating that defects in autophagy contribute to the pathogenesis of VAPB-mediated ALS [159].

SigR1

Sigma receptor-1 (SigR1, also known as ALS16) is an ER chaperone protein involved in calcium signaling, ion channel activity, synaptic plasticity, and neuronal survival [160]. A mutation in SigR1 (E102Q) was identified as causative of juvenile ALS-FTD [161]. Emerging evidence has shown the association of SigR1 with autophagy. Vollrath et al. reported that knockdown of SigR1 in HEK 293 or NSC34 cells leads to impaired autophagic degradation. Additionally, in cells stably expressing autophagy reporter RFP-GFP-LC3, depletion of SigR1 disrupts the fusion of autophagosome to lysosome [162]. More recently, the SigR1-E102Q protein was found to form aggregates in ER, which alters the structure of the ER and further results in autophagy impairment by affecting the fusion of autophagosomes to lysosomes. Moreover, similar results were found in primary lymphoblastoid cells derived from familial ALS patients harboring the SigR1-E102Q mutation [163]. These studies imply that mutations in SigR1 result in the loss of its function in maintaining ER morphology and in autophagic processing.

Conclusions

While dysfunction in multiple cellular processes can underlie the development of ALS/FTD, an assortment of evidence demonstrates a role of autophagy dysfunction in these diseases. The above evidence suggests that different ALS/FTD linked mutations lead to dysfunction in all aspects of autophagy ranging from initiation and cargo recognition to autophagosome fusion with endosomes and lysosomes (Table 1 and Fig. 1). Dysfunction in any of these steps of autophagy leads to a disruption in protein homeostasis and results in the accumulation of toxic protein aggregates. While general enhancement of autophagy is likely to reduce these protein aggregates, the chronic upregulation of autophagy biogenesis can lead to an imbalance of autophagosome formation and clearance, resulting in neurotoxicity. More directed therapeutic interventions targeted at specific regulation of autophagy receptors or proteins are necessary to combat toxic protein accumulation effectively. For instance, specific compounds (e.g., HSF1 inhibitor) that manipulate p62 protein modifications can alter the ability of p62 to recognize and recruit autophagic cargo [164]. Additionally, targeting the activity of kinases involved in autophagy (e.g., ULK1 or TBK1, which modulate selective autophagy) could also provide benefits in protein quality control. However, these initiatives will require further studies in vivo and in vitro to determine how specific mutations alter autophagy and what potential avenues are available for therapeutic intervention.

Abbreviations

ALS: Amyotrophic lateral sclerosis; Atg: Autophagy-related genes; C9ORF72: Chromosome 9 open reading frame 72; CK2: Casein kinase 2; ER: Endoplasmic reticulum; FTD: Frontotemporal dementia; FTLD: Frontotemporal lobar degeneration; FUS: Fused in sarcoma; GEF: Guanine nucleotide exchange factor; GRD: Glycine-rich domain; HACE1: HECT domain and ankyrin repeat containing E3 Ub ligase 1; IBM: Inclusion body myopathy; IBs: Inclusion bodies; Keap1: Kelch-like ECH-associated protein 1; LC3: Microtubule-associated protein1 light chain 3; LIR: LC3 interacting regain; mTORC1: Mechanistic target of rapamycin complex 1; NBR1: Neighbor of BRCA1 gene 1; OPTN: Optineurin; PTPIP51: Protein tyrosine phosphatase interacting protein 51; RRM: RNA recognition motifs; SigR1: Sigma receptor-1; SMCR8: Smith-Magenis Chromosome Region gene 8; SOD1: Cu-Zn Superoxide Dismutase 1; TBK1: TANK-binding kinase 1; TDP-43: Transactive response DNA-binding protein 43; TFEB: Transcription factor EB; TRIM21: Tripartite motif-containing protein 21; UBA: ubiquitin-binding domain; UBQLN2: Ubiquilin 2; UBXD1: Ubiquitin Regulatory X (Ubx) Domain-Containing Protein 1; ULK1: Unc-51 Like Autophagy Activating Kinase 1; UPS: The ubiquitin-proteasome system; VAPB: Vesicle associated membrane protein associated protein B; VCP: Valosin containing protein; WDR41: WD repeat domain 41; WIPI2: WD-repeat protein interacting with phosphoinositides 2; YOD1: Yeast OTU deubiquinating enzyme 1

Acknowledgements

We are thankful to all members of Yue and Chen laboratories for the critical reading and discussion of the manuscript.

Funding

This work was partially supported by NIH grant R01 NS060123 (ZY); Young One Thousand TalentProgram of China (SC); China Scholarship Council Fellowship (ZD).

Authors' contributions

ZD and PS wrote the manuscript. SC and ZY provided critical feedback. All authors read and approved the final manuscript.

Competing interests

All authors declare that they have no competing interests.

Author details

[1]Brain center, Zhongnan Hospital, Wuhan University, Wuhan, Hubei 430071, China. [2]Taihe Hospital, Hubei University of Medicine, Shiyan, Hubei 442000, China. [3]Department of Neurology, The Friedman Brain Institute, Icahn School of Medicine at Mount Sinai, New York 10029, USA.

References

1. Bozzo F, et al. Oxidative stress and mitochondrial damage in the pathogenesis of ALS: new perspectives. Neurosci Lett. 2017;636:3–8.
2. Ling SC, et al. Converging mechanisms in ALS and FTD: disrupted RNA and protein homeostasis. Neuron. 2013;79:416–38.
3. Al-Chalabi A, Hardiman O. The epidemiology of ALS: a conspiracy of genes, environment and time. Nat Rev Neurol. 2013;9:617–28.
4. Neary D, et al. Frontotemporal dementia. Lancet Neurol. 2005;4:771–80.
5. van Langenhove T, et al. The molecular basis of the frontotemporal lobar degeneration–amyotrophic lateral sclerosis spectrum. Ann Med. 2012;44: 817–28.
6. Arai T, et al. TDP-43 is a component of ubiquitin-positive tau-negative inclusions in frontotemporal lobar degeneration and amyotrophic lateral sclerosis. Biochem Biophys Res Commun. 2006;351:602–11.
7. Blokhuis AM, et al. Protein aggregation in amyotrophic lateral sclerosis. Acta Neuropathol. 2013;125:777–94.
8. Gotzl JK, et al. Impaired protein degradation in FTLD and related disorders. Ageing Res Rev. 2016;32:122–39.
9. Ravid T, Hochstrasser M. Diversity of degradation signals in the ubiquitin-proteasome system. Nat Rev Mol Cell Biol. 2008;9:679–90.
10. Klionsky DJ, Emr SD. Autophagy as a regulated pathway of cellular degradation. Science. 2000;290(5497):1717–21.
11. Rubinsztein DC. The roles of intracellular protein-degradation pathways in neurodegeneration. Nature. 2006;443:780–6.
12. Ferrucci M, Fulceri F., Toti L, Soldani P, Siciliano G, Paparelli A, Fornai F. (2011) Protein clearing pathways in ALS. Arch Italiennesde Biol 149(1): 121-149.
13. Pasquali L, Ruggieri S, Murri L, Paparelli A, Fornai F. Does autophagy worsen or improve the survival of dopaminergic neurons? Parkinsonism Relat Disord. 2009;15:S24–7.
14. Ferguson CJ, et al. Defective autophagy in neurons and astrocytes from mice deficient in PI(3,5)P2. Hum Mol Genet. 2009;18:4868–78.
15. Madeo F, et al. Autophagy for the avoidance of neurodegeneration. Genes Dev. 2009;23:2253–9.
16. Settembre C, et al. Signals from the lysosome: a control centre for cellular clearance and energy metabolism. Nat Rev Mol Cell Biol. 2013;14:283–96.
17. Russell RC, et al. ULK1 induces autophagy by phosphorylating Beclin-1 and activating VPS34 lipid kinase. Nat Cell Biol. 2013;15:741–50.
18. Wold MS, et al. ULK1-mediated phosphorylation of ATG14 promotes autophagy and is impaired in Huntington's disease models. Mol Neurodegener. 2016;11:76.
19. Mizushima N, et al. The role of Atg proteins in autophagosome formation. Ann Rev Cell Dev Biol. 2011;27:107–32.
20. Lamb CA, et al. The autophagosome: origins unknown, biogenesis complex. Nat Rev Mol Cell Biol. 2013;14:759–74.
21. Itakura E, et al. The hairpin-type tail-anchored SNARE syntaxin 17 targets to autophagosomes for fusion with endosomes/lysosomes. Cell. 2012;151: 1256–69.
22. Kraft C, et al. Selective types of autophagy in yeast. Biochim Biophys Acta. 2009;1793:1404–12.
23. Khaminets A, et al. Ubiquitin-dependent and independent signals in selective Autophagy. Trends Cell Biol. 2016;26:6–16.
24. Rogov V, et al. Interactions between autophagy receptors and ubiquitin-like proteins form the molecular basis for selective autophagy. Mol Cell. 2014;53:167–78.
25. Deng Z, et al. Autophagy receptors and neurodegenerative diseases. Trends Cell Biol. 2017;27:491–504.
26. Lee JK, et al. Role of autophagy in the pathogenesis of amyotrophic lateral sclerosis. Biochim Biophys Acta. 2015;1852:2517–24.
27. DeJesus-Hernandez M, et al. Expanded GGGGCC hexanucleotide repeat in noncoding region of C9ORF72 causes chromosome 9p-linked FTD and ALS. Neuron. 2011;72:245–56.
28. Belzil VV, et al. Reduced C9orf72 gene expression in c9FTD/ALS is caused by histone trimethylation, an epigenetic event detectable in blood. Acta Neuropathol. 2013;126:895–905.
29. Gendron TF, et al. Mechanisms of toxicity in C9FTLD/ALS. Acta Neuropathol. 2014;127:359–76.
30. Zhang YJ, et al. Aggregation-prone c9FTD/ALS poly(GA) RAN-translated proteins cause neurotoxicity by inducing ER stress. Acta Neuropathol. 2014; 128:505–24.
31. Lee YB, et al. C9orf72 poly GA RAN-translated protein plays a key role in amyotrophic lateral sclerosis via aggregation and toxicity. Hum Mol Genet. 2017;26(24):4765–77.
32. Su Z, et al. Discovery of a biomarker and lead small molecules to target r(GGGGCC)-associated defects in c9FTD/ALS. Neuron. 2014;83:1043–50.
33. Cooper-Knock J, et al. Clinico-pathological features in amyotrophic lateral sclerosis with expansions in C9ORF72. Brain J Neurol. 2012;135:751–64.
34. Al-Sarraj S, et al. p62 positive, TDP-43 negative, neuronal cytoplasmic and intranuclear inclusions in the cerebellum and hippocampus define the pathology of C9orf72-linked FTLD and MND/ALS. Acta Neuropathol. 2011; 122:691–702.
35. Mackenzie IR, et al. The neuropathology associated with repeat expansions in the C9ORF72 gene. Acta Neuropathol. 2014;127:347–57.
36. Yang M, Liang C, Swaminathan K, et al. A C9ORF72 SMCR8-containing complex regulates ULK1 and plays a dual role in autophagy. Sci Adv. 2016; 2(9):e1601167.
37. Sullivan PM, et al. The ALS/FTLD associated protein C9orf72 associates with SMCR8 and WDR41 to regulate the autophagy-lysosome pathway. Acta Neuropathol Commun. 2016;4:51.
38. Sellier C, et al. Loss of C9ORF72 impairs autophagy and synergizes with polyQ Ataxin-2 to induce motor neuron dysfunction and cell death. EMBO J. 2016;35:1276–97.
39. Webster CP, et al. The C9orf72 protein interacts with Rab1a and the ULK1 complex to regulate initiation of autophagy. EMBO J. 2016;35:1656–76.
40. Kim J, et al. AMPK and mTOR regulate autophagy through direct phosphorylation of Ulk1. Nat Cell Biol. 2011;13:132–41.
41. Hosokawa N, et al. Nutrient-dependent mTORC1 association with the ULK1-Atg13-FIP200 complex required for autophagy. Mol Biol Cell. 2009; 20:1981–91.
42. Jung CH, et al. ULK-Atg13-FIP200 complexes mediate mTOR signaling to the autophagy machinery. Mol Biol Cell. 2009;20:1992–2003.
43. Amick J, et al. C9orf72 binds SMCR8, localizes to lysosomes, and regulates mTORC1 signaling. Mol Biol Cell. 2016;27:3040–51.
44. Ugolino J, et al. Loss of C9orf72 enhances Autophagic activity via deregulated mTOR and TFEB signaling. PLoS Genet. 2016;12:e1006443.
45. Cirulli ET, Lasseigne BN, Petrovski S, Sapp PC, Dion PA, Leblond CS, Couthouis J, et al. Exome sequencing in amyotrophic lateral sclerosis identifies risk genes and pathways. Science. 2015;347:1436–41.
46. Freischmidt A, et al. Haploinsufficiency of TBK1 causes familial ALS and fronto-temporal dementia. Nat Neurosci. 2015;18:631–6.
47. Loo YM, Gale M Jr. Immune signaling by RIG-I-like receptors. Immunity. 2011;34:680–92.
48. Wild P, et al. Phosphorylation of the autophagy receptor optineurin restricts salmonella growth. Science. 2011;333:228–33.
49. Richter B, et al. Phosphorylation of OPTN by TBK1 enhances its binding to Ub chains and promotes selective autophagy of damaged mitochondria. Proc Natl Acad Sci U S A. 2016;113:4039–44.
50. Pilli M, et al. TBK-1 promotes autophagy-mediated antimicrobial defense by controlling autophagosome maturation. Immunity. 2012;37:223–34.
51. Matsumoto G, et al. TBK1 controls autophagosomal engulfment of polyubiquitinated mitochondria through p62/SQSTM1 phosphorylation. Hum Mol Genet. 2015;24:4429–42.
52. Moore AS, Holzbaur EL. Dynamic recruitment and activation of ALS-associated TBK1 with its target optineurin are required for efficient mitophagy. Proc Natl Acad Sci U S A. 2016;113:E3349–58.
53. Li F, et al. Structural insights into the interaction and disease mechanism of neurodegenerative disease-associated optineurin and TBK1 proteins. Nat Commun. 2016;7:12708.
54. Richter B, Sliter DA, Herhaus L, Stolz A, Wang C, Beli P, Zaffagnini G, Wild P, Martens S, Wagner SA, Youle RJ, Dikic I. Phosphorylation of OPTN by TBK1 enhances its binding to Ub chains and promotes selective autophagy of damaged mitochondria. PNAS. 2016;113:4039–44.
55. Korac J, et al. Ubiquitin-independent function of optineurin in autophagic clearance of protein aggregates. J Cell Sci. 2013;126:580–92.
56. Gurney ME, Pu H, Chiu AY, Dal Canto MC, Polchow CY, Alexander DD, Caliendo J, Hentati A, Kwon YW, Deng H-X, Chen W, Zhai P, Sufit RL, Siddique T. Motor neuron degeneration in mice that express a human cu Zn superoxide dismutase mutation. Science. 1994;264:1772–5.
57. Ito Y, et al. RIPK1 mediates axonal degeneration by promoting inflammation and necroptosis in ALS. Science. 2016;353(6299):603–8.

58. Maruyama H, Kawakami H. Optineurin and amyotrophic lateral sclerosis. Geriatr Gerontol Int. 2013;13:528–32.
59. Kamada M, et al. Clinicopathologic features of autosomal recessive amyotrophic lateral sclerosis associated with optineurin mutation. Neuropathology. 2014;34:64–70.
60. Kachaner D, et al. Toward an integrative view of Optineurin functions. Cell Cycle. 2012;11:2808–18.
61. Li C, et al. Optineurin mutations in patients with sporadic amyotrophic lateral sclerosis in China. Amyotroph Lateral Sclerosis Frontotemporal Degeneration. 2015;16:485–9.
62. Pottier C, et al. Whole-genome sequencing reveals important role for TBK1 and OPTN mutations in frontotemporal lobar degeneration without motor neuron disease. Acta Neuropathol. 2015;130:77–92.
63. Deng Z, et al. Autophagy receptors and neurodegenerative diseases. Trends Cell Bio. 2017;27:491–504.
64. Sundaramoorthy V, et al. Defects in optineurin- and myosin VI-mediated cellular trafficking in amyotrophic lateral sclerosis. Hum Mol Genet. 2015;24:3830–46.
65. Blokhuis AM, et al. Comparative interactomics analysis of different ALS-associated proteins identifies converging molecular pathways. Acta Neuropathol. 2016;132(2):175–96.
66. Liu Z, et al. Ubiquitylation of autophagy receptor Optineurin by HACE1 activates selective autophagy for tumor suppression. Cancer Cell. 2014;26:106–20.
67. Shen WC, et al. Mutations in the ubiquitin-binding domain of OPTN/ optineurin interfere with autophagy-mediated degradation of misfolded proteins by a dominant-negative mechanism. Autophagy. 2015;11:685–700.
68. Lim J, et al. Proteotoxic stress induces phosphorylation of p62/SQSTM1 by ULK1 to regulate selective autophagic clearance of protein aggregates. PLoS Genet. 2015;11:e1004987.
69. Ohtsuka S, et al. SQSTM1/p62/A170 regulates the severity of Legionella pneumophila pneumonia by modulating inflammasome activity. Eur J Immunol. 2014;44:1084–92.
70. Kang C, et al. The DNA damage response induces inflammation and senescence by inhibiting autophagy of GATA4. Science. 2015;349:aaa5612.
71. Linares JF, et al. Amino acid activation of mTORC1 by a PB1-domain-driven Kinase complex Cascade. Cell Rep. 2015;12:1339–52.
72. Mizuno Y, et al. Immunoreactivities of p62, an ubiqutin-binding protein, in the spinal anterior horn cells of patients with amyotrophic lateral sclerosis. J Neurol Sci. 2006;249:13–8.
73. Arai T, et al. Neuronal and glial inclusions in frontotemporal dementia with or without motor neuron disease are immunopositive for p62. Neurosci Lett. 2003;342:41–4.
74. Hiji M, et al. White matter lesions in the brain with frontotemporal lobar degeneration with motor neuron disease: TDP-43-immunopositive inclusions co-localize with p62, but not ubiquitin. Acta Neuropathol. 2008; 116:183–91.
75. Matsumoto G, et al. Serine 403 phosphorylation of p62/SQSTM1 regulates selective autophagic clearance of ubiquitinated proteins. Mol Cell. 2011;44:279–89.
76. Pan JA, et al. TRIM21 Ubiquitylates SQSTM1/p62 and suppresses protein sequestration to regulate Redox homeostasis. Mol Cell. 2016;61:720–33.
77. Lee Y, et al. Keap1/Cullin3 modulates p62/SQSTM1 activity via UBA domain Ubiquitination. Cell Rep. 2017;19:188–202.
78. Peng H, et al. Ubiquitylation of p62/sequestosome1 activates its autophagy receptor function and controls selective autophagy upon ubiquitin stress. Cell Res. 2017;27:657–74.
79. Rea SL, et al. SQSTM1 mutations–bridging Paget disease of bone and ALS/ FTLD. Exp Cell Res. 2014;325:27–37.
80. van der Zee J, et al. Rare mutations in SQSTM1 modify susceptibility to frontotemporal lobar degeneration. Acta Neuropathol. 2014;128:397–410.
81. Rea SL, et al. New insights into the role of sequestosome 1/p62 mutant proteins in the pathogenesis of Paget's disease of bone. Endocr Rev. 2013; 34:501–24.
82. Cirulli ET, Lasseigne BN, Goldstein DB. Exome sequencing in amyotrophic lateral sclerosis identifies risk genes and pathways. Science. 2015;347:1436–41.
83. Lattante S, et al. Sqstm1 knock-down causes a locomotor phenotype ameliorated by rapamycin in a zebrafish model of ALS/FTLD. Hum Mol Genet. 2015;24:1682–90.
84. Goode A, et al. Defective recognition of LC3B by mutant SQSTM1/p62 implicates impairment of autophagy as a pathogenic mechanism in ALS-FTLD. Autophagy. 2016;12:1–11.
85. Brady OA, et al. Regulation of TDP-43 aggregation by phosphorylation and p62/SQSTM1. J Neurochem. 2011;116:248–59.
86. Hadano S, et al. Functional links between SQSTM1 and ALS2 in the pathogenesis of ALS: cumulative impact on the protection against mutant SOD1-mediated motor dysfunction in mice. Hum Mol Genet. 2016;25(15):3321–40.
87. Kleijnen MF, et al. The ubiquitin-associated domain of hPLIC-2 interacts with the proteasome. Mol Biol Cell. 2003;14:3868–75.
88. N'Diaye EN, et al. PLIC proteins or ubiquilins regulate autophagy-dependent cell survival during nutrient starvation. EMBO Rep. 2009;10:173–9.
89. Rothenberg C, et al. Ubiquilin functions in autophagy and is degraded by chaperone-mediated autophagy. Hum Mol Genet. 2010;19:3219–32.
90. Deng HX, et al. Mutations in UBQLN2 cause dominant X-linked juvenile and adult-onset ALS and ALS/dementia. Nature. 2011;477:211–5.
91. Dillen L, et al. Explorative genetic study of UBQLN2 and PFN1 in an extended Flanders-Belgian cohort of frontotemporal lobar degeneration patients. Neurobiol Aging. 2013;34(1711):e1711–5.
92. Wu Q, et al. Pathogenic Ubqln2 gains toxic properties to induce neuron death. Acta Neuropathol. 2015;129:417–28.
93. Osaka M, et al. Disturbance of proteasomal and autophagic protein degradation pathways by amyotrophic lateral sclerosis-linked mutations in ubiquilin 2. Biochem Biophys Res Commun. 2016;472:324–31.
94. Hjerpe R, et al. UBQLN2 mediates Autophagy-independent protein aggregate clearance by the Proteasome. Cell. 2016;166:935–49.
95. Ayala YM, Zago P, Ambrogio AD', Xu Y-F, Petrucelli L, Buratti E, Baralle FE. Structural determinants of the cellular localization and shuttling of TDP-43. J Cell Sci. 2008;121:3778–85.
96. Neumann M, Sampathu DM, Kwong LK, Truax AC, Micsenyi MC, Chou TT, Bruce J, Schuck T, Grossman M, Clark CM, LF MC, Miller BL, Masliah E, Mackenzie IR, Feldman H, Feiden W, Kretzschmar HA, Trojanowski JQ, Lee VM. Ubiquitinated TDP-43 in frontotemporal lobar degeneration and amyotrophic lateral sclerosis. Science. 2006; 314:130–3.
97. Lagier-Tourenne C, Cleveland DW. Rethinking ALS: the FUS about TDP-43. Cell. 2009;136:1001–4.
98. Scotter EL, et al. Differential roles of the ubiquitin proteasome system and autophagy in the clearance of soluble and aggregated TDP-43 species. J Cell Sci. 2014;127:1263–78.
99. Wang X, et al. Degradation of TDP-43 and its pathogenic form by autophagy and the ubiquitin-proteasome system. Neurosci Lett. 2010; 469:112–6.
100. Wang I-F, G.B.-S., Liu Y-C, Wu C-C, Yang C-H, Tsai K-J, Shen C-KJ (2012) Autophagy activators rescue and alleviate pathogenesis of a mouse model with proteinopathies of the TAR DNA-binding protein 43. Proc Natl Acad Sci U S A 109: 15024 –15029.
101. Caccamo A, et al. Reduced protein turnover mediates functional deficits in transgenic mice expressing the 25 kDa C-terminal fragment of TDP-43. Hum Mol Genet. 2015;24:4625–35.
102. Bose JK, et al. Regulation of autophagy by neuropathological protein TDP-43. J Biol Chem. 2011;286:44441–8.
103. Xia Q, et al. TDP-43 loss of function increases TFEB activity and blocks autophagosome-lysosome fusion. EMBO J. 2016;35:121–42.
104. Li YR, et al. Stress granules as crucibles of ALS pathogenesis. J Cell Biol. 2013;201:361–72.
105. Monahan Z, et al. Stress granules at the intersection of autophagy and ALS. Brain Res. 2016;1649:189–200.
106. Bosco DA, et al. Mutant FUS proteins that cause amyotrophic lateral sclerosis incorporate into stress granules. Hum Mol Genet. 2010;19:4160–75.
107. Colombrita C, et al. TDP-43 is recruited to stress granules in conditions of oxidative insult. J Neurochem. 2009;111:1051–61.
108. Vance C, et al. Mutations in FUS, an RNA processing protein, cause familial amyotrophic lateral sclerosis type 6. Science. 2009;323:1208–11.
109. Kwiatkowski TJ, Bosco DA, Leclerc AL, Tamrazian E, Vanderburg CR, Russ C, et al. Mutations in the FUS TLS gene on chromosome 16 cause familial amyotrophic lateral sclerosis. Science. 2009;323:1205–8.
110. Ryu HH, et al. Autophagy regulates amyotrophic lateral sclerosis-linked fused in sarcoma-positive stress granules in neurons. Neurobiol Aging. 2014; 35:2822–31.

111. Baron DM, et al. Amyotrophic lateral sclerosis-linked FUS TLS alters stress granule assembly and dynamics. Mol Neurodegener. 2013;8:30.
112. Buchan JR, et al. Eukaryotic stress granules are cleared by autophagy and Cdc48/VCP function. Cell. 2013;153:1461–74.
113. Thomas MG, et al. RNA granules: the good, the bad and the ugly. Cell Signal. 2011;23:324–34.
114. Kim HJ, et al. Therapeutic modulation of eIF2alpha phosphorylation rescues TDP-43 toxicity in amyotrophic lateral sclerosis disease models. Nat Genet. 2014;46:152–60.
115. Stolz A, et al. Cdc48: a power machine in protein degradation. Trends Biochem Sci. 2011;36:515–23.
116. Chapman E, et al. The complexities of p97 function in health and disease. Mol bio Syst. 2011;7:700–10.
117. Uchiyama K, Kondo H. p97/p47-mediated biogenesis of Golgi and ER. J Biochem. 2005;137:115–9.
118. Meyer H, et al. Emerging functions of the VCP/p97 AAA-ATPase in the ubiquitin system. Nat Cell Biol. 2012;14:117–23.
119. Watts GD, et al. Inclusion body myopathy associated with Paget disease of bone and frontotemporal dementia is caused by mutant valosin-containing protein. Nat Genet. 2004;36:377–81.
120. Johnson JO, et al. Exome sequencing reveals VCP mutations as a cause of familial ALS. Neuron. 2010;68:857–64.
121. Hubbers CU, et al. Pathological consequences of VCP mutations on human striated muscle. Brain J Neurol. 2007;130:381–93.
122. Schroder R, et al. Mutant valosin-containing protein causes a novel type of frontotemporal dementia. Ann Neurol. 2005;57:457–61.
123. Custer SK, et al. Transgenic mice expressing mutant forms VCP/p97 recapitulate the full spectrum of IBMPFD including degeneration in muscle, brain and bone. Hum Mol Genet. 2010;19:1741–55.
124. Ju JS, et al. Valosin-containing protein (VCP) is required for autophagy and is disrupted in VCP disease. J Cell Biol. 2009;187:875–88.
125. Dargemont C, Ossareh-Nazari B. Cdc48/p97, a key actor in the interplay between autophagy and ubiquitin/proteasome catabolic pathways. Biochim Biophys Acta. 2012;1823:138–44.
126. Krick R, et al. Cdc48/p97 and Shp1/p47 regulate autophagosome biogenesis in concert with ubiquitin-like Atg8. J Cell Biol. 2010;190:965–73.
127. Ching JK, et al. mTOR dysfunction contributes to vacuolar pathology and weakness in valosin-containing protein associated inclusion body myopathy. Hum Mol Genet. 2013;22:1167–79.
128. Papadopoulos C, et al. VCP/p97 cooperates with YOD1, UBXD1 and PLAA to drive clearance of ruptured lysosomes by autophagy. EMBO J. 2017;36:135–50.
129. Tanaka A, et al. Proteasome and p97 mediate mitophagy and degradation of mitofusins induced by Parkin. J Cell Biol. 2010;191:1367–80.
130. Renton AE, et al. State of play in amyotrophic lateral sclerosis genetics. Nat Neurosci. 2013;17:17–23.
131. Kato S. Amyotrophic lateral sclerosis models and human neuropathology: similarities and differences. Acta Neuropathol. 2008;115:97–114.
132. Galaleldeen A, et al. Structural and biophysical properties of metal-free pathogenic SOD1 mutants A4V and G93A. Arch Biochem Biophys. 2009; 492:40–7.
133. Schmidlin T, et al. Structural changes to monomeric CuZn superoxide dismutase caused by the familial amyotrophic lateral sclerosis-associated mutation A4V. Biophys J. 2009;97:1709–18.
134. Kabuta T, et al. Degradation of amyotrophic lateral sclerosis-linked mutant cu,Zn-superoxide dismutase proteins by macroautophagy and the proteasome. J Biol Chem. 2006;281:30524–33.
135. Meissner F, Molawi K, Zychlinsky A. Mutant superoxide dismutase 1-induced IL-1beta accelerates ALS pathogenesis. PNAS. 2010;107:13046–50.
136. Hadano S, et al. Functional links between SQSTM1 and ALS2 in the pathogenesis of ALS: cumulative impact on the protection against mutant SOD1-mediated motor dysfunction in mice. Hum Mol Genet. 2016;25:3321–40.
137. Rudnick ND, Griffey CJ, Guarnieri P, Gerbino V, Wang X, Piersaint JA, Tapia JC, Rich MM, Maniatis T. Distinct roles for motor neuron autophagy early and late in the SOD1G93A mouse model of ALS. PNAS. 2017;114:E8294–303.
138. Keiko Imamura YI, Inoue H. The Src c-Abl pathway is a potential therapeutic target in amyotrophic lateral sclerosis. Sci Transl Med. 2017;9:eaaf 3962.
139. Xie Y, et al. Endolysosomal deficits augment mitochondria pathology in spinal motor neurons of asymptomatic fALS mice. Neuron. 2015;87:355–70.
140. Nassif M, et al. Pathogenic role of BECN1/Beclin 1 in the development of amyotrophic lateral sclerosis. Autophagy. 2014;10:1256–71.
141. Chen Y, Liu H, Guan Y, Wang Q, Zhou F, Jie L, Ju J, Pu L, Du H, Wang X. The altered autophagy mediated by TFEB in animal and cell models of amyotrophic lateral sclerosis. Am J Transl Res. 2015;7(9):1574–87.
142. Bandyopadhyay U, et al. Absence of lipofuscin in motor neurons of SOD1-linked ALS mice. Proc Natl Acad Sci U S A. 2014;111:11055–60.
143. Morimoto N, et al. Increased autophagy in transgenic mice with a G93A mutant SOD1 gene. Brain Res. 2007;1167:112–7.
144. Hadano S, et al. Molecular and cellular function of ALS2/alsin: implication of membrane dynamics in neuronal development and degeneration. Neurochem Int. 2007;51:74–84.
145. Eker HK, et al. A novel homozygous mutation in ALS2 gene in four siblings with infantile-onset ascending hereditary spastic paralysis. Eur J Med Genet. 2014;57:275–8.
146. Wakil SM, et al. Infantile-onset ascending hereditary spastic paraplegia with bulbar involvement due to the novel ALS2 mutation c.2761C>T. Gene. 2014; 536:217–20.
147. Topp JD, et al. Alsin is a Rab5 and Rac1 guanine nucleotide exchange factor. J Biol Chem. 2004;279:24612–23.
148. Kunita R, et al. The Rab5 activator ALS2/alsin acts as a novel Rac1 effector through Rac1-activated endocytosis. J Biol Chem. 2007;282:16599–611.
149. Otomo A. ALS2, a novel guanine nucleotide exchange factor for the small GTPase Rab5, is implicated in endosomal dynamics. Hum Mol Genet. 2003; 12:1671–87.
150. Otomo A, et al. Defective relocalization of ALS2/alsin missense mutants to Rac1-induced macropinosomes accounts for loss of their cellular function and leads to disturbed amphisome formation. FEBS Lett. 2011;585:730–6.
151. Kanekura K, et al. Alsin, the product of ALS2 gene, suppresses SOD1 mutant neurotoxicity through RhoGEF domain by interacting with SOD1 mutants. J Biol Chem. 2004;279:19247–56.
152. Lev S, et al. The VAP protein family: from cellular functions to motor neuron disease. Trends Cell Biol. 2008;18:282–90.
153. Kuijpers M, et al. The ALS8 protein VAPB interacts with the ER-Golgi recycling protein YIF1A and regulates membrane delivery into dendrites. EMBO J. 2013;32:2056–72.
154. De Vos KJ, et al. VAPB interacts with the mitochondrial protein PTPIP51 to regulate calcium homeostasis. Hum Mol Genet. 2012;21:1299–311.
155. Gomez-Suaga P, et al. The ER-mitochondria tethering complex VAPB-PTPIP51 regulates Autophagy. Curr Biol. 2017;27:371–85.
156. Nishimura, A.L. (2004) A novel locus for late onset amyotrophic lateral sclerosis/motor neurone disease variant at 20q13. J Med Genet 41, 315-320.
157. Kabashi E, et al. Investigating the contribution of VAPB/ALS8 loss of function in amyotrophic lateral sclerosis. Hum Mol Genet. 2013;22:2350–60.
158. Chattopadhyay D, Sengupta S. First evidence of pathogenicity of V234I mutation of hVAPB found in amyotrophic lateral sclerosis. Biochem Biophys Res Commun. 2014;448:108–13.
159. Larroquette F, et al. Vapb/amyotrophic lateral sclerosis 8 knock-in mice display slowly progressive motor behavior defects accompanying ER stress and autophagic response. Hum Mol Genet. 2015;24:6515–29.
160. Hayashi T, Su TP. Sigma-1 receptor chaperones at the ER-mitochondrion interface regulate ca(2+) signaling and cell survival. Cell. 2007;131:596–610.
161. Al-Saif A, et al. A mutation in sigma-1 receptor causes juvenile amyotrophic lateral sclerosis. Ann Neurol. 2011;70:913–9.
162. Vollrath JT, et al. Loss of function of the ALS protein SigR1 leads to ER pathology associated with defective autophagy and lipid raft disturbances. Cell Death Dis. 2014;5:e1290.
163. Dreser A, et al. The ALS-linked E102Q mutation in sigma receptor-1 leads to ER stress-mediated defects in protein homeostasis and dysregulation of RNA-binding proteins. Cell Death Differ. 2017;24:1655–71.
164. Watanabe Y, et al. HSF1 stress response pathway regulates autophagy receptor SQSTM1/p62-associated proteostasis. Autophagy. 2017;13:133–48.
165. Soo KY, et al. ALS-associated mutant FUS inhibits macroautophagy which is restored by overexpression of Rab1. Cell Death Discov. 2015;1:15030.

7

Genetic ablation of dynactin p150^{Glued} in postnatal neurons causes preferential degeneration of spinal motor neurons in aged mice

Jia Yu[1,2], Chen Lai[2,5], Hoon Shim[2,6], Chengsong Xie[2], Lixin Sun[2], Cai-Xia Long[2,7], Jinhui Ding[3], Yan Li[4] and Huaibin Cai[2*]

Abstract

Background: Dynactin p150^{Glued}, the largest subunit of the dynactin macromolecular complex, binds to both microtubules and tubulin dimers through the N-terminal cytoskeleton-associated protein and glycine-rich (CAP-Gly) and basic domains, and serves as an anti-catastrophe factor in stabilizing microtubules in neurons. P150^{Glued} also initiates dynein-mediated axonal retrograde transport. Multiple missense mutations at the CAP-Gly domain of p150^{Glued} are associated with motor neuron diseases and other neurodegenerative disorders, further supporting the importance of microtubule domains (MTBDs) in p150^{Glued} functions. However, most functional studies were performed in vitro. Whether p150^{Glued} is required for neuronal function and survival in vivo is unknown.

Methods: Using Cre-loxP genetic manipulation, we first generated a line of p150^{Glued} knock-in mice by inserting two *LoxP* sites flanking the MTBD-coding exons 2 to 4 of p150^{Glued}–encoding *Dctn1* gene (*Dctn1*$^{LoxP/}$), and then crossbred the resulting *Dctn1*$^{LoxP/}$ mice with *Thy1-Cre* mice to generate the bigenic p150^{Glued} (*Dctn1*$^{LoxP/LoxP}$; *Thy1-Cre*) conditional knockout (cKO) mice for the downstream motor behavioral and neuropathological studies.

Results: P150^{Glued} expression was completely abolished in Cre-expressing postnatal neurons, including corticospinal motor neurons (CSMNs) and spinal motor neurons (SMNs), while the MTBD–truncated forms remained. P150^{Glued} ablation did not affect the formation of dynein/dynactin complex in neurons. The p150^{Glued} cKO mice did not show any obvious developmental phenotypes, but exhibited impairments in motor coordination and rearing after 12 months of age. Around 20% loss of SMNs was found in the lumbar spinal cord of 18-month-old cKO mice, in company with increased gliosis, neuromuscular junction (NMJ) disintegration and muscle atrophy. By contrast, no obvious degeneration of CSMNs, striatal neurons, midbrain dopaminergic neurons, cerebellar granule cells or Purkinje cells was observed. Abnormal accumulation of acetylated α-tubulin, and autophagosome/lysosome proteins was found in the SMNs of aged cKO mice. Additionally, the total and cell surface levels of glutamate receptors were also substantially elevated in the p150^{Glued}-depleted spinal neurons, in correlation with increased vulnerability to excitotoxicity.

Conclusion: Overall, our findings demonstrate that p150^{Glued} is particularly required to maintain the function and survival of SMNs during aging. P150^{Glued} may exert its protective function through regulating the transportation of autophagosomes, lysosomes, and postsynaptic glutamate receptors in neurons.

Keywords: Dynactin p150^{Glued}, Dynein, Microtubule binding domain, Motor neuron, Neurodegeneration, Autophagy, Lysosome, Glutamate receptor, Excitotoxicity

* Correspondence: caih@mail.nih.gov
[2]Transgenic Section, Laboratory of Neurogenetics, National Institute on Aging, National Institutes of Health, Building 35, Room 1A112, MSC 3707, 35 Convent Drive, Bethesda, MD 20892–3707, USA
Full list of author information is available at the end of the article

Background

Impairments in intracellular transport are often associated with neurological disorders, including Alzheimer's disease, Huntington's disease, Parkinson's disease and amyotrophic lateral sclerosis (ALS) [1]. Dynein mediates the retrograde transport of cargos from microtubule plus ends to the minus ends, while the dynactin protein complex is proposed to promote the processivity of dynein motor proteins moving along the microtubules, as well as expand the variety of dynein cargoes [2, 3]. Dynactin consists of more than 20 subunits, with its largest subunit p150^{Glued} to interact with both microtubules and dynein motor protein complex [2]. P150^{Glued}, encoded by the full-length *DCTN1* gene, weights around 150 kD and contains the N-terminal CAP-Gly and basic domains, followed by the coiled-coil 1 (CC1) and CC2 domains [2]. Both the CAP-Gly and basic domains exhibit microtubule binding affinity, and together form the tandem MTBDs [4]. On the other hand, the CC1 and CC2 domains mediate the interactions with dynein intermediate chain (DIC) and the other dynactin subunits [2]. The MTBDs of p150^{Glued} are required for cell division by providing essential attachment to the microtubules in spindle formation and chromosome movement [5], p150^{Glued} inhibition causes cell proliferation arrest [6] and germline deletion of p150^{Glued} leads to early embryonic lethality [7]. Multiple missense mutations in the CAP-Gly domain of p150^{Glued} have been linked to a slowly progressive, autosomal dominant form of lower motor neuron disease without sensory symptoms [8]; Perry syndrome, which consists of parkinsonism with severe mental depression and central hypoventilation [9]; and progressive supranuclear palsy [10]. P150^{Glued} is proposed as an anti-catastrophe factor in maintaining the stability of microtubules in neurons, and facilitate the dynein-mediated axonal retrograde transport in neuronal cultures [11]. These disease-causal mutations seem to weaken the microtubule binding affinity of p150^{Glued} [3]. However, the functional significance of p150^{Glued} has not been critically evaluated in neurons in living animals.

In addition to p150^{Glued}, *DCTN1* also encodes p135 and other short splicing variants [12]. P135 lacks the coding exons 2 to 5, resulting in a complete loss of the CAP-Gly domain and a large portion of basic domain. P150^{Glued} is expressed in all types of mammalian cells, while p135 is more abundant in neurons [13]. Dynein/dynactin is required for the mitosis as germline deletion of p150^{Glued} caused early embryonic lethality and apoptosis in p150^{Glued} knockout mice [7]. However, p135 can compensate for the most dynactin activity in p150^{glued}-deficient post-mitotic cells [12]. These observations raise questions about the overall importance of p150^{Glued} in neurons, despite mutations in its CAP-Gly domain are associated with multiple neurological disorders. One possible scenario is that p150^{Glued} proteins are particularly needed to maintain the integrity of microtubule network and the efficiency of axonal retrograde transport in the large projection neurons with long axons, such as the CSMNS and SMNs.

In this study, we utilized Cre-loxP system [14] to selectively deplete p150^{Glued} but keep p135 expression in CSMNs and SMNs. To our surprise, genetic ablation of p150^{Glued} in postnatal neurons did not cause overt behavioral and neuropathological phenotypes in mice. Only moderate motor deficits and SMN loss were observed in aged p150^{Glued} cKO mice. The p150^{Glued}-lacking neurons appeared to be more susceptible to excitotoxicity in correlation with abnormal augmentations of total and surface expression of glutamate receptors, a potential pathogenic mechanism of SMN degeneration in p150^{Glued} cKO mice.

Methods

Generation of *Dctn1*$^{LoxP/}$ knock-in mice and *Dctn1*$^{LoxP/LoxP}$; *Cre* conditional knockout mice

Genomic DNA fragments containing *Dctn1* gene locus were isolated from a mouse genomic DNA library (Stratagene). A 9.3 kb KpnI/AflII fragment carrying exons 2–4 of *Dctn1* was subcloned into the pBluescript vector for later modifications. To construct the targeting vector, the *Dctn1* clone was modified by inserting the first loxP site and a neomycin (Neo) selection cassette flanked with two Frt sites in intron 1, and the second loxP site in intron 4 (Fig. 1a). The targeting vector was linearized at a unique NotI site and transfected into 129/SvJ ES cells. After neomycin resistance (Neo) positive selection with G418 for 7 days, ES clones that had undergone homologous recombination were picked and screened by PCR, Southern blot analysis and partial genome sequencing (Fig. 1b). Two positive ES clones were expanded and injected into blastocysts. The resulting male chimera mice were bred with wild-type C57BL/6 J female mice to obtain *Dctn1*$^{LoxP\text{-}Frt\text{-}Neo\text{-}Frt}$ mice. The *Dctn1*$^{LoxP\text{-}Frt\text{-}Neo\text{-}Frt}$ mice were then cross-bred with FLPe knock-in mice [15] (JAX, stock number: 003946) to remove Neo selection marker and get *Dctn1*$^{LoxP/}$ mice. Finally, the *Dctn1*$^{LoxP/}$ mice were crossed with *Thy1-Cre* [16] (JAX, Stock Number: 006143) or *Cre/Esr1* [17] (JAX, Stock Number: 004682) mice to delete exons 2 to 4 and thereby the MTBD-containing p150^{Glued} from the Cre-expressing cells. The mice were housed in a 12 h light/dark cycle and fed regular diet ad libitum. All mouse work followed the guidelines approved by the Institutional Animal Care and Use Committees of the National Institute on Aging, NIH.

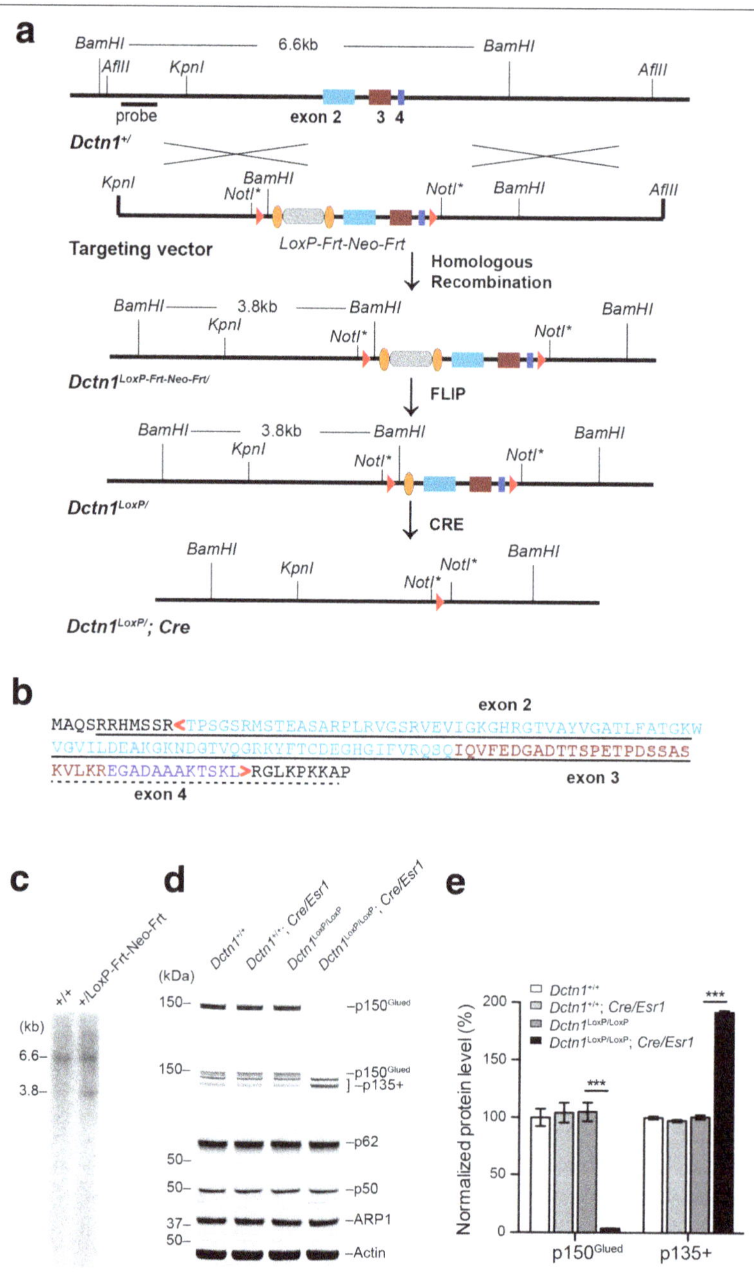

Fig. 1 Genetic deletion of p150^{Glued} in *Dctn1*$^{LoxP/}$; *Cre* mice. **a** The schematic diagram depicts the generation of *Dctn1*$^{LoxP/}$; *Cre* mice in which the exon 2–4 of *Dctn1* gene is deleted. **b** Amino acid sequence highlights residues encoded by exon 2 (light blue), exon 3 (brown), and exon 4 (navy blue). The CAP-Gly domain was marked by solid line. The basic domain was indicated by dash line. **c** Southern blot of genomic DNAs isolated from mouse embryonic stem (ES) cell clones shows a correct gene targeting of the *Dctn1* gene locus in *Dctn1*$^{+/LoxP\text{-}Frt\text{-}Neo\text{-}Frt}$ ES cell clones. As predicted, the insertion of the LoxP-Frt-Neo-Frt gene-targeting cassette into the *Dctn1* gene locus generated a new 3.8 kb *BamHI* fragment in *Dctn1*$^{+/LoxP\text{-}Frt\text{-}Neo\text{-}Frt}$ ES cell clones. **d-e** Western blot analysis shows the protein levels of p150^{Glued}, p135+, p62, p50 and ARP1 in cultured *Dctn1*$^{+/+}$, *Dctn1*$^{+/+}$; *Cre/Esr1*, *Dctn1*$^{LoxP/LoxP}$ and *Dctn1*$^{LoxP/LoxP}$; *Cre/Esr1* cortical neurons at 7 days in vitro (DIV). Actin was used as loading control. Bar graphs show the quantification of p150^{Glued} and p135+ levels normalized with actin ($n = 3$ per genotype). Data were presented as mean ± SEM. One-way ANOVA plus Tukey's post hoc test was used for statistical analysis. $^{***}p < 0.001$ for difference against *Dctn1*$^{LoxP/LoxP}$; *Cre/Esr1*, while no difference was found among *Dctn1*$^{+/+}$, *Dctn1*$^{+/+}$; *Cre/Esr1 and Dctn1*$^{LoxP/LoxP}$

Genotyping

Genomic DNA was prepared from tail biopsy using DirectPCR Lysis Reagent (Viagen Biotech) and subjected to PCR amplification using specific sets of PCR primers for each genotype, including *Dctn1*$^{LoxP/}$ knock-in mice (mDCTN1-Ex4-F, CAG CTG CAA AGA CCA GCA AA; mDCTN1-Ex5-R: CAC ACC ACC TTC TTA GGC TTC A), *Cre* transgenic mice (CRE-F, CAT TTG GGC

CAG CTA AAC AT; CRE-R, TGC ATG ATC TCC GGT ATT GA).

Sucrose density gradient fractionation and sedimentation analysis

Neuronal cells or neural tissues were homogenized in 50 mM Tris-HCl, pH 7.5, containing 150 mM NaC1, 1 mM EDTA and Protease Inhibitor Cocktail (Thermo Scientific). The cytosolic extracts were prepared by centrifugation at 16,000 × g for 15 min at 4 °C, and further clarified at 100,000 × g for 15 min. The resulting supernatant was layered over a 12 ml, 5–20% sucrose density gradient and centrifuged at 120,000 × g for 18 h at 4 °C. 1-ml gradient fractions were collected and equal volumes of all fractions analyzed by SDS-PAGE followed by Western blotting.

Behavior tests

Open-field test. As described previously [18], the ambulatory and rearing activities of male mice were measured by the Flex-Field Activity System (San Diego Instruments). Flex-Field software was used to trace and quantify mouse movement in the unit as the number of beam breaks per 30 min.

Rotarod test. As described previously [19], male mice were placed onto a rotating rod with auto-acceleration from 0 rpm to 40 rpm for 1 min (San Diego Instruments). The length of time the mouse stayed on the rotating rod was recorded. Three measurements were taken for each animal during each test.

Hindlimb clasping test. In the hindlimb clasping test, male mice were suspended by the tail and observed for 10 s. The severity of hindlimb clasping phenotype was scored as follows: 0 = both hindlimbs consistently spread outward and away from the abdomen, 1 = one hindlimb retracted toward the abdomen, 2 = both hindlimbs partially retracted toward the abdomen, 3 = both hindlimbs completely retracted toward the abdomen. For each mouse, three separate tests were taken over 3 h, and the averaged hindlimb clasping severity score of the three tests was calculated.

Histology, immunohistochemistry and light microscopy

For neuropathology study, mice were perfused with 4% paraformaldehyde (PFA) in cold phosphate buffered saline (PBS), brains and spinal cords were collected, post-fixed overnight, submerged in 30% sucrose in PBS for at least 72 h, and sectioned at 40–50 μm thickness using CM1950 cryostat (Leica). For muscle pathology analysis, mice were euthanized, gastrocnemius muscles were dissected, snap frozen in 2-methylbutane (Sigma-Aldrich) cooled in dry ice, sectioned at 20 or 40 μm thickness, and fixed in 4% PFA in PBS for 15 min. For Nissl staining, sections were stained with 0.1% Cresyl Violet (Sigma-Aldrich). For HE staining, hematoxylin and eosin stain kit (Vector Laboratories) were used as suggested by manufacturers. For immunostaining, antibodies specific to p150^{Glued} N-terminus (amino acid 3–202, 1:200, BD Biosciences), p150^{Glued} C-terminus (amino acid 1266–1278, 1:500, Abcam), neuron-specific nuclear protein (NeuN, 1:1000, Millipore), CTIP2 (1:200, Abcam), choline acetyltransferase (CHAT, 1:500, Millipore), Glial Fibrillary Acidic Protein (GFAP, 1:1000, Abcam), Ionized calcium-Binding Adaptor Molecule-1 (IBA1, 1:1000, Wako Chemicals), acetylated α-tubulin (ac-TUBA, 1:500, Abcam), Lysosomal Associated Membrane Protein 2 (LAMP2, 1:200, Abcam), Tyrosine Hydroxylase (TH, 1:500, Pel-Freeze) and Calbindin D28K (1:200, Abcam) were used as suggested by manufacturers. For immunofluorescence study, Alexa Fluor 488-, 546- or 647-conjugated secondary antibody (1:500, Invitrogen) was used to visualize the staining. Alexa Fluor 488-conjugated α-bungarotoxin (1:500, Invitrogen) was applied to label postsynaptic acetylcholine receptors of NMJs. Fluorescence images were captured using LSM 780 laser-scanning confocal microscope (Zeiss). The paired images in all the figures were collected at the same gain and offset settings. Post collection processing was applied uniformly to all paired images. The images were presented as either a single optic layer after acquisition in z-series stack scans at 1.0 μm intervals from individual fields or displayed as maximum-intensity projections to represent confocal stacks. For immunohistochemistry study, Vectastain Elite ABC Kit and DAB Kit (Vector Laboratories) were used to visualize the staining. Bright field images were captured by Axio microscope Imager A1 (Zeiss).

Image analysis

For the quantitative assessment of various marker protein distributions, images were taken using identical settings and exported to ImageJ (NIH) for imaging analysis. Images were converted to an 8-bit color scale (fluorescence intensity from 0 to 255) using ImageJ. The areas of interest were first selected with Polygon or Freehand selection tools and then subjected to measurement by mean optical intensities or area fractions. The mean intensity for the background area was subtracted from the selected area to determine the net mean intensity.

Stereology

Stereology for CSMNs, striatal neurons, SMNs and midbrain dopaminergic neurons was performed as described previously [19, 20]. To examine the number of CSMNs and striatal neurons, series of sagittal brain sections (40 μm per section thickness, every ninth section, nine sections per case) were processed for Nissl staining or CTIP2 immunohistochemistry. The motor cortex was designated as layer V neurons in the anteromedial cortex, and outlined according to the mouse brain in stereotaxic coordinates. To examine the number of SMNs, series of coronal spinal cord sections (50 μm per section, every tenth section from L3 to L5, ten sections per case) were processed for Nissl staining or CHAT immunohistochemistry. To examine the number of midbrain dopaminergic neurons, series of coronal sections across the midbrain (40 μm per section, every fourth section from Bregma − 2.54 to − 4.24 mm, ten sections per case) were processed for TH immunohistochemistry. For the unbiased stereological estimation of CSMNs, striatal neurons, SMNs and midbrain dopaminergic neurons, the number of CTIP2 positive or Nissl-stained large (>15 μm in diameter) cortical neurons in layer V, Nissl-stained neurons in stratum, CHAT positive or Nissl-stained large (>35 μm in diameter) spinal neurons in ventral horn, and TH-positive neurons in substantia nigra pars compacta (SNpc) were assessed using the Optical Fractionator function of Stereo Investigator 10 (MicroBrightField). Six mice were used per genotype at each time point. Counters were blinded to the genotypes of the samples. The sampling scheme was designed to have a coefficient of error less than 10% in order to obtain reliable results.

Preparation of postsynaptic density (PSD) fraction

PSD fractions were prepared from mouse brains as described previously [18]. All procedures were performed at 4 °C. Mouse brains were isolated and homogenized in 10 volumes of ice-cold Buffer A (0.32 M sucrose, 5 mM HEPES, pH 7.4, 1 mM $MgCl_2$, 0.5 mM $CaCl_2$, Protease and Phosphatase Inhibitor Cocktail) with Teflon homogenizer (12 strokes). The homogenate was spun at 1400 × *g* for 10 min. Supernatant (S1') was saved and pellet (P1') was homogenized again with Teflon homogenizer in another 10 volumes of Buffer A (5 strokes). After centrifugation at 700 × *g* for 10 min, the supernatant (S1') was collected and pooled with S1, and the pellet (P1') were saved as crude nuclear fraction. Pooled S1 and S1' were centrifuged at 13,800 × *g* for 10 min to collect the crude synaptosomal pellet (P2) and the supernatant (S2), which contains the cytosol and light membranes. S2 was centrifuged at 100,000 × g for 15 min to separate the cytosolic fraction (Cyt) and the light membrane fraction (LM). P2 was resuspended in 10 volumes of Buffer B (0.32 M sucrose, 6 mM Tris, pH 8.0, supplemented with Protease and Phosphatase Inhibitor Cocktail) with Teflon homogenizer (5 strokes). The P2 suspension was loaded onto a discontinuous sucrose gradient (0.85 M/1 M/1.15 M sucrose solution in 6 mM Tris, pH 8.0), and centrifuged at 82,500 × *g* for 2 h. Synaptosome fraction (Syn) was collected from the layer between 1 M and 1.15 M sucrose, supplemented with 0.5% Triton X-100 and mixed for 15 min. The suspension was spun at 32,800 × *g* for 20 min, and the resulting pellet was saved as PSD fraction (PSD). P1', LM and PSD fractions were lysed in 1% SDS buffer. SDS were added into Cyt and Syn fraction to 1% final concentration. Equal amount of total protein from each fraction were resolved in SDS-PAGE and applied to western blot analysis.

Primary neuron culture

Mouse primary neuron cultures were prepared from the cortex or spinal cord of newborn (postnatal day 0, P0) pups, as described previously [21, 22]. Briefly, individual cortex or spinal cord was dissected and subjected to papain digestion (5 U/ml, Worthington Biochemicals) for 40 min at 37 °C. The digested tissue was carefully triturated into single cells using increasingly smaller pipette tips. The cells were then centrifuged at 250 × g for 5 min and resuspended in warm Basal Medium Eagle (BME, Sigma-Aldrich) supplemented with 5% heat-inactivated fetal bovine serum (FBS; Invitrogen), 1× N2/B27 supplement (100× stock, Invitrogen), 1× GlutaMax (100× stock, Invitrogen), 0.45% D-glucose (Sigma-Aldrich), 10 U/ml penicillin (Invitrogen), and 10 μg/ml streptomycin (Invitrogen). The dissociated neurons were seeded in plated in Biocoat Poly-D-Lysine Cellware plate (BD Biosciences), and maintained at 37 °C in a 95% O_2 and 5% CO_2 humidified incubator. Twenty-four hours after seeding, the cultures were switched to serum-free medium supplemented with 1 μM cytosine β-D-arabinofuranoside (Sigma-Aldrich) to suppress the proliferation of glia and 1 μM 4-hydroxytamoxifen (4-OHT, Sigma-Aldrich) to induce CRE recombinase activity. Starting from 5 days in vitro (DIV), culture medium was changed twice every week.

Biotinylation of neuronal surface proteins

Spinal neurons were cultured at the density of 1.2 × 10^6 per well in Poly-D-Lysine coated 6-Well plate (BD Biosciences) and treated with 0 or 10 μM glutamate (Sigma-Aldrich) on 20 DIV. After 24-h treatment, neurons were washed with PBS containing 0.1 mM $CaCl_2$ and 1 mM $MgCl_2$ (PBS/CM), and then incubated with 1 ml biotin solution (0.5 mg/ml Sulfo-NHS-SS-Biotin in cold PBS/CM, Thermo Fisher Scientific) for 20 min at 4 °C and then washed subsequently with PBS/CM, 0.1 M glycine solution, and TBS (25 mM Tris-HCl, pH 7.4, containing 137 mM NaCl) buffer. Cells were harvested in 250 μl RIPA buffer (Sigma) supplemented with protease inhibitor and phosphatase inhibitor cocktail, lysed on ice for 30 min, and centrifuged at 16,000 × g for 15 min at 4 ° C. Resulting supernatant containing equal amount of total protein was incubated with 50 μl neutral-avidin agarose (Pierce) at 4 °C for 2 h with gently rotating.

After washing in RIPA buffer for 5 times, the biotin-labeled surface protein was eluted with SDS sample buffer by heating at 70 °C for 10 min. Total proteins and isolated biotinylated surface proteins were analyzed by western blotting.

Assessment of cell survival by 3-(4, 5-Dimethylthiazol-2-yl)-2, 5-diphenyl-tetrazolium bromide (MTT) assay

Spinal neurons were cultured at the density of 1.0×10^5 per well in Poly-D-Lysine coated 96-Well plate (BD Biosciences) and treated with 0 or 10 μM glutamate (Sigma-Aldrich) on 20 DIV. After 24-h treatment, the cells were incubated with 0.5 mg/ml MTT (Sigma-Aldrich) at 37 ° C for 4 h. After the media were removed, dimethyl sulfoxide (DMSO, 100 μl) was added to each well to solubilize the formazan crystals generated by viable mitochondrial succinate dehydrogenase from MTT. The absorbance at 570 nm was measured using a SpectraMax M5 Multi-Mode Microplate Reader (Molecular Devices) as the MTT reducing activity of the cells.

Western blot analysis

Neurons or tissues were homogenized and sonicated in RIPA buffer (Sigma-Aldrich) or 1% SDS lysis buffer (50 mM Tris–HCl, 150 mM NaCl, 2 mM EDTA, pH 7.5, and 1% SDS) supplemented with Protease Inhibitor Cocktails (Thermo Scientific). Lysates were clarified by centrifugation at 15000 × g for 15 min at 4 °C. The supernatants were quantified for protein content using the bicinchoninic acid (BCA) assay kit (Thermo Fisher Scientific) and separated by 4–12% NuPage BisTris-PAGE (Invitrogen) using MES or MOPS running buffer (Invitrogen). The separated proteins were then transferred to nitrocellulose membranes using the iBlot Dry Blotting system (Invitrogen) and incubated with specific primary antibodies. The antibodies used for western blot analysis included p150^{Glued} N-terminus (amino acid 3–202, 1:1000, BD Biosciences), p150^{Glued} C-terminus (amino acid 1266–1278, 1:1000, Abcam), dynactin subunit p62 (1:1000, Abcam), dynactin subunit p50 (1:5000, BD Biosciences), dynactin subunit Actin Related Protein 1 (ARP1, 1:1000, Sigma-Aldrich), dynein heavy chain (DHC, 1:500, Santa Cruz Biotechnology), dynein intermediate chain (DIC, 1:1000, Sigma-Aldrich), dynein light chain (DLC, 1:500, Santa Cruz Biotechnology), α-tubulin (TUBA, 1:10000, Abcam), acetylated α-tubulin (ac-TUBA, 1:10000, Abcam), tyrosinated α-tubulin (tyro-TUBA, 1:10000, Abcam), detyrosinated α-tubulin (detyro-TUBA, 1:10000, Abcam), Autophagy Related Protein ATG3 (ATG3, 1:1000, Cell Signaling), ATG5 (1:1000, Cell Signaling), ATG7 (1:1000, Cell Signaling), autophagy related protein LC3 (1:1000, Abcam), Lysosomal Associated Membrane Protein 1 (LAMP1, 1:1000, BD Biosciences), LAMP2 (1:1000, Abcam), synaptophysin (SYP, 1:10000, Millipore), Postsynaptic Density Protein 95 (PSD95, 1:1000, Sigma-Aldrich), AMPA receptor subunit GLUR1 (1:1000, Abcam), GLUR2 (1:1000, BD Biosciences), NMDA receptor subunit NR2A (1:250, BD Biosciences), NR2B ((1:500, BD Biosciences), and β-actin (1:5000, Sigma-Aldrich). Protein signals were visualized by IRDye secondary antibodies and Odyssey system (LI-COR Biosciences), and quantified with NIH ImageJ software.

Statistical analysis

Statistical analysis was performed using GraphPad Prism 5 (GraphPad Software). Data were presented as mean ± SEM. Statistical significance was determined by comparing means of different groups using unpaired t-test, one-way or two-way ANOVA followed by the post hoc test. $^{*}p < 0.05$, $^{**}p < 0.01$, $^{***}p < 0.001$, $^{****}p < 0.0001$.

Results

Selective depletion of p150^{Glued} expression in neurons

To selectively disrupt the expression of p150^{Glued}, we initially generated *Dctn1*^{LoxP} knock-in mice by inserting two *LoxP* sites in the first and fourth introns of mouse *Dctn1* gene locus, respectively, resulting in a complete loss CAP-Gly domain and partial loss of basic domain (Fig. 1a-c). The *Dctn1*^{LoxP} knock-in mice were then crossbred with *Cre/Esr1* mice to generate *Dctn1*$^{LoxP/LoxP}$; *Cre/Esr1* pups and littermate controls for neuronal cultures. The administration of tamoxifen activated the estrogen receptor (ESR) tagged-Cre and removed the floxed exons, resulting in a selective ablation of p150^{Glued} expression in cortical neurons cultured from postnatal day 0 (P0) *Dctn1*$^{LoxP/LoxP}$; *Cre/Esr1* pups (Fig. 1d, e). P150^{Glued} proteins were identified by an antibody against the N-terminal 200 amino acids of p150^{Glued}. By contrast, the levels of p135 and other N-terminal truncated p150^{Glued}, called collectively as p135+, were substantially increased (Fig. 1d, e). The p135+ proteins were recognized by an antibody against the C-terminus of p150^{Glued}. On the other hand, the other dynactin subunits–p62, p50, and ARP1 showed comparable expression levels in *Dctn1*$^{LoxP/LoxP}$; *Cre/Esr1* and control neuronal cultures (Fig. 1d, e). Therefore, genetic depletion of p150^{Glued} increases p135+ expression, but does not affect the other dynactin subunit levels in neurons.

A lack of p150^{Glued} does not affect the formation of dynein and dynactin complexes

To evaluate the impact of p150^{Glued} on the formation of dynein/dynactin complexes, we fractionated the cell lysates from *Dctn1*$^{LoxP/LoxP}$; *Cre/Esr1* and control *Dctn1*$^{LoxP/LoxP}$ cortical neuron cultures in a sucrose gradient column and compared the distribution patterns of dynein and dynactin subunits in different fractions. In

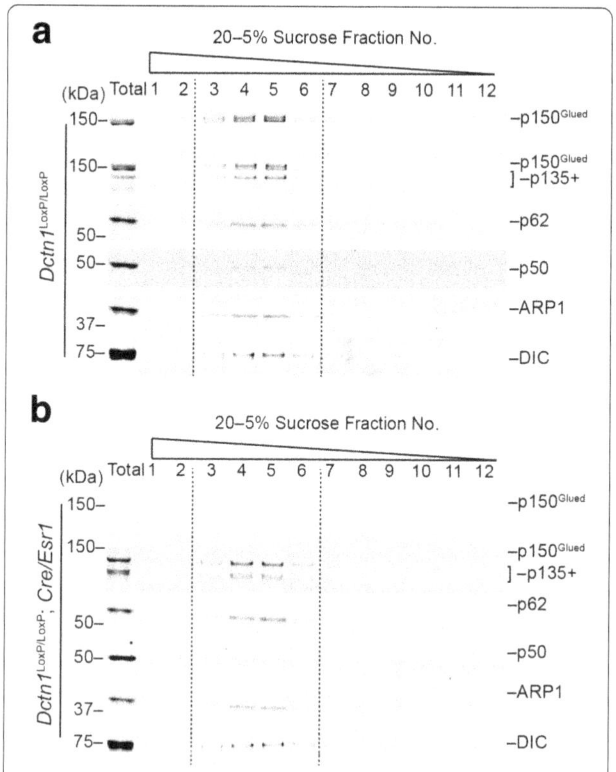

Fig. 2 Dynein/dynactin complex remains intact in *Dctn1*$^{LoxP/LoxP}$; *Cre/Esr1 neurons.* **a-b** Sucrose density gradient centrifugation shows p150^{Glued} and p135+ predominantly migrate at fraction 4 and 5 in a 5–20% sucrose gradient similar to the other dynactin subunits p62, p50, and ARP1, as well as the dynactin-interacting dynein subunit DIC in the control *Dctn1*$^{LoxP/LoxP}$ (**a**) and p150^{Glued} cKO *Dctn1*$^{LoxP/LoxP}$; *Cre/Esr1* cortical neuron cultures (**b**) at 7 DIV

control cell lysates, all the dynactin subunits and dynein DIC subunit concentrated in fractions 3 to 6 (Fig. 2a). The same distribution pattern of dynein and dynactin subunits was also observed in the p150^{Glued}-lacking cell lysates (Fig. 2b). Thus, a lack of p150^{Glued} does not affect the formation of dynein/dynactin complexes.

Generation of p150^{Glued} conditional knockout mice that lack p150^{Glued} expression in the postnatal forebrain and spinal neurons

Our previous study suggests the G59S missense mutation in the MTBDs of p150^{Glued} might cause the autosomal dominant motor neuron disease through a dominant-negative mechanism [7]. On the one hand, the G59S substitution disrupts the normal folding and destabilizes the mutant p150^{Glued} proteins. On the other hand, the residual mutant proteins might dimerize with the wild-type proteins and thereby compromises the overall function of p150^{Glued}. However, the exact pathogenic mechanisms of G59S mutation remain controversial [1]. To test the hypothesis that p150^{Glued} is required for the survival of motor neurons, we decided to remove p150^{Glued} from both CSMNs in the frontal cortex and SMNs in the ventral spinal cords by generating *Dctn1*$^{LoxP/LoxP}$; *Thy1-Cre* cKO mice. In line with the early study [16], Cre was widely expressed by neurons in the forebrain regions (Additional file 1: Figure S1A), including olfactory bulb, frontal cortex, striatum, and hippocampus, as well as in the spinal cord (Additional file 1: Figure S1B). Although the expression of Cre was detectable in the brain extracts of P0 pups, a substantial reduction of p150^{Glued} expression became apparent in 2-month-old *Dctn1*$^{LoxP/LoxP}$; *Thy1-Cre* mice (Additional file 1: Figure S1C). The depletion of p150^{Glued} restrictive to adult neurons may avoid any potential developmental defects in the p150^{Glued} cKO mice.

Immuno-staining showed endogenous p150^{Glued} proteins were highly expressed by neurons in the olfactory bulb, cerebral cortex, hippocampus, midbrain, and hindbrain regions of control *Dctn1*$^{LoxP/LoxP}$ mice (Fig. 3a). Following the expression pattern of Cre (Additional file 1: Figure S1A), the levels of p150^{Glued} were substantially depleted in the olfactory bulb, frontal cortex, and hippocampus of *Dctn1*$^{LoxP/LoxP}$; *Thy1-Cre* cKO mice (Fig. 3a). More importantly, p150^{Glued} was absent in the CSMNs of cKO mouse brains, while the p135+ remained (Fig. 3b). Here the CSMNs were indicated by staining with CSMN-specific marker protein CTIP2 [23]. P150^{Glued} was also abundantly expressed by spinal neurons, including the SMNs in the ventral horns, but disappeared in the cKO spinal cords (Fig. 3c, d). In contrast, the p135+ proteins were still present in the SMNs of cKO mice (Fig. 3d). Therefore, we generated a line of p150^{Glued} cKO mice that depleted the expression of p150^{Glued} in the adult CSMNs and SMNs, while kept p135 and other MTBD-lacking variants.

P150^{Glued} conditional knockout mice develop late-onset motor impairments

The *Dctn1*$^{LoxP/LoxP}$; *Thy1-Cre* p150^{Glued} cKO mice were born at a normal Mendelian ratio, developed normally, and had similar body weights as littermate controls (Fig. 4a). The cKO mice also displayed normal ambulatory movement in the open-field tests (Fig. 4b), but showed markedly reduced rearing at 18 months of age (Fig. 4c), and stayed less time on the rotating rods compared to the controls starting at 12 months of age (Fig. 4d). These data suggest that a lack of p150^{Glued} affects the motor control of aged animals.

P150^{Glued} conditional knockout mice develop late-onset, selective degeneration of SMNs

To investigate whether p150^{Glued} depletion causes motor neuron loss, we used the unbiased stereology approach to count the numbers of lumbar SMNs and CSMNs in 9 and 18-month-old control *Dctn1*$^{LoxP/LoxP}$ mice and *Dctn1*$^{LoxP/LoxP}$; *Thy1-Cre* cKO mice. Series of evenly

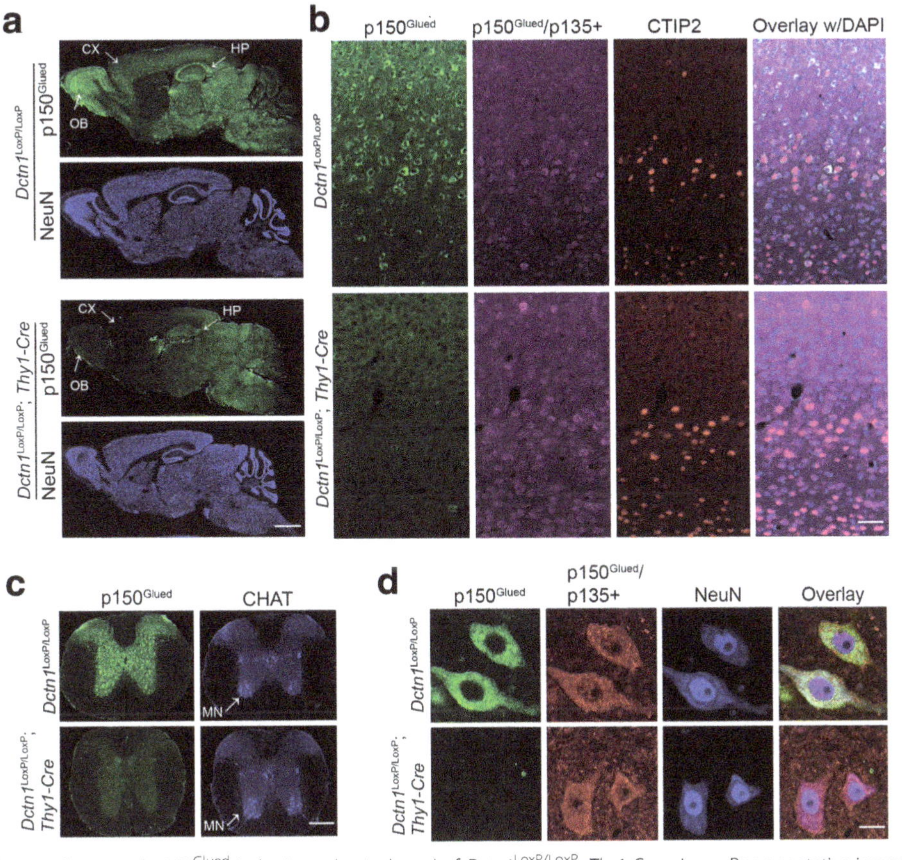

Fig. 3 Selective deletion of neuronal p150^{Glued} in brain and spinal cord of *Dctn1*$^{LoxP/LoxP}$; *Thy1-Cre* mice. **a** Representative images show p150^{Glued} (green) and NeuN (blue) staining in the sagittal brain sections of 3-month-old *Dctn1*$^{LoxP/LoxP}$ and *Dctn1*$^{LoxP/LoxP}$; *Thy1-Cre* mice. Arrows point to olfactory bulb (OB), cortex (CX) and hippocampus (HP) with intense p150^{Glued} staining in *Dctn1*$^{LoxP/LoxP}$ mice and weak p150^{Glued} staining in *Dctn1*$^{LoxP/LoxP}$; *Thy1-Cre* mice. Scale bar: 500 μm. **b** Representative images show p150^{Glued} (green) and p150^{Glued}/p135+ (purple) expression in the CTIP2-positive (red) CSMNs of 3-month-old *Dctn1*$^{LoxP/LoxP}$ and *Dctn1*$^{LoxP/LoxP}$; *Thy1-Cre* mice. Scale bar: 500 μm. **c** Representative images show p150^{Glued} (green) and CHAT (blue) staining in the lumbar spinal cord sections of 3-month-old *Dctn1*$^{LoxP/LoxP}$ and *Dctn1*$^{LoxP/LoxP}$; *Thy1-Cre* mice. Arrows point to the CHAT-positive SMNs. Scale bar: 500 μm. **d** Representative images show p150^{Glued} (green) and p150^{Glued}/p135+ (red) expression in the NeuN-positive SMNs of 3-month-old *Dctn1*$^{LoxP/LoxP}$ and *Dctn1*$^{LoxP/LoxP}$; *Thy1-Cre* mice. Scale bar: 20 μm

sampled lumbar spinal sections were stained with SMN marker CHAT or histological dye Nissl for neuron counting (Fig. 5a). There was modest but statistically significant reduction of CHAT-positive SMN numbers in the lumbar spinal cord of 18-month-old cKO mice (Fig. 5b). The decrease of lumbar SMN numbers in 18-month-old cKO mice was also observed in the Nissl-stained sections (Fig. 5b). On the other hand, no significant alterations of lumbar SMN numbers were found in 9-month-old cKO mice (Fig. 5b). Additionally, no apparent changes of CTIP2-positive or Nissl-stained CSMN numbers were detected in the motor cortex of 18-month-old cKO mice (Fig. 5c, d). Given that endogenous p150^{Glued} are ubiquitously expressed throughout central neuronal system, we investigated whether p150^{Glued} depletion led to neurodegeneration in other motor function-related brain regions, including midbrain, striatum and cerebellum. Unbiased stereology revealed that no obvious loss of TH-positive dopaminergic (DA) neurons in substantia nigra pars compacta (SNpc) (Additional file 1: Figure S2A, B) and striatal neurons in 18-month-old cKO mice (Additional file 1: Figure S2C-E). Furthermore, neither the thickness of molecular layer (ML) and granule cell layer (GCL), or the density of Calbindin D28K-positive Purkinje cells in the cerebellum of 18-month-old cKO mice was obviously altered (Additional file 1: Figure S2C, F-I). These results demonstrate that p150^{Glued} depletion in adult neurons causes preferentially SMN loss in aged animals.

P150^{Glued} depletion induces astrogliosis and microgliosis in the spinal cord of aged p150^{Glued} cKO mice

Given that astrogliosis and microgliosis are often in accompany with motor neurodegeneration in the spinal cord [24], we stained the lumbar spinal sections with

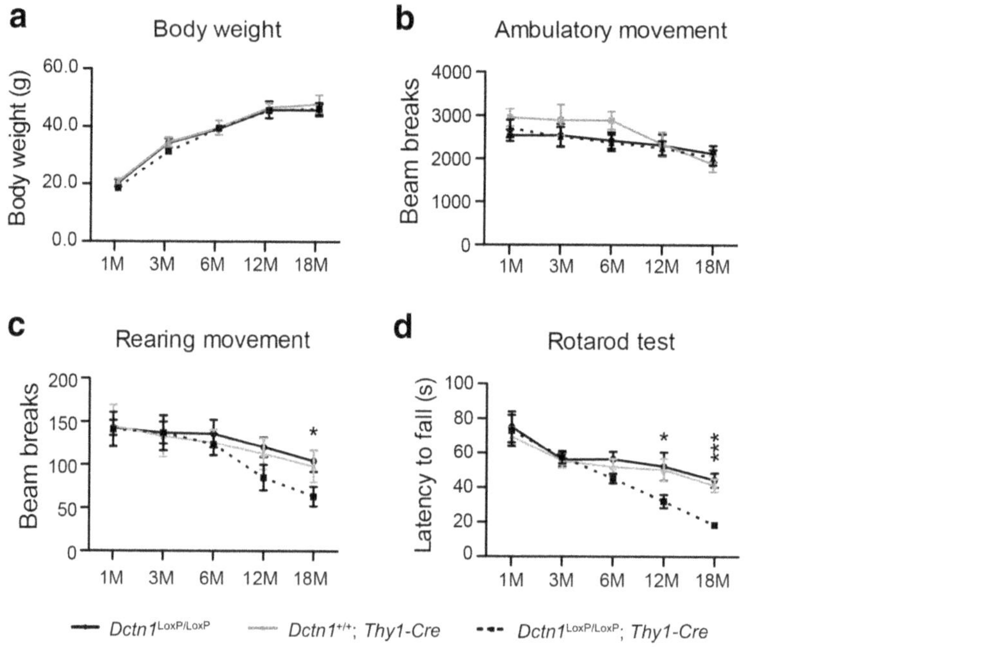

Fig. 4 *Dctn1*$^{LoxP/LoxP}$; *Thy1-Cre* mice develop abnormal motor phenotypes. **a-d** Male *Dctn1*$^{LoxP/LoxP}$, *Dctn1*$^{+/+}$; *Thy1-Cre* and *Dctn1*$^{LoxP/LoxP}$; *Thy1-Cre* mice ($n \geq 10$ per genotype per time point) were measured for body weight (**a**); tested for the ambulatory movement (**b**) and rearing movement (**c**) in Open-field; and examined for the latency to fall in Rotarod test (**d**) at 1, 3, 6, 12 and 18 months of age. Data were presented as mean ± SEM. One-way ANOVA plus Tukey's post hoc test was used for statistical analysis. **c** At 18 months of age, $^{*}p < 0.05$ for difference against *Dctn1*$^{LoxP/LoxP}$; *Thy1-Cre*, while no difference was found between *Dctn1*$^{LoxP/LoxP}$ and *Dctn1*$^{+/+}$; *Thy1-Cre*. **d** At 12 or 18 months of age, $^{*}p < 0.05$ or $^{***}p < 0.001$ for difference against *Dctn1*$^{LoxP/LoxP}$; *Thy1-Cre*, respectively, while no difference was found between *Dctn1*$^{LoxP/LoxP}$ and *Dctn1*$^{+/+}$; *Thy1-Cre*

antibodies against astrogliosis marker GFAP and microgliosis marker IBA1. In line with previous findings [24], we observed a substantial induction of astrogliosis and microgliosis in the spinal cord of 18-month-old cKO mice (Fig. 5e, f).

P150^{Glued} ablation causes severe neuromuscular defects in aged p150^{Glued} cKO mice

To investigate whether p150^{glued} depletion impairs the connections between SMN axon terminals and the innervated muscles, we examined the neuromuscular junctions (NMJs) of gastrocnemius muscles of 18-month-old control and p150^{Glued} cKO mice. α-Bungarotoxin (BTX), which specifically labels acetylcholine receptors at the postsynaptic sites, was applied to label the NMJs (Fig. 6a). Meanwhile, acetylated α-tubulin (ac-TUBA), which is enriched in axons, was used to mark the axon terminals (Fig. 6a). While the NMJs in control mice remained mostly intact, the majority of NMJs in p150^{Glued} cKO mice were either partially or fully fragmented, in company with severe denervation (Fig. 6a, b). The hindlimb clasping test has been used to rate the extent of neuromuscular function impairment in rodent models of motor neuron diseases [25]. 18-month-old male control and p150^{Glued} cKO mice were suspended by the tail for 10 s and the severity of hindlimb clasping was scored. Control mice splayed their hindlimbs outward and away from the abdomen with no clasping reflex, while p150^{Glued} cKO mice retracted their hindlimbs toward the abdomen with substantially higher hindlimb clasping severity score than control mice (Fig. 6c, d). Given that denervation often induce skeletal muscle atrophy in motor neuron diseases, we measured muscle weight and examined gross muscle pathology of control and p150^{Glued} cKO mice. We observed a substantial decrease of gastrocnemius muscle weight in 24-month-old male p150^{Glued} cKO mice (Fig. 6e). Hematoxylin and eosin (HE) staining of gastrocnemius cross sections revealed that 24-month-old male control mice had a polygonal shaped muscle fibers with homogenous fiber size, whereas p150^{Glued} cKO mice exhibited significantly smaller size of muscle fiber in accompany with pathological hallmarks of myofiber de-/regenerating and inflammatory cells infiltration (Fig. 6f, g). These results demonstrate that a loss of p150^{glued} caused substantial NMJ disruption and muscle atrophy in aged mice.

A loss of p150^{Glued} increases α-tubulin acetylation

Microtubules are formed by the polymerization of α- and β-tubulin dimers [26]. Various post-translational modifications (PTMs) of α-tubulin affect the

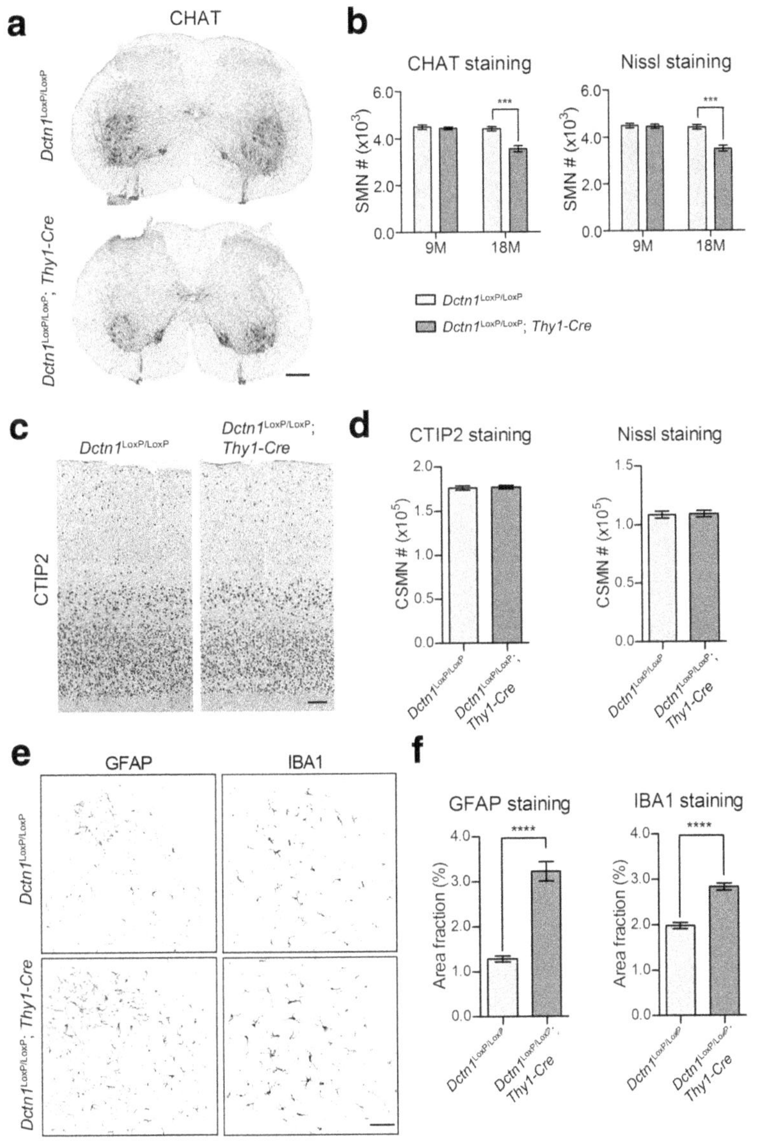

Fig. 5 *Dctn1*$^{LoxP/LoxP}$; *Thy1-Cre* mice display loss of spinal motor neurons and gliosis. **a** Representative images show CHAT staining in the lumbar spinal cord of *Dctn1*$^{LoxP/LoxP}$ and *Dctn1*$^{LoxP/LoxP}$; *Thy1-Cre* mice at 18 months of age. Scale bar: 500 μm. **b** Unbiased stereological estimation of the number of CHAT-positive SMNs and Nissl-stained SMNs in the lumbar spinal cord of 9 and 18-month-old *Dctn1*$^{LoxP/LoxP}$ and *Dctn1*$^{LoxP/LoxP}$; *Thy1-Cre* mice ($n = 6$ per genotype per time point). Data were presented as mean ± SEM. Two-way ANOVA plus Bonferroni's post hoc test was used for statistical analysis. At 18 months of age, $^{***}p < 0.001$ for difference between *Dctn1*$^{LoxP/LoxP}$ and *Dctn1*$^{LoxP/LoxP}$; *Thy1-Cre*. There were significant main effects for age (CHAT staining: $F_{(1,\ 20)} = 25.51$, $p < 0.0001$; Nissl staining: $F_{(1,\ 20)} = 25.18$, $p < 0.0001$), genotype (CHAT staining: $F_{(1,\ 20)} = 22.46$, $p = 0.0001$; Nissl staining: $F_{(1,\ 20)} = 21.85$, $p = 0.0001$) and age-genotype interaction (CHAT staining: $F_{(1,\ 20)} = 17.08$, $p = 0.0005$; Nissl staining: $F_{(1,\ 20)} = 18.47$, $p - 0.0004$). **c** Representative images show CTIP2 staining in the motor cortex of *Dctn1*$^{LoxP/LoxP}$ and *Dctn1*$^{LoxP/LoxP}$; *Thy1-Cre* mice at 18 months of age. Scale bar: 500 μm. **d** Unbiased stereological estimation of the number of CTIP2-positive and Nissl-stained large pyramidal neurons in the layer V motor cortex of 18-month-old *Dctn1*$^{LoxP/LoxP}$ and *Dctn1*$^{LoxP/LoxP}$; *Thy1-Cre* mice ($n = 6$ per genotype per time point). Data were presented as mean ± SEM. Unpaired t-test showed no statistical significance ($p > 0.05$). **e** Representative images show GFAP and IBA1 staining in the ventral horn of lumbar spinal cord of *Dctn1*$^{LoxP/LoxP}$ and *Dctn1*$^{LoxP/LoxP}$; *Thy1-Cre* mice at 18 months of age. Scale bar: 500 μm. **f** The areas occupied by GFAP-positive astrocytes and IBA1-positive microglia in the ventral horn of lumbar spinal cord of *Dctn1*$^{LoxP/LoxP}$ and *Dctn1*$^{LoxP/LoxP}$; *Thy1-Cre* mice at 18 months of age ($n = 6$ animals and 10 sections per animal). Data were presented as mean ± SEM; $^{****}p < 0.0001$. Unpaired t-test was used for statistical analysis

microtubule dynamics [27]. To assess the impact of p150^{Glued} depletion on α-tubulin PTMs, we examined the levels of α-tubulin acetylation, tyrosination, and detyrosination by western blots in the spinal cord homogenates of 9-month-old *Dctn1*$^{LoxP/LoxP}$; *Thy1-Cre* cKO mice and littermate *Dctn1*$^{LoxP/LoxP}$ mice (Fig. 7a). We observed a substantial increase of acetylated α-tubulin levels in the p150^{Glued} cKO samples (Fig. 7a, b).

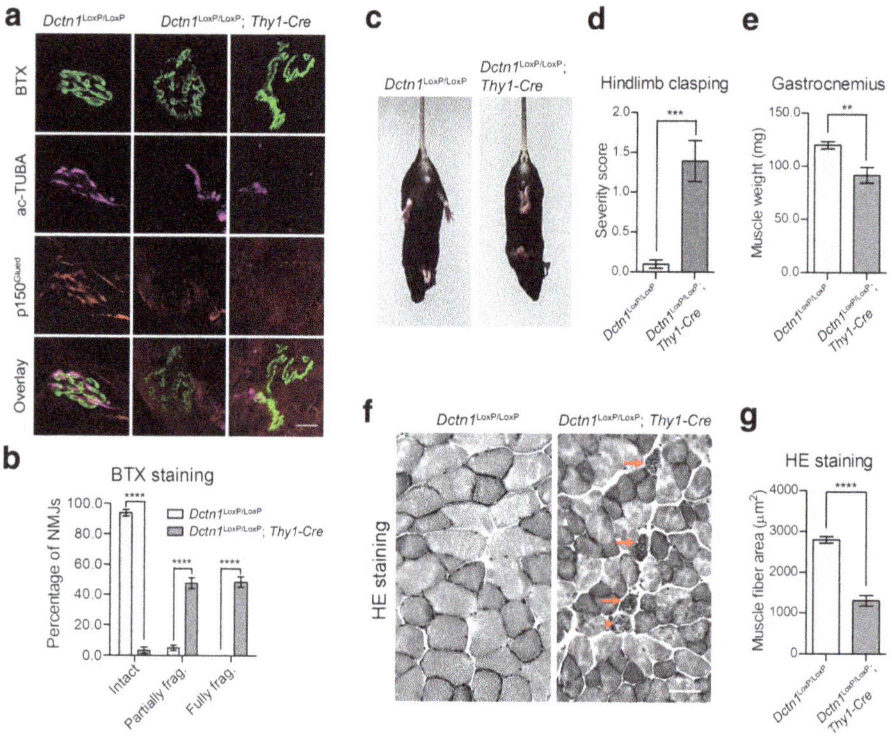

Fig. 6 *Dctn1*$^{LoxP/LoxP}$; *Thy1-Cre* mice show NMJ fragmentation. **a** Representative images show α-bungarotoxin (BTX, green), p150^{Glued} (red) and ac-TUBA (purple) staining in the gastrocnemius muscles of *Dctn1*$^{LoxP/LoxP}$ and *Dctn1*$^{LoxP/LoxP}$; *Thy1-Cre* mice at 18 months of age. Scale bar: 20 μm. **b** Bar graph shows the percentage of intact, partially fragmented, and fully fragmented NMJs in the gastrocnemius muscles of *Dctn1*$^{LoxP/LoxP}$ and *Dctn1*$^{LoxP/LoxP}$; *Thy1-Cre* mice at 18 months of age (n = 6 animals and 10 sections per animal). Data were presented as mean ± SEM; $^{****}p < 0.0001$. Unpaired t-test was used for statistical analysis. **c** Photographs display posture of 18-month-old male *Dctn1*$^{LoxP/LoxP}$ and *Dctn1*$^{LoxP/LoxP}$; *Thy1-Cre* mice in the hindlimb clasping test. **d** Bar graph shows the hindlimb clasping severity score of 18-month-old male *Dctn1*$^{LoxP/LoxP}$ and *Dctn1*$^{LoxP/LoxP}$; *Thy1-Cre* mice (*n* = 10–11 per genotype). Data were presented as mean ± SEM; $^{***}p < 0.001$. Unpaired t-test was used for statistical analysis. **e** Quantification of gastrocnemius muscle weight from 24-month-old male *Dctn1*$^{LoxP/LoxP}$ and *Dctn1*$^{LoxP/LoxP}$; *Thy1-Cre* mice (n = 10–11 per genotype). Data were presented as mean ± SEM; $^{**}p < 0.01$. Unpaired t-test was used for statistical analysis. **f** Representative images show hematoxylin and eosin (HE) staining of gastrocnemius cross sections from 24-month-old male *Dctn1*$^{LoxP/LoxP}$ and *Dctn1*$^{LoxP/LoxP}$; *Thy1-Cre* mice. Note the very high amount of small muscle fibers as well as myofiber de–/regeneration (arrow head) and inflammatory cells infiltration (arrow) in *Dctn1*$^{LoxP/LoxP}$; *Thy1-Cre* mice. Scale bar: 50 μm. **g** Quantification of gastrocnemius muscle fiber areas from 24-month-old male *Dctn1*$^{LoxP/LoxP}$ and *Dctn1*$^{LoxP/LoxP}$; *Thy1-Cre* mice (n = 6 mice per genotype and 6 sections per mouse). Data were presented as mean ± SEM; $^{****}p < 0.0001$. Unpaired t-test was used for statistical analysis

We further confirm this finding by immuno-staining the lumbar spinal sections of 9-month-old mice. There were a few spots in the ventral root SMN axon bundles positive to acetylated α-tubulin staining in the control spinal cords (Fig. 7c). By contrast, a drastic upregulation of acetylated α-tubulin was found in the SMN axons of cKO mice (Fig. 7d). These data demonstrate that p150^{Glued} depletion leads to substantial increase of acetylated α-tubulin levels in the SMN axons, suggesting potential alterations of microtubule stability in p150^{Glued}-lacking SMNs.

A loss of p150^{Glued} promotes autophagosome and lysosome protein accumulation

Dynein/dynactin complexes mediate the transport of autophagosomes and lysosomes in cells [28]. Early studies show impairments of autophagosome and lysosome trafficking in the SMNs of transgenic mice overexpressing disease-related p150^{Glued} G59S mutation, resulting in cytoplasmic accumulation of autophagosome and lysosome-enriched proteins [29, 30]. Accordingly, we examined the levels of autophagosome and lysosome marker proteins in the spinal cord lysates of 9-month-old p150^{Glued} control and cKO mice by western blots. Substantial increases of autophagosome protein LC3II [31] and lysosome proteins LAMP1 and LAMP2 [32] were found in the cKO spinal cords (Fig. 8a, b). However, no apparent alterations of other autophagosome proteins ATG3, ATG5, ATG7, and LC3I were detected (Fig. 8a, b). Since the LAMP2 antibody also works well in immunostaining of brain tissues, we further checked the distribution pattern of LAMP2-postive signals in the SMNs of 9-month-old control and cKO mice. We observed markedly

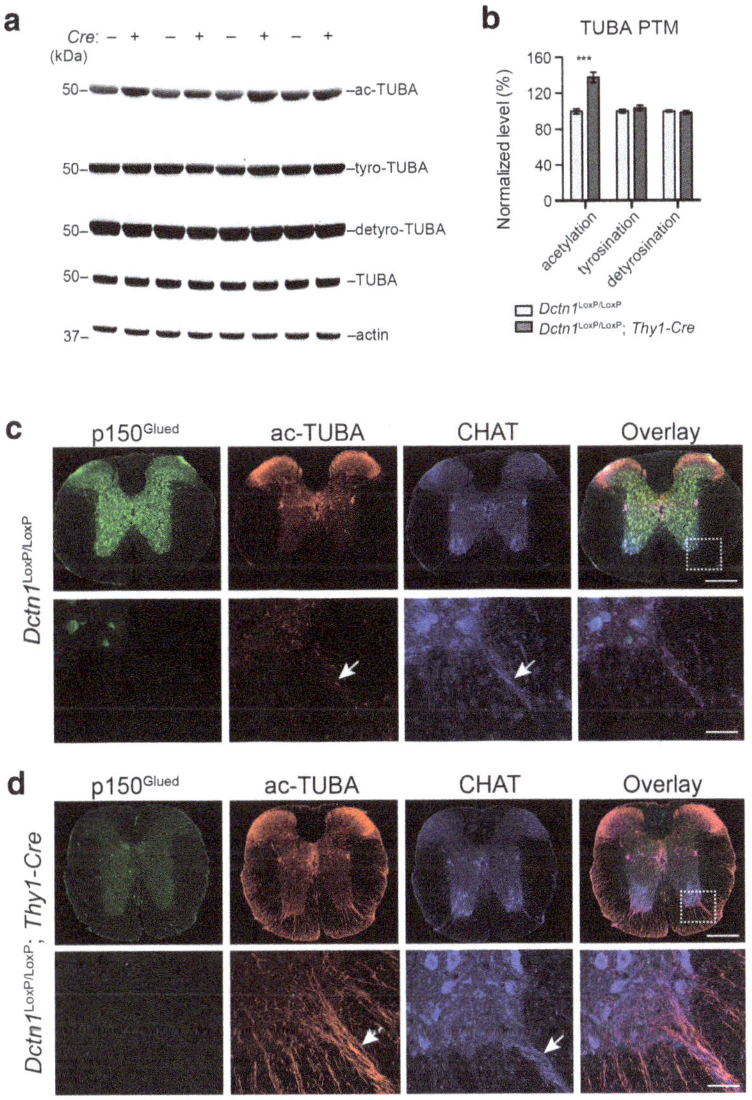

Fig. 7 P150^{Glued} deficiency enhances tubulin acetylation in spinal motor neurons. **a-b** Western blot analysis shows the expression of acetylated (ac-), tyrosinated (tyro-), detyrosinated (detyro-) and total alpha tubulin (TUBA) in the spinal cord homogenate of 9-month-old *Dctn1*$^{LoxP/LoxP}$ and *Dctn1*$^{LoxP/LoxP}$; *Thy1-Cre* mice. Actin was used as loading control. Bar graphs show the quantification of ac-TUBA, tyro-TUBA and detyro-TUBA level normalized with total TUBA ($n = 8$ per genotype). Data were presented as mean ± SEM, $^{***}p < 0.001$. Unpaired t-test was used for statistical analysis. **c**, **d** Representative images show p150^{Glued} (green), ac-TUBA (red) and CHAT (blue) staining in the lumbar spinal cord of 9-month-old *Dctn1*$^{LoxP/LoxP}$ (**c**) and *Dctn1*$^{LoxP/LoxP}$; *Thy1-Cre* (**d**) mice. Four mice per genotype and 10 sections per mouse were examined. Arrows point to CHAT-positive ventral roots with weak ac-TUBA staining in *Dctn1*$^{LoxP/LoxP}$ mice and substantial ac-TUBA staining in *Dctn1*$^{LoxP/LoxP}$; *Thy1-Cre* mice. Scale bars: 500 μm (low-magnification images), 20 μm (high-magnification images)

increased LAMP2 signals in the perinuclear regions of cKO SMNs (Fig. 8c). Together, our results reveal the impairments of autophagosome and lysosome transportation in the p150^{Glued}-depleted SMNs.

P150^{Glued} and other dynactin subunits are more enriched in the postsynaptic sites compared to dynein motor proteins

Neurons communicate with each other through synapses, where the transmitters released from the presynaptic axon terminals bind to the receptors located in the opposite postsynaptic sites in dendritic spines, small protrusions from dendritic shaft [33]. P150^{Glued} is enriched in the axon terminals and facilitate the loading of cargos to dynein-mediated axonal retrograde transport in developing neurons [34]. To investigate whether p150^{Glued} plays any role in the postsynaptic sites, we purified postsynaptic density (PSD)-enriched fractions from control mouse brains. The purity of extracted PSD fractions was verified by the presence of high levels of PSD95 proteins, but not the presynaptic protein synaptophysin (Fig. 9). Interestingly, p150^{Glued}, p135, and

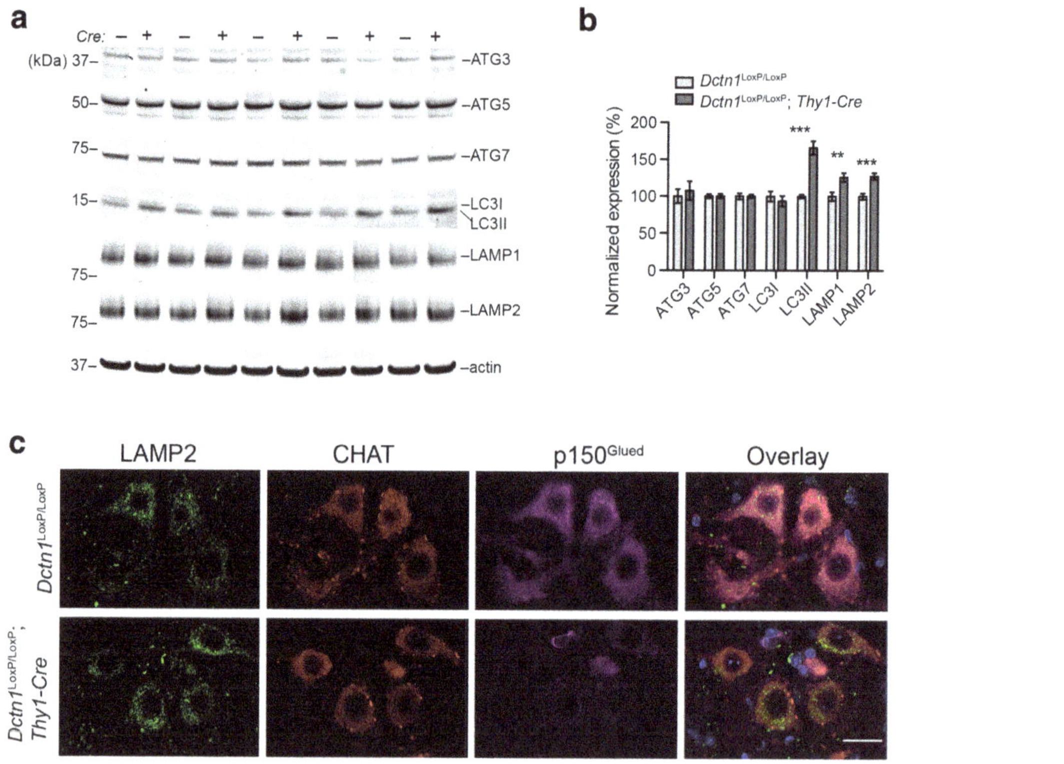

Fig. 8 P150^{Glued} deficiency alters autophagosome and lysosome marker protein expression in spinal motor neurons. **a** Western blot analysis shows the expression of ATG3, ATG5, ATG7, LC3, LAMP1 and LAMP2 in the spinal cord homogenate of 9-month-old *Dctn1*$^{LoxP/LoxP}$ and *Dctn1*$^{LoxP/LoxP}$; *Thy1-Cre* mice. Actin was used as loading control. **b** Bar graphs show the quantification of ATG3, ATG5, ATG7, LC3, LAMP1 and LAMP2 level normalized with actin ($n = 10$ per genotype). Data were presented as mean ± SEM; $^{**}p < 0.01$, $^{***}p < 0.001$. Unpaired t-test was used for statistical analysis. **c** Representative images show LAMP2 (green), CHAT (red) and p150^{Glued} (purple) staining in the lumbar spinal cord of 9-month-old *Dctn1*$^{LoxP/LoxP}$ and *Dctn1*$^{LoxP/LoxP}$; *Thy1-Cre* mice. Four mice per genotype and 10 sections per mouse were examined. Scale bar: 20 μm

other dynactin subunits were found in the PSD fractions, whereas dynein heavy chain (DHC), DIC, and tubulins were undetectable (Fig. 9). On the other hand, low levels of dynein light chain (DLC) were present in the PSD fraction (Fig. 9). These data suggest that p150^{Glued} and dynactin may mediate the transport of postsynaptic cargos from the postsynaptic sites to dynein motor complex associated with microtubules in the dendrites.

P150^{Glued} depletion leads to increased cell surface targeting of glutamate receptors and increased vulnerability to glutamate-induced excitotoxicity

Excitotoxicity mediated by glutamate and its receptors has been implicated in the pathogenesis of motor neuron diseases [35]. Using western blots, we found the levels of glutamate receptors GLUR1, GLUR2, NR2A, and NR2B, as well as postsynaptic density protein 95 (PSD95) were all substantially elevated in the spinal cord lysates of 9-month-old *Dctn1*$^{LoxP/LoxP}$; *Thy1-Cre* cKO mice (Fig. 10a, b). By contrast, we did not observe any obvious changes of presynaptic protein synaptophysin expression (Fig. 10a, b). To investigate whether more glutamate receptors are transported to the synapses, we isolated the biotin-labeled cell surface proteins from cultured spinal neurons, and found substantial elevation of glutamate receptor GLUR1, GLUR2, NR2A and NR2B present at the membrane fractions (Fig. 10c, d). In correlation with the increased cell surface targeting of glutamate receptors, p150^{Glued} cKO neurons showed more severe cell death after treated with 10 μm glutamate (Fig. 10e). Therefore, p150^{Glued} depletion causes more postsynaptic accumulation of glutamate receptors, making p150^{Glued}-lacking neurons more susceptible to excitotoxicity.

Discussion

In the current study, we generated and characterized a line of p150^{Glued} cKO mice to critically evaluate the roles of CAP-Gly domain-containing dynactin p150^{Glued} in postnatal neurons. A loss of p150^{Glued} in postnatal neurons did not affect the assembly of dynein/dynactin motor protein complex in neurons, but caused rather selective SMN degeneration and movement impairments in aged mice. The depletion of p150^{Glued} also led to substantial elevation of acetylated α-tubulin, glutamate receptors, and proteins involved in autophagosome and

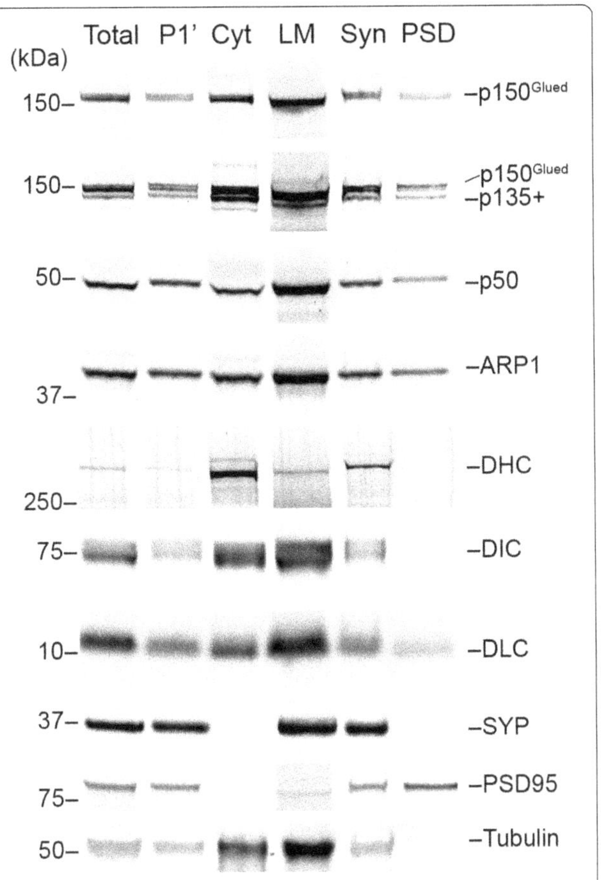

Fig. 9 P150^{Glued} and other dynactin subunits are present in the postsynaptic sites. Subcellular fractionation of 3-month-old wild-type mouse brains shows the distribution of dyanctin subunits p150^{Glued}, p135+, p50 and ARP1, dynein subunits DHC, DIC and DLC, synaptophysin (SYP), postsynaptic density protein 95 (PSD95), and α-tubulin in total brain lysates (Total), crude nuclear fraction (P1'), cytosol (Cyt), light membrane fraction (LM), synaptosomes (Syn), and postsynaptic density (PSD)

lysosome pathways in the cKO neurons. Finally, p150^{Glued} ablation rendered spinal neurons more susceptible to excitotoxicity. Considering all the disease-causative mutations compromise the MTBD functions of p150^{Glued}, increased excitotoxicity may underlie a common pathogenic mechanism of p150^{Glued} mutations in diverse neurodegenerative diseases.

The absence of more drastic morphological and functional phenotypes in p150^{Glued} cKO neurons suggests that p135 and other MTBD-lacking p150^{Glued} splicing variants may largely substitute the functions of p150^{Glued} in neurons. The CC1 domain of p150^{Glued} mediates the interaction with DIC and other dynein motor protein complex [2]. Since p135 and other p150^{Glued} short forms contain the CC1 domain, it is not surprising that dynein and dynactin complex remains intact and appears mostly functional in neurons. P150^{Glued} thereby is likely devoted to some special tasks in neurons. Neurons, especially the large projection neurons like CSMNs and SMNs, contain long axons. Microtubules form the backbone of these axons. P150^{Glued} is proposed to play a critical role in maintaining the stability of microtubules by serving as an anti-catastrophe factor in neuronal cultures [11]. However, we did not observe any substantial loss of axons in brain and spinal cord of presyptomatic p150^{Glued} cKO mice. Instead, we found a substantial augmentation of acetylated α-tubulin in neural tissues, including the axons of SMNs. It has been well documented that the acetylation of α-tubulin improves the stability of microtubules [36]. Therefore, the increased acetylation of α-tubulin may serve as a compensatory mechanism to maintain the integrity of microtubules in the absence of p150^{Glued}. It will be interesting to delineate the signaling pathways leading to the increased α-tubulin acetylation in p150^{Glued} cKO neurons.

In addition to maintaining microtubule stability, p150^{Glued} is also proposed as a key player in uploading various cargos to the dynein motor complex in the axon terminals before being transported to the soma [34]. For example, live imaging studies show p150^{Glued} captures the cargos and loads to the microtubule plus ends for the minus-end-directed transport [37]. Accordingly, we found a lack of p150^{Glued} caused substantial disruption of NMJ structures in p150^{Glued} cKO mice. Moreover, our studies suggest that p150^{Glued} also plays a role in uploading postsynaptic glutamate receptors to dynein-mediated transport in dendrites. As results, p150^{Glued} depletion led to increased accumulation of glutamate receptors in the postsynaptic sites, which makes the p150^{Glued} cKO neurons more vulnerable to glutamate stimulation, suggesting increased excitotoxicity may contribute to the eventual loss of SMNs in p150^{Glued} cKO mice. Future studies will be needed to investigate whether the disease-causative mutations also make neurons subject to excitotoxicity.

The dynein/dynactin complex is critical for organelle transport from cell periphery to the perinuclear sites along the microtubule networks, such as the centripetal movement of autophagosomes, lysosomes and endosomes [2]. It has been shown in the previous studies that overexpressing the motor neuron disease–causative G59S mutant p150^{Glued} impairs the autophagosome and lysosome pathways [1, 30]. In line with these earlier findings, we observed similar defects in abnormal accumulation of autophagosome and lysosome proteins in p150^{Glued}-lacking SMNs. The disruption of autophagosome and lysosome-mediated protein turnover thereby could also lead to the SMN loss in aging.

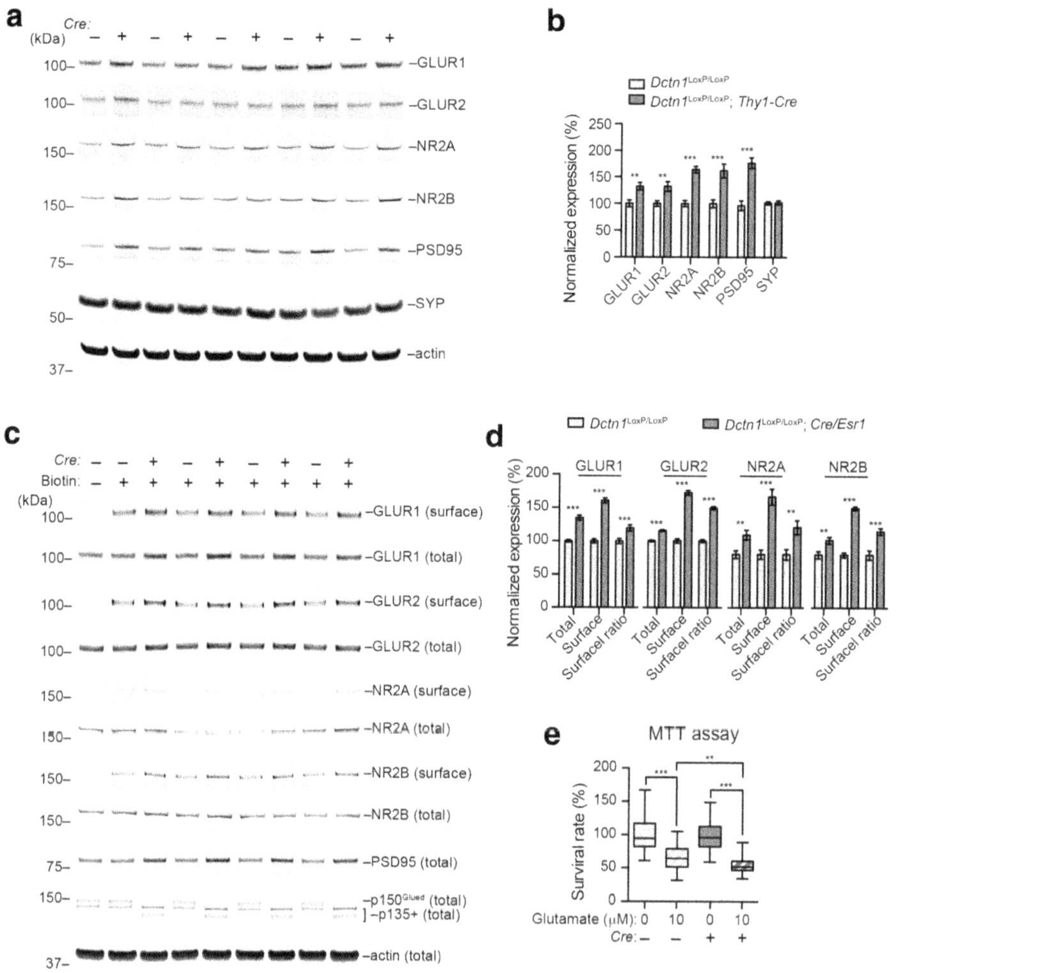

Fig. 10 P150[Glued] deficiency increases protein expression of glutamate receptors and vulnerability to glutamate-mediated excitotoxicity in spinal neurons. **a** Western blot analysis shows the expression of AMPAR subunits GLUR1 and GLUR2, NMDAR subunits NR2A and NR2B, postsynaptic density protein 95 (PSD95) and synaptophysin (SYP) in the spinal cord homogenate of 9-month-old *Dctn1*[LoxP/LoxP] and *Dctn1*[LoxP/LoxP]; *Thy1-Cre* mice. Actin was used as loading control. **b** Bar graphs show the quantification of GLUR1, GLUR2, NR2A, NR2B, PSD95 and SYP level normalized with actin (n = 10 per genotype). Data were presented as mean ± SEM; $^{**}p < 0.01$, $^{***}p < 0.001$. Unpaired t-test was used for statistical analysis. **c** Western blot analysis shows the levels of biotinylated cell surface and total AMPAR subunits GLUR1 and GLUR2, NMDAR subunits NR2A and NR2B in cultured *Dctn1*[LoxP/LoxP] and *Dctn1*[LoxP/LoxP]; *Cre/Esr1* spinal neurons at 21 DIV. Actin was used as loading control. **d** Bar graphs show the quantification of total and surface GLUR1, GLUR2, NR2A and NR2B level normalized with actin, and the ratio of GLUR1, GLUR2, NR2A and NR2B at cell surface versus total proteins (n = 8 per genotype). Data were presented as mean ± SEM; $^{**}p < 0.01$, $^{***}p < 0.001$. Unpaired t-test was used for statistical analysis. (E) Primary spinal neurons were treated with glutamate, and the viability of these neurons was measured by the MTT assay. Box & whiskers graphs show survival rate (percentage) of cultured *Dctn1*[LoxP/LoxP] and *Dctn1*[LoxP/LoxP]; *Cre/Esr1* spinal neurons (21 DIV) treated with 0 or 10 μM glutamate for 24 h (*N* = 40 per genotype per condition). Data were presented as mean ± SEM. One-way ANOVA plus Tukey's post hoc test was used for statistical analysis. $^{***}p < 0.001$ for difference between *Dctn1*[LoxP/LoxP] neurons treated with 0 and 10 μM glutamate, $^{***}p < 0.001$ for difference between *Dctn1*[LoxP/LoxP]; *Cre/Esr1* neurons treated with 0 and 10 μM glutamate, $^{**}p < 0.01$ for difference between *Dctn1*[LoxP/LoxP] and *Dctn1*[LoxP/LoxP]; *Cre/Esr1* neurons treated with 10 μM glutamate, while no difference was found between *Dctn1*[LoxP/LoxP] and *Dctn1*[LoxP/LoxP]; *Cre/Esr1* neurons treated with 0 μM glutamate

While in this study we focused on the roles of p150[Glued] in CSMNs and SMNs, the floxed MTBD of p150[Glued] can also be removed from the other neuron and cell types at different time points based on the spatial and temporal expression pattern of Cre DNA recombinase. The availability of p150[Glued] cKO mice therefore provides a useful tool to study the functional significance of the CAP-Gly domain of p150[Glued] in vivo.

Conclusions

Multiple missense mutations in the CAP-Gly domain of dynactin p150[Glued] have been linked to lower motor neuron disease, and other degenerative neurological disorders. These disease-causative mutations seem to weaken the microtubule binding affinity of p150[Glued]. However, the functional significance of p150[Glued] has not been critically evaluated in vivo. In the present study, we generated and characterized a line of $p150^{Glued}$ cKO mice to critically evaluate the roles of CAP-Gly domain-containing dynactin $p150^{Glued}$ in postnatal neurons. The depletion of $p150^{Glued}$ caused selective spinal motor neuron degeneration and movement impairments in aged mice. Substantial elevation of acetylated α-tubulin, proteins involved in autophagosome and lysosome pathways, and glutamate receptors were observed in the cKO neurons, while higher glutamate receptor levels were correlated with increase susceptibility of spinal neurons to excitotoxicity. Increased excitotoxicity may underlie a common pathogenic mechanism of $p150^{Glued}$ mutations in diverse neurodegenerative diseases.

Acknowledgements
The authors thank Cai lab members for their various supports, China Scholarship Council (CSC) for its International Exchange Program, and Beijing Municipal Administration of Hospitals for its High-level Talents Program.

Funding
This work was supported in part by the intramural research programs of National Institute on Aging (AG000946), National Natural Science Foundation of China (No. 81601117), Beijing Natural Science Foundation (No. 7152077 and 7184221), Beijing Hundreds and Thousands of Talents Project (No. 2017A14), and Beijing Nova Program (No. xx2018099).

Authors' contributions
HC, JY, CL. HS conceived the research and designed the experiments. JY, CL, HS, CX, LS, C-XL, JD, and YL performed experiments. HC and JY analyzed data and wrote manuscript. CL critically reviewed manuscript. All authors read and approved the final manuscript.

Competing interests
The authors declare that they have no competing interests.

Author details
[1]Institute for Geriatrics and Rehabilitation, Beijing Geriatric Hospital, Beijing University of Chinese Medicine, Beijing 100095, People's Republic of China. [2]Transgenic Section, Laboratory of Neurogenetics, National Institute on Aging, National Institutes of Health, Building 35, Room 1A112, MSC 3707, 35 Convent Drive, Bethesda, MD 20892–3707, USA. [3]Computational Biology Core, Laboratory of Neurogenetics, National Institute on Aging, National Institutes of Health, Bethesda, MD 20892, USA. [4]NINDS Protein/Peptide Sequencing Facility, National Institute of Neurological Disorders and Stroke, National Institutes of Health, Bethesda, MD 20892, USA. [5]Present address: Symptom Management Branch, National Institute of Nursing Research, National Institutes of Health, Bethesda, MD 20892, USA. [6]Department of Anesthesiology, Albert Einstein College of Medicine, Bronx, New York 10467, USA. [7]Dendrite Morphogenesis and Plasticity Unit, National Institute of Neurological Disorders and Stroke, National Institutes of Health, Bethesda, MD 20892, USA.

References
1. Levy JR, Holzbaur EL. Cytoplasmic dynein/dynactin function and dysfunction in motor neurons. Int J Dev Neurosci. 2006;24(2–3):103–11.
2. Schroer TA. Dynactin. Annu Rev Cell Dev Biol. 2004;20:759–79.
3. Ayloo S, Lazarus JE, Dodda A, Tokito M, Ostap EM, Holzbaur EL. Dynactin functions as both a dynamic tether and brake during dynein-driven motility. Nat Commun. 2014;5:4807.
4. Culver-Hanlon TL, Lex SA, Stephens AD, Quintyne NJ, King SJ. A microtubule-binding domain in dynactin increases dynein processivity by skating along microtubules. Nat Cell Biol. 2006;8(3):264–70.
5. Robinson RW, Snyder JA. Colocalization studies of Arp1 and p150Glued to spindle microtubules during mitosis: the effect of cytochalasin on the organization of microtubules and motor proteins in PtK1 cells. Cell Biol Int. 2006;30(7):631–9.
6. Zhapparova ON, Bryantseva SA, Dergunova LV, Raevskaya NM, Burakov AV, Bantysh OB, Shanina NA, Nadezhdina ES. Dynactin subunit p150Glued isoforms notable for differential interaction with microtubules. Traffic. 2009; 10(11):1635–46.
7. Lai C, Lin X, Chandran J, Shim H, Yang WJ, Cai H. The G59S mutation in p150(glued) causes dysfunction of dynactin in mice. J Neurosci. 2007;27(51): 13982–90.
8. Puls I, Jonnakuty C, LaMonte BH, Holzbaur EL, Tokito M, Mann E, Floeter MK, Bidus K, Drayna D, Oh SJ, et al. Mutant dynactin in motor neuron disease. Nat Genet. 2003;33(4):455–6.
9. Farrer MJ, Hulihan MM, Kachergus JM, Dachsel JC, Stoessl AJ, Grantier LL, Calne S, Calne DB, Lechevalier B, Chapon F, et al. DCTN1 mutations in Perry syndrome. Nat Genet. 2009;41(2):163–5.
10. Gustavsson EK, Trinh J, Guella I, Szu-Tu C, Khinda J, Lin CH, Wu RM, Stoessl J, Appel-Cresswell S, McKeown M *et al*: DCTN1 p.K56R in progressive supranuclear palsy. Parkinsonism Relat Disord 2016, 28:56–61.
11. Lazarus JE, Moughamian AJ, Tokito MK, Holzbaur EL. Dynactin subunit p150(glued) is a neuron-specific anti-catastrophe factor. PLoS Biol. 2013; 11(7):e1001611.
12. Dixit R, Levy JR, Tokito M, Ligon LA, Holzbaur EL. Regulation of dynactin through the differential expression of p150Glued isoforms. J Biol Chem. 2008;283(48):33611–9.
13. Tokito MK, Howland DS, Lee VM, Holzbaur EL. Functionally distinct isoforms of dynactin are expressed in human neurons. Mol Biol Cell. 1996;7(8):1167–80.
14. Austin S, Ziese M, Sternberg N. A novel role for site-specific recombination in maintenance of bacterial replicons. Cell. 1981;25(3):729–36.
15. Farley FW, Soriano P, Steffen LS, Dymecki SM. Widespread recombinase expression using FLPeR (flipper) mice. Genesis. 2000;28(3–4):106–10.
16. Dewachter I, Reverse D, Caluwaerts N, Ris L, Kuiperi C, Van den Haute C, Spittaels K, Umans L, Serneels L, Thiry E, et al. Neuronal deficiency of presenilin 1 inhibits amyloid plaque formation and corrects hippocampal long-term potentiation but not a cognitive defect of amyloid precursor protein [V717I] transgenic mice. J Neurosci. 2002;22(9):3445–53.
17. Hayashi S, McMahon AP. Efficient recombination in diverse tissues by a tamoxifen-inducible form of Cre: a tool for temporally regulated gene activation/inactivation in the mouse. Dev Biol. 2002;244(2):305–18.
18. Parisiadou L, Yu J, Sgobio C, Xie C, Liu G, Sun L, Gu XL, Lin X, Crowley NA, Lovinger DM, et al. LRRK2 regulates synaptogenesis and dopamine receptor activation through modulation of PKA activity. Nat Neurosci. 2014;
19. Lin X, Parisiadou L, Sgobio C, Liu G, Yu J, Sun L, Shim H, Gu XL, Luo J, Long CX, et al. Conditional expression of Parkinson's disease-related mutant alpha-synuclein in the midbrain dopaminergic neurons causes progressive neurodegeneration and degradation of transcription factor nuclear receptor related 1. J Neurosci. 2012;32(27):9248–64.
20. Aliaga L, Lai C, Yu J, Chub N, Shim H, Sun L, Xie C, Yang WJ, Lin X, O'Donovan MJ, et al. Amyotrophic lateral sclerosis-related VAPB P56S mutation differentially affects the function and survival of corticospinal and spinal motor neurons. Hum Mol Genet. 2013;22(21):4293–305.
21. Cai H, Lin X, Xie C, Laird FM, Lai C, Wen H, Chiang HC, Shim H, Farah MH, Hoke A, et al. Loss of ALS2 function is insufficient to trigger motor neuron degeneration in knock-out mice but predisposes neurons to oxidative stress. J Neurosci. 2005;25(33):7567–74.
22. Lai C, Xie C, McCormack SG, Chiang HC, Michalak MK, Lin X, Chandran J, Shim H, Shimoji M, Cookson MR, et al. Amyotrophic lateral sclerosis 2-deficiency leads to neuronal degeneration in amyotrophic lateral sclerosis through altered AMPA receptor trafficking. J Neurosci. 2006; 26(45):11798–806.
23. Arlotta P, Molyneaux BJ, Chen J, Inoue J, Kominami R, Macklis JD. Neuronal subtype-specific genes that control corticospinal motor neuron development in vivo. Neuron. 2005;45(2):207–21.
24. Bruijn LI, Miller TM, Cleveland DW. Unraveling the mechanisms involved in motor neuron degeneration in ALS. Annu Rev Neurosci. 2004;27:723–49.
25. McGoldrick P, Joyce PI, Fisher EM, Greensmith L. Rodent models of amyotrophic lateral sclerosis. Biochim Biophys Acta. 2013;1832(9):1421–36.
26. Weisenberg RC. Microtubule formation in vitro in solutions containing low calcium concentrations. Science. 1972;177(4054):1104–5.

27. Janke C, Bulinski JC. Post-translational regulation of the microtubule cytoskeleton: mechanisms and functions. Nat Rev Mol Cell Biol. 2011; 12(12):773–86.
28. Fu MM, Nirschl JJ, Holzbaur EL. LC3 binding to the scaffolding protein JIP1 regulates processive dynein-driven transport of autophagosomes. Dev Cell. 2014;29(5):577–90.
29. Levy JR, Sumner CJ, Caviston JP, Tokito MK, Ranganathan S, Ligon LA, Wallace KE, LaMonte BH, Harmison GG, Puls I, et al. A motor neuron disease-associated mutation in p150Glued perturbs dynactin function and induces protein aggregation. J Cell Biol. 2006;172(5):733–45.
30. Laird FM, Farah MH, Ackerley S, Hoke A, Maragakis N, Rothstein JD, Griffin J, Price DL, Martin LJ, Wong PC. Motor neuron disease occurring in a mutant dynactin mouse model is characterized by defects in vesicular trafficking. J Neurosci. 2008;28(9):1997–2005.
31. Wang QJ, Ding Y, Kohtz DS, Mizushima N, Cristea IM, Rout MP, Chait BT, Zhong Y, Heintz N, Yue Z. Induction of autophagy in axonal dystrophy and degeneration. J Neurosci. 2006;26(31):8057–68.
32. Cuervo AM, Dice JF. A receptor for the selective uptake and degradation of proteins by lysosomes. Science. 1996;273(5274):501–3.
33. Blanpied TA, Ehlers MD. Microanatomy of dendritic spines: emerging principles of synaptic pathology in psychiatric and neurological disease. Biol Psychiatry. 2004;55(12):1121–7.
34. Moughamian AJ, Holzbaur EL. Dynactin is required for transport initiation from the distal axon. Neuron. 2012;74(2):331–43.
35. Rothstein JD. Current hypotheses for the underlying biology of amyotrophic lateral sclerosis. Ann Neurol. 2009;65(Suppl 1):S3–9.
36. Portran D, Schaedel L, Xu Z, Thery M, Nachury MV. Tubulin acetylation protects long-lived microtubules against mechanical ageing. Nat Cell Biol. 2017;19(4):391–8.
37. Vaughan PS, Miura P, Henderson M, Byrne B, Vaughan KT. A role for regulated binding of p150(glued) to microtubule plus ends in organelle transport. J Cell Biol. 2002;158(2):305–19.

8

Amyloid-beta modulates microglial responses by binding to the triggering receptor expressed on myeloid cells 2 (TREM2)

Li Zhong[1†], Zongqi Wang[1†], Daxin Wang[1†], Zhe Wang[1†], Yuka A. Martens[2†], Linbei Wu[1], Ying Xu[1], Kai Wang[1], Jianguo Li[1], Ruizhi Huang[1], Dan Can[1], Huaxi Xu[1,3], Guojun Bu[1,2*] and Xiao-Fen Chen[1,4*]

Abstract

Background: TREM2 is an innate immune receptor specifically expressed in microglia. Coding variations in TREM2 have been reported to increase the risk for Alzheimer's disease (AD) and other neurodegenerative diseases. While multiple studies support a role for TREM2 in microglial recruitment to amyloid plaques, the chemoattractant factor modulating TREM2-dependent microglial responses has not been defined.

Methods: Potential binding of oligomeric amyloid-β 1–42 ($oA\beta_{1-42}$) to TREM2 was tested by complementary approaches including solid phase binding, surface plasmon resonance and immunoprecipitation assays. The ability of $oA\beta_{1-42}$ to activate TREM2 signaling pathways was examined by analyzing the phosphorylation of Syk and Akt in primary microglia as well as TREM2-mediated signaling in a reporter cell system. Lastly, the functional outcome of $oA\beta_{1-42}$-TREM2 interaction was tested by examining impacts on microglial migration in vitro and clustering around $oA\beta_{1-42}$-bearing brain areas in vivo.

Results: We found that $oA\beta_{1-42}$ bound to TREM2 with high affinity and activated TREM2-dependent signaling pathway. Neither monomeric nor scrambled Aβ bound to TREM2 supporting a specific interaction between oAβ and TREM2. The disease-associated mutations of TREM2 reduced its binding affinity to $oA\beta_{1-42}$. Furthermore, we identified several positively charged amino acids within residues 31–91 of TREM2 that were crucial for its interaction with $oA\beta_{1-42}$. Importantly, $oA\beta_{1-42}$ promoted microglial migration in vitro and clustering in vivo in a TREM2-dependent manner.

Conclusions: Our data establish a critical link between $oA\beta_{1-42}$, a major pathological component of AD, and TREM2, a strong genetic risk factor for AD expressed in microglia, and suggest that such interaction contributes to the pathogenic events in AD by modulating microglial responses.

Keywords: β-amyloid, microglia, migration, TREM2, Alzheimer's disease

* Correspondence: bu.guojun@mayo.edu; chenxf@xmu.edu.cn
†Equal contributors
[1]Fujian Provincial Key Laboratory of Neurodegenerative Disease and Aging Research, Institute of Neuroscience, Medical College, Xiamen University, Xiamen 361102, China
Full list of author information is available at the end of the article

Background

Alzheimer's disease (AD) is the most common form of dementia with histopathological hallmarks of amyloid-β (Aβ) plaques and tau neurofibrillary tangles in the brain [1, 2]. While the mechanism by which neurodegeneration occurs in AD is not entirely clear, disturbed Aβ clearance and plaque removal by microglia likely contribute to Aβ accumulation and neuritic dystrophy [3, 4]. As the brain resident innate immune cells, microglia constantly survey the microenvironment and become activated in response to pathogenic components that disrupt the homeostasis of the nervous system [5]. Intriguingly, microglia have been identified to constitute a protective barrier that prevents the outward extension of amyloid fibrils [6, 7]. The involvement of microglia in AD is further supported by recent genome-wide association and genome sequencing studies showing that rare coding variants in genes highly expressed in microglia as risk factors for late-onset AD [8–15]. Single-cell RNA-sequencing in AD mouse model has also identified a novel microglia type that is associated with AD and restricts its development [16]. Therefore, mounting evidence supports a causal role of microglial dysfunction in AD.

TREM2 is a cell surface receptor of the Ig superfamily that is specifically expressed by microglia within the central nervous system (CNS) [17]. Interest in TREM2 stems from its genetic mutations associated with several neurodegenerative disorders [18]. Homozygous missense mutations of *TREM2* including Y38C or T66 M have been identified to be associated with Nasu-Hakola disease (NHD) [19]. The R47H mutation in *TREM2* constitutes one of the strongest single allele genetic risk factors for AD, with an odds ratio similar to that of carrying an apolipoprotein E (*APOE*) ε4 allele [8, 9, 19]. The R62H, D87N and T96 K mutations in *TREM2* were also linked to AD after extensive analyses of *TREM2* polymorphisms [8, 10, 20]. However, the precise effects of TREM2 mutations on AD pathogenesis remain elusive.

TREM2 consists of an ectodomain, a transmembrane region and a short cytoplasmic tail. By coupling with DNAX-activating protein of 12 kDa (DAP12), TREM2 regulates a wide array of functions in microglia including cell survival, proliferation, phagocytosis, and inflammation [21–24]. Recent studies in *Trem2*-deficient AD mouse models have showed contradictory results regarding the amounts of Aβ plaques accumulation [21, 25, 26]. A later study indicated that *Trem2* deficiency has opposing effects on amyloid pathology at early and late stages of AD progression [27]. Nevertheless, it has been consistently reported that *Trem2* deficiency leads to reduced number of microglia around amyloid plaques, allowing greater amount of plaque pathology and related toxicity [26, 28]. However, it remains unknown how TREM2 affects the recruitment of microglia to the vicinity of plaque.

A diverse set of potential TREM2 ligands that are anionic or lipidic in nature have been proposed [29]. Bacteria and poly-anionic molecules were the first ligands proposed for TREM2 [30, 31]. TREM2 was also found to bind macrophages [32], astrocytes [33] and neurons [34]. Recently, TREM2 was shown to bind phospholipids [21], apolipoproteins (including apoE, apoJ and apoA) and lipoprotein particles (including low-density lipoprotein or "LDL") [35–37]. The binding of apolipoproteins to TREM2 was shown to facilitate either the phagocytosis of apoptotic neurons or the uptake of Aβ by microglia [35, 37]. Interestingly, the AD risk-associated variants, including R47H, R62H and D87N, have reduced affinity to these ligands. While multiple TREM2 ligands have been proposed, the identification of bona fide endogenous TREM2 ligands and the exploration of their physiological and pathological roles remain elusive. In this study, we found that $oA\beta_{1-42}$, but not monomeric or scrambled Aβ, bound to TREM2 with high affinity. The disease-associated mutations of TREM2 reduced its binding affinity to $oA\beta_{1-42}$. We further identified the specific region of TREM2 encompassing the arginine 47 and 62 residues that is critical for binding to $oA\beta_{1-42}$. Functional analyses revealed that $oA\beta_{1-42}$ activated TREM2 signaling pathway, promoted microglial migration and clustering in $oA\beta_{1-42}$-bearing brain regions via a TREM2-dependent manner. Our data provide mechanistic insight by which microglia recognize Aβ-related pathologies in AD.

Methods

Reagents and antibodies

Granulocyte-macrophage colony-stimulating factor (GM-CSF, 415-ML-010), RAGE-Fc recombinant protein (1145-RG-050) and anti-Fc antibody (MAB110) were purchased from R&D systems. Anti-Phospho-Syk (Tyr525/526) (2711 s), anti-total-Syk (13,198 s), anti-Phospho-Akt (Ser473) (4060 s), anti-total-Akt (4685 s) and anti-β-actin antibody (4970 s) were purchased from Cell Signaling Technology. Anti-Aβ antibody (MOAB-2, ab126649) was from Abcam. Unlabeled $A\beta_{1-42}$ (AS-20276), FAM-labeled $A\beta_{1-42}$ (AS-23525-05) and scrambled $A\beta_{42}$ (AS-25382) were from AnaSpec. The $mA\beta_{1-42}$ and $oA\beta_{1-42}$ were prepared as previously described with minor modification [38, 39]. Dissolved peptides in DMSO (5 mM) were diluted to 100 μM with cold phenol-free F-12 cell culture media (Gibco) and sonicated for 10 min to make $mA\beta_{1-42}$ which was used freshly. Part of the peptides were then incubated at 22 °C for 16 h followed by 24 h incubation at 4 °C, centrifuged at 16,000×g for 15 min, and the collected supernatant was used as $oA\beta_{1-42}$.

Western blotting

Cells were lysed with NP-40 lysis buffer (1% NP-40, 50 mM Tris-HCl, pH 8.0, 150 mM sodium chloride containing protease inhibitor mixture from Roche Applied Science) 24 h post transfection. Protein concentrations were determined using the BCA protein assay kit (Thermo Fisher Scientific, 23,225). Equal amounts of samples were subjected to sodium dodecyl sulfate-polyacrylamide gel electrophoresis (SDS-PAGE). Proteins were transferred onto PVDF membranes and probed with specific antibodies. Detection was performed using corresponding secondary antibodies and immunoreactive bands were quantified using ImageJ.

Immunoprecipitation assay

Two micrograms of $oA\beta_{1-42}$ were added into 400 μL of 1% solution of Tween-20 in TBS (1% TBST) with protease inhibitor cocktail. Two micrograms of sTREM2-Fc, sTREM1-Fc or Fc protein was pre-bound to 25 μL of protein A beads (Thermo Fisher Scientific, 20,334). The beads were then incubated with $oA\beta_{1-42}$ in 1% TBST at 4 °C overnight. Beads were washed 5 times with 1% TBST for 3 min, resuspended in 20 μL 2 × SDS loading buffer and subjected to electrophoresis on 4–12% Bis--Tris NuPAGE precast gels (Thermo Fisher Scientific, NP0322PK2).

Immunofluorescence staining

Human embryonic kidney 293 T cells (HEK 293 T) were transfected with pmCherry-N1, pmCherry-TREM1 or pmCherry-TREM2 plasmid. Twenty-four hours after transfection, cells were washed 3 times with DMEM and incubated with 1.0 μM FAM-labeled $oA\beta_{1-42}$ for 2 h at 4 °C. After 3 washes with PBS, cells were fixed with 4% paraformaldehyde for 15 min. Cells were then stained with DAPI for 3 min and then washed twice with PBS for 15 min. Coverslips were mounted on the glass slide using antifade reagent (Thermo Fisher Scientific, P36935) and observed using NIKON A1R Plus confocal microscope.

Expression and purification of sTREM2-Fc fusion proteins

The human TREM2 extracellular domain tagged with Fc that carries different fragments and mutations were cloned and purified from the conditioned medium of HEK 293 T cells as previously described [35]. Purified proteins were quantified with the BCA protein assay kit and the purity was determined on silver-stained SDS-PAGE gels.

Solid phase binding assay

A 96-well plate (Corning Incorporated) was coated with 100 nM $oA\beta_{1-42}$ in PBS overnight at 4 °C. Wells were washed with 0.05% PBST and blocked with 4% BSA for 1 h at 37 °C. Purified Fc or sTREM2-Fc proteins diluted in PBST containing 0.5% BSA were added and incubated for 30 min at 37 °C. After washing, the bound proteins were detected with biotinylated-anti-Fc antibody for 1 h at 37 °C. Plates were washed and then incubated with avidin-HRP for 30 min at 37 °C, washed again, and developed with TMB substrate solution (Sigma Aldrich, T5569), and read at 620 nm.

Mouse primary microglial culture

All animal experiments were conducted in compliance with the protocols of the Institutional Animal Care and Use Committee at Xiamen University. *Trem2*-knockout mice (KO, on C57BL/6 N background) and wild-type (WT) C57BL/6 N mice were obtained from the UC Davis Knockout Mouse Project (KOMP) repository as described previously [35]. Primary microglial cultures were prepared as previously described [35, 40]. WT or *Trem2*-KO mice at postnatal day 1–3 were used to prepare mixed glial cultures. Cells were plated onto poly-lysine coated flasks and grown in fresh DMEM (Gibco) supplemented with 10% FBS (Gibco). Medium was changed after 3 days to that contains 25 ng/mL GM-CSF and 10% FBS. Primary microglial cells were harvested after 10–12 days in culture and once every 3 days thereafter (up to two harvests).

Transwell assay

Cell migration assay was performed with Transwell cell culture inserts comprised of two chambers separated by an 8.0 μm polycarbonate membrane (Costar, 3422). Primary microglial cells (5×10^4) suspended in serum-free DMEM were added to the upper chamber of the inserts with serum-free DMEM in the bottom chamber. After 30 min incubation at 37 °C, the bottom medium was replaced with DMEM containing vehicle, 0.5 μM $oA\beta_{1-42}$ or 10% FBS. After 20 h, cells remained on the upper surface of the membrane were removed by scraping with a cotton swab. Cells that migrated through the membrane were fixed with 4% paraformaldehyde, stained with hematoxylin and eosin, and counted under Nikon inverted microscope.

TREM2 reporter assay

BWZ thymoma reporter cells (WT and TD4) were a generous gift from Dr. William E. Seaman (UCSF). BWZ cells express lacZ under control of the promoter for nuclear factor of activated T cells (NFAT) [41]. The TD4 cells are stably transfected to co-express TREM2 and DAP12 [34]. TD4 or WT cells were seeded in 96-well plates at 10^5 cells/well in RPMI media supplemented with 10 ng/mL phorbol 12-myristate 13-acetate (PMA). Ionomycin was added to a final concentration of 1 μM to serve as a positive control. Reporter cells were stimulated with different concentrations of $oA\beta_{1-42}$, $mA\beta_{1-42}$ or $scA\beta_{42}$ for 16 h at 37 °C, washed once with PBS, and lysed in a buffer containing 100 mM 2-mercaptoethanol, 9 mM $MgCl_2$, 0.125% NP-40, and 0.3 mM chlorophenol red-β-D-galactopyranoside. After 4 h at 37 °C, absorbance was measured at 595 nm, with correction for background absorbance at 630 nm.

Surface Plasmon Resonance assay

Surface Plasmon Resonance (SPR) analysis was performed at 25 °C using the Biacore T200 (GE Healthcare). Purified sTREM2-Fc and Fc protein were immobilized onto Biacore CM5 (GE Healthcare, BR-1005-30) chip using amine coupling kit (GE Healthcare, BR-1000-50). $oA\beta_{1-42}$, $mA\beta_{1-42}$ or $scA\beta_{42}$ was tested with a gradient concentration of 1.25 μM, 2.5 μM, 5.0 μM and 10.0 μM respectively.

Stereotactic injection of $oA\beta_{1-42}$

WT or *Trem2*-KO male mice at 6 months of age were anesthetized and placed in a stereotaxic frame. Investigators were blind to the condition of each animal during the experimental procedure and the quantification and analysis stages. A skin incision was made and holes were drilled at defined x (± 2.0 mm from bregma) and y (– 2.2 mm from bregma) positions. The left and the right hemisphere were injected with FAM-$oA\beta_{1-42}$ (a total of 1.5 μg in 3.0 μL) or vehicle at 0.30 μL/min with z-depths of 2.0 mm, respectively. Before being withdrawn slowly, the syringe was left in place for 10 min after each injection. Four or sixteen hours after injection, mice were anesthetized and perfused with ice-cold PBS. Brains were fixed in 4% PFA overnight at 4 °C, transferred to 30% sucrose for 48 h before embedded for cryostat sectioning.

Immunohistochemistry and microscopy

Twelve-μm thick cryosections were washed in PBS for 15 min, permeabilized in 5% normal donkey serum and 0.2% Triton X-100 for 1 h, followed by 48 h' incubation with Iba1 antibodies at 4 °C. The cryosections were washed with PBS for 30 min and treated with the Alexa-fluorophore-conjugated secondary antibodies for 2 h at RT. Sections were stained with DAPI (5 μg/mL), washed and mounted with anti-fade reagent. For confocal microscopy, 6 μm z-stacks (consisting of 13 optical slices of 0.5 μm thickness) were acquired using a NIKON A1R Plus confocal microscope.

Statistics

Data were obtained from at least three independent experiments, and presented as mean ± standard deviation (SD). Statistical analyses were performed using Graphpad Prism 5.0 software or SPSS software. Statistical significance was determined by one-way ANOVA or two-way ANOVA when more than two groups were compared and unpaired Student's *t*-test for single comparisons. $p < 0.05$ was considered significant.

Results

Oligomeric $A\beta_{1-42}$ binds to TREM2 and activates TREM2 signaling pathway

TREM2 deficiency was found to reduce the number of microglia clustering around Aβ plaques [21, 25, 26], suggesting a role of TREM2 in bridging the interaction between microglia and plaque. This prompts us to hypothesize that Aβ aggregates serve as chemoattractant for microglia by binding to cell surface TREM2. To test this hypothesis, we used a soluble TREM2-Fc (sTREM2-Fc) construct that consists of the extracellular domain of TREM2 spanning the N-terminal amino acids 1–171 fused to the Fc region of human IgG1 (Fig. 1a) as previously described [42]. The fusion protein was purified from the conditioned medium of transfected human embryonic kidney 293 T (HEK 293 T) cells (Fig. 1b). The extracellular domain of another TREM family member TREM1 fused to Fc (sTREM1-Fc) was also purified and served as a control (Fig. 1b). Soluble $oA\beta_{1-42}$ was assembled from synthetic Aβ peptides as previously described [38, 39] and exhibited heterogeneous distribution as low-n and high-n oligomers (Fig. 1c). In the solid phase protein binding assay, we found a specific binding of $oA\beta_{1-42}$ to sTREM2-Fc with a K_D of 86.50 nM, but not to the Fc region alone or sTREM1-Fc (Fig. 1d). Furthermore, in vitro immunoprecipitation assay revealed that soluble $oA\beta_{1-42}$ species in the form of both low-n and high-n aggregates were captured by bead-bound sTREM2-Fc but not sTREM1-Fc or Fc alone control (Fig. 1e), indicating a specific interaction between Aβ oligomers and sTREM2. Consistent with the binding of synthetic Aβ to TREM2, the endogenous Aβ from the brain lysates of 5xFAD amyloid mice model also bound to TREM2 immobilized on beads (Additional file 1: Figure S1A). As a negative control, endogenous Aβ was not detected when TREM1 was used as bait. Therefore, TREM2 specifically interacts with both synthetic and in vivo brain-derived Aβ. Co-localization between TREM2 and $oA\beta_{1-42}$ on the cell surface was observed when HEK 293 T cells were transfected with TREM2-Cherry and incubated with FAM-$oA\beta_{1-42}$; whereas, co-localization was not observed between TERM1 and $oA\beta_{1-42}$ (Additional file 1: Figure S1B and Additional file 1: Figure S1C). The interaction between TREM2 and $oA\beta_{1-42}$ was further confirmed by a surface plasmon resonance (SPR) assay which showed a dose-dependent binding of $oA\beta_{1-42}$ to sTREM2-Fc fusion protein but not Fc alone (Fig. 1f and g). Since our $oA\beta_{1-42}$ was prepared without separation of monomeric $A\beta_{1-42}$ ($mA\beta_{1-42}$), we further tested whether $mA\beta_{1-42}$ binds to TREM2. An SPR assay with

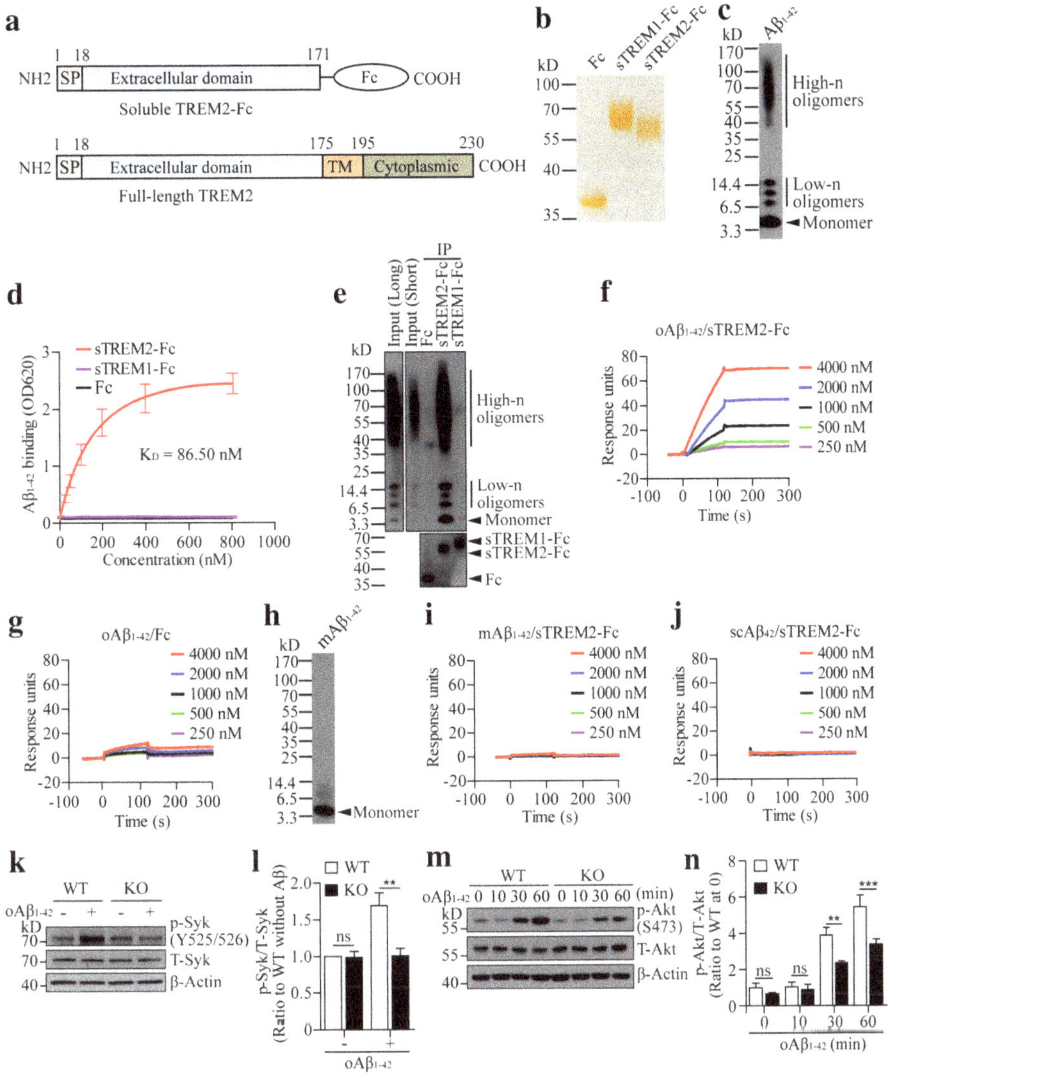

Fig. 1 Oligomeric $A\beta_{1-42}$ specifically binds to TREM2 and activates TREM2 signaling pathway. **a** Schematic representation of human TREM2 extracellular domain (sTREM2, amino acid residues 1–171) tagged with human IgG1 Fc. SP: signal peptide. **b** The cDNA encoding sTREM2-Fc, sTREM1-Fc or Fc alone was transfected into HEK 293 T cells. Each protein was purified from the conditioned medium and analyzed by silver stained SDS-PAGE. **c** The prepared $oA\beta_{1-42}$ peptides were analyzed by Western blotting using 4–12% Bis-Tris NuPAGE gel. **d** Solid phase binding assay showing the saturation binding curve and equilibrium dissociation constant (K_D) of $oA\beta_{1-42}$ binding to sTREM2-Fc. Fc and sTREM1-Fc served as negative controls ($n = 3$). **e** The Fc, sTREM2-Fc or sTREM1-Fc control was pre-bound to protein A agarose beads and used as baits for immunoprecipitation of $oA\beta_{1-42}$. The precipitated products were separated on 4–12% Bis-Tris NuPAGE gel and further subjected to Western blotting. (**f** and **g**) The binding profiles of $oA\beta_{1-42}$ to different concentrations of sTREM2-Fc **f** or Fc **g** were generated by SPR assay. **h** The prepared monomeric $A\beta_{1-42}$ ($mA\beta_{1-42}$) peptides were analyzed by Western blotting using 4–12% Bis-Tris NuPAGE gel. **i** The binding profiles of $mA\beta_{1-42}$ to different concentrations of sTREM2-Fc were generated by SPR assay. **j** The binding profiles of scrambled $A\beta_{42}$ ($scA\beta_{42}$) to different concentrations of sTREM2-Fc were generated by SPR assay. **k** Wild-type (WT) or *Trem2*-knockout (KO) microglia were stimulated with 1.0 μM $oA\beta_{1-42}$ for 1 h. Cell lysates were analyzed by Western blotting using antibodies specific for either total (T-Syk) or phosphorylated form (p-Syk) of Syk. **l** Quantification of Western blots as ratios of p-Syk/T-Syk. β-Actin was used as an internal control ($n = 3$, two-way ANOVA). **m** WT or *Trem2*-KO microglia were stimulated with 1.0 μM $oA\beta_{1-42}$ for the indicated time. Cell lysates at each time point were analyzed by Western blotting using antibodies specific for either total (T-Akt) or phosphorylated form (p-Akt) of Akt. **n** Quantification of Western blots as ratios of p-Akt/T-Akt. β-Actin was used as an internal control (n = 3, two-way ANOVA). Data information: Data represent mean ± SD. **, $p < 0.01$; ***, $p < 0.001$; ns, not significant

$mA\beta_{1-42}$ was performed and showed that $mA\beta_{1-42}$ had minimal binding to TREM2 (Fig. 1h and i). The lack of interaction between scrambled $A\beta_{42}$ ($scA\beta_{42}$) and sTREM2-Fc further confirmed the specific binding of $oA\beta_{1-42}$ to sTREM2-Fc (Fig. 1j). However, we did not include the characterization of fibrillar Aβ in the binding assay due to its structural heterogeneity, limited solubility, and sticky nature. The binding efficiency of $oA\beta_{1-42}$ to sTREM2-Fc was compared to that of the receptor for advanced glycosylation endproducts (RAGE), a microglial surface receptor that has been reported to induce microglial activation and chemotaxis upon binding to soluble Aβ [43]. We found TREM2 showed a higher binding affinity for $oA\beta_{1-42}$ than RAGE (Additional file 1: Figure S1D), supporting a potentially predominant role of TREM2 in mediating microglial-amyloid interaction. Taken together, our data revealed a specific interaction between TREM2 and $oA\beta_{1-42}$, supporting $oA\beta_{1-42}$ as a novel ligand for TREM2.

To determine if $oA\beta_{1-42}$ can functionally engage TREM2 and initiate intracellular signaling, we utilized TREM2 reporter cells (TD4) which express both TREM2 and DAP12 and produce β-galactosidase upon TREM2 engagement [34]. As a positive control, ionomycin stimulated the expression of reporter β-galactosidase in both wild-type (WT) and TREM2 reporter cells (Additional file 1: Figure S2A and Additional file 1: Figure S2B). Consistent with $oA\beta_{1-42}$ as a specific ligand for TREM2, it selectively activated TREM2 reporter cells but not WT cells in a dose-dependent manner, suggesting the requirement of TREM2 engagement. Consistent with the binding data, neither $mA\beta_{1-42}$ nor $scA\beta_{42}$ stimulated the reporter activity in TD4 cells. To gain more direct evidence that $oA\beta_{1-42}$ stimulates TREM2 signaling, we compared the levels of phosphorylated Syk (p-Syk) and Akt (p-Akt) known to represent TREM2 activation in microglia [44]. The stimulation with $oA\beta_{1-42}$ induced significantly higher level of p-Syk in WT but not *Trem2*-KO microglia (Fig. 1k and l). Furthermore, $oA\beta_{1-42}$ increased to a greater extent of p-Akt in WT than *Trem2*-KO microglia at both the 30- and 60-min time points (Fig. 1m and n). Taken together, these results indicate that $oA\beta_{1-42}$ binds to TREM2 and activates TREM2-dependent signaling pathway in microglia.

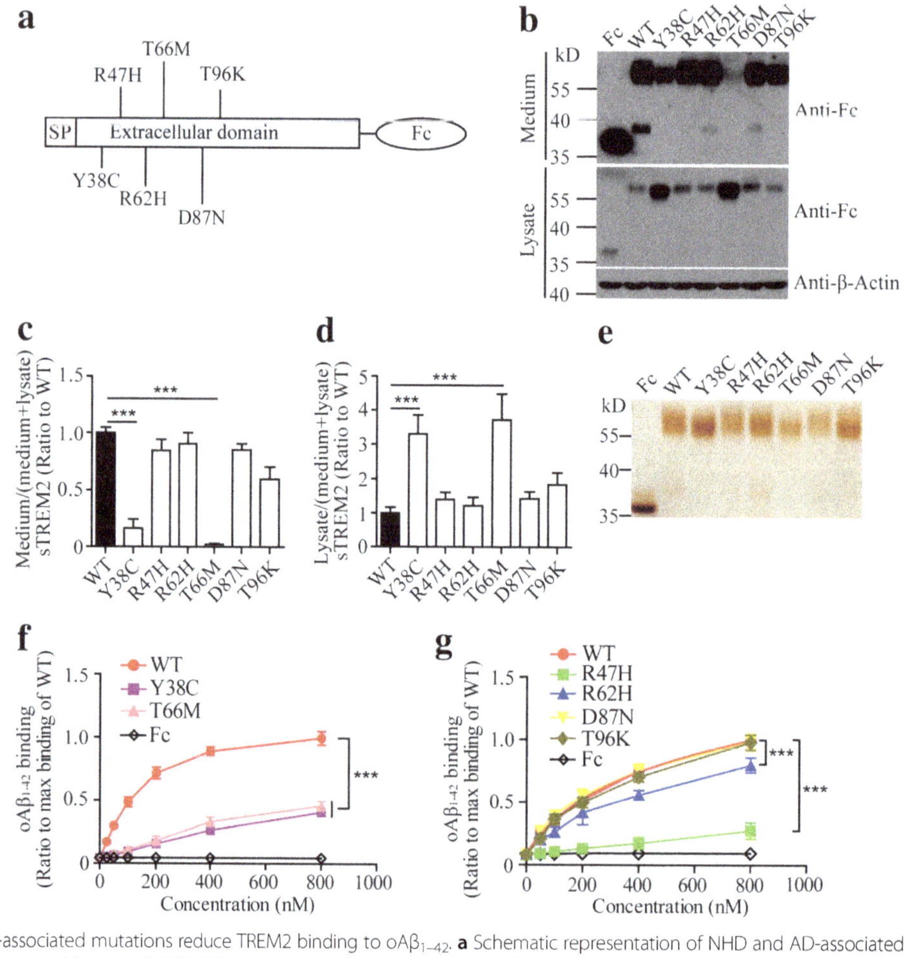

Fig. 2 The disease-associated mutations reduce TREM2 binding to $oA\beta_{1-42}$. **a** Schematic representation of NHD and AD-associated sTREM2 variants tagged with Fc. **b** Immunoblotting of sTREM2-Fc in the conditioned medium or cell lysate from HEK 293 T cells expressing AD-associated TREM2 mutations (R47H, R62H, D87N and T96 K) or NHD-associated TREM2 mutations (Y38C and T66 M). (**c** and **d**) Bar graphs show the quantification of Western blots from panel B (n = 3, one-way ANOVA). **e** The purified Fc, wild-type sTREM2 WT-Fc (WT) and sTREM2-Fc with disease-associated mutations were analyzed by silver staining. (**f** and **g**) Solid phase binding assay showing the binding affinity of $oA\beta_{1-42}$ to WT and different variants of TREM2-Fc (n = 3, two-way ANOVA). Data information: Data represent mean ± SD. ***, $p < 0.001$

The disease-associated mutations reduce TREM2 binding to $oA\beta_{1-42}$

The majority of disease-associated mutations are clustered within the putative ligand binding region of TREM2 ectodomain. With this in mind, we investigated how TREM2 variants affect its binding to $oA\beta_{1-42}$. We focused on two NHD-causing mutations (Y38C and T66 M) and four AD risk variants (R47H, R62H, D87N and T96 K) by generating sTREM2-Fc constructs carrying corresponding point mutations (Fig. 2a). Expression of Y38C and T66 M mutants in HEK 293 T cells resulted in a strong retention of sTREM2-Fc within the cytoplasm, thereby leading to reduced levels of both proteins in the conditioned medium (Figs. 2b-d). In contrast, none of the four AD risk-associated variants affected surface transport of sTREM2. Nevertheless, all proteins were purified to near homogeneity (Fig. 2e) and subjected to the solid phase protein binding assay using the same amount of each sTREM2-Fc variant. Compared to the wild-type (WT) protein, both NHD mutants exhibited dramatically decreased binding to $oA\beta_{1-42}$ (Fig. 2f). Among the four AD risk-associated variants, the D87N and T96 K mutants bound to $oA\beta_{1-42}$ with comparable affinity to WT protein (Fig. 2g). However, the R47H variant exhibited a large reduction (72%) in binding to $oA\beta_{1-42}$; while the binding of R62H mutant to $oA\beta_{1-42}$ was impaired to a lesser degree (20%).

Residues 31–91 of TREM2, in particular the positively charged amino acids within this region, are crucial for its interaction with $oA\beta_{1-42}$

In an attempt to map the critical region on TREM2 for its association with $oA\beta_{1-42}$, we constructed a series of C-terminally truncated mutants of sTREM2-Fc (Fig. 3a). Expression of the mutants carrying residues 1–71 and 1–91 resulted in a significantly increased secretion of sTREM2 fragments into the medium (Figs. 3b-d). The truncation mutants were purified and subjected to $oA\beta_{1-42}$ binding assay (Fig. 3e). Interestingly, mutants carrying residues 1–31 showed no detectable binding to

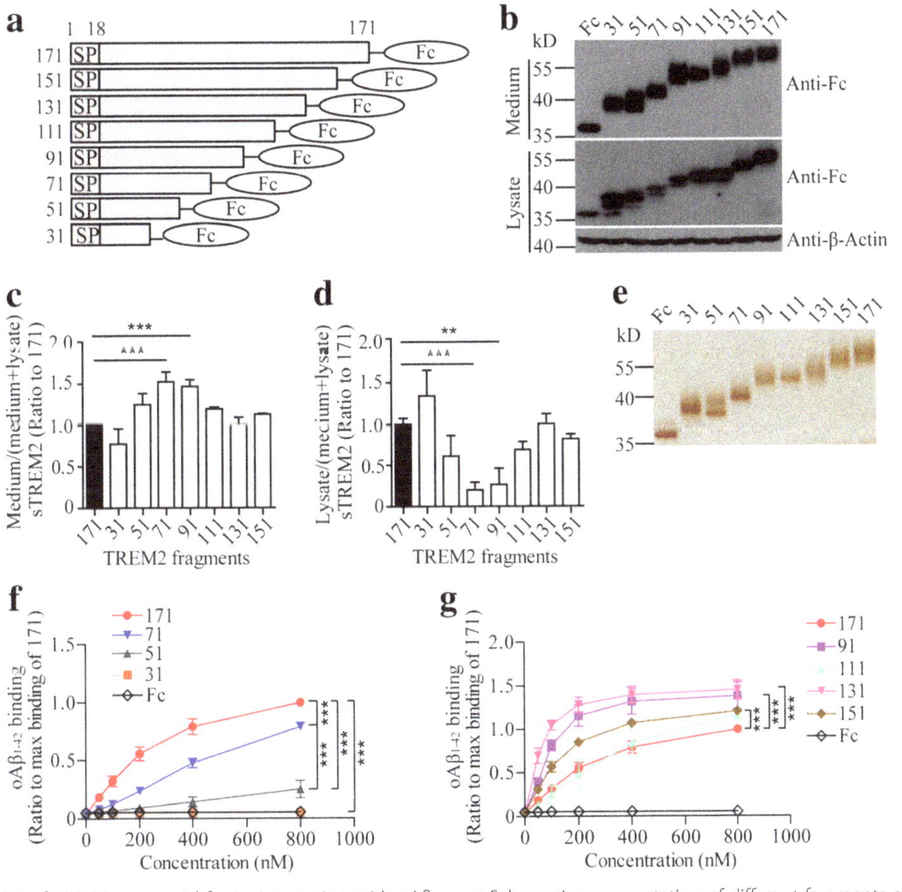

Fig. 3 Residues 31–91 of TREM2 are crucial for its interaction with $oA\beta_{1-42}$. **a** Schematic representation of different fragments of sTREM2-Fc. **b** Immunoblotting of sTREM2-Fc fragments in the conditioned medium or cell lysate from HEK 293 T cells. (**c** and **d**) Bar graphs showing the quantification of Western blots from panel B (n = 3, one-way ANOVA). **e** The purified Fc and sTREM2-Fc fragments were analyzed by silver staining. (**f** and **g**) Solid phase binding assay showing the binding affinity of $oA\beta_{1-42}$ to sTREM2-Fc fragments (n = 3, two-way ANOVA). Data information: Data represent mean ± SD. **, $p < 0.01$; ***, $p < 0.001$

$oA\beta_{1-42}$, while both fragments spanning 1–51 and 1–71 residues exhibited a statistically significant reduction in binding to $oA\beta_{1-42}$ as compared to the 1–171 fragment (Fig. 3f). For other truncation mutants, the binding affinity of the 1–111 fragment to $oA\beta_{1-42}$ was similar to the 1–171 fragment. However, fragments carrying 1–91, 1–131 and 1–151 residues showed significantly higher affinity to $oA\beta_{1-42}$ than the 1–171 fragment (Fig. 3g). Therefore, we conclude that residues 31–91 of TREM2 are necessary for its interaction with $oA\beta_{1-42}$.

Based on our observation that both R47H and R62H mutants significantly impaired the interaction between TREM2 and $oA\beta_{1-42}$, we sought to examine whether the positively charged amino acids (arginine and lysine) within residues 31–91 play important roles in TREM2 binding to $oA\beta_{1-42}$. Mutant forms of sTREM2-Fc carrying K42A, R46A, R47A, K48A, R52A, K57A, R62A, R76A or R77A mutation were constructed and expressed in HEK 293 T cells (Fig. 4a). The K42A, R47A, K57A, R62A, R76A and R77A mutants exhibited similar surface transport to WT sTREM2-Fc (Figs. 4b-d). However, the mutations in the forms of R46A, K48A or R52A led to significantly decreased levels of sTREM2 in the medium. Remarkably, the K48A mutation almost completely abolished the secretion of sTREM2 into the extracellular space, therefore preventing the follow-up protein purification for further analysis (Fig. 4e). Interestingly, all the mutations significantly reduced the binding affinity of TREM2 to $oA\beta_{1-42}$ (Fig. 4f), indicating that the interaction between TREM2 and $oA\beta_{1-42}$ relies on the positively charged amino acids within residues 31-91of TREM2.

Oligomeric $A\beta_{1-42}$ modulates microglial responses dependent on TREM2 receptor

Both $oA\beta_{1-42}$ and TREM2 have been reported to modulate the migration of microglial cells [45, 46]. We explored whether $oA\beta_{1-42}$-induced cell migration in microglia relies on endogenous TREM2. Primary microglia were isolated from both WT and *Trem2*-knockout (KO) mice and subjected to the transwell migration assay in the presence or absence of $oA\beta_{1-42}$ (Figs. 5a and b). Consistent with previous reports, the deficiency of *Trem2* led to a significant

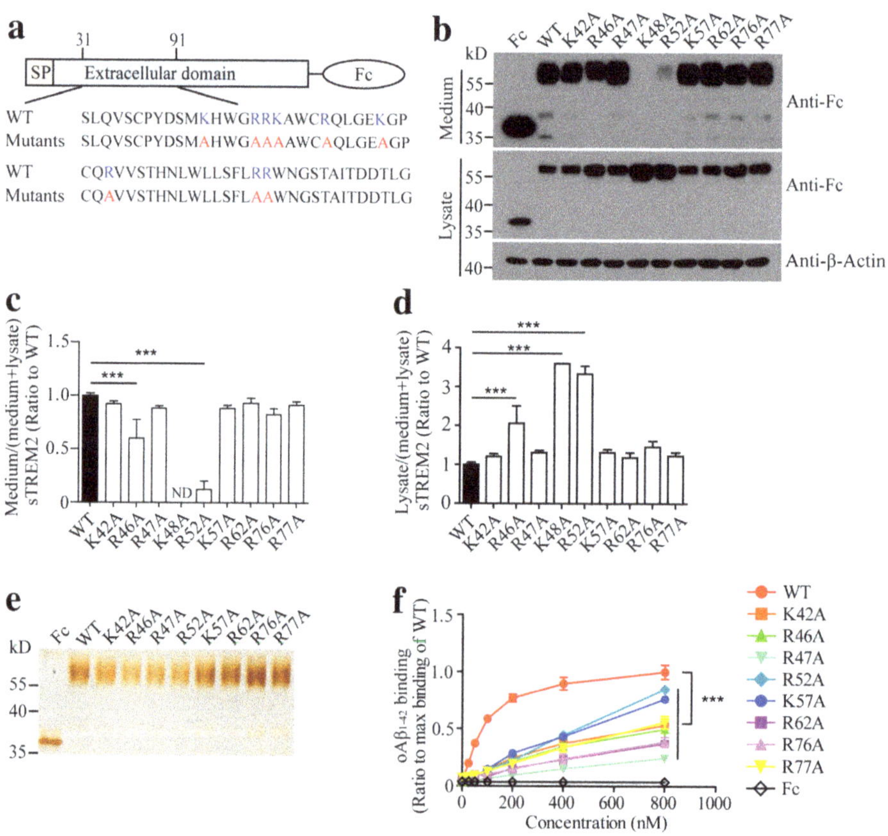

Fig. 4 The positively charged amino acids in TREM2 mediate its interaction with $oA\beta_{1-42}$. **a** Schematic representation of mutagenesis of positively charged amino acids on sTREM2-Fc. **b** Immunoblotting of sTREM2-Fc mutants in the conditioned medium or cell lysate from HEK 293 T cells. (**c** and **d**) Bar graphs showing the quantification of Western blots from panel B (n = 3, one-way ANOVA). ND: not determined. **e** The purified Fc and sTREM2-Fc mutants were analyzed by silver staining. **f** Solid phase binding assay showing the binding affinity of $oA\beta_{1-42}$ to sTREM2-Fc mutants (n = 3, two-way ANOVA). Data information: Data represent mean ± SD. ***, $p < 0.001$

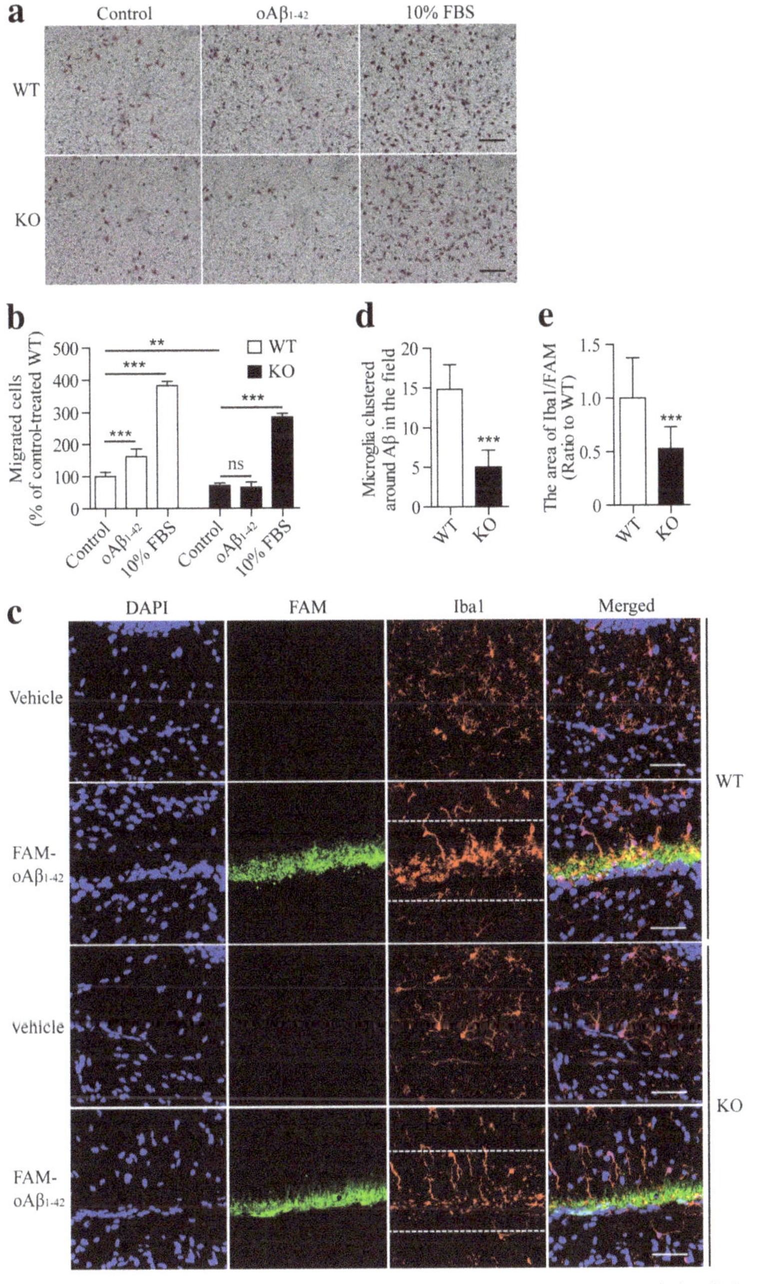

Fig. 5 Oligomeric $A\beta_{1-42}$ modulates microglial responses dependent on TREM2 receptor. **a** Primary microglial cells (5×10^4) from WT or *Trem2*-knockout (KO) mice were plated onto transwell chamber inserts. Following 20 h incubation with vehicle, $oA\beta_{1-42}$ (0.5 μM), or 10% FBS, cells migrated through the membrane were stained with hematoxylin and eosin and imaged under Nikon inverted microscope. Scale bar, 100 μm. **b** At least 24 different fields from three independent experiments of transwell tests were selected for quantifying the number of migrated cells (two-way ANOVA). **c** WT or *Trem2*-KO (KO) mice brain was harvested after FAM-$oA\beta_{1-42}$ injection for 4 h. Coronal sections from these mice were stained with DAPI (blue) for nuclei, and Iba1 (red) for microglia. Representative z stack images of $oA\beta_{1-42}$-bearing regions are shown. Scale bar, 50 μm. **d** At least 16 fields (212 μm × 100 μm, marked by white dotted lines in the panel C) from four mice were selected for quantifying the number of microglia (co-stained with DAPI and Iba1) clustered in the $oA\beta_{1-42}$-bearing regions (unpaired, Student's *t*-test). **e** The Iba1-positive area within the white dotted lines in the panel C was normalized to that of FAM-$oA\beta_{1-42}$-positive area (unpaired, Student's *t*-test). Data information: Data represent mean ± SD. **, $p < 0.01$; ***, $p < 0.001$; ns, not significant

decrease in cell migration across the transwell membrane [45]. Treatment with $oA\beta_{1-42}$ aggregates caused an increase in the migration of WT microglia as compared to the vehicle control. In contrast, $oA\beta_{1-42}$ was incapable of inducing migration of *Trem2*-KO microglial cells. Notably, the 10% FBS (Fig. 5a and b) and ATP (Additional file 1:

Figure S3A and Additional file 1: Figure S3B) dramatically stimulated the migration of both WT and *Trem2*-KO microglial cells, suggesting that the lack of response to $oA\beta_{1-42}$ in *Trem2*-KO microglia is likely specific. To further test whether TREM2 modulates the clustering of microglia around $oA\beta_{1-42}$ aggregates in vivo, we stereotactically injected FAM-$oA\beta_{1-42}$ into the hippocampi of adult WT and *Trem2*-KO mice and quantified the number of microglia in the vicinity of $oA\beta_{1-42}$. A significantly increased number of microglia accumulated around the injected Aβ in WT mouse brain as early as 4 h postinjection; however, the effect was diminished in the absence of *Trem2* (Figs. 5c-e). Similar results were obtained 16 h postinjection (Additional file 1: Figure S3C, Additional file 1: Figure S3D and Additional file 1: Figure S3E), further supporting a key role of TREM2 in microglial clustering around amyloid in vivo. Taken together, our data revealed that $oA\beta_{1-42}$ promotes microglial migration in vitro and clustering in vivo in a TREM2-dependent manner.

Discussion

Human genetic association studies increasingly highlight microglial genes, such as *TREM2*, *CD33*, and *CR1* playing important roles in the pathogenesis of AD [47]. Although mechanistic understanding of TREM2 action remains elusive, TREM2 presumably carries out its function in AD by binding to endogenous ligand(s). The many diverse ligands reported for TREM2 suggest that TREM2 is a highly promiscuous receptor. In this study, we found that oAβ specifically bound to TREM2 with high affinity. The interaction is functionally relevant to the pathogenesis of AD as evidenced by the observation that oAβ triggers microglial migration in vitro and microglial clustering around oAβ-bearing regions in vivo in a TREM2-dependent manner. Therefore, different ligands of TREM2 likely trigger ligand-specific events to accomplish the multi-functions reported for TREM2, in the case of oAβ microglial migration.

Interestingly, the disease-associated mutations of TREM2 reduced its binding affinity to Aβ. Although coding variants of TREM2 are linked to the risk of neurodegenerative diseases, the underlying mechanisms remain unknown. Several recent studies have shed light on how TREM2 missense mutations affect TREM2 function. First, the disease-associated mutations of TREM2 have impaired cell surface expression as reported previously [48, 49] and in our current study. Second, TREM2 missense mutations have been reported to reduce its shedding by ADAM proteases and impair the phagocytic activity of TREM2-expressing cells [48]. Furthermore, AD risk-associated mutations abrogate the function of soluble TREM2 in both suppressing apoptosis and triggering inflammatory responses [42]. Importantly, TREM2 variants exhibited deficits in binding to a wide array of ligands, including phospholipids, apolipoproteins, lipoprotein particles [21, 35–37] and $oA\beta_{1-42}$ as reported in the current study. Taken together, the disease-associated mutations of TREM2 likely modify the disease progression via multiple pathways.

Although our current study emphasizes a critical role of membrane-bound TREM2 which associates with DAP12 for downstream signaling, we could not rule out a potential contribution by sTREM2, a shed product of membrane-bound TREM2, that binds to a yet identified microglial receptor [42]. Hence, both full-length TREM2 and sTREM2 might be involved in microglial recruitment to the vicinity of plaques. Although the molecular mechanism underlying each pathway remains to be defined in future, our data suggest that the membrane-bound TREM2 signals through Syk and Akt, while sTREM2 might act on a separate microglial cell-surface receptor [42].

One striking feature of microglia in AD brain is their universal clustering around amyloid plaque. It was consistently reported that the number of microglia around amyloid plaques was reduced in *Trem2*-deficient amyloid mouse models, leading to an increase in less compact plaques [26, 28]. A critical function of microglia is thought to remove Aβ deposits via phagocytosis [50]. Indeed, loss of *Trem2* has been reported to impair the phagocytosis of Aβ by microglia in vitro [48]. Therefore, the physical interaction between TREM2 and Aβ likely regulates microglial mobility, potentially contributing to both the barrier function of microglia to compact the plaques and the phagocytic activity of microglia in removing the plaques. Future studies elucidating the biological function of their interaction might uncover targetable pathways for AD therapy.

Conclusions

Our current study demonstrates that oAβ binds to TREM2 with high affinity and activates TREM2-dependent signaling pathways in microglia. The absence of TREM2 impairs the oAβ-induced microglial migration in vitro and microglial clustering around oAβ-bearing brain regions in vivo. The identification of Aβ as a novel TREM2 ligand links TREM2 to the most prominent pathological features of AD and provides a critical mechanism by which microglia recognize and react to Aβ pathology.

Abbreviations

AD: Alzheimer's Disease; CNS: Central Nervous System; DAP12: DNAX-activating Protein of 12 kDa; GM-CSF: Granulocyte-Macrophage Colony-stimulating Factor; $oA\beta_{1-42}$: Oligomeric Amyloid-β 1–42; RAGE: Receptor for Advanced Glycosylation Endproducts; SPR: Surface Plasmon Resonance; sTREM2: soluble TREM2; TREM1: Triggering Receptor expressed on Myeloid Cells 1; TREM2: Triggering Receptor expressed on Myeloid Cells 2

Acknowledgements
The authors thank Junjie Chen from the Analysis and Measurement Center, School of Pharmaceutical Sciences, Xiamen University for kindly performing the data analysis on surface plasmon resonance assay.

Author contributions
X.C., G.B., L.Z., Z.W. and H.X. designed research; L.Z., Z.W., D.W., Z.W., Y.M., L.W., K.W., Y.X., J.L., R.H. and D.C. performed experiments; L.Z., Z.W., D.W., Z.W., Y.M. and X.C. analyzed data; X.C., Z.W. L.Z. and G.B. wrote the manuscript. All authors read and approved the final manuscript.

Funding
Research by the authors was supported by a grant from the Natural Science Foundation of Guangdong Province 2016A030306005 (to X.C.), grants from the National Natural Science Foundation of China 81370459, 31400914 (to X.C.), U1505227 (to G.B.), U1405222, 81771163 (to H.X.), 81701079 (to L.Z.), a grant from the Fundamental Research Funds for the Central Universities (20720180055, to X.C.), NIH grants RF1AG056130 (to G.B. and H.X.), R01AG035355 (to G.B.), R37AG027924 (to G.B.), RF1AG056114 (to H.X.); grants from the Postdoctoral Science Foundation of China 2016 M600503 and 2017 T100469 (to L.Z.), and the Cure Alzheimer's Fund (to G.B. and H.X.).

Competing interests
The authors declare that they have no competing interests.

Author details
[1]Fujian Provincial Key Laboratory of Neurodegenerative Disease and Aging Research, Institute of Neuroscience, Medical College, Xiamen University, Xiamen 361102, China. [2]Department of Neuroscience, Mayo Clinic, Jacksonville, FL 32224, USA. [3]Neuroscience Initiative, Sanford Burnham Prebys Medical Discovery Institute, La Jolla, CA 92037, USA. [4]Shenzhen Research Institute of Xiamen University, Shenzhen 518063, China.

References

1. Holtzman DM, Morris JC, Goate AM. Alzheimer's disease: the challenge of the second century. Sci Transl Med. 2011;3:77–1.
2. Huang Y, Mucke L. Alzheimer mechanisms and therapeutic strategies. Cell. 2012;148:1204–22.
3. Mandrekar S, Jiang Q, Lee CY, Koenigsknecht-Talboo J, Holtzman DM, Landreth GE. Microglia mediate the clearance of soluble Abeta through fluid phase macropinocytosis. J Neurosci. 2009;29:4252–62.
4. El Khoury J, Toft M, Hickman SE, Means TK, Terada K, Geula C, Luster AD. Ccr2 deficiency impairs microglial accumulation and accelerates progression of Alzheimer-like disease. Nat Med. 2007;13:432–8.
5. Hanisch UK, Kettenmann H. Microglia: active sensor and versatile effector cells in the normal and pathologic brain. Nat Neurosci. 2007;10:1387–94.
6. Condello C, Yuan P, Schain A, Grutzendler J. Microglia constitute a barrier that prevents neurotoxic protofibrillar Abeta42 hotspots around plaques. Nat Commun. 2015;6:6176.
7. Zhao R, Hu W, Tsai J, Li W, Gan WB. Microglia limit the expansion of beta-amyloid plaques in a mouse model of Alzheimer's disease. Mol Neurodegener. 2017;12:47.
8. Guerreiro R, Wojtas A, Bras J, Carrasquillo M, Rogaeva E, Majounie E, Cruchaga C, Sassi C, Kauwe JS, Younkin S, et al. TREM2 variants in Alzheimer's disease. N Engl J Med. 2013;368:117–27.
9. Jonsson T, Stefansson H, Steinberg S, Jonsdottir I, Jonsson PV, Snaedal J, Bjornsson S, Huttenlocher J, Levey AI, Lah JJ, et al. Variant of TREM2 associated with the risk of Alzheimer's disease. N Engl J Med. 2013;368:107–16.
10. Jin SC, Benitez BA, Karch CM, Cooper B, Skorupa T, Carrell D, Norton JB, Hsu S, Harari O, Cai Y, et al. Coding variants in TREM2 increase risk for Alzheimer's disease. Hum Mol Genet. 2014;23:5838–46.
11. Korvatska O, Leverenz JB, Jayadev S, McMillan P, Kurtz I, Guo X, Rumbaugh M, Matsushita M, Girirajan S, Dorschner MO, et al. R47H Variant of TREM2 Associated With Alzheimer Disease in a Large Late-Onset Family: Clinical, Genetic, and Neuropathological Study. JAMA Neurol. 2015;72:920–7.
12. Bertram L, Lange C, Mullin K, Parkinson M, Hsiao M, Hogan MF, Schjeide BM, Hooli B, Divito J, Ionita I, et al. Genome-wide association analysis reveals

9. Jonsson T, Stefansson H, Steinberg S, Jonsdottir I, Jonsson PV, Snaedal J, Bjornsson S, Huttenlocher J, Levey AI, Lah JJ, et al. Variant of TREM2 associated with the risk of Alzheimer's disease. N Engl J Med. 2013;368:107–16.
10. Jin SC, Benitez BA, Karch CM, Cooper B, Skorupa T, Carrell D, Norton JB, Hsu S, Harari O, Cai Y, et al. Coding variants in TREM2 increase risk for Alzheimer's disease. Hum Mol Genet. 2014;23:5838–46.
11. Korvatska O, Leverenz JB, Jayadev S, McMillan P, Kurtz I, Guo X, Rumbaugh M, Matsushita M, Girirajan S, Dorschner MO, et al. R47H Variant of TREM2 Associated With Alzheimer Disease in a Large Late-Onset Family: Clinical, Genetic, and Neuropathological Study. JAMA Neurol. 2015;72:920–7.
12. Bertram L, Lange C, Mullin K, Parkinson M, Hsiao M, Hogan MF, Schjeide BM, Hooli B, Divito J, Ionita I, et al. Genome-wide association analysis reveals

putative Alzheimer's disease susceptibility loci in addition to APOE. Am J Hum Genet. 2008;83:623–32.
13. Naj AC, Jun G, Beecham GW, Wang LS, Vardarajan BN, Buros J, Gallins PJ, Buxbaum JD, Jarvik GP, Crane PK, et al. Common variants at MS4A4/MS4A6E, CD2AP, CD33 and EPHA1 are associated with late-onset Alzheimer's disease. Nat Genet. 2011;43:436–41.
14. Hollingworth P, Harold D, Sims R, Gerrish A, Lambert JC, Carrasquillo MM, Abraham R, Hamshere ML, Pahwa JS, Moskvina V, et al. Common variants at ABCA7, MS4A6A/MS4A4E, EPHA1, CD33 and CD2AP are associated with Alzheimer's disease. Nat Genet. 2011;43:429–35.
15. Huang KL, Marcora E, Pimenova AA, Di Narzo AF, Kapoor M, Jin SC, Harari O, Bertelsen S, Fairfax BP, Czajkowski J, et al. A common haplotype lowers PU.1 expression in myeloid cells and delays onset of Alzheimer's disease. Nat Neurosci. 2017;20:1052–61.
16. Keren-Shaul H, Spinrad A, Weiner A, Matcovitch-Natan O, Dvir-Szternfeld R, Ulland TK, David E, Baruch K, Lara-Astaiso D, Toth B, et al. A Unique Microglia Type Associated with Restricting Development of Alzheimer's Disease. Cell. 2017;169:1276–90. e1217
17. Schmid CD, Sautkulis LN, Danielson PE, Cooper J, Hasel KW, Hilbush BS, Sutcliffe JG, Carson MJ. Heterogeneous expression of the triggering receptor expressed on myeloid cells-2 on adult murine microglia. J Neurochem. 2002;83:1309–20.
18. Jay TR, von Saucken VE, Landreth GE. TREM2 in Neurodegenerative Diseases. Mol Neurodegener. 2017;12:56.
19. Guerreiro R, Hardy J. TREM2 and neurodegenerative disease. N Engl J Med. 2013;369:1569–70.
20. Jin SC, Carrasquillo MM, Benitez BA, Skorupa T, Carrell D, Patel D, Lincoln S, Krishnan S, Kachadoorian M, Reitz C, et al. TREM2 is associated with increased risk for Alzheimer's disease in African Americans. Mol Neurodegener. 2015;10:19.
21. Wang Y, Cella M, Mallinson K, Ulrich JD, Young KL, Robinette ML, Gilfillan S, Krishnan GM, Sudhakar S, Zinselmeyer BH, et al. TREM2 lipid sensing sustains the microglial response in an Alzheimer's disease model. Cell. 2015;160:1061–71.
22. Zheng H, Jia L, Liu CC, Rong Z, Zhong L, Yang L, Chen XF, Fryer JD, Wang X, Zhang YW, et al. TREM2 Promotes Microglial Survival by Activating Wnt/beta-Catenin Pathway. J Neurosci. 2017;37:1772–84.
23. Takahashi K, Rochford CD, Neumann H. Clearance of apoptotic neurons without inflammation by microglial triggering receptor expressed on myeloid cells-2. J Exp Med. 2005;201:647–57.
24. Zhong L, Chen XF, Zhang ZL, Wang Z, Shi XZ, Xu K, Zhang YW, Xu H, Bu G. DAP12 Stabilizes the C-terminal Fragment of the Triggering Receptor Expressed on Myeloid Cells-2 (TREM2) and Protects against LPS-induced Pro-inflammatory Response. J Biol Chem. 2015;290:15866–77.
25. Jay TR, Miller CM, Cheng PJ, Graham LC, Bemiller S, Broihier ML, Xu G, Margevicius D, Karlo JC, Sousa GL, et al. TREM2 deficiency eliminates TREM2 + inflammatory macrophages and ameliorates pathology in Alzheimer's disease mouse models. J Exp Med. 2015;212:287–95.
26. Wang Y, Ulland TK, Ulrich JD, Song W, Tzaferis JA, Hole JT, Yuan P, Mahan TE, Shi Y, Gilfillan S, et al. TREM2-mediated early microglial response limits diffusion and toxicity of amyloid plaques. J Exp Med. 2016;213:667–75.
27. Jay TR, Hirsch AM, Broihier ML, Miller CM, Neilson LE, Ransohoff RM, Lamb BT, Landreth GE. Disease Progression-Dependent Effects of TREM2 Deficiency in a Mouse Model of Alzheimer's Disease. J Neurosci. 2017;37:637–47.
28. Yuan P, Condello C, Keene CD, Wang Y, Bird TD, Paul SM, Luo W, Colonna M, Baddeley D, Grutzendler J. TREM2 Haplodeficiency in Mice and Humans Impairs the Microglia Barrier Function Leading to Decreased Amyloid Compaction and Severe Axonal Dystrophy. Neuron. 2016;92:252–64.
29. Kober DL, Brett TJ. TREM2-Ligand Interactions in Health and Disease. J Mol Biol. 2017;429:1607–29.

30. Daws MR, Sullam PM, Niemi EC, Chen TT, Tchao NK, Seaman WE. Pattern recognition by TREM-2: binding of anionic ligands. J Immunol. 2003;171:594–9.
31. Quan DN, Cooper MD, Potter JL, Roberts MH, Cheng H, Jarvis GA. TREM-2 binds to lipooligosaccharides of Neisseria gonorrhoeae and is expressed on reproductive tract epithelial cells. Mucosal Immunol. 2008;1:229–38.
32. Hamerman JA, Jarjoura JR, Humphrey MB, Nakamura MC, Seaman WE, Lanier LL. Cutting edge: inhibition of TLR and FcR responses in macrophages by triggering receptor expressed on myeloid cells (TREM)-2 and DAP12. J Immunol. 2006;177:2051–5.
33. Stefano L, Racchetti G, Bianco F, Passini N, Gupta RS, Bordignon PP, Meldolesi J. The surface-exposed chaperone, Hsp60, is an agonist of the microglial TREM2 receptor. J Neurochem. 2009;110:284–94.
34. Hsieh CL, Koike M, Spusta SC, Niemi EC, Yenari M, Nakamura MC, Seaman WE. A role for TREM2 ligands in the phagocytosis of apoptotic neuronal cells by microglia. J Neurochem. 2009;109:1144–56.
35. Atagi Y, Liu CC, Painter MM, Chen XF, Verbeeck C, Zheng H, Li X, Rademakers R, Kang SS, Xu H, et al. Apolipoprotein E Is a Ligand for Triggering Receptor Expressed on Myeloid Cells 2 (TREM2). J Biol Chem. 2015;290:26043–50.
36. Bailey CC, DeVaux LB, Farzan M. The Triggering Receptor Expressed on Myeloid Cells 2 Binds Apolipoprotein E. J Biol Chem. 2015;290:26033–42.
37. Yeh FL, Wang Y, Tom I, Gonzalez LC, Sheng M. TREM2 Binds to Apolipoproteins, Including APOE and CLU/APOJ, and Thereby Facilitates Uptake of Amyloid-Beta by Microglia. Neuron. 2016;91:328–40.
38. Stine WB Jr, Dahlgren KN, Krafft GA, LaDu MJ. In vitro characterization of conditions for amyloid-beta peptide oligomerization and fibrillogenesis. J Biol Chem. 2003;278:11612–22.
39. Kim T, Vidal GS, Djurisic M, William CM, Birnbaum ME, Garcia KC, Hyman BT, Shatz CJ. Human LilrB2 is a beta-amyloid receptor and its murine homolog PirB regulates synaptic plasticity in an Alzheimer's model. Science. 2013;341:1399–404.
40. Zhu X, Wang S, Yu L, Yang H, Tan R, Yin K, Jin J, Zhao H, Guan D, Xu Y. TL-2 attenuates beta-amyloid induced neuronal apoptosis through the AKT/GSK-3beta/beta-catenin pathway. Int J Neuropsychopharmacol. 2014;17:1511–9.
41. Sanderson S, Shastri N. LacZ inducible, antigen/MHC-specific T cell hybrids. Int Immunol. 1994;6:369–76.
42. Zhong L, Chen XF, Wang T, Wang Z, Liao C, Wang Z, Huang R, Wang D, Li X, Wu L, et al. Soluble TREM2 induces inflammatory responses and enhances microglial survival. J Exp Med. 2017;214:597–607.
43. Yan SD, Chen X, Fu J, Chen M, Zhu H, Roher A, Slattery T, Zhao L, Nagashima M, Morser J, et al. RAGE and amyloid-beta peptide neurotoxicity in Alzheimer's disease. Nature. 1996;382:685–91.
44. Peng Q, Malhotra S, Torchia JA, Kerr WG, Coggeshall KM, Humphrey MB. TREM2- and DAP12-dependent activation of PI3K requires DAP10 and is inhibited by SHIP1. Sci Signal. 2010;3:ra38.
45. Mazaheri F, Snaidero N, Kleinberger G, Madore C, Daria A, Werner G, Krasemann S, Capell A, Trumbach D, Wurst W, et al. TREM2 deficiency impairs chemotaxis and microglial responses to neuronal injury. EMBO Rep. 2017;18:1186–98.
46. Kim HJ, Ajit D, Peterson TS, Wang Y, Camden JM, Gibson Wood W, Sun GY, Erb L, Petris M, Weisman GA. Nucleotides released from $A\beta_{1-42}$-treated microglial cells increase cell migration and $A\beta_{1-42}$ uptake through $P2Y_2$ receptor activation. J Neurochem. 2012;121:228–38.
47. Malik M, Parikh I, Vasquez JB, Smith C, Tai L, Bu G, MJ LD, Fardo DW, Rebeck GW, Estus S. Genetics ignite focus on microglial inflammation in Alzheimer's disease. Mol Neurodegener. 2015;10:52.
48. Kleinberger G, Yamanishi Y, Suarez-Calvet M, Czirr E, Lohmann E, Cuyvers E, Struyfs H, Pettkus N, Wenninger-Weinzierl A, Mazaheri F, et al. TREM2 mutations implicated in neurodegeneration impair cell surface transport and phagocytosis. Sci Transl Med. 2014;6:243–86.
49. Sirkis DW, Bonham LW, Aparicio RE, Geier EG, Ramos EM, Wang Q, Karydas A, Miller ZA, Miller BL, Coppola G, Yokoyama JS. Rare TREM2 variants associated with Alzheimer's disease display reduced cell surface expression. Acta Neuropathol Commun. 2016;4:98.
50. Lee CY, Landreth GE. The role of microglia in amyloid clearance from the AD brain. J Neural Transm (Vienna). 2010;117:949–60.

Apolipoprotein E4 impairs spontaneous blood brain barrier repair following traumatic brain injury

Bevan S. Main[1], Sonia Villapol[1], Stephanie S. Sloley[1], David J. Barton[1], Maia Parsadanian[1], Chinyere Agbaegbu[1], Kathryn Stefos[1], Mondona S. McCann[1], Patricia M. Washington[1], Olga C. Rodriguez[2] and Mark P. Burns[1,3*]

Abstract

Background: Traumatic Brain Injury (TBI) is a major cause of disability and mortality, to which there is currently no comprehensive treatment. Blood Brain Barrier (BBB) dysfunction is well documented in human TBI patients, yet the molecular mechanisms that underlie this neurovascular unit (NVU) pathology remains unclear. The apolipoprotein-E (apoE) protein has been implicated in controlling BBB integrity in an isoform dependent manner, via suppression of Cyclophilin A (CypA)–Matrix metallopeptidase-9 (MMP-9) signaling cascades, however the contribution of this pathway in TBI-induced BBB permeability is not fully investigated.

Methods: We exposed C57Bl/6 mice to controlled cortical impact and assessed NVU and BBB permeability responses up to 21 days post-injury. We pharmacologically probed the role of the CypA-MMP-9 pathway in BBB permeability after TBI using Cyclosporin A (CsA, 20 mg/kg). Finally, as the apoE4 protein is known to be functionally deficient compared to the apoE3 protein, we used humanized APOE mice as a clinically relevant model to study the role of apoE on BBB injury and repair after TBI.

Results: In C57Bl/6 mice there was an inverse relationship between soluble apoE and BBB permeability, such that damaged BBB stabilizes as apoE levels increase in the days following TBI. TBI mice displayed acute pericyte loss, increased MMP-9 production and activity, and reduced tight-junction expression. Treatment with the CypA antagonist CsA in C57Bl/6 mice attenuates MMP-9 responses and enhances BBB repair after injury, demonstrating that MMP-9 plays an important role in the timing of spontaneous BBB repair after TBI. We also show that *apoe* mRNA is present in both astrocytes and pericytes after TBI.

We report that APOE3 and APOE4 mice have similar acute BBB responses to TBI, but APOE3 mice display faster spontaneous BBB repair than APOE4 mice. Isolated microvessel analysis reveals delayed pericyte repopulation, augmented and sustained MMP-9 expression at the NVU, and impaired stabilization of Zonula Occludens-1, Occludin and Claudin-5 expression at tight junctions in APOE4 mice after TBI compared to APOE3 mice.

Conclusions: These data confirm apoE as an important modulator of spontaneous BBB stabilization following TBI, and highlights the APOE4 allele as a risk factor for poor outcome after TBI.

Keywords: Apolipoprotein E, Blood brain barrier, Neurovascular unit, Pericyte, MMP-9, CD31, Lectin, TBI

* Correspondence: mpb37@georgetown.edu
[1]Laboratory for Brain Injury and Dementia, Department of Neuroscience, Georgetown University Medical Center, Washington, DC 20057, USA
[3]Department of Neuroscience, Georgetown University Medical Center, New Research Building-EG11, 3970 Reservoir Rd, NW, Washington, D.C 20057, USA
Full list of author information is available at the end of the article

Background

Traumatic Brain Injury (TBI) is defined as a head injury sustained from an external physical force, resulting in the disruption of normal brain function. It represents a significant socio-economic and public health burden, with an estimated 2.5 million Americans sustaining a TBI per year, placing an extremely high economic cost on the community, currently estimated at $76.5 billion annually. It is well established that changes in blood brain barrier (BBB) function are a major determinant of TBI severity and recovery timeframes [1]. In addition to primary damage resulting from the initial impact, alterations in BBB integrity can also be influenced by deleterious secondary injury responses, including inflammatory cascades and abnormal metabolic processes within the central nervous system [2].

The human apolipoprotein-E protein (apoE) is a protein produced primarily by astrocytes and serves as a major lipid transport molecule in the central nervous system [3]. ApoE deficient mice have greater cell death, axonal pathology, and behavioral deficits after brain injury [4, 5], and apoE infusion reduces neuronal cell death in experimental ischemia [6]. Severe human TBI patients show a 70% decrease in cerebrospinal fluid apoE acutely post-injury [7], and we see a similar acute decrease in soluble apoE protein levels in mouse TBI brain [8]. Critically, the apoE protein regulates BBB permeability by regulating the activity of an LRP1-Cyclophilin A (CypA)–Matrix Metallopeptidase-9 (MMP-9) signaling pathway in pericytes located at the neurovascular unit (NVU) [9].

The human apolipoprotein-E gene (APOE) and its 3 associated polymorphisms (APOE2, APOE3, and APOE4) are hypothesized to contribute to several secondary injury processes [8], including influencing BBB breakdown [10, 11]. Clinically, the APOE4 gene polymorphism is associated with unfavorable outcomes following TBI [12], with the presence of at least one E4 allele associated with increased mortality [13], prolonged coma [14], poor prognosis [15], and an enhanced risk of late-onset Alzheimer's disease [16]. These features are recapitulated in animal models of TBI, with APOE4 mice displaying increased mortality [17], impaired cognition [18], and exacerbated secondary injury pathways including amyloid beta accumulation [19] and neuroinflammation [20] compared to APOE3 mice. In non-injured APOE mice, APOE4 mice have enhanced BBB permeability compared to APOE3 and APOE2 mice [9]. Additionally, human APOE4 carriers exhibit increased cerebral spinal fluid MMP-9 expression, correlating with enhanced BBB dysfunction [21], while APOE4 post-mortem AD brains have increased CypA and MMP-9 in cortical pericytes [22]. This suggests that apoE isoforms may play a key role in regulating BBB integrity; however, the contribution of respective apoE isoforms to TBI-induced BBB permeability has not been investigated.

We hypothesized that apoE influences BBB permeability and subsequent stabilization following TBI. To test this hypothesis, we used multiple techniques to demonstrate the normal timecourse of BBB breakdown and repair after controlled cortical impact (CCI) in mice. We examined the protein levels and activity of MMP-9 in isolated microvessels after TBI, and also probed these microvessels for mRNA expression of *Apoe*, *Mmp-9*, and tight junction proteins. As the human apoE4 protein is known to be functionally deficient compared to the apoE3 protein, we also used humanized APOE mice as a clinically relevant model to study the role of apoE on BBB injury and repair after TBI. We report an inverse relationship between soluble apoE and BBB permeability after TBI, such that BBB permeability decreases as apoE levels increase over time post-injury. Additionally, we demonstrate that APOE4 mice display enhanced MMP-9 profiles and reduced tight junction protein expression, resulting in impaired BBB stabilization following TBI compared to APOE3 mice.

Methods

Animals

Wildtype C57Bl/6 male mice were purchased from Jackson Laboratories (Bar Harbor, ME) and were 3–4 months old at the time of injury. Male human APOE targeted replacement mice with the human APOE3 or APOE4 inserted at the endogenous murine APOE promoter on a C57BL/6 J background were 3–4 months old at the time of injury. A limitation of the work in this study is that it only included male mice. Further research will be needed to determine if these results translate to female mice.

Animals were group housed under a 12 h light/dark cycle with ad libitum access to food and water. All mice were euthanized via carbon dioxide inhalation followed by saline perfusion. All procedures were conducted in accordance with protocols approved by the Georgetown University Animal Care and Use Committee. Experiments adhered to guidelines from the Guide for the Care and Use of Laboratory Animals, U.S. Department of Health and Human Services.

Controlled cortical impact (CCI) mouse model of TBI

CCI was conducted as previously described [8, 19]. Briefly, surgical anesthesia was induced using 4% isoflurane with maintenance in 2%, at flow rate of 1–1.5 L/min in freely breathing oxygen. The anesthetized animal was mounted in a stereotaxic frame and the surgical site clipped and aseptically sterilized. A 10 mm midline incision was made over the skull, the skin and fascia reflected and craniotomy performed (4 mm) on the central aspect of the left parietal bone. The impounder tip of a Leica StereoOne Impactor was sterilized, positioned to the surface of the exposed dura, and set to impact the cortical surface at 5.25-m/s velocity, 1.5 mm tissue deformation as previously described [23]. Sham animals received isoflurane anesthesia, skin incision, and reflection, but no impact. After injury, the incision was closed with wound clips, anesthesia discontinued, 1 ml saline administered by intraperitoneal (i.p) injection and the mouse placed in a heated cage to maintain normothermia for a 45 min recovery period. All animals monitored carefully for 4 h after surgery and then daily.

Pharmacological treatments

For cyclosporine A (CsA) experiments, wildtype mice were randomly assigned in a blinded manner to receive either cyclosporine A (Sigma-Aldrich, St Louis, MO) or vehicle (5% ethanol, 25% cremaphor oil, and 70% saline), at 15 min post-injury. CsA was administered i.p. at 20 mg/kg in 10 mL/kg initially, with repeat doses administered at 10 mg/kg at 10 mL/kg, i.p. at 24 h intervals. The safety and efficacy of this dosing regimen in rodents has previously been established [24].

Magnetic resonance imaging

Magnetic resonance imaging (MRI) was performed using the 7 Tesla horizontal bore Bruker Magnetic Resonance Imager in the Lombardi Comprehensive Cancer Center's Preclinical Imaging Research Laboratory, at Georgetown University. Animals were anesthetized using 1.5% isoflurane and 30% nitrous oxide, positioned in a custom-made mouse stereotaxic device, and monitored for temperature and respiration. Following a pre-injection scan, the mice were withdrawn from the scanner and 200 μl of the gadolinium (Gd)-enhanced contrast dye gadopentetate dimeglumine ((GdDTPA), 10% in phosphate-buffered saline (PBS)) was subcutaneously injected. Imaging was performed with a 35 mm mouse brain volume coil. Images were then obtained after injection, and dye was visualized with T1-weighted RARE sequencing with the following parameters: FOV: 3.0 cm × 3.0 cm, matrix: 256 × 256, TR: 1650 ms, TE: 10. 6 ms, Inversion Time: 650 ms, averages: 1, Rare Factor: 2, slice thickness: 1 mm, inter-slice distance: 1 mm. Since Gd-DPTA clears quickly from the body and is non-toxic, we used the same animals ($n = 3$) to longitudinally analyze BBB permeability, allowing for minimization of inter-subject variability. On each MRI day, we performed a prescan prior to GdDTPA injection to ensure that no residual signal remained from the prior GdDTPA injections. Multiple scans were collected for each mouse up to 90 min post-GDDTPA injection, and the scans shown in this manuscript were collected 1 h after the GdDTPA injection. Sequential images through the lesion site were analyzed using ImageJ software (National Institutes of Health, Bethesda, MD). Total Gd signal through the lesion was quantified for each mouse from the ipsilateral cortex and expressed as percent of the corresponding Gd signal from the contralateral cortex.

BBB integrity assay- Evans blue

Evans blue (EB) extravasation assessed BBB permeability following CCI. Two hours before euthanasia, animals were administered 200 μL of EB dye (2% *w*/*v*, i.p., Sigma-Aldrich, St Louis, MO) in saline. After euthanasia, animals were immediately transcardially perfused with ice-cold PBS, brains extracted and micro-dissected to obtain the cortex and thalamus/striatum in both the ipsilateral and contralateral hemispheres. Samples were weighed and placed in ice-cold trichloroacetic acid (50% w/v in distilled water), before homogenization by sonication. Homogenates were incubated at 4 °C for 30 min, followed by centrifugation at 16,000×g for 30 min at 4 ° C. The supernatant of each sample was removed and absorbance measured at an excitation of 540 nm and an emission of 680 nm. Absorbance measurements were adjusted for tissue weight and subsequent levels of EB in each sample was calculated relative to a standard curve of known EB concentrations.

Protein extraction

Subcellular fractions containing soluble and membrane bound proteins were separated by sequential centrifugation. Mice were perfused with ice-cold PBS; brain removed and a 5 mm-diameter region of tissue surrounding the cortex lesion, or tissue corresponding to the area of lesion in sham mice, was excised by punch extraction. Ipsilateral cortex punches were homogenized in PBS with protease and phosphatase inhibitors using a glass dounce (88668, Pierce, Waltham, MA), then centrifuged at 135,000 x g for 45 min at 4 °C. Following centrifugation, the supernatant containing PBS soluble proteins was removed and stored at – 80 ° C. The remaining pellet was resuspended in ice-cold RIPA buffer containing protease and phosphatase inhibitors (20–188, Millipore, Billerica, MA), sonicated and centrifuged at 14,000 x g for 15 min at 4 °C. The subsequent RIPA supernatant containing membrane bound proteins was removed and stored at – 80 °C.

Western blot analysis

Protein concentrations were measured using the BCA protein assay kit (23227, Pierce), with 20 μg of protein added to a 1:1 *v*/*v* of reducing buffer (2× Laemmli sample buffer (1610737, BioRad, Hercules, CA), 5% v/v β-mercaptoethanol (1610710, BioRad)) and heated at 95 °C for 5 min. Proteins were separated using SDS-PAGE gel electrophoresis and transferred to nitrocellulose membranes. Following transfer, membranes were blocked in

5% *w/v* skim milk powder in PBS-T (PBS, 0.05% v/v Tween-20, pH 7.6) for 1 h. Blots were then incubated with primary antibodies in 2% w/v skim milk/TBS-T, overnight at 4 °C. Primary antibodies used were PDGFRβ (1:1000, #3169, Cell Signaling, Danvers, MA), apoE (1:1000, ab1907, Abcam, Cambridge, MA), MMP-9 (1:800, 38898, Abcam) and β-Actin (1:5000, A5441, Sigma-Aldrich). Following primary antibody incubation, membranes were washed for 3 × 10 min in PBS-T at RT, before incubation with HRP-conjugated goat anti-rabbit, goat anti-mouse or rabbit anti-goat (Jackson ImmunoResearch, Westgrove, PA, 1:1000 in 2% w/v skim milk powder in PBS-T) secondary antibodies, for 90 min at RT. Membranes then washed for 3 × 10 min in PBS-T before detection using SuperSignal West Pico Chemiluminescent Substrate detection kit (34580, ThermoScientific, Waltham, MA) and visualization with Amersham 600 imaging machine (GE healthcare, Chicago, IL). Raw pixel intensities of bands from Western blots were quantified by densitometry using Image J software (Version 1.47, NIH, Bethesda, MD).

Immunohistological analysis

Free-floating parallel brain sections (20 μm thickness) from wildtype, APOE3, and APOE4 mice were cut using a microtome (Microm HM 430, Thermo Fisher Scientific, Tusin, CA), and washed three times with PBS, before staining and incubated with blocking buffer (5% normal goat serum (NGS) in PBS) and 0.3% Triton X-100 (PBST) for 2 h at room temperature. Brain sections were incubated overnight at 4 °C with the following primary antibodies: rabbit polyclonal PDGFRβ antibody for pericytes (1:200, #3169, Cell Signaling), dylight 488 labeled *Lycopersicon Esculentum* (tomato lectin) (1:1000, DL-1174, Vector Laboratories, Burlingame, CA) for blood vessels, rabbit anti-CD31 (1:500, ab28364, Abcam) for microvessels, mouse monoclonal anti-Claudin-5 antibody (1:500, 35–2500, Invitrogen, Carlsbad, CA) and rabbit anti-Zonula Occludens 1 (1:500, 21,773–1-AP, Proteintech, Rosemont, IL) for tight junctions in the epithelial cells. After three 5 min washes in PBS, sections were incubated for 2 h with a corresponding anti-rabbit Alexa Fluor 568-conjugated or anti-mouse Alexa Fluor 594-conjugated IgG secondary antibodies (1:1000, S11227, Invitrogen) for 2 h at room temperature. As negative controls, sections were incubated without primary antibody. Sections were rinsed with PBS and distilled water and coverslipped with Fluoro-Gel with Tris Buffer mounting medium (Electron Microscopy Sciences, Hatfield, PA). Quantitative image analysis of the PDGFRβ Claudin-5, Zonula Occludens-1 and CD31 immunoreactive cortical regions were performed on five fields (× 20, 151.894 mm^2), and three cortical sections per animal through the level of impact site using the same densitometric analysis method as previously described [23]. Image J software was used for analysis as previously described [23].

In-situ Zymography

Following euthanasia and transcardial perfusion with ice-cold PBS, brains were harvested and flash frozen on dry ice. Brains were cryosectioned into 20 μm sections in series that encompass the ipsilateral lesion, as well as the contralateral hemisphere. Fluorescein conjugated, dye-quenched gelatin (DQ-gelatin, 1 mg/ml, D12054, Molecular Probes, Invitrogen) was prepared in reaction buffer (50 mM Tris HCl, Tris Base $NH_2C(CH_2OH)_3$, 150 mM NaCl, 5 mM $CaCl_2$, 0.2 mM NaN_3, pH 7.6) and stored at 4 °C. Sections were incubated in DQ-gelatin reaction buffer in the dark for 1 h at 37 °C. Following incubation, reaction buffer was removed and coverslips placed over the tissue using vectashield. Fluorescence visualized using an Olympus BX51 microscope (Olympus American, Center Valley, PA) equipped with Olympus DP72 camera, and cell Sens Standard software.

In situ hybridization combined with immunohistochemistry

Coronal brain sections (20 μm thickness) were washed three times in PBS before mounting on gelatin-coated glass slides (Superfrost Plus, Thermo Fisher Scientific) and stored at – 80 °C until use. Tissue was allowed to dry at room temperature (RT) and then stored at -20 °C until use. Fluorescent in situ hybridization (FISH) was performed using RNAscope® Technology 2.0 (Advanced Cell Diagnostics (ACD), Hayward, CA), as previously described [23, 25]. In short, mounted tissue sections were serially dehydrated in 50%, 70%, 95%, 100% and 100% ethanol for 5 min each. In between all pretreatment steps, tissue sections were briefly washed with ultra-pure water. The pretreat solution 1 (hydrogen peroxide reagent) was applied for 10 min at RT, and then the tissue sections were boiled in pretreat solution 2 (target retrieval reagent) for 15 min. Mounted slices were treated with pretreat solution 3 (protease reagent) for 30 min at 40 °C on the HybEz™ hybridization system (ACD). Mouse Apoe probe (Cat. No. 313278, ACD) targets the region 83–1245 (Accession number: NM_009696.3) of the Apoe sequence with 19 pairs of ZZ-target probes. In addition, the negative (Cat. No. 310043, ACD) and positive (Cat. No. 313911, ACD) control probes were applied and let hybridized for 2 h at 40 °C. The amplification steps were performed according to manufacturer's directions. In between every amplification step, sections were washed with 1× wash buffer. Detection was performed using a mixture ratio of the Red-A to the Red-B solution of 1:60. Sections were incubated for 10 min at RT and rinsed with ultra-pure water. Following in situ hybridization, the sections were processed for immunohistochemistry. Briefly, following the blocking step with 5% NGS in PBS for 1 h at RT, post-hybridized slides were incubated with an antibody against anti-mouse GFAP (glial fibrillary acidic protein, 1:1000, EMD Millipore, Temecula, CA) or anti-rabbit PDGFRβ in the presence of 2% NGS in PBS overnight at 4 °C. After three washes with PBS, the slides were incubated with corresponding anti-mouse or anti-rabbit Alexa Fluor® 488 secondary antibodies (1:500; Molecular probes®, ThermoFisher Scientific, Grand Island, NY) for 2 h at RT. Brain sections were rinsed with PBS three times and incubated for 5 min in PBS with DAPI solution (1: 50,000, Sigma-Aldrich) for counterstained nuclei. Fluorescent images were acquired on an Olympus XB51 microscope equipped with Olympus DP72 camera, and cell Sens Standard software.

Microvessel isolation

Microvessels were isolated as previously described [26]. Briefly, sham and CCI mice were euthanized and ipsilateral and contralateral brain tissue punch excised and rinsed in sucrose buffer (S.B, 0.32 mol/L sucrose, 3 mmol/L HEPES, pH 7.4). Samples were homogenized in a glass dounce homogenizer containing 2 ml S.B., then centrifuged for 10 min × 1000 *g* at 4 °C. Following centrifugation, the supernatant (containing the visible white upper myelin layer) was discarded and remaining pellet resuspended in 2 ml S.B., re-homogenized using glass dounce and centrifuged again for 10 min × 1000 *g* at 4 °C. Supernatant was discarded and the sediment pellet was resuspended in a further 2 ml S.B. and centrifuged (30s × 100 *g*, 4 °C). Following centrifugation, supernatant was removed and kept, and the resulting pellet underwent a second resuspension (in 2 ml S.B) and centrifuged (30s × 100 *g*, 4 °C). The supernatant was removed and pooled together, before a final centrifugation for 2 min × 200 *g* at 4 °C. The resulting pellet was resuspended (25 μl, 0.1% BSA in PBS) and microvessels confirmed by Toluidin Blue staining and brightfield microscopy, before being prepared for RNA extraction.

RNA isolation and cDNA synthesis

RNA was extracted from microvessels using TRIzol® reagent (15596026, Invitrogen) as per manufacturer's guidelines. Concentration and purity of the RNA was assessed using the NanoDrop 1000 spectrophotometer (ThermoScientific). One microgram of RNA was reverse transcribed into cDNA using a High-Capacity RNA-to-cDNA Reverse Transcription Kit (4368814, Applied Biosystems, Foster City, CA) in accordance with manufacturer's guidelines. The resulting cDNA was diluted 1:3 in diethylpyrocarbonate (DEPC) treated H_2O for use in RT-QPCR. Samples were stored at – 80 °C until use.

Real time quantitative polymerase chain reaction (RT-QPCR)

RT-QPCR was conducted as described previously [27, 28]. Briefly, RT-QPCR was performed in triplicate in standard 384-well plates using the Prism 7900HT fast sequence detection system (Applied Biosystems). Taqman probes were used to analyze *GAPDH* (Mm99999915_m1), *apoe* (Mm01307193_g1), *APOE* (Hs00171168_m1), *Mmp-9* (Mm01317678_m1), *Claudin-5* (Mm00727012_s1), *Occludin* (Mm00500912_m1), *Zonula Occludens-1* (Mm00493699_m1) and *Pdgfrβ* (Mm00435546_m1) under the following cycle conditions, 50 °C for 2 min, 95 °C for 20 s, (95 °C for 1 s, 60 °C for 20 s) × 40 repeats. The SDS 2.4 software (Applied Biosystems) was used to generate threshold cycle (Ct) values, and fold change in mRNA expression calculated using the ΔΔCt method (2-ΔΔCt) as previously described [29].

Statistical analysis

All data is presented as mean ± SEM. Data was analyzed using a One-way ANOVA with Dunnett's post hoc test or a Two-way ANOVA with Bonferroni multiple comparison post-hoc tests where appropriate. All statistical analysis was carried out using Graph Pad Prism™ Software (version 7.0), with $^*p < 0.05$ considered statistically significant for all experiments.

Results

Characterization of BBB permeability and stabilization following TBI

It has been well established that BBB dysfunction occurs following TBI, contributing to secondary injury processes and the overall degree of injury severity [30]. To characterize the time course of BBB permeability following primary impact, wildtype mice were subject to TBI before BBB permeability assessed by EB analysis. Levels of EB extravasation were increased by 411% in the ipsilateral cortex at day 1 ($P < 0.001$) and remained elevated by 201% at day 3 post-injury ($P < 0.05$) compared to sham animals (Fig. 1a). Full closure of the BBB to EB permeability was observed approximately 7–10 days post-injury. No change in BBB permeability was observed in the contralateral cortex (Fig. 1b) or the ipsilateral or contralateral thalamus/striatum at any timepoint post-TBI (Fig. 1c-d).

We also assessed BBB permeability using GdDTPA enhanced MRI. Consistent with EB observations, T1-weighted MRI with Gadolinium-enhanced contrast displayed increased leakage in the pericontusional area of the ipsilateral cortex that extended approximately 5 mm from the rostral to the caudal aspect of the lesion (Fig. 1e). We assessed GdDTPA leakage into the mouse brain at multiple timepoints up to 21 days post-TBI and observed GdDTPA signal at 1, 3, and 7 days post-injury compared to pre-injection scans, but not at 14 or 21 days post-injury (Fig. 1f). We quantified this signal and confirmed that the

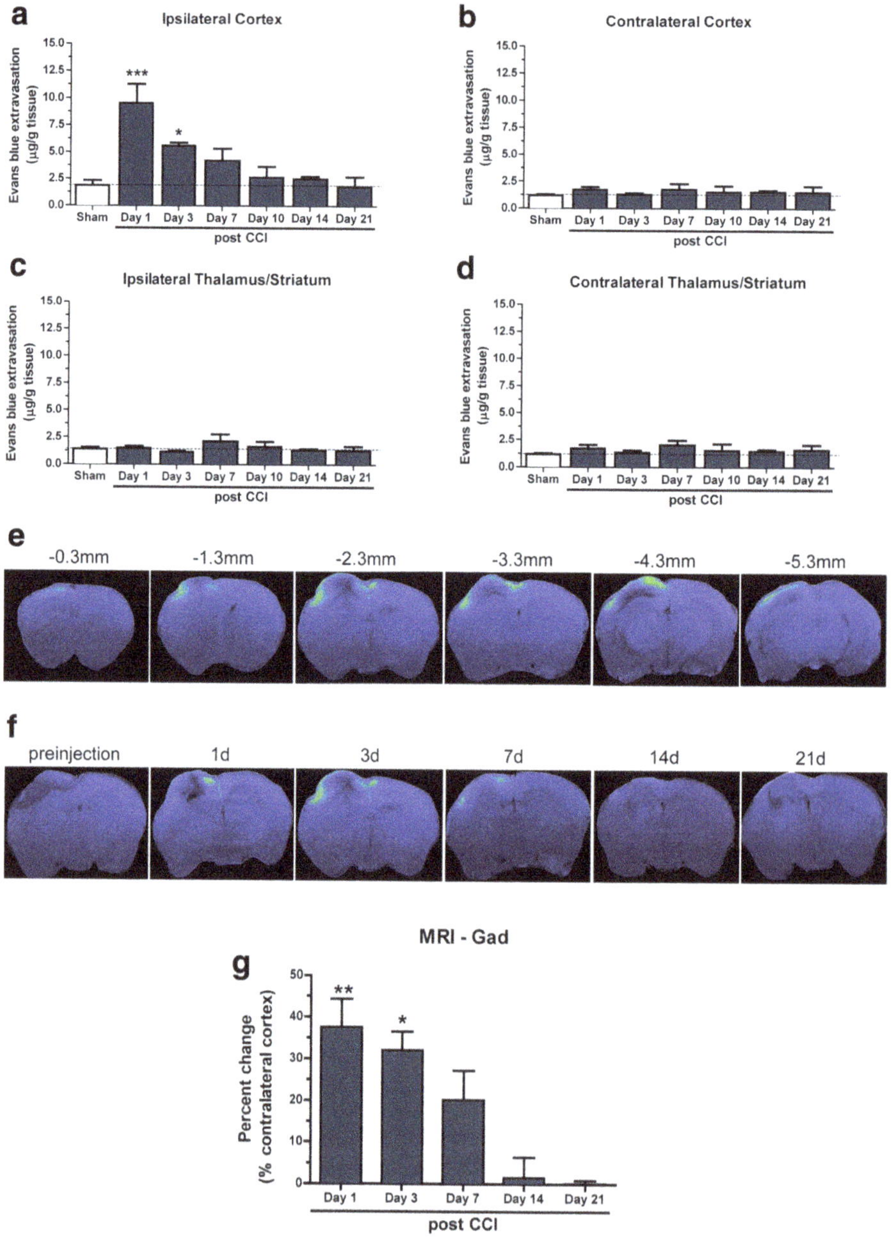

Fig. 1 Characterization of BBB permeability following TBI. (**a**) Increased EB extravasation in the ipsilateral cortex of wildtype mice at 1 (***$p < 0.001$, *$p < 0.05$; $n = 4$) and 3 days post-injury compared to sham. No change is observed in the (**b**) contralateral cortex ($n = 4$), (**c**) ipsilateral Thalamus/Striatum ($n = 4$) or (**d**) contralateral Thalamus/Striatum ($n = 4$) compared to sham. (**e**) T1-weighted MRI images representing the range of pericontusional leakage across bregma brain coordinates of a single wildtype mouse, at 3 days post-TBI. (**f**) T1-weighted MRI images displaying wildtype mice pre injection and at 1, 3, 7, 14 and 21 days post-TBI. (**g**) Quantification of the T1-weighted MRI time course of BBB leakage post TBI ((**$p < 0.01$, *$p < 0.05$ vs Day 14 and Day 21; $n = 3$ per group). The intensity of signal increases from blue<green. Data expressed as mean ± S.E.M. One way ANOVA with Dunnett post hoc test

BBB was fully closed to GdDTPA leakage at 14d post-TBI (Fig. 1g).

Levels of soluble apoE are inversely associated with MMP-9 activation

The apoE protein has been demonstrated to modulate cerebrovascular integrity at the NVU via an apoE-LRP1 mediated suppression of MMP-9 [9]. To characterize the apoE and MMP-9 response following TBI stimulus, wildtype mice were subject to TBI before a micropunch of the ipsilateral cortex was extracted and analyzed at 1, 3 and 7 days post-injury. TBI induced a biphasic response in PBS-soluble apoE protein (Fig. 2a), with protein levels significantly reduced by 73% at day 1 ($P < 0.$

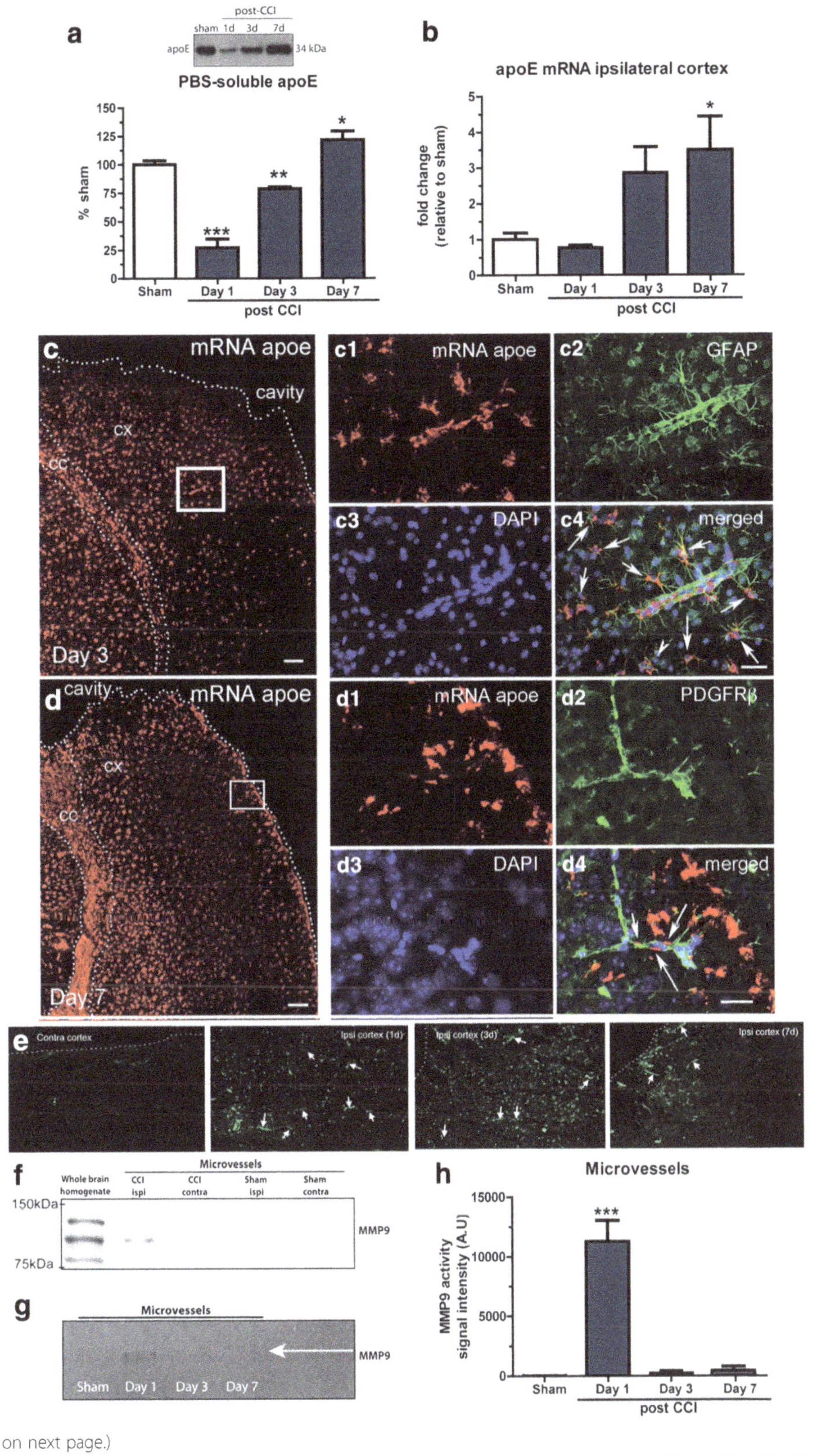

Fig. 2 (See legend on next page.)

(See figure on previous page.)

Fig. 2 TBI-induced apoE and MMP-9 responses in the ipsilateral cortex of wildtype mice. Wildtype mice were subject to TBI before whole ipsilateral cortex punches collected at 1, 3, and 7 days post-injury for protein and RNA analysis. (**a**) Western blot and densitometry analysis of PBS-soluble apoE in the ipsilateral cortex of wildtype mice following TBI ($n = 3$, $*p < 0.05$, $**p < 0.01$, $***p < 0.001$). (**b**) *apoe* mRNA expression post-injury ($n = 4$, $*p < 0.05$). (**c-d**) Fluorescent in situ hybridization analysis of apoe expression at 3 and 7 days post-TBI. (**c1–4**) *apoe* mRNA and GFAP immunofluorescence surrounding a cortical microvessel. (**d1–4**) *apoe* mRNA with PDGFRβ immunofluorescence. Scale bars C-D images 50 μm, inset C1-D4 images 20 μm. (**e**) In-situ zymography evidencing MMP-9 activity after TBI. (**f**) Western blot of MMP-9 in whole brain ipsilateral cortex and ipsilateral microvessels from wildtype mice 24 h post-injury (representative of n = 3). (**g**) In-gel zymography of MMP-9 activity in ipsilateral microvessels isolated from wildtype mice following TBI. (**h**) Densitometry analysis of in-gel MMP-9 zymography ($n = 3$, $***p < 0.001$). Data expressed as mean ± S.E.M. One way ANOVA with Dunnett post hoc test

001) and by 21% at day 3 ($P < 0.01$) post-injury compared to sham (Fig. 2a). At 7 days post-injury, apoE protein levels were significantly increased by 22% compared to sham levels ($P < 0.05$; Fig. 2a). *Apoe* mRNA expression in cortical punch was elevated by 3.5-fold in the ipsilateral cortex at 7 days post-injury (P < 0.05) (Fig. 2b). To explore the source of *apoe* mRNA after TBI, we used *apoe* mRNA FISH alongside markers of astrocytes and pericytes. We found widespread expression of apoe in our mice, with the majority of expression found in GFAP-positive astrocytes (Fig. 2c). Fig. 2C1–4 show *apoe* mRNA and GFAP immunofluorescence surrounding a cortical microvessel. The astrocytic projections and endfeet surrounding the microvessel are clear, however it is also apparent that cells associated with the microvessel are also producing *apoe* mRNA. To investigate this further, we repeated our *apoe* mRNA FISH with PDGFRβ immunofluorescence. We found colocalization of the PDGFRβ positive cells with *apoe* mRNA (Fig. 2d, D1–4).

To determine if microvessels were locally producing MMP, we used in-situ zymography. We report that MMP activity was greatly increased in the ipsilateral cortex at 1 days post-TBI, and that microvessel-related MMP activity was clearly visible in the ipsilateral cortex using this technique (Fig. 2e, arrows indicate microvessel-associated activity). At 3 days post-injury MMP activity was still visible, but there were noticeably less microvessel-associated activity compared to 1 day post-TBI. At 7 days post-injury there was still ongoing microvessel associated activity, but this was spatially limited to the area directly adjacent to the lesion (Fig. 2e). We next isolated microvessels from micropunches of the ipsilateral and contralateral cortex of TBI and sham mice and analyzed these vessels for the presence of MMP-9 protein. MMP-9 protein was detectable in the ipsilateral cortex microvessels from TBI mice, but not from the contralateral microvessels, or from sham microvessels (Fig. 2f). We further performed gel zymography on isolated microvessels from the ipsilateral cortex at 1, 3, and 7 days post-TBI, and found that while TBI substantially increased microvessel MMP-9 activity at 1 day post-TBI, but that this activity was below detection threshold at 3 and 7 days post-injury (Fig. 2g-h).

Characterization of the NVU response in wildtype mice following TBI

The NVU is a crucial structure that regulates BBB vascular integrity, stability and maintenance. To further elucidate the specific TBI mediated BBB response at the NVU, wildtype mice were subject to TBI before ipsilateral cortex microvessels were isolated and analyzed by RT-QPCR. Baseline characterization of microvessel preparations from sham mice revealed elevated *Glut1* and *PDGFRβ* mRNA expression, indicative of enriched endothelial and pericyte populations compared to whole cortex tissue (Fig. 3a). Furthermore, these microvessels contain minimal astrocytic presence, with reduced levels *GFAP* and *S100β* observed compared to whole cortex fractions (Fig. 3a). Following TBI, *apoe* mRNA expression was significantly increased at 3 and 7 days post-injury compared to sham ($P < 0.05$; Fig. 3b). *Mmp-9* expression was significantly increased 1 day post-injury ($P < 0.001$; Fig. 3c), but returned towards baseline by 3 days post-injury. There was a time-dependent decrease in *Pdgfrβ* mRNA, a pericyte marker, until 3 days post-TBI (P < 0.05), before recovering at day 7 post-injury (Fig. 3d). At the tight-junction protein level, we observed significant decreases in mRNA for *Zonula Occludens-1* and *Occludin* at 1 and 3 days post-injury ($P < 0.05$; Fig. 3e, f), with a similar trend in the mRNA for *Claudin-5* (Fig. 3g). All tight-junction protein mRNA returned to baseline expression by 7 days post-injury. We confirmed that PDGFRβ is found on vessels by examining protein co-localization with vessel specific lectin and examining vessel size and morphology. PDGFRβ colocalizes with lectin, and was found primarily on vessels with a diameter of 5–20μM (Fig. 3h).

Treatment with the Cyclophilin A (CypA) antagonist Cyclosporine A (CsA) improves BBB repair after TBI

To investigate the role of CypA–MMP-9 in BBB stabilization and repair, wildtype mice were subject to TBI, followed by administration of either CsA or vehicle. We assessed acute BBB permeability at 1 day to establish if CypA was involved in the acute response to trauma, and at 5 days post-injury to assess if inhibition of CypA could induce faster BBB stabilization than the 7–10 day spontaneous closure window we observed in untreated mice. At 1 day following TBI, EB extravasation from the ipsilateral cortex was significantly elevated in both vehicle and CsA

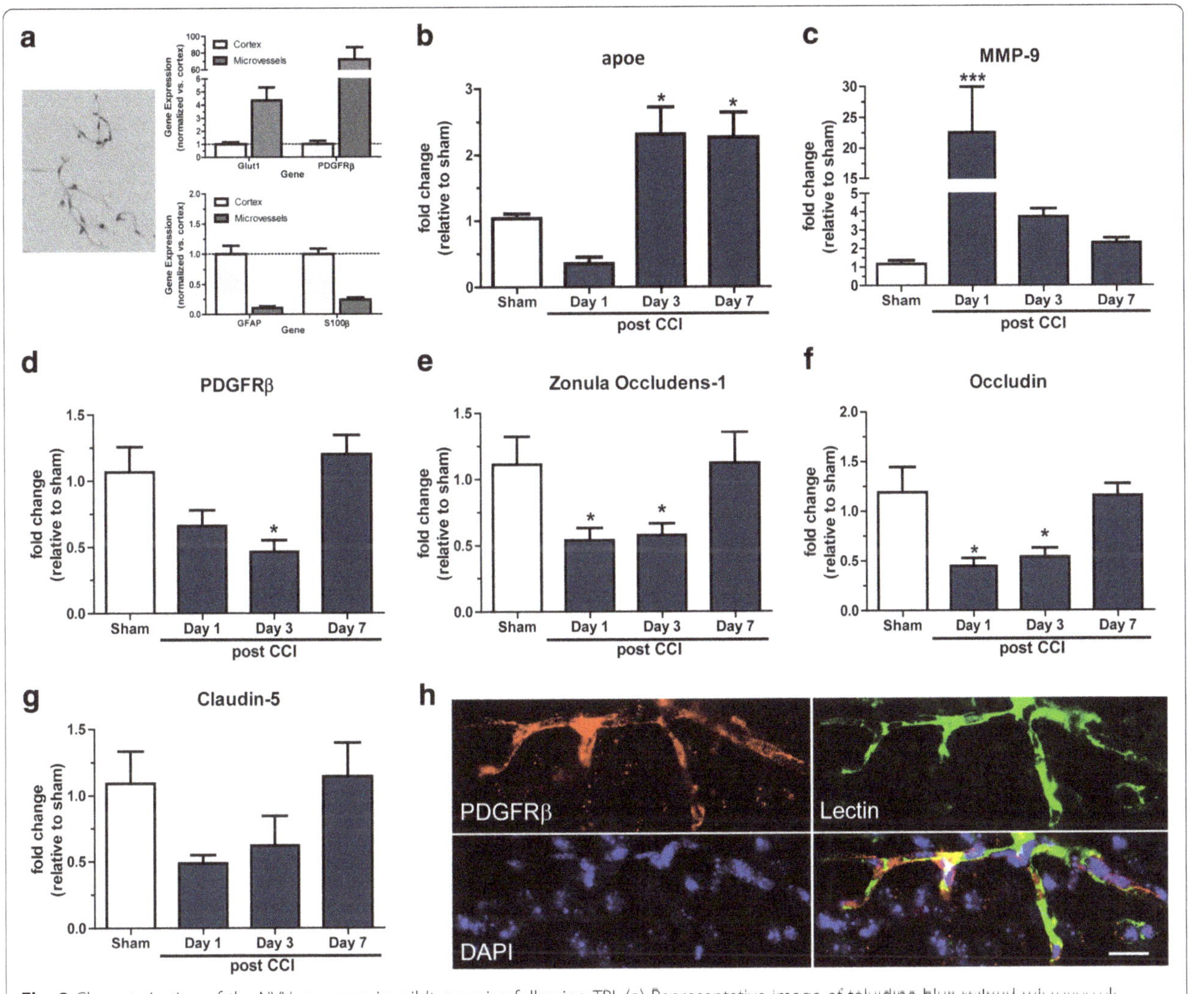

Fig. 3 Characterization of the NVU response in wildtype mice following TBI. (**a**) Representative image of toluidine blue stained microvessels isolated from the ipsilateral cortex. RT-QPCR analysis shows the purity of microvessel preparations, consisting of enriched endothelial (Glut1) and pericyte (PDGFRβ) markers with minimal astrocytic expression (GFAP/S100β) in comparison to whole cortex punch fractions. Wildtype mice were subject to TBI before microvessels isolated at 1, 3 and 7 days post-injury and subject to RNA analysis. RT-QPCR analysis of the mRNA expression for (**b**) *apoe* ($n = 3$, *$p < 0.05$), (**c**) *Mmp-9* ($n = 5$–6, ***$p < 0.001$), (**d**) *Pdgfrβ* ($n = 6$, *$p < 0.05$), (**e**) *Zonula Occludens-1* ($n = 5$–6, *$p < 0.05$), (**f**) *Occludin* ($n = 5$–6, *$p < 0.05$) and (**g**) *Claudin-5* (Sham, day 1, day 3 $n = 5$–6, day 7 $n = 3$). (**h**) Immunohistochemistry analysis assessing the co-localization of the respective microvessel and pericyte markers, Lectin and PDGFRβ. Scale bar: 20 μm. Data expressed as mean ± S.E.M. One way ANOVA with Dunnett post hoc test

treated mice ($P < 0.001$). At 5 days post-injury, BBB permeability remained significantly elevated by 135% in vehicle treated mice ($P < 0.01$ vs vehicle sham), but had returned to sham levels in CsA treated animals ($P < 0.05$ vs. CsA sham mice, Fig. 4a). In a separate cohort of mice, the effect of CsA on NVU responses was investigated by isolating microvessels from the ipsilateral cortex of CsA and vehicle treated wildtype mice after TBI. RT-QPCR analysis showed *Mmp-9* expression was increased in the vehicle group at 1 and 5 days post-injury, a response that is significantly attenuated by CsA administration ($P < 0.01$; Fig. 4b). Pericyte expression was unchanged, with *Pdgfrβ* mRNA reduced in both groups at 1 day post-TBI ($P < 0.001$, Fig. 4c), before rebounding by day 5 post-injury. At the tight junction level, we observed significant decreases in mRNA for *Zonula Occludens-1* and *Occludin* in both CsA and vehicle groups at 1 day post-TBI ($P < 0.001$; Fig. 4d, e). However, at 5 days post injury, CsA treatment resulted in a 20% increase in *Zonula Occludens-1* ($P < 0.001$; Fig. 4d), whilst *Occludin* levels were unchanged to that observed in sham animals.

APOE4 mice exhibit impaired closure of the BBB and delayed pericyte recovery after TBI

The human apoE4 protein is known to be functionally deficient compared to the apoE3 protein, and we used humanized APOE mice as a clinically relevant model to

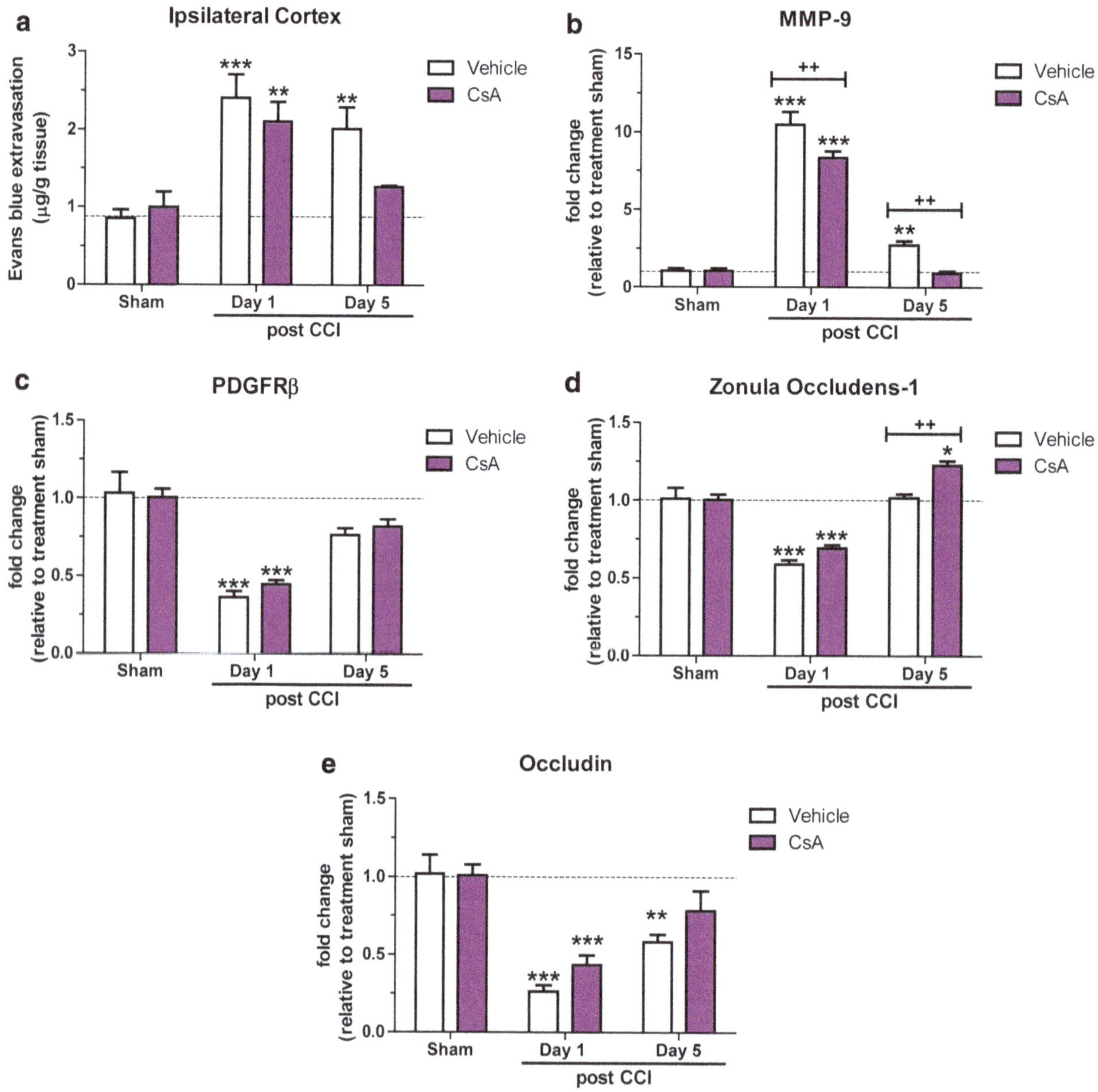

Fig. 4 Cyclosporine A (CsA) treatment improves BBB stabilization and closure in wildtype mice. Wildtype mice were subject to TBI before administration of 20 mg/kg CsA or vehicle at 15 min post-injury. (**a**) Evans blue analysis of BBB permeability in the ipsilateral cortex analyzed at 1 and 5 days post-injury ($n = 5$ per group and timepoint, $^{***}p < 0.001$, $^{**}p < 0.05$). Isolated microvessels analyzed by RT-QPCR for (**b**) *Mmp-9* ($n = 4$, $^{***}p < 0.001$, $^{**}p < 0.01$ vs treatment sham, $^{++}p < 0.01$ vs relevant timepoint), (**c**) *Pdgfrβ* ($n = 4$, $^{***}p < 0.001$) (**d**) *Zonula Occludens-1* ($n = 4$, $^{***}p < 0.001$, $^{*}p < 0.05$ vs treatment sham, $^{++}p < 0.01$ vs relevant timepoint) and (**e**) *Occludin* ($n = 4$, $^{***}p < 0.001$, $^{*}p < 0.05$) mRNA expression. All data expressed as mean ± S.E.M. Two-way ANOVA with Bonferroni post hoc test

study the role of apoE on BBB injury and repair after TBI. APOE3 and APOE4 mice were subject to TBI and their BBB permeability assessed using the EB method. 3 days following TBI, EB extravasation from the ipsilateral cortex was increased by 202% in APOE3 mice ($P < 0.0001$ vs APOE3 sham) and by 174% in APOE4 mice ($P < 0.001$ vs APOE4 sham) (Fig. 5a). Similar to wildtype mice, BBB permeability in APOE3 TBI mice had returned to within 5% of APOE3 sham levels by 10 days post-TBI, and was significantly reduced compared to APOE3 mice at 3 days post-TBI ($P < 0.001$). In contrast, BBB closure to EB was not achieved in APOE4 mice at 10 days post-TBI. At 10 days post-injury, BBB permeability in APOE4 mice remained significantly elevated by 94% compared to APOE4 sham mice ($P < 0.05$), and was not significantly decreased compared to APOE4 3 day

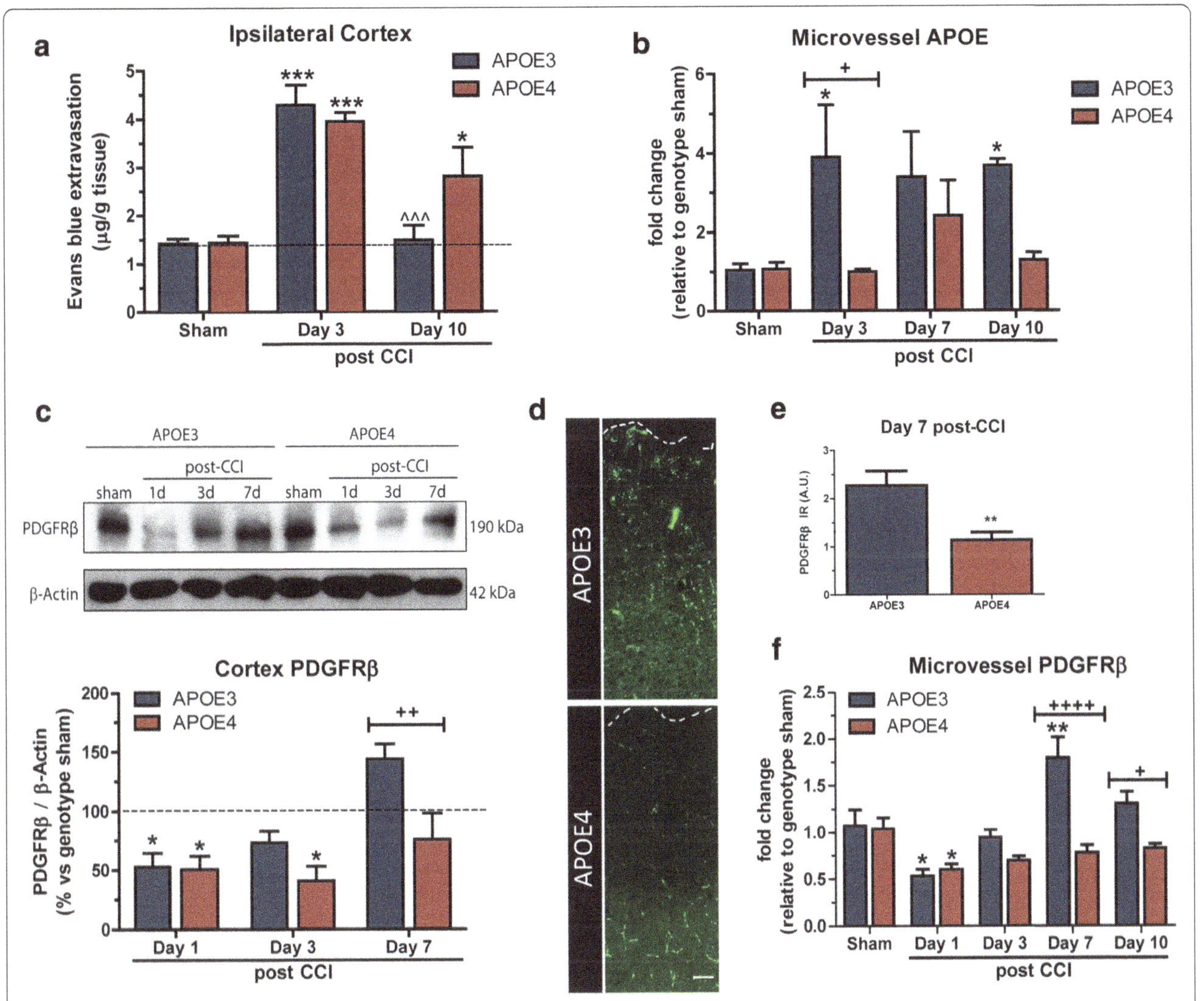

Fig. 5 APOE4 mice exhibit impaired closure of the BBB and delayed pericyte recovery after TBI. (**a**) APOE3 and APOE4 mice were subject to TBI, before BBB permeability in the ipsilateral cortex analyzed at 3 and 10 days post-injury using Evans Blue extravasation ($n = 5$, ***$p < 0.001$, *$p < 0.05$ vs genotype sham, ^^^$p < 0.001$ vs APOE3 day 3). (**b**) APOE mRNA expression in isolated microvessels ($n = 4$–6, *$p < 0.05$ vs genotype sham; $^{+}p < 0.05$ vs relevant timepoint). (**c**) Western blot and densitometry analysis of PDGFRβ expression in the ipsilateral cortex of APOE3 and APOE4 mice following TBI ($n = 4$, *$p < 0.05$ vs genotype sham; $^{++}p < 0.01$ vs relevant timepoint). (**d-e**) Immunohistochemistry displaying reduced PDGFRβ expression in the ipsilateral cortex of APOE4 compared with APOE3 mice at 7-days post-TBI. Scale bar: 200 µm. ($n = 4$ per genotype, **$p < 0.01$). (**f**) *Pdgfrβ* mRNA expression in microvessels isolated from ipsilateral cortex of APOE3 and APOE4 mice after TBI ($n = 4$–6, **$p < 0.01$, *$p < 0.05$ vs genotype sham; $^{++++}p < 0.0001$, $^{+}p < 0.05$ vs relevant timepoint). Data expressed as mean ± S.E.M. Two-way ANOVA with Bonferroni post-hoc test

mice (Fig. 5a). Previously we have demonstrated reduced levels of soluble apoE in the ipsilateral cortex of APOE4 mice compared to APOE3, up to 7 days post-TBI [8]. To investigate the NVU specific *apoe* response, ipsilateral microvessels were isolated and assessed after TBI. APOE3 microvessels displayed significantly elevated a*poe* mRNA expression at 3 and 10 days post-injury compared to APOE4 counterparts (P < 0.05; Fig. 5b). Given the role of brain pericytes in maintaining and regulating the integrity of the BBB [31, 32], we investigated the pericyte response to TBI in APOE3 and APOE4 mice. Western blot analysis of the ipsilateral cortex revealed that both APOE3 and APOE4 exhibit acute pericytes loss, with a 47% loss of PDGFRβ protein in APOE3 mice at 1 day post-TBI, and a 49% loss in APOE4 mice at the same timepoint (P < 0.05 vs genotype sham; Fig. 5c). PDGFRβ expression recovers by 3 days post-TBI in APOE3 mice, and is elevated by 44% at 7d post-TBI. In contrast, PDGFRβ remains significantly depressed at 3 days in APOE4 mice (*P* < 0.05 vs APOE4 sham), and remains 47% below APOE3 PDGFRβ levels at 7 days post-TBI (Fig. 5c, P < 0.01). In support of this finding, we found that immunohistochemistry for PDGFRβ was reduced in the pericontusional cortex of APOE4 mice compared to APOE3 mice at 7 days post injury (Fig. 5d-e). Furthermore, RT-QPCR analysis of the pericyte marker *Pdgfrβ* in isolated microvessels, revealed APOE4 animals exhibit decreased expression at 7 ($P < 0.001$, Fig. 5f) and 10 days post-injury ($P < 0.05$, Fig. 5f) in comparison to APOE3 mice.

APOE4 mice display impaired BBB stabilization at the NVU following TBI

To investigate the genotype specific effects of APOE on BBB dynamics, APOE3 and APOE4 mice were subject to TBI before cerebrovascular integrity assessed. We used lectin and CD31 to determine if the number of blood vessels was impacted in the perilesion area 7 days post-TBI. In sham mice, we found no effect of genotype using either lectin or CD31. However we found that in TBI mice, lectin is no longer specific for blood vessels, with widespread cellular staining through the glial scar that had the morphological characteristics of glial cells (Fig. 6a). CD31 immunohistochemistry remained specific for blood vessels, and we found that neither APOE genotype nor TBI caused a significant change in the area of blood vessel coverage in the pericontusional area (Fig. 6a). At the tight junction level, immunohistochemistry analysis showed APOE4 mice display reduced levels of Claudin-5 and Zonula Occludens-1 at 7 days post-TBI compared to APOE3 mice (Fig. 6b, c). In support of our protein analysis, APOE4 microvessels isolated from a micropunch of the ipsilateral cortex display significantly reduced mRNA expression of *Claudin-5* ($P < 0.05$, Fig. 6d), *Zonula Occludens-1* (Day 3 and 10, $P < 0.05$, Fig. 6e) and *Occludin* ($P < 0.05$, Fig. 6f) after TBI compared to APOE3 counterparts. Furthermore, increased levels of *Mmp-9* is observed in APOE4 microvessels at day 1 ($P < 0.01$, Fig. 6g) and day 3 ($P < 0.05$, Fig. 6g) post-TBI compared to APOE3 microvessels. In addition, *Mmp-9* expression remained elevated in APOE4 microvessels at day 7 and day 10 ($P < 0.05$, Fig. 6g) post-injury, relative to genotype control.

Discussion

In this study, we characterized the extent of BBB permeability after TBI, and investigated the cellular and molecular processes underlying this pathology. Here we report TBI induces acute BBB dysfunction in C57Bl/6 mice, before stabilization at 7–10 days post-injury, a response that is inversely associated with soluble apoE levels. We used multiple techniques to demonstrate BBB dysfunction, including EB extravasation and GdDTPA MRI imaging. Cortical punch analysis of the ipsilateral cortex revealed an acute decrease in PBS-soluble apoE protein that rebounded to be significantly higher at 7d post-TBI, a timecourse that was inversely related to MMP-9 activity in microvessels isolated from the same area. RT-PCR analysis of isolated microvessels also revealed pericyte loss at 1 day post-TBI that corresponded with increased MMP-9 expression and a loss of tight junction protein expression. At 3-7d post-TBI we found that apoE expression is found locally at the NVU, and that this increase in expression corresponds with a return of pericytes to the NVU, decreased MMP-9 expression and activity, and stabilization and production of tight junction proteins (Fig. 7). FISH co-localization revealed that both astrocytes associated with the microvessel, and pericytes on the microvessel, express *apoe* mRNA. We report similar NVU responses to TBI in APOE3 mice, however we found that BBB stabilization was significantly delayed in APOE4 mice with a delayed pericyte repopulation, augmented and sustained MMP-9 expression at the NVU, and impaired stabilization of Zonula Occludens-1, Occludin and Claudin-5 expression at tight junctions after TBI, compared to APOE3 mice. Finally, we report prolonged BBB permeability in APOE4 but not APOE3 mice, showing that the E4 isoform prolongs BBB impairments following TBI.

It is clear that TBI can result in a loss cerebrovascular structure/integrity in both human and experimental TBI models. Post-mortem clinical evidence shows defined lesion alterations and reduced lumen vessels in cortical zones between 24 h-20 days post TBI [33]. Similar microvascular injury is observed almost universally in experimental TBI [34], including fluid percussion injury [35–38] and CCI models [39–42]. Ultrastructural and 3D microscopy analysis show pyknotic neurons, irreversible mechanically induced vascular damage, and morphological vessel alterations at the site of contusion acutely after injury [38, 43]. Indeed, the temporal progression of tissue loss at the cortical lesion is well characterized [41], however the impact of TBI on remaining pericontusional vascular structures is less well defined.

In remaining blood vessels, the importance of BBB repair in regaining vascular integrity is a well-established factor in reducing the impact of mediating secondary injury responses, disease severity and recovery timeframes [2]. Despite this, the extent and time course of TBI-associated BBB permeability remains poorly understood. In limited clinical studies, BBB permeability measurements after TBI are diverse. Increased CSF to serum albumin quotients suggests acute BBB dysfunction at 12 h–76 h [44–47], with some cases remaining elevated up to 22 days post-injury compared to control patients [47, 48]. Furthermore, higher resolution imaging demonstrates BBB disruption persisting for months/years at the site of injury following TBI [49, 50]. Consistent with clinical studies, conflicting data on the time course of BBB disruption is also reflected in animal models. Crucially, the effect of experimental TBI on brain permeability is likely to differ according to species, injury model, severity of impact and post-injury interval time. Indeed, rat TBI models (using variants of open or closed head injuries, mostly report BBB

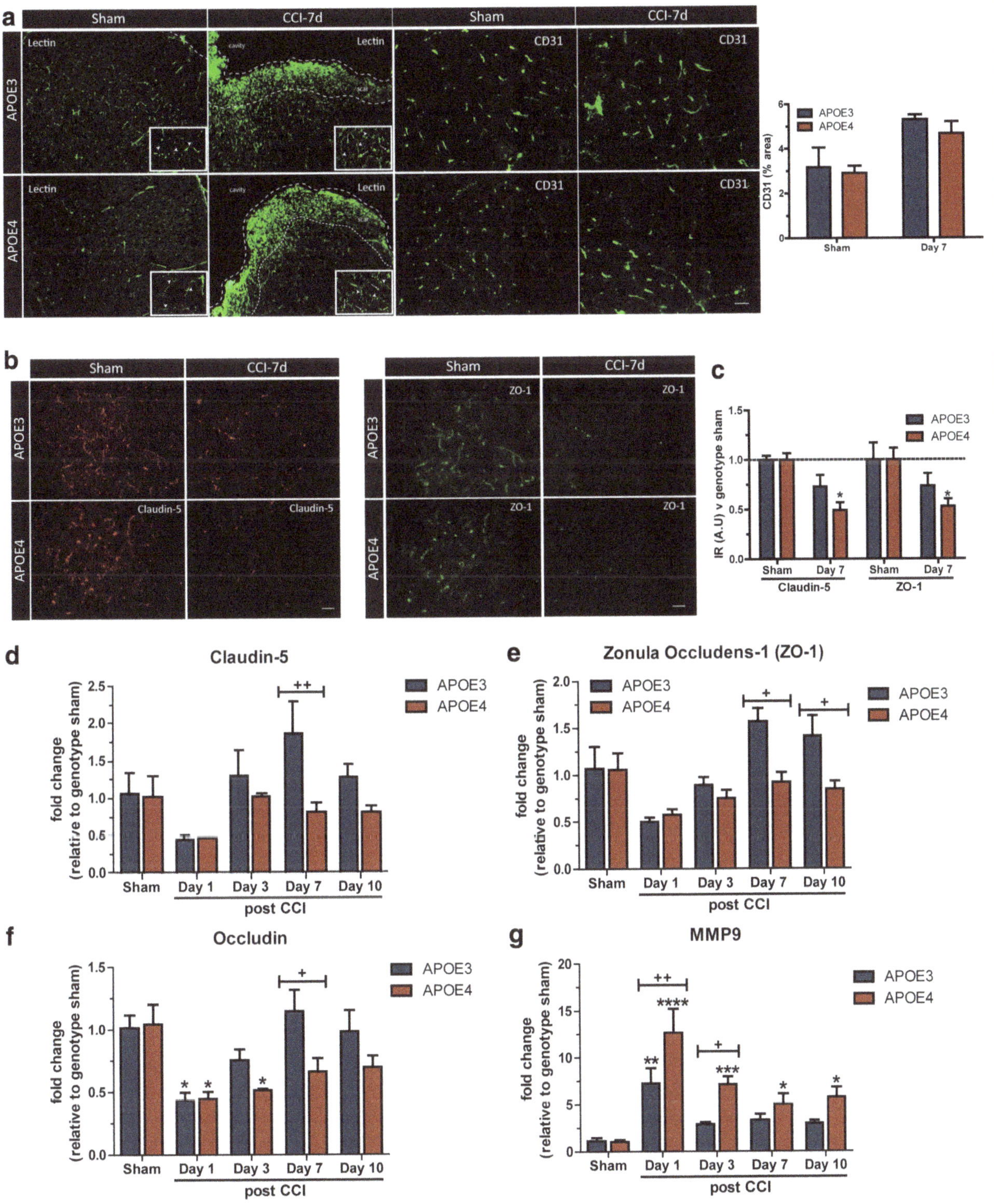

Fig. 6 APOE4 mice display prolonged BBB dysfunction at the NVU following TBI. (**a**) Immunohistochemistry analysis of lectin (inset: arrowheads = vessel, arrows = glial) and CD31 staining in the ipsilateral pericontusional cortex following TBI ($n = 3–4$). (**b-c**) Quantitative immunohistochemistry showing the expression of Claudin-5 and Zonula Occludens-1 (ZO-1) in the ipsilateral pericontusional cortex of APOE3 and APOE4 sham and injured mice. ($n = 4$, $^{*}p < 0.05$ vs genotype sham). APOE3 and APOE4 mice were subject to TBI, before ipsilateral microvessels were isolated at 1, 3, 7 and 10 days post-injury. mRNA analysis of (**d**) *Claudin-5* ($n = 4–6$, $^{++}p < 0.01$ vs relevant timepoint), (**e**) *Zonula Occludens-1* ($n = 4–6$, $^{+}p < 0.05$ vs relevant timepoint), (**f**) *Occludin* ($n = 4–6$, $^{*}p < 0.05$ vs genotype sham; $^{+}p < 0.05$ vs relevant timepoint) and (**g**) *Mmp-9* ($n = 4–6$, $^{***}p < 0.001$, $^{**}p < 0.01$, $^{*}p < 0.05$, vs genotype sham. $^{+}p < 0.05$, $^{++}p < 0.01$ vs relevant timepoint). All data expressed as mean ± S.E.M. Two-way ANOVA with Bonferroni post hoc test

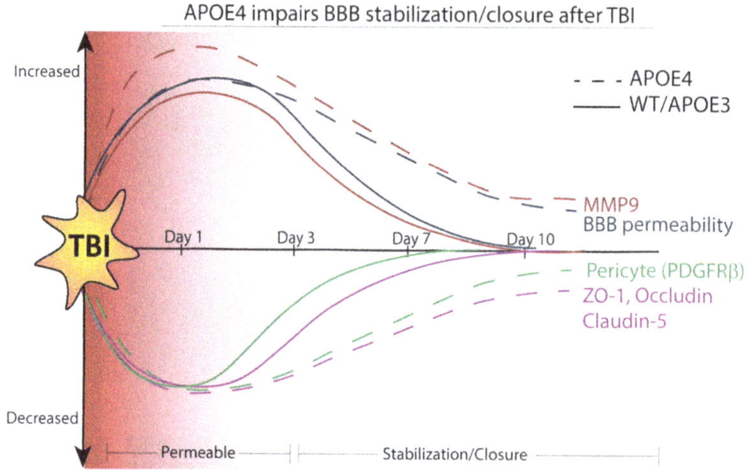

Fig. 7 APOE isoforms influence the time course of BBB dysfunction following TBI. Diagram summarizing the time course of TBI-induced BBB disruption, stabilization and closure in Wildtype, APOE3 and APOE4 mice. Despite Wildtype, APOE3 and APOE4 mice all displaying similar acute BBB responses to TBI, such as elevated permeability and pericyte loss, APOE4 mice display a significantly extended period of BBB leakage following injury. This enhanced time-course of BBB permeability in APOE4 mice occurs in parallel with reduced pericyte repopulation back to the NVU after injury, as well as sustained MMP-9 responses that may cumulatively contribute to the prolonged levels of tight junction degradation

permeability at acute time points (30 min-24 h) [51–56], with few extending out to 3-days post injury [57]. Similarly, mouse models of TBI focus on BBB assessment acutely (6 h-3 days), with many comparing pharmacological treatments at a single time point, most often 24 h post injury [58–63]. These studies all share common limitations, as most do not verify the overall time-course of BBB permeability specific to their TBI model. It is important to note that BBB permeability is more complex than simply an open or closed state. It's dynamic structure exists in a continuum after TBI, ranging from primary injury rupture to various states of permeability due to secondary injury-induced biochemical alterations, which can change functional profile over time [64]. As such we sought to comprehensively characterize the time-course of BBB permeability following TBI. To the best of our knowledge, this study is the first to report the overall time course (24 h-21 days) of BBB permeability, including BBB rupture, stabilization and closure, in a CCI mouse model of TBI. Using serum albumin detection and MRI visualization, our findings demonstrate dynamically increased BBB permeability at the ipsilateral lesion for the first 3 days post-TBI, before resolution 7–10 days post-injury. We also used pharmacological intervention to show that CypA is a functional target, with CypA inhibition shifting the BBB repair curve towards a faster resolution.

The APOE gene encodes for the 34 kDa protein apoE, which serves as a major lipid transport molecule in the CNS [65]. Transcriptomic analysis of TBI-induced alterations in genomic profiles, has revealed elevated apoE signatures after injury. Moreover, translational integration analysis of this apoE response demonstrates a significant profile overlap between experimental TBI and human GWAS neurodegeneration studies [66], enhancing the notion that apoE plays a pertinent role after brain injury. Indeed, apoE$^{-/-}$ mice display progressive, age-dependent BBB leakage [10, 11] which appears to be exacerbated with injury [10], suggesting that a lack of apoE may increase BBB dysfunction and edema following brain trauma. Despite this, time-course analysis of how apoE may mediate BBB integrity after TBI has largely been unexplored. In the present study, we report what appears to be a biphasic, inverse relationship between apoE (mRNA and protein expression) and BBB dysfunction, such that BBB permeability decreases as apoE levels increase over time post-TBI. This biphasic pattern of a reduction in PBS-soluble apoE followed by an increase is consistent with our previous finding with diethylamine-soluble apoE following experimental TBI [8], and with clinical reports documenting a 70% reduction in CSF derived apoE acutely following severe TBI [7]. The mechanisms by which apoE is degraded or removed from the soluble fraction after TBI remain unclear. *Apoe* expression is controlled by an LXR/RXR responsive element, and we have shown that levels of the CYP46 enzyme responsible for production of the endogenous LXR agonist 24S-hydroxycholesterol are increased after TBI [67]. Furthermore, both apoE and another LXR-responsive protein, ABCA1, are increased at 3 and 7 days after experimental TBI in mice and rats [67, 68]. While we have not directly measured the lipidation status of apoE produced after TBI, all of the elements are in place to rapidly produce and lipidated apoE in the sub-acute phase post-TBI.

ApoE is primarily produced in astrocytes [69] and with robust gliosis in our model of TBI, our FISH and protein imaging show that astrocytes remain the primary site of *apoe* production after injury. However, we also detect *apoe* mRNA signal from pericytes. Isolated brain pericytes have previously been shown to be capable of producing apoE [70, 71], and here we provide evidence that this also happens in vivo. Brain pericytes play a crucial role in maintaining and regulating the integrity of the BBB, through their ability to modulate endothelial tight junction expression and transcytosis of blood-derived macromolecules [31, 32]. ApoE regulates BBB integrity within the NVU by signaling through LRP1 on pericytes, suppressing downstream CypA-MMP-9 responses that degrade tight junction proteins in the vascular endothelium [9]. Critically, this pathway is controlled in an isoform-specific manner, with MMP-9 responses not suppressed by apoE4, resulting in enhanced BBB dysfunction [9]. We have also previously shown that APOE4 mice have less soluble apoE than APOE3 mice up to 7 days post-TBI [8], which could interfere with the ability of apoE4 to suppress MMP-9 production in microvessels after TBI.

In the present study, we sought to comprehensively characterize the TBI induced NVU response in C56Bl/6 mice, before moving into the clinically relevant APOE3 and APOE4 mouse model. Unlike previous studies that employ whole brain methodologies to analyze BBB properties, here we utilized isolated microvessels to analyze specific NVU cell types. This approach has been previously demonstrated to provide an isolation containing with enriched pericyte and endothelial expression, with minimal transcripts derived from astrocytic end feet suggesting glial cells have negligible contributions to the responses observed in microvessel preparations [72]. In the current study, ipsilateral microvessels from C57Bl/6 mice exhibit increased MMP-9 expression up to 3 days post-injury, even in the presence of concurrent pericyte loss as demonstrated by reduced PDGFRβ expression. Given pericytes are key producers of MMP-9 at the NVU [73], this data highlights that despite TBI induced pericyte loss, those that do remain at the NVU following injury are still capable of robust MMP-9 production. Consequentially, this response appears to contribute to endothelial dysfunction within the NVU, with reduced expression of key tight junction elements Zonula Occludens-1 and Occludin up to 3 days post-TBI. Significantly these NVU injury responses are attenuated in the presence of microvessel specific apoE, with the time dependent increase in apoE (3–7 days) corresponding with reduced MMP-9 and restored expression of tight junction proteins, indicative of BBB stabilization.

Recent research indicates that apoE is not having a direct signaling effect on endothelial cells, as targeted deletion of LRP1 from brain endothelial cells does not affect BBB integrity [74]. Rather, we believe that microvessel-derived apoE exerts its effects through LRP1 mediated inhibition of MMP-9 responses in remaining pericytes after injury, subsequently suppressing a stimulus which contributes to tight junction degradation following TBI. Supporting this, our experiments using the CypA antagonist CsA, demonstrate reduced microvessel specific MMP-9 levels with no change in pericyte expression, resulting in greater stabilization of BBB integrity.

The role of APOE polymorphisms regulating BBB function is rapidly becoming an emerging field of interest in the development of genotype-specific therapies. In non-injury paradigms, APOE4 but not APOE3 mice display dysfunctional BBB properties that contributes to exacerbated secondary injury and cognitive decline [9, 75]. Furthermore, individuals carrying the APOE4 gene in Alzheimer's Disease display accelerated pericyte degeneration [22]. A recent experimental TBI paper also found that whole cortex homogenates from APOE4 mice have reduced tight protein compared to APOE3 mice at 7 days post-injury, alongside increased MMP-9 activity [76]. Our results show that at 10 days post-injury, closure of the BBB has occurred in APOE3 mice. In contrast, APOE4 mice do not display significant reductions in BBB permeability at 10 days compared to 3 days post-injury when BBB leakage is evident. This demonstrates that the E4 isoform impairs the closure of the BBB following TBI. Mechanistically, our data suggests differential roles of APOE polymorphisms in regulating multiple pericyte-derived responses, which may cumulatively combine to be key determinants of BBB permeability after TBI. We observe a time dependent loss of PDGFRβ expression acutely after TBI. This is pertinent given previous studies evidencing its critical role, with PDGFRβ deficiency resulting in pericyte loss, increased BBB permeability and enhanced secondary injury processes [31, 32, 77]. Both APOE3 and APOE4 mice display reduced PDGFRβ expression up to 3 days post-TBI, consistent with a recent study utilizing similar trauma parameters showing rapid pericyte loss (PDGFRβ staining) in wildtype mice, starting at 6 h and lasting for 3 days post-injury [78]. However, in comparison to C57Bl/6 and APOE3 mice that display recovery of PDGFRβ expression at 7 days, APOE4 mice exhibit significantly prolonged reductions in PDGFRβ. This may be indicative of either reduced pericyte proliferation or delayed pericyte recruitment and/or migration back to the site of the pericontusional lesion following injury, as has been previously reported [79].

Given pericytes are considered a key source of MMP-9 production/release at the NVU following injury stimuli [73, 80], our results demonstrating augmented and sustained MMP-9 expression in APOE4 microvessels suggests that altered signaling in remaining pericytes contributes to the isoform dependent regulation of BBB integrity following TBI. Consistent with our data, not only is MMP-9 rapidly upregulated in human TBI patients [81, 82], clinical evidence suggests that this may be exacerbated in the presence of the APOE4 allele. Cognitively normal human apoE4 carriers exhibit increased CSF expression of MMP-9 correlating with BBB dysfunction, whilst post-mortem AD brains display elevated MMP-9 in cortical pericytes, in an isoform dependent manner (APOE4 > APOE3) [22]. At the vascular level, there was no difference between genotypes in the total density of regenerating/surviving microvessels in the pericontusional area after TBI, as identified by CD31 staining. Tomato-lectin is widely used to stain blood vessels through its binding to *N*-acetylglucosamine oligomers, trimers and tetramers expressed in the endothelium. However, *N*-acetylglucosamine is also expressed in glial cells [83], including those that are involved in the formation of the glial scar after TBI [84, 85]. As a result lectin stains glial cells [86, 87], and in our experiments we found wide-spread lectin staining in the glial scar and surrounding cortex that made it impossible to quantify lectin-positive blood vessels in this area – even though these blood vessels were still clearly visible. What we do find is that APOE polymorphisms differentially regulate tight junction mRNA recovery at the NVU after TBI. APOE4 mice displayed reduced levels of Zonula Occludens-1, Occludin and Claudin-5 compared to APOE3 post-injury, enhancing the notion that APOE4 significantly prolongs BBB dysfunction after TBI. Importantly we have shown that inhibition of the CypA-MMP-9 pathway can enhance BBB repair after TBI. As this step is downstream of the apoE-LRP interaction, this remains a plausible target for reversing the detrimental effect of apoE4 on BBB repair after TBI.

Conclusion

In conclusion, we have identified a role for apoE in contributing to BBB permeability, stabilization and closure after TBI. Specifically, the presence of APOE4 allele prolongs a variety of deleterious cellular responses that results in the overall delay of spontaneous BBB closure after injury. This data may help explain the mechanisms underlying the unfavorable recoveries of APOE4 carriers following TBI. Future studies investigating genotype-specific therapies targeting the BBB may prove beneficial to improving outcomes after TBI.

Abbreviations

APOE: apolipoprotein-E; BBB: Blood-brain barrier; CCI: controlled cortical impact; CNS: Central nervous system; CsA: Cyclosporine A; CSF: Cerebrospinal fluid; CypA: Cyclophilin A; EB: Evans blue; GWAS: Genome wide association study; LRP1: Low density lipoprotein receptor-related protein-1; MMP: Matrix metalloproteinase; MRI: Magnetic resonance imaging; NVU: Neurovascular Unit; RT-QPCR: Real time quantitative polymerase chain reaction; TBI: Traumatic Brain Injury

Acknowledgements

The authors would like to thank the Preclinical Imaging Research Laboratory (PIRL) at Georgetown University Medical Center for their technical assistance with MRI studies.

Funding

This work was supported by R01NS067417 (MPB) and R03NS095038 (SV) from the National Institute for Neurological Disorders and Stroke (NINDS). The Advanced Rehabilitation Research and Training Program (90AR5005) funded by The Department of Health and Human Services provided fellowship support for BSM and a T32 NS041218 Neural Injury and Plasticity pre-doctoral fellowship supported SSS.

Authors' contributions

BSM, SV, SSS, DJB, MP, CA, KS, MSM, PMW, OCR, and MPB conducted experiments. BSM and MPB designed experiments, analyzed the data and interpreted the results. BSM and MPB wrote the manuscript. All authors contributed to editing the manuscript. The authors declare that outside of the funding agencies outlined above, they have no conflict of interests to declare. All authors read and approved the final manuscript.

Authors' information

OCR is from the Department of Oncology, Georgetown University Medical Center, Washington, DC, 20057, USA. All other authors are in the Laboratory for Brain Injury and Dementia, Department of Neuroscience, Georgetown University Medical Center, Washington, DC, 20057, USA.

Competing interests

The authors declare that they have no competing interests.

Author details

[1]Laboratory for Brain Injury and Dementia, Department of Neuroscience, Georgetown University Medical Center, Washington, DC 20057, USA. [2]Lombardi Comprehensive Cancer Center, Department of Oncology, Georgetown University Medical Center, Washington, DC 20057, USA. [3]Department of Neuroscience, Georgetown University Medical Center, New Research Building-EG11, 3970 Reservoir Rd, NW, Washington, D.C 20057, USA.

References

1. Neuwelt E, et al. Strategies to advance translational research into brain barriers. The Lancet Neurology. 2008;7(1):84–96.
2. Shlosberg D, et al. Blood-brain barrier breakdown as a therapeutic target in traumatic brain injury. Nat Rev Neurol. 2010;6(7):393–403.

3. Mahley RW. Apolipoprotein E: cholesterol transport protein with expanding role in cell biology. Science. 1988;240(4852):622–30.
4. Chen Y, et al. Motor and cognitive deficits in apolipoprotein E-deficient mice after closed head injury. Neuroscience. 1997;80(4):1255–62.
5. Namjoshi DR, et al. The liver X receptor agonist GW3965 improves recovery from mild repetitive traumatic brain injury in mice partly through apolipoprotein E. PLoS One. 2013;8(1):e53529.
6. Horsburgh K, et al. Intraventricular infusion of apolipoprotein E ameliorates acute neuronal damage after global cerebral ischemia in mice. J Cereb Blood Flow Metab. 2000;20(3):458–62.
7. Kay AD, et al. Alterations in cerebrospinal fluid apolipoprotein E and amyloid beta-protein after traumatic brain injury. J Neurotrauma. 2003; 20(10):943–52.
8. Washington PM, Burns MP. The effect of the APOE4 gene on accumulation of Abeta40 after brain injury cannot be reversed by increasing apoE4 protein. J Neuropathol Exp Neurol. 2016;
9. Bell RD, et al. Apolipoprotein E controls cerebrovascular integrity via cyclophilin a. Nature. 2012;485(7399):512–6.
10. Methia N, et al. ApoE deficiency compromises the blood brain barrier especially after injury. Mol Med. 2001;7(12):810–5.
11. Hafezi-Moghadam A, Thomas KL, Wagner DD. ApoE deficiency leads to a progressive age-dependent blood-brain barrier leakage. Am J Physiol Cell Physiol. 2007;292(4):C1256–62.
12. Jordan B. Apolipoprotein E ϵ4 associated with chronic traumatic brain injury in boxing. JAMA. 1997;278(2):136.
13. Teasdale G, et al. Association of apolipoprotein E polymorphism with outcome after head injury. Lancet. 1997;350(9084):1069–71.
14. Sorbi S, et al. ApoE as a prognostic factor for post-traumatic coma. Nat Med. 1995;1(9):852.
15. Friedman G, et al. Apolipoprotein E-epsilon4 genotype predicts a poor outcome in survivors of traumatic brain injury. Neurology. 1999;52(2):244–8.
16. Mayeux R, et al. Synergistic effects of traumatic head injury and apolipoprotein-epsilon 4 in patients with Alzheimer's disease. Neurology. 1995;45(3 Pt 1):555–7.
17. Sabo T, et al. Susceptibility of transgenic mice expressing human apolipoprotein E to closed head injury: the allele E3 is neuroprotective whereas E4 increases fatalities. Neuroscience. 2000;101(4):879–84.
18. Mannix R, et al. Age-dependent effect of apolipoprotein E4 on functional outcome after controlled cortical impact in mice. J Cereb Blood Flow Metab. 2011;31(1):351–61.
19. Washington P, et al. Experimental traumatic brain injury induces rapid aggregation and oligomerization of amyloid-Beta in an Alzheimer's disease mouse model. J Neurotrauma. 2014;31(1):125–34.
20. Loane D, et al. Progressive neurodegeneration after experimental brain trauma: association with chronic microglial activation. J Neuropathol Exp Neurol. 2014;73(1):14–29.
21. Halliday MR, et al. Relationship between cyclophilin a levels and matrix metalloproteinase 9 activity in cerebrospinal fluid of cognitively normal apolipoprotein e4 carriers and blood-brain barrier breakdown. JAMA Neurol. 2013;70(9):1198–200.
22. Halliday MR, et al. Accelerated pericyte degeneration and blood-brain barrier breakdown in apolipoprotein E4 carriers with Alzheimer's disease. J Cereb Blood Flow Metab. 2016;36(1):216–27.
23. Villapol S, Loane DJ, Burns MP. Sexual dimorphism in the inflammatory response to traumatic brain injury. Glia. 2017;65(9):1423–38.
24. Sullivan PG, et al. Dose-response curve and optimal dosing regimen of cyclosporin a after traumatic brain injury in rats. Neuroscience. 2000; 101(2):289–95.
25. Fe Lanfranco M, et al. Combination of fluorescent in situ hybridization (FISH) and immunofluorescence imaging for detection of cytokine expression in microglia/macrophage cells. Bio Protoc. 2017;7(22)
26. Yamakawa H, et al. Normalization of endothelial and inducible nitric oxide synthase expression in brain microvessels of spontaneously hypertensive rats by angiotensin II AT1 receptor inhibition. J Cereb Blood Flow Metab. 2003;23(3):371–80.
27. Main B, et al. Type-1 interferons contribute to the neuroinflammatory response and disease progression of the MPTP mouse model of Parkinson's disease. Glia. 2016;64(9):1590–604.
28. Main BS, et al. Type-I interferons mediate the neuroinflammatory response and neurotoxicity induced by rotenone. J Neurochem. 2017;141(1):75–85.
29. Winer J, et al. Development and validation of real-time quantitative reverse transcriptase-polymerase chain reaction for monitoring gene expression in cardiac myocytes in vitro. Anal Biochem. 1999;270(1):41–9.
30. Alves JL. Blood-brain barrier and traumatic brain injury. J Neurosci Res. 2014;92(2):141–7.
31. Armulik A, et al. Pericytes regulate the blood-brain barrier. Nature. 2010; 468(7323):557–61.
32. Bell RD, et al. Pericytes control key neurovascular functions and neuronal phenotype in the adult brain and during brain aging. Neuron. 2010;68(3):409–27.
33. Rodriguez-Baeza A, et al. Morphological features in human cortical brain microvessels after head injury: a three-dimensional and immunocytochemical study. Anat Rec A Discov Mol Cell Evol Biol. 2003; 273((1):583–93.
34. Kenney, K., et al., Cerebral vascular injury in traumatic brain injury. Exp Neurol, 2016 275 Pt 3: p. 353–366.
35. Lin Y, et al. Blood-brain barrier permeability is positively correlated with cerebral microvascular perfusion in the early fluid percussion-injured brain of the rat. Lab Investig. 2012;92(11):1623–34.
36. Park E, et al. An analysis of regional microvascular loss and recovery following two grades of fluid percussion trauma: a role for hypoxia-inducible factors in traumatic brain injury. J Cereb Blood Flow Metab. 2009; 29(3):575–84.
37. Dixon CE, Lighthall JW, Anderson TE. Physiologic, histopathologic, and cineradiographic characterization of a new fluid-percussion model of experimental brain injury in the rat. J Neurotrauma. 1988;5(2):91–104.
38. Dietrich WD, Alonso O, Halley M. Early microvascular and neuronal consequences of traumatic brain injury: a light and electron microscopic study in rats. J Neurotrauma. 1994;11(3):289–301.
39. Glushakova OY, Johnson D, Hayes RL. Delayed increases in microvascular pathology after experimental traumatic brain injury are associated with prolonged inflammation, blood-brain barrier disruption, and progressive white matter damage. J Neurotrauma. 2014;31(13):1180–93.
40. Li S, et al. Enoxaparin ameliorates post-traumatic brain injury edema and neurologic recovery, reducing cerebral leukocyte endothelial interactions and vessel permeability in vivo. J Trauma Acute Care Surg. 2015;79(1):78–84.
41. Villapol S, Byrnes KR, Symes AJ. Temporal dynamics of cerebral blood flow, cortical damage, apoptosis, astrocyte-vasculature interaction and astrogliosis in the pericontusional region after traumatic brain injury. Front Neurol. 2014;5:82.
42. Cherian L, Goodman JC, Robertson C. Improved cerebrovascular function and reduced histological damage with darbepoietin alfa administration after cortical impact injury in rats. J Pharmacol Exp Ther. 2011;337(2):451–6.
43. Sangiorgi S, et al. Early-stage microvascular alterations of a new model of controlled cortical traumatic brain injury: 3D morphological analysis using scanning electron microscopy and corrosion casting. J Neurosurg. 2013; 118(4):763–74.
44. Blyth BJ, et al. Validation of serum markers for blood-brain barrier disruption in traumatic brain injury. J Neurotrauma. 2009;26(9):1497–507.
45. Ho KM, et al. Prognostic significance of blood-brain barrier disruption in patients with severe nonpenetrating traumatic brain injury requiring decompressive craniectomy. J Neurosurg. 2014;121(3):674–9.
46. Saw MM, et al. Differential disruption of blood-brain barrier in severe traumatic brain injury. Neurocrit Care. 2014;20(2):209–16.
47. Stahel PF, et al. Intrathecal levels of complement-derived soluble membrane attack complex (sC5b-9) correlate with blood-brain barrier dysfunction in patients with traumatic brain injury. J Neurotrauma. 2001;18(8):773–81.
48. Csuka E, et al. IL-10 levels in cerebrospinal fluid and serum of patients with severe traumatic brain injury: relationship to IL-6, TNF-alpha, TGF-beta1 and blood-brain barrier function. J Neuroimmunol. 1999;101(2):211–21.
49. Tomkins O, et al. Blood-brain barrier breakdown following traumatic brain injury: a possible role in posttraumatic epilepsy. Cardiovasc Psychiatry Neurol. 2011;2011:765923.
50. Hay JR, et al. Blood-brain barrier disruption is an early event that may persist for many years after traumatic brain injury in humans. J Neuropathol Exp Neurol. 2015;74(12):1147–57.
51. Barzo P, et al. Magnetic resonance imaging-monitored acute blood-brain barrier changes in experimental traumatic brain injury. J Neurosurg. 1996; 85(6):1113–21.
52. Beaumont A, et al. Bolus tracer delivery measured by MRI confirms edema without blood-brain barrier permeability in diffuse traumatic brain injury. Acta Neurochir Suppl. 2006;96:171–4.

53. Higashida T, et al. The role of hypoxia-inducible factor-1alpha, aquaporin-4, and matrix metalloproteinase-9 in blood-brain barrier disruption and brain edema after traumatic brain injury. J Neurosurg. 2011;114(1):92–101.
54. Shapira Y, et al. Blood-brain barrier permeability, cerebral edema, and neurologic function after closed head injury in rats. Anesth Analg. 1993; 77(1):141–8.
55. Baldwin SA, et al. Blood-brain barrier breach following cortical contusion in the rat. J Neurosurg. 1996;85(3):476–81.
56. Si D, et al. Progesterone protects blood-brain barrier function and improves neurological outcome following traumatic brain injury in rats. Exp Ther Med. 2014;8(3):1010–4.
57. Baskaya MK, et al. The biphasic opening of the blood-brain barrier in the cortex and hippocampus after traumatic brain injury in rats. Neurosci Lett. 1997;226(1):33–6.
58. Yuan F, et al. SIRT2 inhibition exacerbates neuroinflammation and blood-brain barrier disruption in experimental traumatic brain injury by enhancing NF-kappaB p65 acetylation and activation. J Neurochem. 2016;136(3):581–93.
59. Li H, et al. Sodium butyrate exerts neuroprotective effects by restoring the blood-brain barrier in traumatic brain injury mice. Brain Res. 2016;1642:70–8.
60. Tao X, et al. Protective actions of PJ34, a poly(ADP-ribose)polymerase inhibitor, on the blood-brain barrier after traumatic brain injury in mice. Neuroscience. 2015;291:26–36.
61. Dash PK, et al. Activation of alpha 7 cholinergic nicotinic receptors reduce blood-brain barrier permeability following experimental traumatic brain injury. J Neurosci. 2016;36(9):2809–18.
62. Yao X, et al. Mildly reduced brain swelling and improved neurological outcome in Aquaporin-4 knockout mice following controlled cortical impact brain injury. J Neurotrauma. 2015;32(19):1458–64.
63. Chen CC, et al. Wogonin improves histological and functional outcomes, and reduces activation of TLR4/NF-kappaB signaling after experimental traumatic brain injury. PLoS One. 2012;7(1):e30294.
64. Price L, Wilson C, Grant G. Chapter 4: Blood-brain barrier pathophysiology following traumatic brain injury. In: Laskowitz D, Grant G, editors. Translational Research in Traumatic Brain Injury. Boca Raton: CRC Press/ Taylor and Francis Group; 2016.
65. Cao F, et al. Apolipoprotein E-mimetic COG1410 reduces acute Vasogenic edema following traumatic brain injury. J Neurotrauma. 2016;33(2):175–82.
66. Meng Q, et al. Traumatic brain injury induces genome-wide transcriptomic, Methylomic, and network perturbations in brain and blood predicting neurological disorders. EBioMedicine. 2017;16:184–94.
67. Cartagena CM, et al. Cortical injury increases cholesterol 24S hydroxylase (Cyp46) levels in the rat brain. JNeurotrauma. 2008;25(9):1087–98.
68. Loane DJ, et al. Modulation of ABCA1 by an LXR agonist reduces beta-amyloid levels and improves outcome after traumatic brain injury. J Neurotrauma. 2011;28(2):225–36.
69. Xu Q, et al. Profile and regulation of apolipoprotein E (ApoE) expression in the CNS in mice with targeting of green fluorescent protein gene to the ApoE locus. J Neurosci. 2006;26(19):4985–94.
70. Wilhelmus MM, et al. Apolipoprotein E genotype regulates amyloid-beta cytotoxicity. J Neurosci. 2005;25(14):3621–7.
71. Casey CS, et al. Apolipoprotein E inhibits cerebrovascular Pericyte mobility through a RhoA protein-mediated pathway. J Biol Chem. 2015;290(22): 14208–17.
72. Enerson BE, Drewes LR. The rat blood-brain barrier transcriptome. J Cereb Blood Flow Metab. 2006;26(7):959–73.
73. Zozulya A, Weidenfeller C, Galla HJ. Pericyte-endothelial cell interaction increases MMP-9 secretion at the blood-brain barrier in vitro. Brain Res. 2008;1189:1–11.
74. Storck SE, et al. Endothelial LRP1 transports amyloid-beta(1-42) across the blood-brain barrier. J Clin Invest. 2016;126(1):123–36.
75. Alata W, et al. Human apolipoprotein E varepsilon4 expression impairs cerebral vascularization and blood-brain barrier function in mice. J Cereb Blood Flow Metab. 2015;35(1):86–94.
76. Teng Z, et al. ApoE influences the blood-brain barrier through the NF-kappaB/MMP-9 pathway after traumatic brain injury. Sci Rep. 2017;7(1):6649.
77. Winkler EA, et al. Blood-spinal cord barrier pericyte reductions contribute to increased capillary permeability. J Cereb Blood Flow Metab. 2012;32(10): 1841–52.
78. Zehendner CM, et al. Traumatic brain injury results in rapid pericyte loss followed by reactive pericytosis in the cerebral cortex. Sci Rep. 2015;5:13497.
79. Dore-Duffy P, et al. Pericyte migration from the vascular wall in response to traumatic brain injury. Microvasc Res. 2000;60(1):55–69.
80. Takata F, et al. Brain pericytes among cells constituting the blood-brain barrier are highly sensitive to tumor necrosis factor-alpha, releasing matrix metalloproteinase-9 and migrating in vitro. J Neuroinflammation. 2011;8:106.
81. Vilalta A, et al. Moderate and severe traumatic brain injury induce early overexpression of systemic and brain gelatinases. Intensive Care Med. 2008; 34(8):1384–92.
82. Suehiro E, et al. Increased matrix metalloproteinase-9 in blood in association with activation of interleukin-6 after traumatic brain injury: influence of hypothermic therapy. J Neurotrauma. 2004;21(12):1706–11.
83. Tsuji D, et al. Specific induction of macrophage inflammatory protein 1-alpha in glial cells of Sandhoff disease model mice associated with accumulation of N-acetylhexosaminyl glycoconjugates. J Neurochem. 2005; 92(6):1497–507.
84. Zhang H, et al. N-Acetylglucosamine 6-O-sulfotransferase-1 is required for brain keratan sulfate biosynthesis and glial scar formation after brain injury. Glycobiology. 2006;16(8):702–10.
85. Zhang H, Uchimura K, Kadomatsu K. Brain keratan sulfate and glial scar formation. Ann N Y Acad Sci. 2006;1086:81–90.
86. Colton CA, et al. Lectin staining of cultured CNS microglia. J Histochem Cytochem. 1992;40(4):505–12.
87. Kelley BJ, Lifshitz J, Povlishock JT. Neuroinflammatory responses after experimental diffuse traumatic brain injury. J Neuropathol Exp Neurol. 2007; 66(11):989–1001.

TMEM106B haplotypes have distinct gene expression patterns in aged brain

Yingxue Ren[1], Marka van Blitterswijk[2], Mariet Allen[2], Minerva M. Carrasquillo[2], Joseph S. Reddy[1], Xue Wang[1], Thomas G. Beach[3], Dennis W. Dickson[2], Nilüfer Ertekin-Taner[2,4], Yan W. Asmann[1] and Rosa Rademakers[2*]

Abstract

Background: Single nucleotide polymorphisms (SNPs) inherited as one of two common haplotypes at the *transmembrane protein 106B* (*TMEM106B*) locus are associated with the risk of multiple neurodegenerative diseases, including frontotemporal lobar degeneration with pathological inclusions of TDP-43. Among the associated variants, rs3173615 (encoding p.T185S) is the only coding variant; however, non-coding variants may also contribute to disease risk. It has been reported that the risk haplotype is associated with higher levels of TMEM106B and increased levels of TMEM106B cause cytotoxicity; however, the precise mechanism through which *TMEM106B* haplotypes contribute to neurodegeneration is unclear.

Methods: We utilized RNA sequencing data derived from temporal cortex (TCX) and cerebellum (CER) from 312 North American Caucasian subjects neuropathologically diagnosed with Alzheimer's disease, progressive supranuclear palsy, pathological aging or normal controls to analyze transcriptome signatures associated with the risk (TT) and protective (SS) *TMEM106B* haplotypes. In cohorts matched for disease phenotype, we used Analysis of Variance (ANOVA) to identify differentially expressed genes and Weighted Gene Co-expression Network Analysis (WGCNA) to identify gene networks associated with the risk and protective *TMEM106B* haplotypes.

Results: A total of 110 TCX and 116 CER samples were included in the analyses. When comparing TT to SS carriers, we detected 593 differentially expressed genes in TCX and 7 in CER. Gene co-expression network analyses further showed that in both TCX and CER the SS haplotype was positively correlated with gene networks involved in synaptic transmission, whereas the TT haplotype was positively correlated with gene networks enriched for immune response. Gene expression patterns of 5 cell-type-specific markers revealed significantly reduced expression of the neuronal marker and relative increases in all other cell markers in TT as compared to SS carriers in TCX with a similar but non-significant trend in CER.

Conclusions: By comparing the common *TMEM106B* risk and protective haplotypes we identified significant and partly conserved transcriptional differences across TCX and CER and striking changes in cell-type composition, especially in TCX. These findings illustrate the profound effect of *TMEM106B* haplotypes on brain health and highlight the importance to better understand TMEM106B's function and dysfunction in the context of neurodegenerative diseases.

Keywords: TMEM106B, Frontotemporal dementia, Co-expression networks, Differential expression, Synaptic transmission, Immune response, Progranulin

* Correspondence: Rademakers.Rosa@mayo.edu
[2]Department of Neuroscience, Mayo Clinic, Jacksonville, FL, USA
Full list of author information is available at the end of the article

Background

Given the world's aging population, neurodegenerative diseases have become a major cause of disability and death. While the disease mechanisms differ, neurodegeneration often results from the accumulation of misfolded aggregated proteins in different areas of the aging brain, and this process yields cell death and inflammatory damage in those brain regions [1]. Recent studies have revealed that two common haplotypes in transmembrane protein 106B (*TMEM106B*) are associated with risk of multiple neurodegenerative diseases, most notably with frontotemporal lobar degeneration with pathological inclusions of TDP-43 (FTLD-TDP) [2–4], progranulin (*GRN*)-related FTLD [3, 5], chromosome 9 open reading frame 72 (*C9ORF72*)-mediated FTLD [6, 7] and hippocampal sclerosis of aging [8, 9]. *TMEM106B* haplotypes were also shown to associate with the development of cognitive impairment in amyotrophic lateral sclerosis (ALS) [10] and with the presence of TDP-43 pathology in Alzheimer's disease (AD) [11] and elderly individuals without FTLD [12]. The broad involvement of *TMEM106B* in neurodegenerative diseases makes it an important gene to characterize and a promising target for potential therapies.

As with most risk loci identified by genome-wide association studies (GWAS), the functional variant(s) in the *TMEM106B* locus associated with the reported associations remains elusive. Within the associated linkage disequilibrium (LD) block, rs3173615 is the only variant encoding an amino acid change from the more common, highly conserved, threonine (Thr185; risk allele) to a serine (Ser185; protective allele) at position 185. In vitro, the protective (Ser185) TMEM106B isoform was consistently expressed at lower levels than the risk (Thr185) TMEM106B isoform due to an increased rate of protein degradation, possibly resulting from changes in TMEM106B glycosylation [13]. In addition to the coding variant (rs3173615) numerous non-coding variants also differentiate the *TMEM106B* haplotypes and at least one of these variants (rs1990620) was suggested to affected higher-order chromatin architecture at the *TMEM106B* locus and changes in mRNA expression [14]. Indeed, expression studies in FTLD-TDP brains have shown increased *TMEM106B* mRNA levels in carriers of the risk haplotype [2]. Regardless of the identity of the specific functional variant(s), these findings suggest the presence of higher levels of TMEM106B in carriers of the risk haplotype and lower levels of TMEM106B in carriers of the protective haplotype. These findings are in line with cell biological studies which showed that increased TMEM106B levels were cytotoxic and led to an increase in lysosomal size and reduced lysosomal acidification [4]. Importantly, however, the specific mechanism by which *TMEM106B* haplotypes and changes in its expression contribute to neurodegeneration remains unknown.

In this study, we utilized RNA sequencing data of temporal cortex (TCX) and cerebellum (CER) samples from 312 North American Caucasian subjects to identify transcriptome signatures associated with the *TMEM106B* haplotypes. By comparing homozygote rs3173615 TT (risk) and SS (protective) carriers, we discovered differentially expressed genes in both TCX and CER regions, and identified shared gene co-expression networks between TCX and CER through which the *TMEM106B* haplotypes may contribute to brain function and brain health.

Materials and methods

Dataset description

We used RNA sequencing data of 268 TCX and 266 CER brain samples from 312 North American Caucasian subjects with neuropathological diagnosis of AD, progressive supranuclear palsy (PSP), pathologic aging (PA; defined as aging in nondemented elderly humans that is associated with moderate to marked cerebral amyloid deposition in the absence of significant neurofibrillary degeneration) [15] or elderly controls (CON) without clinically-significant neurodegenerative diseases [16]. The tissue processing, RNA extraction, RNA sequencing, quality control and data normalization were previously described [16, 17]. To differentiate individuals with the *TMEM106B* risk and protective haplotypes we used rs3173615 as the tagging variant. Genotypes of rs3173615 for the 312 individuals were extracted by PLINK using data generated from Illumina Omni2.5 BeadChips [17].

Differential gene expression analysis

Conditional Quantile Normalization (CQN) was previously performed on the raw gene counts to correct for GC bias and gene length differences, and to obtain similar quantile-by-quantile distributions of gene expression levels across samples [17]. Based on the bi-modal distribution of the CQN normalized and log2-transformed reads per kb per million (RPKM) gene expression values, for both TCX and CER samples, protein-coding genes with average log2 RPKM $> = -1$ in at least one haplotype group were considered expressed above detection threshold and were included in further analysis. Using this selection threshold, 16,868 genes were included for the TCX analysis and 14,994 were included for the CER analysis.

Differential gene expression analyses were performed using Partek Genomics Suite (Partek Inc., St. Louis, MO). Gene expression between the rs3173615 SS and TT individuals were compared using Analyses of Variance models (ANOVA), while correcting for RNA integrity number (RIN), age at death, sex and disease type. The selection of these covariates was based on the source of variation analyses from which factors with mean F ratio > 1.25 were considered confounding factors that needed to be adjusted for. The *Benjamini–Hochberg* procedure was performed to adjust for multiple testing and control false discovery rate (FDR). Differentially expressed genes (DEG) were defined by thresholds of |fold change| (FC) >= 1.5 and adjusted p value < 0.05. The significance of DEG overlap between TCX and CER was tested by calculating empirical p-value based on 100,000 simulations. Pathway analyses of differentially expressed genes were performed using MetaCore pathway analysis (Thomson Reuters) (Version 6.25).

Weighted gene co-expression network analysis

To identify groups of genes that are correlated with the *TMEM106B* haplotype, we performed Weighted Gene Co-expression Network Analysis (WGCNA) [18] using residual expression values calculated from adjusting for RIN, age at death, sex, and disease type. Separate WGCNA analyses were performed for the TCX and CER datasets. Signed hybrid co-expression networks were built for both WGCNA analyses. For each set of genes, a pairwise correlation matrix was computed and an adjacency matrix was calculated by raising the correlation matrix to a power. Based on the relationships between power and scale independence, the power of 4 was chosen for the TCX dataset, and the power of 14 was chosen for CER dataset. We used hybrid dynamic tree cutting, a minimum module size of 40 genes, and a minimum height for merging modules at 0.25 for both TCX and CER. Each module was summarized by the first principal component of the scaled (standardized) module expression profiles (module eigengene). For each module, the module membership measure (MM) was defined as the correlation between gene-expression values and the module eigengene. Hub genes from relevant modules, which have the highest connectivity to other genes within the module, were selected using the WGCNA function "chooseTopHubInEachModule". Each module was assigned a unique color identifier, and genes that did not fulfil these criteria for any of the modules were assigned to the gray module. To assess the correlation of modules to the *TMEM106B* protective (SS) haplotype, we defined the TT genotype as 0, and SS as 1. Modules significantly associated with TT or SS were annotated using WGCNA R function GOenrichmentAnalysis. Modules were also tested for enrichment of the respective DEG signatures using the anRichment R package.

Results

Selection of study population and basic characteristics

In our available dataset, we identified 77 individuals homozygous for the C allele at rs3173615 corresponding to Thr185 (16 AD, 29 PSP, 8 PA and 24 CON; further referred to as TT) and 65 individuals homozygous for the G allele at rs3171615 corresponding to Ser185 (26 AD, 16 PSP, 5 PA and 18 CON, further referred to as SS) in the TCX. In the CER dataset, 80 individuals were TT (21 AD, 29 PSP, 5 PA and 25 CON) and 64 individuals were SS (26 AD, 16 PSP, 6 PA and 16 CON). Since our cohort comprised samples from cases with different neurodegenerative disease as well as neuropathologically normal individuals, we further matched TT and SS study groups on pathological diagnosis and subsequently on sex and age at death, where possible. In sum, we included 55 TT and 55 SS TCX samples ($n = 110$) with equal numbers of AD, PSP, PA and CON in each group (Additional file 1: Table S1). In the CER, we selected 58 TT and 58 SS samples ($n = 116$) with equal numbers of AD, PSP, PA and CON in each group. The 110 TCX and 116 CER samples were from 133 individual subjects (93 individuals had both CER and TCX samples). The general characteristics of the TT and SS study groups included in the analyses are presented in Table 1. TT and SS individuals were of comparable composition in terms of sex and age at death (by study design) and postmortem interval (PMI), and were also found to be similar in terms of Braak stage and brain weight.

Transcriptional differences between TMEM106B TT and SS carriers in TCX and CER

We first compared transcriptome-wide gene expression between TT and SS carriers. In the TCX dataset, we identified 593 DEGs between TT and SS carriers (Additional file 1: Table S2). In the CER dataset, we only identified 7 DEGs (Additional file 1: Table S3), none of which overlapped with the TCX DEGs. The large difference between TCX and CER suggests that the impact of *TMEM106B* is more prominent in a brain region affected by neurodegeneration. To further study potential similarities in the expression changes in CER and TCX we compared the top 500 genes with |FC| ≥ 1.2 between SS and TT ranked by unadjusted p value in the TCX and CER dataset, which showed significant overlap in genes ($n = 28$; $p = 0.0008$) (Additional file 1: Table S4).

Table 1 Characteristics of the subjects included in this study

Traits	TT	SS	*P* value
Sex (male %)	0.41	0.55	NA
Age at death	81.79 ± 9.31	81.15 ± 9.10	0.69
Post-mortem interval	4.43 ± 5.95	5.29 ± 7.39	0.53
Braak stage	3.63 ± 1.89	3.78 ± 1.99	0.72
Brain weight (g)	1116.60 ± 133.42	1144.13 ± 158.82	0.37

Sex and Age at death are known for all 133 subjects; Braak stage and post-mortem interval (PMI) are known for 98 subjects and brain weight is known for 93 subjects

Most of these genes are involved in neurotransmitter formation and regulation and interestingly *GAD1* (FC_{CER} 1.44; FC_{TCX} 1.90), *GAD2* (FC_{CER} 1.49; FC_{TCX} 2.14) and *SLC32A1* (FC_{CER} 1.39; FC_{TCX} 2.25), all critical for GABAergic neurotransmission, are among the shared genes.

Next we performed pathway enrichment analysis on the DEGs. In TCX, 9 out of the 10 top enriched gene ontology (GO) terms were related to synaptic signaling or cell communication (Table 2). In the CER, since only 7 genes passed the thresholds of $|FC| >= 1.5$ and adjusted p values < 0.05, we loosened the threshold to $|FC| >= 1.2$ and unadjusted p values < 0.05 to allow the study of sufficient genes in the pathway analysis. In CER, we found most top enriched GO processes to be related to immune response; however, signaling was also among the top enriched GOs (Table 3).

Co-expression network analyses reveals gene clusters significantly correlated with TMEM106B TT and SS carrier status in TCX and CER

To gain further insight into the gene networks associated with the TMEM106B T (risk) and S (protection) haplotypes, we applied a gene co-expression network approach, WGCNA, which can functionally probe transcriptomic patterns of change. WGCNA is a computational tool that clusters genes in an unsupervised manner based on their correlated co-expression, and thus defines biologically relevant groups of genes that typically correspond to specific processes. WGCNA analysis of the TCX dataset identified 25 gene clusters (modules). The *TMEM106B* haplotype was significantly correlated with 10 modules: 4 positively correlated with SS and 6 positively correlated with TT (Table 4, Fig. 1a). WGCNA analysis of the CER dataset identified 14 modules. The *TMEM106B* haplotype was significantly correlated with 2 modules: 1 positively correlated with SS and 1 positively correlated with TT (Table 5, Fig. 1b). GO enrichment analysis on the modules significantly correlated with the *TMEM106B* haplotypes showed that synaptic transmission was a highly enriched GO in both TCX and CER from modules significantly positively correlated with the SS haplotype (modules turquoise in TCX and tan in CER). In addition, immune response was a highly enriched GO from modules significantly negatively correlated with the SS haplotype (positively correlated with TT) (modules darkred in TCX and purple in CER). This suggests that the *TMEM106B* haplotypes may influence brain function in multiple brain regions through similar mechanisms. Additionally, the TCX and CER synaptic transmission modules and the CER immune response module were significantly enriched for their respective DEGs, which demonstrated the consistency between the two analytic approaches (Additional file 1: Table S5).

We next identified the intramodular hub genes in the modules significantly correlated with the *TMEM106B* haplotype status. Hub genes are the genes with the highest connectivity to other genes of the same module; therefore, they often have important roles in the network and biological functions even if they do not meet the DEG threshold. Using the WGCNA function "chooseTopHubInEachModule", we identified one hub gene for each significant module (Tables 5 and 6). The expression level of each hub gene in SS and TT carriers is shown in Fig. 2. For the synaptic transmission modules and immune response modules in TCX and CER, we also visualized the connection among hub genes and the top 30 genes with the highest connectivity within the respective modules using VisANT [19] (Fig. 3).

Cell type composition may underlie expression differences observed in TMEM106B TT and SS carriers

The central nervous system (CNS) includes 5 main cell types: neurons, astrocytes, microglia, oligodendrocytes, and endothelial cells. We hypothesized that the relative abundance of different cell types may at least partially

Table 2 Top 10 enriched GO terms from differentially expressed genes in TCX

GO Process	*P* value	FDR	# Genes
single organism signaling	1.801E-20	5.424E-17	253
signaling	1.986E-20	5.424E-17	253
cell communication	5.539E-20	1.008E-16	256
G-protein coupled receptor signaling pathway	3.527E-19	2.908E-16	74
chemical synaptic transmission	4.260E-19	2.908E-16	59
trans-synaptic signaling	4.260E-19	2.908E-16	59
synaptic signaling	4.260E-19	2.908E-16	59
anterograde trans-synaptic signaling	4.260E-19	2.908E-16	59
multicellular organismal process	3.899E-18	2.366E-15	297
cell-cell signaling	3.492E-17	1.907E-14	91

Table 3 Top 10 enriched GO terms from differentially expressed genes in CER

GO Process	P value	FDR	# Genes
immune system process	1.990E-19	1.005E-15	101
defense response	3.083E-17	7.783E-14	69
regulation of multicellular organismal process	1.448E-16	2.438E-13	122
immune response	4.750E-16	5.996E-13	61
inflammatory response	1.576E-15	1.591E-12	38
response to stimulus	6.918E-15	5.822E-12	224
response to lipid	4.419E-14	3.187E-11	61
single organism signaling	1.247E-13	7.520E-11	163
signaling	1.341E-13	7.520E-11	163
positive regulation of multicellular organismal process	5.047E-13	2.548E-10	76

explain the differences in the transcriptional signatures observed in TT and SS carriers. Because the cell type composition can be estimated by cell-type-specific gene expression levels, we adopted the approached described in Allen et al. [17] and used 5 genes to estimate the cell type composition in the brain tissue samples: *ENO2* for neurons (ENSG00000111674), *GFAP* for astrocytes (ENSG00000131095), *CD68* for microglia (ENSG00000129226), *OLIG2* for oligodendrocytes (ENSG00000205927), and *CD34* for endothelial cells (ENSG00000174059). When we compared the expression of these 5 genes in the TT and SS carriers we found, in TCX, that the SS carriers had significantly higher neuronal gene expression and lower astrocyte, endothelium and oligodendrocyte gene expression as compared to the TT carriers. The expression of the microglial marker CD68 was also lower in SS as compared to TT carriers, but this difference was not significant. In CER, the same trends were observed, although none of the differences were significant (Fig. 4).

Discussion

In this study, we used RNA sequencing data of two brain regions to investigate the involvement of the *TMEM106B* risk and protective haplotypes in brain health. We identified large transcriptional differences between the protective SS and risk TT haplotypes in TCX, and much smaller differences in CER, consistent with the higher level of tissue damage and neuronal loss in the TCX region. Importantly, even though not statistically significant in CER, our data suggested similarities in the effects of *TMEM106B* haplotypes on the transcriptional signatures in both brain regions. By comparing the top 500 differentially expressed genes in TCX and CER with $|\text{fold change}| \geq 1.2$ between SS and TT, we found 28 overlapping genes, all with a fold-change in the same direction (25 are increased and 3 are decreased in SS carriers as compared to TT carriers). Some of the biggest increases in SS carriers were seen in *GAD1* and *GAD2*, glutamic acid decarboxylases which are responsible for catalyzing the production of gamma-aminobutyric acid (GABA) from glutamate, and

Table 4 Modules significantly correlated to the *TMEM106B* rs3173615 status in TCX

Module	Correlation	P value	Top GO	FDR	Hub gene
turquoise	0.35	2e-04	synaptic transmission	6.64E-37	*FGF14*
greenyellow	0.27	0.004	Ribonucleoprotein complex biogenesis	1	*OXR1*
darkgrey	0.24	0.01	centriolar satellite	1	*IGSF9B*
midnightblue	0.24	0.01	ribosome binding	0.99	*TRAPPC2L*
brown	−0.37	7e-05	cell-cell adhesion	6.24E-07	*PDLIM5*
tan	−0.25	0.009	cellular response to zinc ion	0.025	*MFSD6*
black	−0.23	0.01	vasculature development	2.01E-19	*ADGRL4*
darkred	−0.22	0.02	humoral immune response	0.0002	*LIMK2*
lightgreen	−0.21	0.03	cytosolic ribosome	2.98E-123	*RPS19*
lightyellow	−0.2	0.04	extracellular matrix organization	9.04E-14	*DSP*

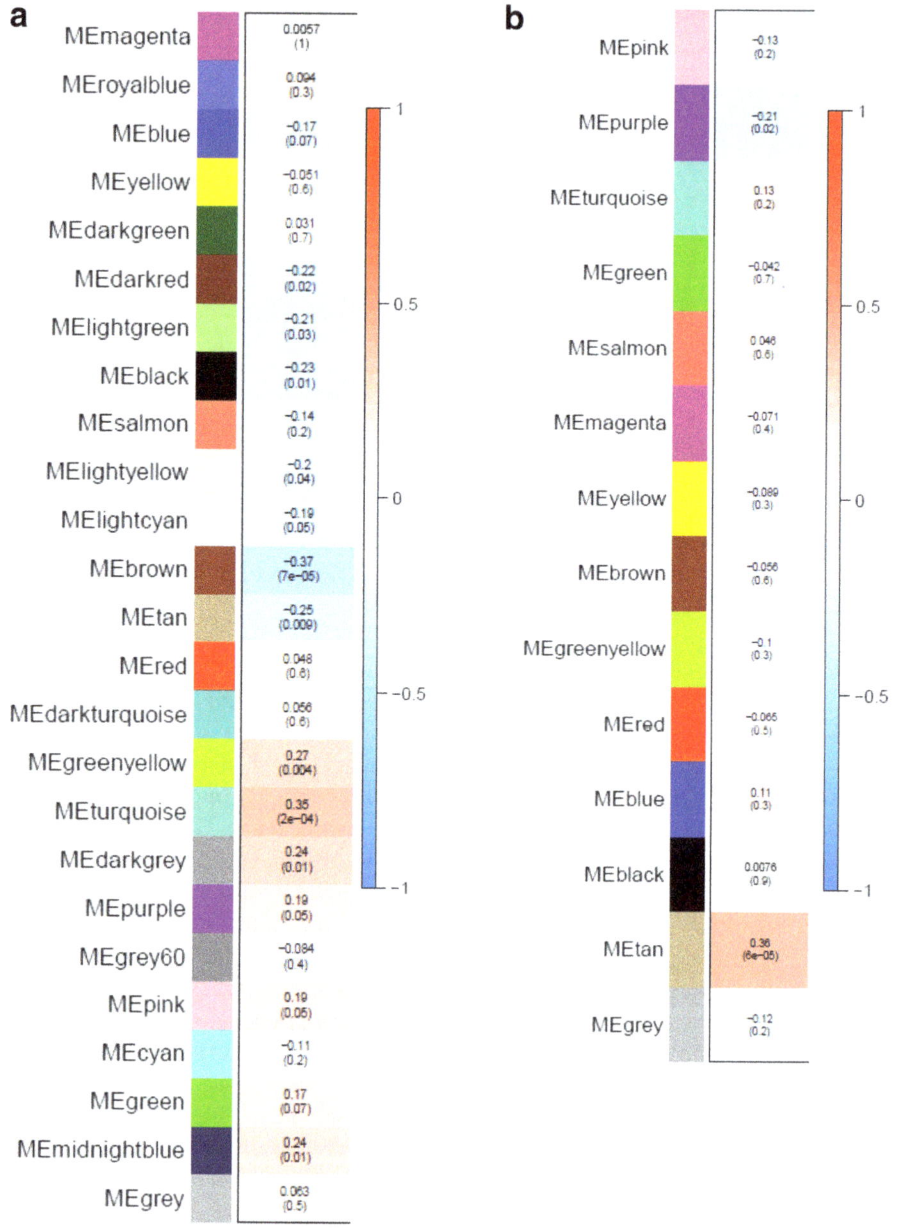

Fig. 1 Module-haplotype correlation in (**a**) TCX and (**b**) CER. Each rectangle represents a module. The top number in each rectangle is the correlation coefficient (r) between the module eigengene to haplotype, and the bottom number is the p value of the correlation. The color orange represents positive correlation to the SS haplotype and blue represents negative correlation to SS (positive correlation to TT)

SLC32A1 (also known as *VGAT*) which is a transporter involved in the uptake of GABA and glycine into synaptic vesicles. The specific changes in GABA-related signaling are interesting in light of a recent study which reported the preferential elimination of inhibitory synapses (defined by VGAT+ immunoreactivity) in the ventral thalamus of *Grn* knock-out mouse brains [20]. This observation raises the possibility that more robust GABAergic signaling or an increase in the number of inhibitory synapses at baseline in SS haplotype carriers

Table 5 Modules significantly correlated to the *TMEM106B* rs3173615 status in CER

Module	Correlation	P value	Top GO	FDR	Hub gene
tan	0.36	6e-05	synaptic transmission	4.74E-05	*PCP4L1*
purple	−0.21	0.02	immune response	1.42E-27	*ITGB2*

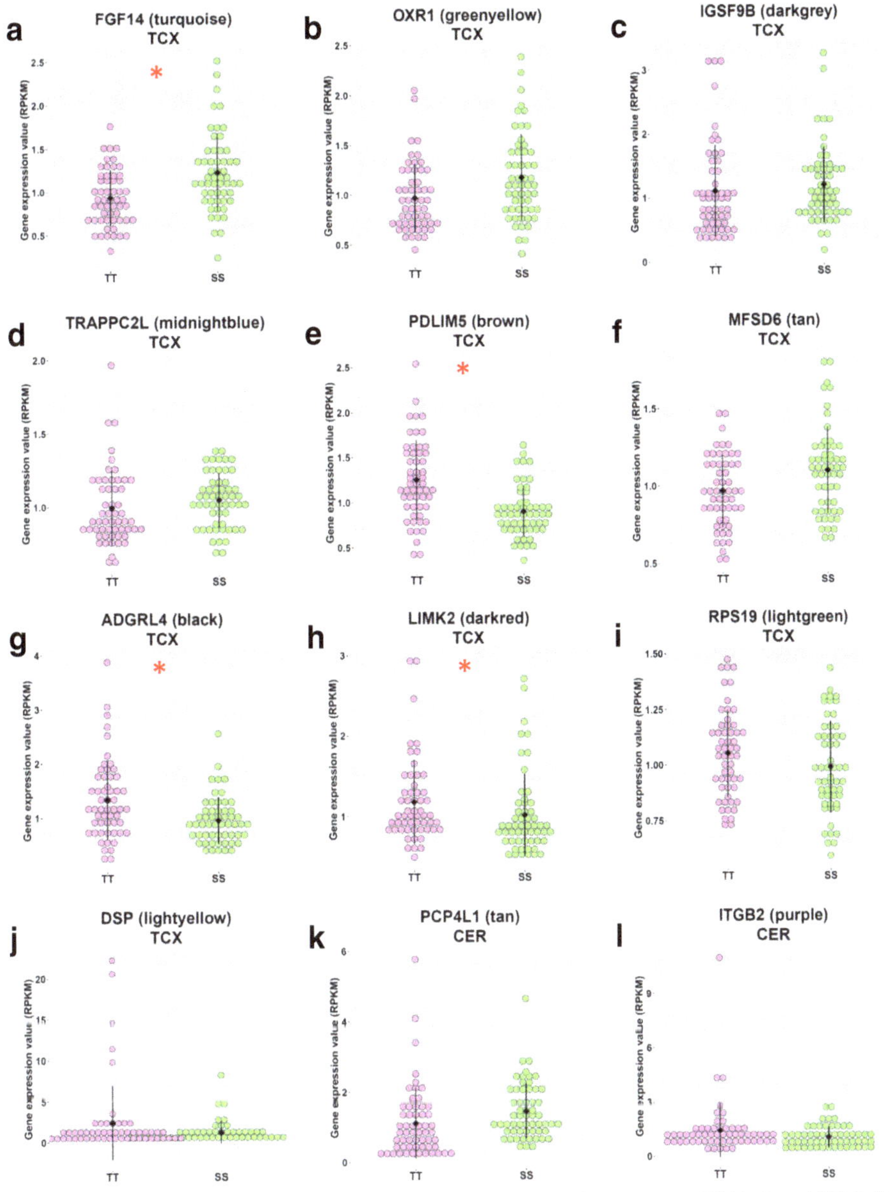

Fig. 2 Expression values of the intramodular hub genes in significant modules in TT and SS carriers in TCX (**a**-**j**) and CER (**k**-**l**). The expression values (RPKM) have been adjusted for RIN, age at death, sex and disease type. The black dots represent the mean; the black lines represent the standard deviation. Red asterisks indicate significant difference between TT and SS (FDR <0.05)

may contribute to the profound protection conferred by this haplotype in patients with *GRN* mutations. Future immunohistochemical studies in human brain samples from SS and TT *TMEM106B* carriers are needed to confirm this hypothesis.

Using gene co-expression network analyses we further identified significant correlations of *TMEM106B* haplotypes with gene expression modules enriched for genes involved in similar biological processes across both brain regions. In TCX and CER, the *TMEM106B* SS haplotype was correlated with gene networks involved in synaptic transmission, whereas the TT haplotype was correlated with immune response networks in both brain regions, in addition to other specific gene networks such as cell-cell adhesion found only in TCX. In a further reference to the *Grn* knock-out mouse model, it is of interest to note that the gene expression modules most significantly correlated with the loss of *Grn* in cerebral cortex, cerebellum and hippocampus in mice were annotated by GO as involved in the innate immune response with *C1qa*, *C1qb*, *C1qc*, and *C3* among the most connected genes in the module, similar to what we observed when we compared SS to TT carriers in the CER (purple module; Fig. 3d) [20]. Finally, using 5 genes as surrogates for

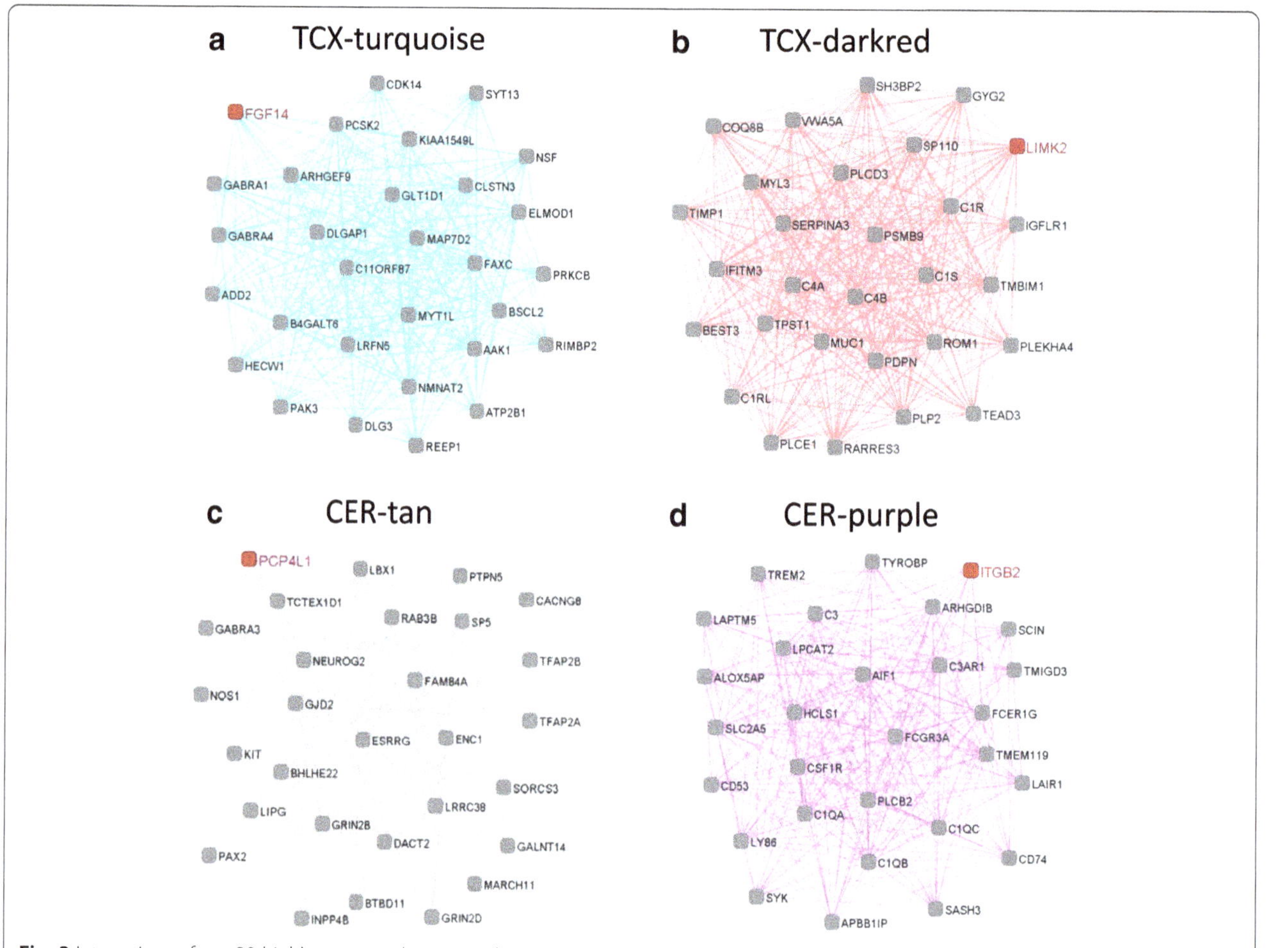

Fig. 3 Interactions of top 30 highly connected genes in the synaptic transmission and immune response modules. **a** and **b** are modules in TCX. **c** and **d** are modules in CER. The red nodes represent hub genes of each module

the 5 major brain cell types, we found that the gene networks were associated with the cell type composition in the TT and SS brains: the SS carriers showed higher neuronal gene expression as compared to the TT carriers, corresponding to an increase in networks related to synaptic transmission in SS brains; the TT carriers showed higher microglial gene expression as compared to SS carriers, in agreement with the observed enrichment for immune response networks in TT brains.

TMEM106B risk variants had previously been reported to be associated with both brain volume and connectivity. Specifically, using imaging studies, the *TMEM106B* risk allele was shown to significantly associate with reduced brain volume in non-demented elderly individuals, particularly in the superior temporal gyrus in the left hemisphere [21]. In addition, *GRN* mutation carriers with two copies of the *TMEM106B* risk allele demonstrated worsened brain connectivity compared to those who carried one or no risk alleles [22]. These authors found that *TMEM106B* haplotypes did not influence grey matter volume directly on its own, but in mutation carriers the protective *TMEM106B* haplotype was able to enhance the benefit of cognitive reserve on brain structure. Similarly, in our study, we found no significant differences in total brain weight between our TT and SS carriers. Instead our data suggest that the SS protective haplotype may confer higher synaptic transmission by strengthening brain connectivity in aged or diseased brain.

TMEM106B has also recently been linked to healthy neurological aging. In frontal cortex, the *TMEM106B* risk haplotype was associated with gene expression patterns suggestive of an older age than the individual's true chronological age [23]. Similar to our study, the *TMEM106B* risk haplotype was further found to be associated with increased inflammation and reduced neuronal expression in these neuropathologically normal elderly individual. Contrary to our findings, however, they did not observe an effect of *TMEM106B* on gene expression in cerebellar tissues. This may be related to the fact that they focused on neurologically normal individuals whereas we included a mixture of neurodegenerative

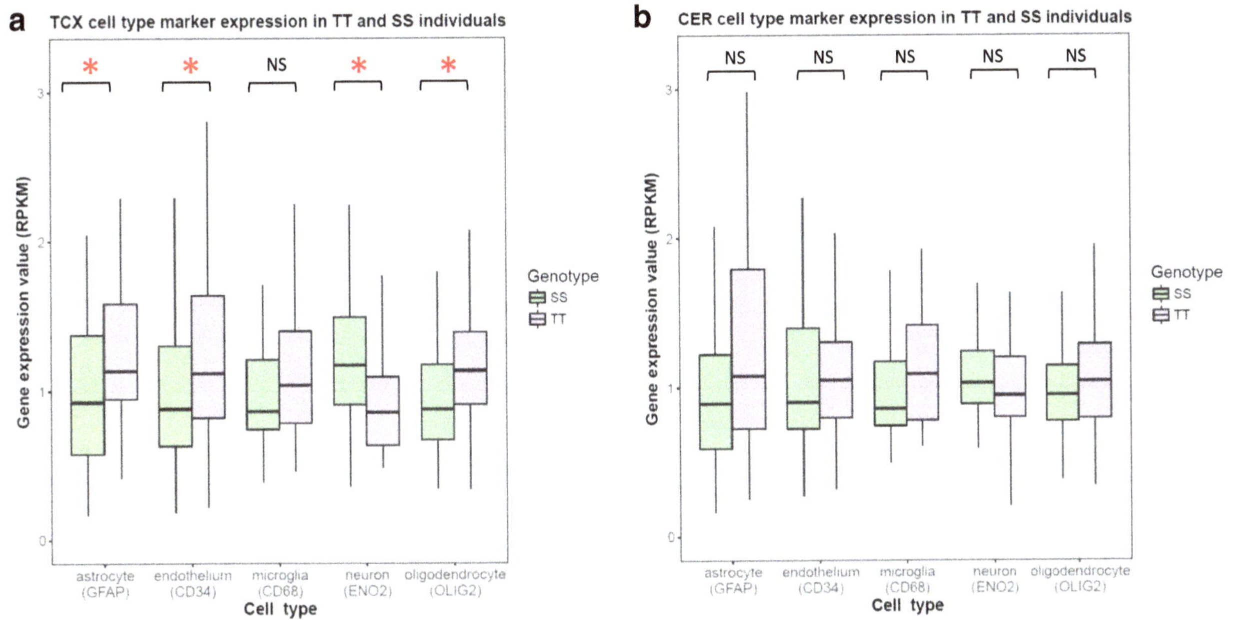

Fig. 4 Expression values (RPKM) of the 5 cell-type marker genes. The expression values (RPKM) have been adjusted for RIN, age at death, sex and disease type. **a** TCX samples. **b** CER samples. Red asterisks represent significant difference between TT and SS (FDR < 0.05)

diseases and normal controls. To determine whether the significant modules we identified were mainly contributed by disease samples or controls, we performed additional WGCNA analyses with only cases in TCX ($n = 74$, 37 TT and 37 SS) or CER ($n = 84$, 42 TT and 42 SS), and using only controls in TCX ($n = 42$: 24 TT and 18 SS) or CER ($n = 41$: 25 TT and 16 SS). In both TCX and CER, analysis of the cases identified similar modules as we did in the full TCX and CER datasets (Additional file 1: Table S6). Furthermore, independent analyses of each disease group: TCX-AD, TCX-PSP, CER-AD and CER-PSP all identified synaptic transmission modules that are significantly correlated with the *TMEM106B* haplotype (Additional file 1: Table S7), suggesting that the effects of the *TMEM106B* haplotype was not specific to disease type. Analysis of only the control samples in TCX and CER identified less modules, and synaptic transmission and immune response modules were not significantly correlated with the *TMEM106B* haplotype in either brain region (Additional file 1: Table S8). While the smaller sample size of the control cohorts may have reduced our power to detect significant difference, these results suggest that the effects of *TMEM106B* haplotypes on the transcriptome are more pronounced in disease tissues than in healthy tissues.

Conclusions

In summary, our study demonstrates significant and partly conserved effects of the *TMEM106B* haplotypes on the transcriptome across multiple brain regions. It is quite remarkable that a variant which is common in the normal population (minor allele frequency = 0.40) can have such profound effects on gene expression and cell type composition, especially since our SS and TT study groups were matched for disease phenotypes and age at death. This suggests that additional genetic and/or environmental factors are likely to modulate the effect of the *TMEM106B* haplotypes on neurological and normal brain aging in individual human subjects. TMEM106B has only begun to be characterized since the discovery of its association to FTLD-TDP several years ago. While its function has mostly been linked to lysosome functions and trafficking, and recently to myelination [24], our results suggest that *TMEM106B* plays a broader role in the CNS response to pathological or age-related insults in multiple brain regions. Continued research into *TMEM106Bs* normal function and dysfunction in the context of neurodegenerative diseases will be critical and holds promise for future therapeutic strategies.

Additional file

Additional file 1: Table S1. Tissue samples available and selected for inclusion in this study. **Table S2.** DEGS in TCX. Positive fold change represents higher gene expression in SS than TT. Negative fold change represents lower gene expression in SS than TT. **Table S3.** DEGS in CER. Positive fold change represents higher gene expression in SS than TT. Negative fold change represents lower gene expression in SS than TT. **Table S4.** Overlapping genes between TCX and CER based on top 500 genes with $|FC| \geq 1.2$ ranked by unadjusted p value. **Table S5.** Enrichment of modules for their respective DEG signatures. **Table S6.** Significant modules identified in the TCX and CER matched cases. **Table S7.** Significant modules identified in separate disease groups in TCX and

CER. **Table S8**. Significant modules identified in the TCX and CER controls.

Abbreviations

AD: Alzheimer's disease; ALS: Amyotrophic lateral sclerosis; AMP-AD: Accelerating Medicines Partnership in Alzheimer's Disease; ANOVA: Analyses of variance; C9ORF72: Chromosome 9 open reading frame 72; CER: Cerebellum; CNS: Central nervous system; CON: Elderly controls; CQN: Conditional Quantile Normalization; DEG: Differentially expressed genes; FC: Fold change; FDR: False discovery rate; FTLD: Frontotemporal lobar degeneration; FTLD-TDP: Frontotemporal lobar degeneration with pathological inclusions of TDP-43; GO: Gene ontology; GRN: Progranulin; GWAS: Genome-wide association studies; LD: Linkage disequilibrium; MM: Module membership; PA: Pathologic aging; PMI: Postmortem interval; PSP: Progressive supranuclear palsy; RIN: RNA integrity number; RPKM: reads per kb per million; TCX: Temporal cortex; TMEM106B: Transmembrane protein 106; WGCNA: Weighted Gene Co-expression Network Analysis

Acknowledgements

The authors thank the patients and their families for their participation, without whom these studies would not have been possible.

Funding

This work was supported by the National Institute on Aging [RF AG051504 to N.E.T.; U01 AG046139 to N.E.T.], the National Institute of Neurological Disorders and Stroke [R01 NS080820 to N.E.T.; R35 NS097261-01 to R.R.], Mayo Clinic and Foundation [R.R. and Y.R.] and Mayo Clinic Center for Individualized Medicine [Y.R. and Y.W.A]. For samples collected through the Sun Health Research Institute Brain and Body Donation Program of Sun City, Arizona: The Brain and Body Donation Program is supported by the National Institute of Neurological Disorders and Stroke (U24 NS072026 National Brain and Tissue Resource for Parkinson's Disease and Related Disorders), the National Institute on Aging (P30 AG19610 Arizona Alzheimer's Disease Core Center), the Arizona Department of Health Services (contract 211002, Arizona Alzheimer's Research Center), the Arizona Biomedical Research Commission (contracts 4001, 0011, 05-901, and 1001 to the Arizona Parkinson's Disease Consortium), and the Michael J. Fox Foundation for Parkinson's Research. The funding body did not play any role in the design of the study and collection, analysis or interpretation of data and in writing the manuscript.

Authors' contributions

YR, YWA and RR designed the study. YR and RR wrote the manuscript. YR and MVB performed data analysis. MA, MMC, JR, XW and NET provided intellectual input, reviewed and edited the manuscript. DWD and TGB provided tissue samples and associated data. All authors read and approved the final manuscript.

Competing interests

The authors declare that they have no competing interests.

Author details

[1]Department of Health Sciences Research, Mayo Clinic, Jacksonville, FL, USA. [2]Department of Neuroscience, Mayo Clinic, Jacksonville, FL, USA. [3]Civin Laboratory for Neuropathology, Banner Sun Health Research Institute, Sun City, AZ, USA. [4]Department of Neurology, Mayo Clinic, Jacksonville, FL, USA.

References

1. Avila J. Common mechanisms in neurodegeneration. Nat Med. 2010;16: 1372.
2. Van Deerlin VM, Sleiman PMA, Martinez-Lage M, Chen-Plotkin A, Wang LS, Graff-Radford NR, et al. Common variants at 7p21 are associated with frontotemporal lobar degeneration with TDP-43 inclusions. Nat Genet. 2010; 42:234–9.
3. Finch N, Carrasquillo MM, Baker M, Rutherford NJ, Coppola G, DeJesus-Hernandez M, et al. TMEM106B regulates progranulin levels and the penetrance of FTLD in GRN mutation carriers. Neurology. 2011;76:467.
4. Nicholson AM, Rademakers R. What we know about TMEM106B in neurodegeneration. Acta Neuropathol. 2016;132:639–51.
5. Cruchaga C, Graff C, Chiang HH, Wang J, Hinrichs AL, Spiegel N, et al. Association of tmem106b gene polymorphism with age at onset in granulin mutation carriers and plasma granulin protein levels. Arch Neurol. 2011;68:581–6.
6. Gallagher MD, Suh E, Grossman M, Elman L, McCluskey L, Van Swieten JC, et al. TMEM106B is a genetic modifier of frontotemporal lobar degeneration with C9orf72 hexanucleotide repeat expansions. Acta Neuropathol. 2014; 127:407–18.
7. van Blitterswijk M, Mullen B, Nicholson AM, Bieniek KF, Heckman MG, Baker MC, et al. TMEM106B protects C9ORF72 expansion carriers against frontotemporal dementia. Acta Neuropathol. 2014;127:397–406.
8. Murray ME, Cannon A, Graff-Radford NR, Liesinger AM, Rutherford NJ, Ross OA, et al. Differential clinicopathologic and genetic features of late-onset amnestic dementias. Acta Neuropathol. 2014;128:411–21.
9. Nelson PT, Wang WX, Partch AB, Monsell SE, Valladares O, Ellingson SR, et al. Reassessment of risk genotypes (GRN, TMEM106B, and ABCC9 variants) associated with hippocampal sclerosis of aging pathology. J Neuropathol Exp Neurol. 2015;74:75–84.
10. Vass R, Ashbridge E, Geser F, Hu WT, Grossman M, Clay-Falcone D, et al. Risk genotypes at TMEM106B are associated with cognitive impairment in amyotrophic lateral sclerosis. Acta Neuropathol. 2011;121: 373–80.
11. Rutherford NJ, Carrasquillo MM, Li M, Bisceglio G, Menke J, Josephs KA, et al. TMEM106B risk variant is implicated in the pathologic presentation of Alzheimer disease. Neurology. 2012;79:717–8.
12. Yu L, De Jager PL, Yang J, Trojanowski JQ, Bennett DA, Schneider JA. The TMEM106B locus and TDP-43 pathology in older persons without FTLD. Neurology. 2015;84:927.
13. Nicholson AM, Finch NA, Wojtas A, Baker MC, Perkerson RB, Castanedes-Casey M, et al. TMEM106B p.T185S regulates TMEM106B protein levels: implications for frontotemporal dementia. J Neurochem. 2013;126:781–91.
14. Gallagher MD, Posavi M, Huang P, Unger TL, Berlyand Y, Gruenewald AL, et al. A dementia-associated risk variant near TMEM106B alters chromatin architecture and gene expression. Am J Hum Genet. 2017;101:643–63.
15. Dickson DW, Crystal HA, Mattiace LA, Masur DM, Blau AD, Davies P, et al. Identification of normal and pathological aging in prospectively studied nondemented elderly humans. Neurobiol Aging. 1992;13:179–89.
16. Allen M, Carrasquillo MM, Funk C, Heavner BD, Zou F, Younkin CS, et al. Human whole genome genotype and transcriptome data for Alzheimer's and other neurodegenerative diseases. Scientific Data. 2016;3:160089.
17. Allen M, Wang X, Burgess JD, Watzlawik J, Serie DJ, Younkin CS, et al. Conserved brain myelination networks are altered in Alzheimer's and other neurodegenerative diseases. Alzheimers Dement. 2018;14:352–66.
18. Langfelder P, Horvath S. WGCNA: an R package for weighted correlation network analysis. BMC Bioinformatics. 2008;9:559.
19. Hu Z, Chang YC, Wang Y, Huang CL, Liu Y, Tian F, et al. VisANT 4.0: integrative network platform to connect genes, drugs, diseases and therapies. Nucleic Acids Res. 2013;41:W225–31.
20. Lui H, Zhang J, Makinson SR, Cahill MK, Kelley KW, Huang HY, et al. Progranulin deficiency promotes circuit-specific synaptic pruning by microglia via complement activation. Cell. 2016;165:921–35.
21. Adams HHH, Verhaaren BF, Vrooman HA, Uitterlinden AG, Hofman A, van Duijn CM, et al. TMEM106B influences volume of left-sided temporal lobe and interhemispheric structures in the general population. Biol Psychiatry. 2014;76:503–8.
22. Premi E, Formenti A, Gazzina S, Archetti S, Gasparotti R, Padovani A, et al. Effect of TMEM106B polymorphism on functional network connectivity in asymptomatic GRN mutation carriers. JAMA Neurology. 2014;71:216–21.

11

Endoplasmic reticulum stress and inflammation in the central nervous system

Neil T. Sprenkle[1], Savannah G. Sims[1], Cristina L. Sánchez[1] and Gordon P. Meares[1,2*]

Abstract

Persistent endoplasmic reticulum (ER) stress is thought to drive the pathology of many chronic disorders due to its potential to elicit aberrant inflammatory signaling and facilitate cell death. In neurodegenerative diseases, the accumulation of misfolded proteins and concomitant induction of ER stress in neurons contributes to neuronal dysfunction. In addition, ER stress responses induced in the surrounding neuroglia may promote disease progression by coordinating damaging inflammatory responses, which help fuel a neurotoxic milieu. Nevertheless, there still remains a gap in knowledge regarding the cell-specific mechanisms by which ER stress mediates neuroinflammation. In this review, we will discuss recently uncovered inflammatory pathways linked to the ER stress response. Moreover, we will summarize the present literature delineating how ER stress is generated in Alzheimer's disease, Parkinson's disease, Amyotrophic Lateral Sclerosis, and Multiple Sclerosis, and highlight how ER stress and neuroinflammation intersect mechanistically within the central nervous system. The mechanisms by which stress-induced inflammation contributes to the pathogenesis and progression of neurodegenerative diseases remain poorly understood. Further examination of this interplay could present unappreciated insights into the development of neurodegenerative diseases, and reveal new therapeutic targets.

Keywords: Endoplasmic reticulum stress, Unfolded protein response, Neuroinflammation, Neurodegeneration

Background

Innate immune activation has emerged as a prominent component in the pathology of many neurodegenerative diseases. Previously, the involvement of immunity in the pathogenesis of neurological disorders had been greatly underappreciated. However, within the last couple decades we have come to realize that an aberrant inflammatory program within the central nervous system (CNS) contributes to neuronal dysfunction [1]. While inflammation is considered a beneficial physiological response, as it promotes debris clearance and aids in tissue repair, sustained inflammatory signaling overwhelms the resolution capabilities of the CNS [2]. This, in turn, is thought to be fundamental to the development of harmful neuroinflammation. Brain-resident microglia and astrocytes are the main source of inflammation in the brain, and under pathological conditions these dysregulated glial cells facilitate the events that promote a neurotoxic microenvironment [3, 4]. Considering that neurons have a limited regenerative capacity, excessive neuronal loss in the CNS has dire consequences on motor and cognitive function. A wealth of data now supports the hypothesis that inflammation in the CNS may contribute to neurodegeneration by establishing a feed-forward inflammatory loop which ultimately leads to sustained neuronal damage [1, 2, 5, 6]. Importantly, this likely reflects impairment of the normal mechanisms involved in immune responses in the brain as inflammation, glial activation and even peripheral immune infiltration are essential elements of normal tissue homeostasis and repair [7, 8].

One of the pathological hallmarks of many neurodegenerative diseases is the accumulation of misfolded proteins within the ER of neurons and neuroglia. In response to ER stress, cells induce a highly conserved cellular stress response called the unfolded protein response (UPR) in an attempt to maintain homeostasis [9]. The UPR program orchestrates transcriptional and translational changes in the cell to minimize stress, while

* Correspondence: gpmeares@hsc.wvu.edu
[1]Department of Microbiology, Immunology and Cell Biology, West Virginia University School of Medicine, One Medical Center Drive, BMRC, Morgantown, WV 311, USA
[2]Blanchette Rockefeller Neurosciences Institute, West Virginia University School of Medicine, Morgantown, WV, USA

concomitantly inducing protein quality control mechanisms in an attempt to reduce protein misfolding. If resolution fails, the temporally-regulated induction of UPR-dependent inflammatory and apoptotic pathways has the potential to exacerbate neuroinflammation and compromise cell fidelity [10–13].

Accumulating evidence suggests that cells under severe ER stress caused by various insults interfere with the immunosuppressive environment of the CNS [10, 11, 14]. These findings imply a heterogeneous cause linking ER stress in neurons, microglia and astrocytes with inflammation in the progression of neurodegeneration. Novel intracellular processes involved in this integrative cellular response continue to emerge. Here, we will introduce recently discovered signaling pathways associated with the UPR and present current findings regarding how chronic ER stress engenders neurological abnormalities. Furthermore, we will discuss how a UPR-induced inflammatory phenotype in CNS-resident cells could promote conditions responsible for impairing neuronal function.

The physiological role of the UPR

The majority of proteins destined for the secretory pathway present a hydrophobic N-terminal signal sequence during the initial stages of translation [15, 16]. This amino acid sequence is recognized by the cytosolic protein signal-recognition particle, which coordinates cotranslational translocation of the nascent polypeptide across the ER membrane and into the ER lumen [17, 18]. Here, the unique environment of the ER lumen facilitates the proper folding events that create a stable protein with functional capabilities.

The ER serves as the cell's largest calcium store owing to the consistent active transport of calcium into the lumen [19]. Intraluminal ER calcium is necessary for the activation of calcium-dependent molecular chaperones, including the ER resident glucose-regulated proteins (GRPs), which go on to stabilize protein folding intermediates [20]. Furthermore, the ER lumen possesses an oxidative environment which allow protein disulphide isomerases (PDIs) to catalyze the formation of disulfide bonds. Reduced PDIs are reoxidized by endoplasmic reticulum oxidoreductase α (Ero1α) to allow for continuous oxidation of free cysteine residues residing on unfolded proteins [21]. Additional post-translational modifications, such as glycosylation, are executed within the ER to produce a mature protein that is packaged into coat protein complex II-coated vesicles and exported out of the ER [22, 23]. ER-derived vesicles then enter the canonical secretory pathway where cargo is either targeted to the plasma membrane or to other cellular compartments.

Features of pathophysiological stress in the form of gene mutations, protein aggregates, inflammatory signals, metabolic alterations, pathogen-associated molecular patterns (PAMPs), danger-associated molecular pattern molecules (DAMPs) and/or reactive oxygen or nitrogen species (ROS/RNS) disrupts efficient protein folding processes in the ER lumen, thus creating an imbalance between the protein load and the folding capabilities of the ER [24]. The UPR responds to cellular stress by triggering effector mechanisms that can be grouped as adaptive, alarming or pro-apoptotic [20]. In the adaptive phase of the UPR, mammalian cells are able to tolerate moderate protein misfolding by upregulating the expression of chaperone proteins to correctly fold and stabilize the increasing amount of polypeptide transported into the ER lumen. In an effort to maintain quality control, the cell also employs ER-associated degradation (ERAD) and attenuates translation of global messenger RNA (mRNA) to alleviate the protein load within the lumen [25, 26]. In more severe situations, the protein folding capacity of the ER fails to keep pace with the increasing influx of polypeptide, as the extensive accumulation of misfolded proteins in the ER lumen begins to overwhelm the compensatory mechanisms of the UPR. If improperly regulated, the buildup of misfolded proteins will compromise normal cellular processes. Under these conditions, the cell initiates signaling pathways associated with cellular stress, most notably the activation of inflammatory pathways, and 'alarms' the extracellular environment of the distress so that the appropriate tissue-wide response is initiated [20]. If all else fails the UPR will trigger cell death through both caspase-dependent and -independent means [27–29].

Signal transducers of the ER stress response

In mammalian cells, the central proteins involved in initiating this evolutionarily conserved response are activating transcription factor 6 (ATF6), inositol-requiring 1α (IRE-1α) and double-stranded RNA dependent protein kinase-like ER kinase (PERK) [24]. GRP78 (also known as binding immunoglobulin protein (BiP)) primarily regulates the initiation of the UPR through its direct interactions with each signal transducing sensor [30–32] (Fig. 1). Physical contact between GRP78 and the luminal domain of the ER-transmembrane proteins stabilizes their inactive state. High demand for chaperone-mediated protein stabilization brought on by increases in protein synthesis or defective protein folding recruits GRP78 away from these proteins [31]. Disrupting this interaction frees the luminal domain of the ER sensors, consequently inducing their functional conformation. Recent evidence has suggested an additional regulatory mechanism by which the sensors become catalytically active. By crystallizing the yeast IRE-1, Credle et al. elucidated a distinct peptide-binding groove in the IRE-1 luminal domain [33, 34]. In this model, unfolded

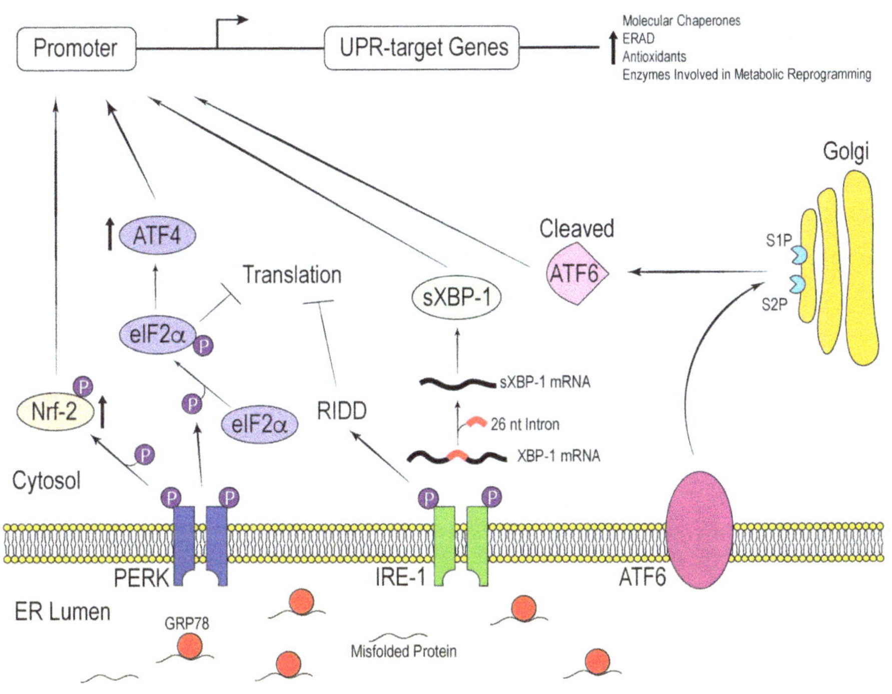

Fig. 1 The Adaptive Signals of the Mammalian UPR. The activation of PERK, IRE-1α and ATF6 in response to protein misfolding stress primarily requires the dissociation of the molecular chaperone GRP78 from each of the ER stress sensors. This initiates signaling cascades which orchestrate the transcriptional and translational landscape of the cell in an effort to maintain homeostasis

polypeptide within the ER lumen may act as a substrate for the peptide-binding groove located in IRE-1. Because of the shared structural homology with that of IRE-1, PERK may also be activated in a similar manner [33]. These findings represent a unique sensing mechanism that regulates the activation of the UPR.

Interplay between active ATF6, IRE-1α and PERK initiate signaling cascades that regulate the transcriptional and translational landscape of the cell to selectively promote the expression UPR-target genes. Each of these mediators promote distinct signaling pathways which converge to produce an effective response to mitigate damage. If overwhelmed, these signaling proteins will initiate apoptosis [35] (Fig. 2).

Mammalian ATF6 is a type II transmembrane protein embedded within the ER membrane [36]. The carboxyl terminus of ATF6 acts as the intraluminal sensor while the amino terminus protrudes into the cytosol and functions as a basic leucine zipper (bZIP) transcription factor [37]. Dissociation of GRP78 from the luminal domain causes ATF6 to translocate to the Golgi apparatus. Located at the Golgi are site-1 and site-2 proteases, both of which have been implicated in the regulation of cholesterol metabolism [38]. It is here that ATF6 is cleaved, resulting in the release of the bZIP transcription factor into the cytosol [36]. From the cytosol, the processed ATF6 fragment localizes into the nucleus and helps upregulate the expression of genes responsible for mediating protein folding and ERAD [36, 39].

IRE-1α is a type 1 transmembrane protein containing an ER-sensing amino terminus, and a cytosolic carboxyl terminal endoribonuclease (RNase) and serine-threonine kinase domain [31, 40, 41]. Detection of unfolded proteins causes IRE-1α to dimerize and/or form higher order oligomers, which in turn activates its kinase domain. Subsequent trans and autophosphorylation stimulates the RNase activity of IRE-1α [42]. Acquisition of RNase catalytic activity enables for the excision of a 26-nucleotide intron within a mature X-box-binding protein 1 (XBP1) mRNA transcript in the cytosol [43]. The spliced XBP1 (sXBP1) mRNA encodes for an XBP1 isoform which, like ATF6, binds upstream cis-elements associated with chaperone and ERAD-mediated genes [39, 44]. Sustained ER stress augments the RNase activity of IRE-1α, thereby causing decreased specificity for XBP1 mRNA and elevated degradation of specific classes of mRNAs, 28S ribosomal RNA and microRNAs through regulated IRE1-dependent decay (RIDD) [45]. The degradation of RNA transcripts destined for the ER and ribosomal RNA is thought to initially help diminish mRNA translation to alleviate the protein load on the ER [46]. Nevertheless, prolonged RIDD activity resulting

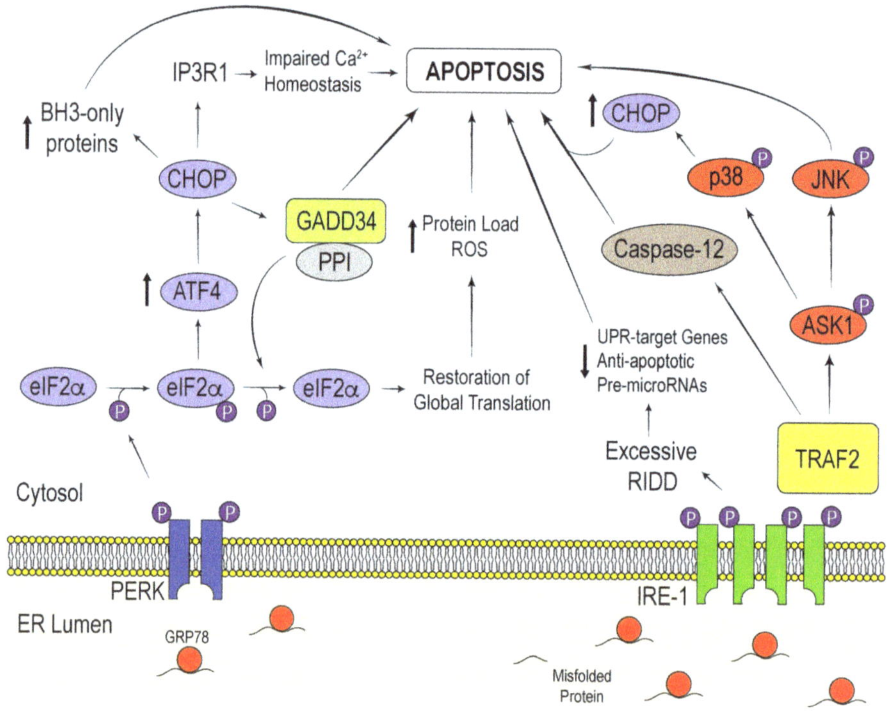

Fig. 2 Apoptotic Signals Associated with Chronic UPR Activation. Persistent ER stress triggers the apoptotic component of the UPR. PERK and IRE-1α drive UPR-induced apoptosis by initiating pathways which facilitate enhanced ROS production, Ca^{2+} dysregulation and caspase activation

from chronic ER stress contributes to cell death by degrading ER-targeted mRNA that encode proteins involved in protein folding and anti-apoptotic micro-RNA, thus pushing cell fate toward apoptosis [47–49].

Lastly, PERK possesses type 1 transmembrane topology and a cytosolic kinase domain [31]. Structural analysis has revealed that the sensing luminal domain of PERK shares a conserved protein sequence with that of IRE-1α [26]. Unsurprisingly, both PERK and IRE-1α respond to ER stress in a similar manner. Along with IRE-1α, PERK indirectly reduces the quantity of unfolded polypeptide within the ER to allow for more efficient chaperone-mediated protein folding in a well-saturated ER lumen. The dimerization of PERK leads to the activation of its cytosolic kinases, which subsequently phosphorylate serine 51 on the α-subunit of eukaryotic initiation factor 2α (eIF2α) [26]. Phosphorylation of eIF2α prevents the translation of many nuclear-encoded mRNA transcripts by compromising the formation of the GTP·eIF2α·Met-$tRNA_i$ ternary complex, which in turn prevents the assembly of the pre-initiation complex at the 5′ end of mRNA [50, 51]. Delaying translation re-initiation in this manner increases the probability that ribosomes will scan past inhibitory upstream open reading frames, resulting in increased translation of a specific subset of mRNAs, most notably mRNA that encodes ATF4 [50, 52]. Like ATF6, ATF4 is a bZIP transcription factor important for maintaining intracellular homeostasis through the upregulation of UPR-target genes involved in efficient protein folding, the antioxidant response and amino acid biosynthesis and transport [53]. In addition to promoting an adaptive response, ATF4 regulates the transcription of the gene encoding pro-apoptotic factor CCAAT-enhancer-binding protein homologous protein (CHOP) [54].

While the role of CHOP in stress-induced apoptosis remains obscure, it is thought that CHOP promotes apoptosis by 1) downregulating the expression of Bcl-2, a pro-survival proto-oncogene, 2) elevating the expression of pro-apoptotic BH3-only Bcl-2 family proteins such as Bad, Bim and p53 upregulated modulator of apoptosis and 3) coordinating intracellular calcium signaling [54, 55]. The latter relies on the involvement of the ER. In addition to its role in mediating stable protein folding, the ER serves an important function in cell signaling due to its ability to release calcium in response to second messengers. During unremitting PERK activation, CHOP accumulates to a point necessary to activate Ero1α, which drives the aperture of the ER calcium release channel inositol 1, 4, 5-triphosphate (IP3) receptor 1 [56, 57]. Prolonged efflux of calcium from the ER promotes the activation of calcium/calmodulin-dependent protein kinase II, which plays a role in promoting cell death [57]. Moreover, free cytosolic calcium leaks into the mitochondrial matrix, causing mitochondrial depolarization [58]. Mitochondrial uptake of calcium released from the ER also elevates the production of ROS through various mechanisms, including activating the mitochondrial permeability transition and stimulating Krebs cycle dehydrogenases [53, 58, 59]. Besides facilitating calcium release, Ero1α contributes to the production of hydrogen peroxide within the ER lumen [60].

Along with targeting Bcl-2 family genes and Ero1α, CHOP binds to promoter elements associated with growth arrest and DNA damage-inducible protein 34 (GADD34). The induction of GADD34 is imperative for attenuating signals downstream of the PERK-eIF2α-ATF4 pathway. This GADD34-dependent negative feedback loop relies on GADD34 recruiting protein phosphatase 1 (PP1) to dephosphorylate eIF2α. Mutating the conserved motifs important for binding PP1 in GADD34 impairs eIF2α dephosphorylation, thus supporting its regulatory role in mediating the phosphorylation state of eIF2α [61]. Moreover, knocking out CHOP diminishes GADD34 protein expression, leading to elevated levels of phosphorylated eIF2α when compared to wild-type (WT) cells experiencing ER stress [62]. Although GADD34-mediated dephosphorylation of eIF2α is essential for cells to restore global mRNA translation after acute insult, the overexpression of GADD34 increases the translation of mRNA transcripts induced during the later stages of prolonged ER stress, thereby elevating the protein load and restoring global translation of proteins involved in ROS production and apoptosis [63]. Additionally, GADD34 may have pro-apoptotic effects that are independent of its role in regulating eIF2α phosphorylation that contribute to ER stress-induced cell death [62, 64].

Another downstream effector of active PERK is the bZIP transcription factor nuclear factor-like 2 (Nrf-2), which is important for the expression of antioxidants [65]. Nrf-2 is normally sequestered within the cytosol by kelch-like ECH-associated protein 1 (Keap1) under basal states, however, the initiation of the UPR allows PERK to act on the Nrf-2-Keap1 complex. PERK-mediated phosphorylation of Nrf-2 promotes its dissociation from Keap1 and translocation into the nucleus where it upregulates the expression of genes essential for redox homeostasis. Cullinan et al. demonstrated that deleting Nrf-2 compromises the ability of mouse embryonic fibroblasts (MEFs) to cope with ER stress, as cells without Nrf-2 were more susceptible to undergoing ER stress-induced apoptosis compared to WT MEFs treated with tunicamycin, a pharmacological ER stress-inducing agent that blocks N-linked glycosylation [66]. The same study also provided evidence showing that PERK phosphorylation was sufficient to disrupt the Nrf-2-Keap1 complex, thereby allowing Nrf-2 to function as a transcription factor independent of the presence of ROS/RNS.

During the UPR, PERK and ATF6 signaling have been shown to upregulate the expression of sXBP1 mRNA (through different mechanisms) to produce an operative transcription factor responsible for inducing the expression of stress-response genes [67, 68]. Furthermore, there is evidence that the transcription of CHOP is also under the control of the active ATF6 transcription factor [69]. This demonstrates that not only do the ER sensors elicit independent signaling cascades in the face of ER stress, but there is cross-talk between the different UPR pathways in an effort to provide a robust response to physiological stress. In addition to ATF6 and IRE-1α regulating the transcription of chaperone proteins and enzymes mediating ERAD, both have also been implicated in the biosynthesis of ER phospholipids, which are used to expand the ER membrane, and in the regulation of other aspects of cellular metabolism [70, 71]. Interestingly, components of the UPR play an essential role in learning, memory and behavior. The eIF2α kinases, including PERK, regulate memory and synaptic plasticity by modulating gene expression and translation [72]. Moreover, a recent study demonstrated an important role for XBP1 in facilitating memory and long-term potentiation through the regulation of brain-derived neurotrophic factor expression [73]. The involvement of the UPR in optimizing the protein folding capacity of the ER as well as modulating cellular metabolism and cognitive function highlights the pleiotropic actions of the ER stress response in maintaining tissue and organismal homeostasis.

UPR-mediated inflammatory pathways

In addition to coordinating the expression of stress-response genes during ER stress, the UPR initiates inflammatory pathways essential for the innate immune response (Fig. 3). The principal inflammatory signaling proteins activated during the UPR are the nuclear factor kappa-light-chain-enhancer of activated B cells (NF-κB) and the mitogen activated protein kinase (MAPK) family proteins c-Jun N-terminal kinase (JNK) and p38. It is important to note that NF-κB and the MAPKs regulate not only inflammatory gene expression, but they also play a role in mediating cell survival in a context-specific manner [74].

The NF-κB family of proteins are made up of homo- and heterodimeric transcription factors composed of proteins in the NF-κB/Rel family [75]. In unstressed cells, NF-κB is sequestered within the cytosol through physical interaction with inhibitors of κB (IκB). Signaling through the canonical NF-κB pathway activates the serine kinase IκB kinase (IKK), which is composed of two catalytic subunits (IKKα and IKKβ) and a regulatory subunit (IKKγ). Site-specific phosphorylation of IκB by IKK signals for its degradation through the ubiquitin-dependent recruitment of the 26S proteasome [76].

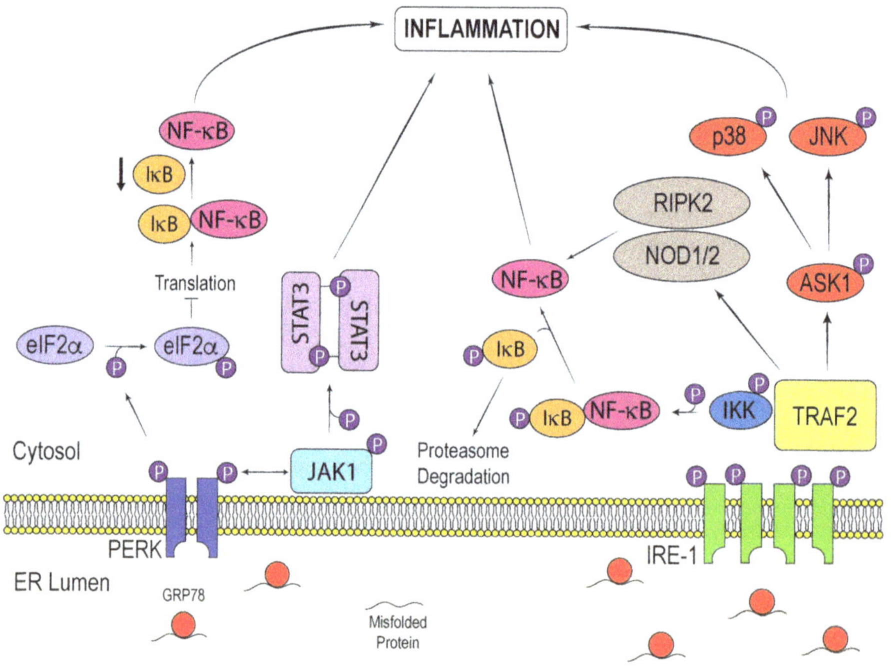

Fig. 3 Inflammatory Pathways Induced by the UPR. The UPR stimulates various inflammatory pathways to alert surrounding cells of potential danger. The transient interaction between impaired proteostasis and inflammation is considered a beneficial feature of the UPR. Nevertheless, sustained UPR-induced inflammation is considered a pathological factor in many chronic disorders, such as neurodegenerative diseases. Inflammatory pathways associated with the UPR include the NF-κB, JAK1/STAT3, NOD1/2-RIPK2, JNK and p38 signaling pathways

Subsequently, free NF-κB is able to localize to the nucleus and bind to κB sites in gene promoters, and drive the expression of cytokines and cell survival proteins. NF-κB can be activated by various forms of cell stress. For example, in addition to ER stress, elevated levels of cytosolic calcium and oxidative stress have been shown to promote NF-κB-mediated transcription [77, 78]. In the context of ER stress, the attenuation of global mRNA translation in response to eIF2α phosphorylation provides a means by which NF-κB is stimulated. Depressing mRNA translation decreases protein levels of IκB and NF-κB within the cytosol [79]. Because IκB has a shorter half-life than NF-κB, the higher proportion of NF-κB to IκB favors the migration of free NF-κB into the nucleus to upregulate the transcription of inflammatory genes.

Along with PERK, IRE-1α elicits inflammatory signaling during the ER stress response. After oligomerization, IRE-1α recruits the adaptor protein tumor-necrosis factor-α (TNF-α)-receptor-associated factor 2 (TRAF2), which couples the activation of IRE-1α with different inflammatory pathways. The formation of the IRE-1α-TRAF2 complex mediates cross-talk between active IRE-1α and the NF-κB and MAPK signaling pathways. TRAF2 directly interacts with IKK and indirectly with JNK by activating apoptosis signal-regulating kinase 1 (ASK1), which then coordinates the activation of JNK [20, 80, 81]. IRE-1α-mediated activation of IKK leads to the phosphorylation of IκB to promote NF-κB-dependent transcriptional regulation, while the IRE-1α-dependent activation of JNK stimulates the bZIP transcription factor activator protein 1 (AP-1). Thereafter, AP-1, a heterodimer composed of a differential combination of Fos, Jun, ATF and Maf sub-family members, binds to enhancer elements which upregulate the transcription of inflammatory genes [82].

Interestingly, the IRE-1α-TRAF2 axis has been shown to stimulate the nucleotide-binding oligomerization domain 1 and 2 (NOD1/2)-receptor-interacting serine/threonine-protein kinase 2 (RIPK2) pathway, resulting in the activation of NF-κB [83]. This proposed mechanism was supported in an in vivo murine model of *Brucella abortus* infection. *Brucella abortus* induces ER stress by injecting host cells with the VceC virulence factor via its type IV secretion system. Here, Keestra-Gounder et al. demonstrated that the resulting ER stress-induced production of interleukin (IL)-6 in infected mice was dependent on TRAF2, NOD1/2 and RIPK2 interplay. These findings provided further evidence of dynamic interactions between innate immunity and UPR-induced inflammation.

In conjunction with its involvement in initiating inflammation, IRE-1α can facilitate cell death through its interactions with the apoptotic proteins during ER stress [84]. IRE-1α-dependent activation of caspase-12 has been reported to be a dispensable contributor in the execution of ER stress-induced apoptosis in mice and rats [85–87]. Nevertheless, many human variants of caspase-12 possess loss-of-function mutations that promote the synthesis of a truncated protein without functional activity, and thus may not be a significant contributor to ER stress-induced cell death in humans [87]. The IRE-1α-TRAF2-JNK pathway coordinates cell death by facilitating Bax-dependent apoptosis and inhibiting the pro-apoptotic protein Bcl-2, while the IRE-1α-TRAF2-p38 branch may enhance CHOP transcriptional activity [20, 88, 89]. This understanding highlights the importance of TRAF2 in linking the UPR to a diverse range of signaling pathways to trigger the appropriate physiological response.

Recently, the interaction between PERK and Janus kinase 1 (JAK1) in the UPR was elucidated in astrocytes. It has been recognized that ER stress influences the JAK-signal transducers and activators of transcription (STAT) pathway [90, 91], however, the molecular mechanisms underlying its involvement in the context of neurodegeneration and how it alters the JAK-STAT pathway in glial cells remained to be clarified. We observed that JAK1-STAT3 signaling in ER stressed astrocytes was dependent on PERK [92]. Transfecting astrocytes with PERK small interfering RNA, followed by treatment with thapsigargin, a non-competitive inhibitor of the sarco/endoplasmic reticulum Ca^{2+} ATPase used to induce ER stress, attenuated JAK1 and STAT3 phosphorylation. Additionally, PERK knockout MEFs incubated with thapsigargin expressed significantly less phosphorylated STAT3 and STAT3-dependent inflammatory cytokines and chemokines relative to their WT counterparts. Mass spectrometry revealed that JAK1 phosphorylates PERK at tyrosine 585 and 619 in vitro. While further investigation is needed to completely unravel how STAT3 is phosphorylated by the PERK/JAK1 complex, these findings present a novel pathway implicating the UPR in driving neuroinflammation.

Each of the three ER stress sensors serves a multifunctional role in maintaining ER protein homeostasis under transient ER stress. If the cell is unable to ameliorate intrinsic protein misfolding stress, the cell will induce apoptotic pathways to avoid continuously secreting distress signals to neighboring cells. The category of stimuli or environmental conditions may be an important determinant regarding whether the cell will trigger a coordinated cell death. One must also consider that certain cell types, such as highly secretory cells, must constantly maintain an optimal ER protein folding environment, making them more susceptible to ER stress.

Chronic ER stress leads to the disproportionate activation of the ATF6, IRE-1α and PERK pathways to amplify the apoptotic component of the UPR [93]. Some experimental models respond to severe ER stress by attenuating ATF6 and IRE-1α signaling and augmenting PERK activation to allow apoptotic signals to dominate [93]. Because CHOP possesses a short half-life, chronic PERK activation is required to overwhelm the adaptive signals of the UPR to promote cell death [94, 95]. Similarly, sustained IRE-1α signaling has the potential to initiate apoptosis in other situations. While various pharmacological approaches have provided invaluable insights into the physiologic role of the UPR, more work must be done to fully appreciate how each of the branches of the UPR respond to specific stimuli and how they integrate to mediate apoptotic events.

ER stress in neurodegenerative diseases

The activation of the UPR plays an essential role in maintaining vital biological processes within the brain during cellular stress. In fact, moderate ER stress enhances cellular protection against subsequent insult by altering the transcriptome and proteome of the cell to increase the adaptive capacity of the ER, a response called the hormetic response [9, 96–99]. However, prolonged ER stress developed in neurodegenerative diseases is believed to disrupt the protective mechanisms of the UPR, leading to the activation of inflammatory and apoptotic programs that promote neurotoxicity. In the following sections we will briefly describe the mechanisms underlying how ER stress is generated in neurodegenerative diseases, such as Alzheimer's disease (AD), Parkinson's disease (PD), Amyotrophic Lateral Sclerosis (ALS) and Multiple Sclerosis (MS), then address its potential contribution to the development of pathological neuroinflammation. In general, ER stress is a consequence of disturbances in protein-quality control machinery, ER Ca^{2+} dysregulation, protein-trafficking impairment or direct defects in UPR components [9].

Alzheimer's disease

AD is a common age-dependent neurodegenerative disease that accounts for a significant number of reported dementia cases [100]. The pathology of AD is characterized by the formation of intracellular neurofibrillary tangles (NFTs) composed of hyperphosphorylated tau and the extracellular parenchymal deposition of amyloid-β (Aβ) aggregates [101, 102]. The cytoplasmic protein tau normally serves to stabilize microtubules which form 'tracks' that facilitate intracellular vesicle trafficking and axonal elongation and maturation. This is highlighted by the finding that knocking down tau leads to severe neurite growth defects in primary cerebellar neurons [103]. However, certain insults cause an imbalance between the activities of tau kinases and phosphatases that lead to the abnormal phosphorylation of tau [104]. In its hyperphosphorylated state, tau becomes soluble and, in turn, polymerizes to form oligomers and/or NFTs [105]. In the case for Aβ pathology, genetic studies have implicated mutations in Aβ precursor protein (APP) and in the transmembrane proteins presenilin-1 (PS1) and presenilin-2 (PS2), which act as subunits for the γ-secretase complex, as the predominant genetic factors contributing to the onset of familial AD [106, 107]. Potentially pathological Aβ is liberated when APP is sequentially cleaved at the plasma membrane by β-secretase, then γ-secretase. [101]. This leads to an extracellular accumulation of either total Aβ or increase relative concentrations of amyloidogenic Aβ, such as Aβ42. Impaired clearance of Aβ has also been implicated in AD, as it creates an imbalance of its turnover in the brain [108].

Chronic ER dysfunction is highly associated with the memory and cognitive manifestations commonly observed in different experimental models of AD [109, 110]. To this point, Ma et al. elucidated that selectively abating the expression of PERK in mice possessing AD-linked mutations in genes encoding APP and PS1 prevented the aberrant phosphorylation of eIF2α [111]. This, in turn, improved synaptic plasticity and spatial memory in AD mice, consistent with the requirement for active protein translation in memory consolidation [112]. Interestingly, sXBP1 overexpression ameliorates cognitive function in the 3× Tg AD mouse model [113]. The eIF2α kinases general control non-derepressible 2 (GCN2) [111] and double stranded RNA-dependent kinase (PKR) have also been implicated in memory impairment [110, 114]. Multiple studies have demonstrated that Aβ oligomers can activate PKR and induce ER stress by eliciting the TNF-α pathway [110, 115]. Additionally, Aβ may stimulate ER Ca^{2+} release through ryanodine receptors and IP3 receptors, which triggers ER stress, neuronal apoptosis and mitochondrial fragmentation [116–118]. Inhibition of both GCN2 and PKR through different mechanisms significantly improves cognitive function in murine AD models [111, 114]. These findings suggest that pathophysiological conditions, not just ER stress, which lead to sustained eIF2α phosphorylation have the potential to aggravate the cognitive abnormalities seen in AD.

Abnormal protein aggregates interfere with the normal processes involved in protein maintenance and trafficking in models of neurodegeneration. Regarding AD, soluble tau has been shown to cause pathological ER stress by targeting and impairing components involved in ERAD [119]. Paradoxically, pre-existing ER stress also promotes NFT formation. It is well known that Aβ oligomer-dependent ER stress responses can lead to the activation of different kinases, such as the serine/threonine kinase glycogen synthase kinase 3 (GSK-3) [120, 121]. This kinase (among others) is capable of subsequently phosphorylating specific epitopes on tau that contribute to the development of NFT [120, 121]. Therefore, ER stress and hyperphosphorylated tau could be induced by each other in a cycle to propagate AD pathology [122]. More recently, however, the correlation between NFT formation and AD severity had been scrutinized [123]. It seems now that soluble oligomers of tau and Aβ may be the primary neurotoxic agents that contribute to AD [123].

It has been suggested that familial AD-linked PS1 mutations suppress the activation of IRE-1α. This predisposes cells to become more susceptible to ER stress due, in part, to decreases in protein chaperone synthesis as a result of reduced UPR induction [124]. A study using SK-N-SH cells and fibroblasts expressing a PS1 mutant associated with familial AD demonstrated that mutant PS1 also disrupts PERK activation, potentially in a similar manner as IRE-1α, and delays nuclear accumulation of processed ATF6 in response to ER stress [125]. The aberrantly spliced isoform of PS2 (PS2V) is also linked to AD. Similar to the PS1 mutations, this isoform increases the vulnerability of the cell to ER stress [126]. Alternatively, the over-expression of PS1 and PS2 mutants in cells perturbs ER calcium homeostasis, implying another mechanism by which genetic mutations in the presenilin genes contribute to AD [127–129]. With this in mind, there is contradictory evidence indicating that neither ablation of PS1 or expression of familial AD-linked PS1 variants impairs the expression of GRP78 mRNA and the activation of IRE1-α [130]. Because of limited knowledge regarding how ER stress is generated during AD, more investigation is needed to fully appreciate how dysregulated UPR signaling contributes to the pathology of AD.

Parkinson's disease

PD is a chronic and progressive movement disorder characterized by the selective loss of dopaminergic neurons in the substantia nigra, and the presence of intraneuronal filamentous inclusion bodies called Lewy bodies. While the development of Lewy bodies is not a definitive causative factor, they are deemed to be a pathological hallmark of PD. A post-mortem study showed that the percentage of Lewy body-containing dopaminergic neurons positive for caspase-3 is significantly higher than the percentage of caspase-3–positive dopaminergic neurons without Lewy bodies, indicating that Lewy body-containing dopaminergic neurons are predisposed to undergo apoptosis [131]. A principal component of Lewy bodies in PD are the abnormal filaments of α-synuclein, which seem to form due to different genetic factors, such as the multiplication of the SCNA locus, or non-genetic factors, such as aberrant post-translational modifications [132–134].

Common mutations implicated in autosomal recessive PD reside within the *Parkin* gene, which encodes for an E3 ubiquitin ligase that is necessary for mitophagy [135, 136]. Studies using post-mortem brain samples and mouse models also suggest that Parkin can be inactivated by post-translational modifications, such as oxidation, nitrosylation and the addition of dopamine [135]. Disrupting the E3 ligase activity of Parkin or defects in PTEN-induced kinase 1, which recruits Parkin to the outer membrane of damaged mitochondria, is thought to play a critical role in the development of familial and sporadic PD, mainly through its failure to maintain mitochondrial fidelity [137]. Similarly, mutations within the gene that encodes leucine-rich repeat kinase 2 (LRRK2) have been shown to promote PD [138]. LRRK2 is a widely expressed protein important for regulating various biological processes. Mutant LRRK2 is highly associated with the onset of inherited and sporadic PD, and the resulting LRRK2-mediated toxicity may be dependent on its kinase activity [139]. Nevertheless, the mechanisms underlying its role in the pathogenesis of PD are still being unraveled.

The notion that prolonged ER stress contributes to PD pathology was first supported with the findings that neurons in toxin-induced models of PD highly expressed genes involved in the UPR [140]. It is now appreciated that α-synuclein-induced neurotoxicity may result from nitrosative stress, accumulation of ERAD substrates and/or defective vesicular trafficking, all of which can lead to ER stress [141]. To this point, under conditions of nitrosative stress, S-nitrosylation directly inactivates PDI [142]. This inactivation impairs proper protein folding and hinders PDI-mediated attenuation of neuronal cell death [142]. Moreover, the concomitant accumulation of toxic α-synuclein oligomers in the ER further exacerbates the severity of ER stress, leading to deleterious UPR signaling [134, 143]. Some findings indicate that α-synuclein-dependent ER stress is the result of blocking ER to Golgi vesicular trafficking, as preventing vesicle mobilization from the ER causes the accumulation of protein cargo within the ER lumen [144]. Targeting pathways associated with these abnormal phenotypes through pharmacological intervention in vitro has been shown to rescue neuronal loss observed in PD models [141].

Post-mortem analysis revealed that human PD patients exhibited greater phosphorylated PERK and eIF2α in neuromelanin containing dopaminergic neurons relative to control cases [145]. In the same study, phosphorylated PERK colocalized with α-synuclein within dopaminergic neurons derived from PD patients. PC12 cells possessing the A53T mutation in the α-synuclein gene, a point mutation that increases the tendency of α-synuclein to form amyloid-like fibrils, exhibit elevated levels of phosphorylated eIF2α, CHOP, GRP78 and active caspase-12 [146]. Treatment with the caspase inhibitor z-VAD or salubrinal, which prevents the de-phosphorylation of eIF2α, improved cell viability of A53T PC12 cells by attenuating apoptotic signaling [146]. Taken together, these findings suggest that pathological α-synuclein may exacerbate disease progression by promoting excessive or unmitigated ER stress responses.

Stress-induced Parkin expression serves as a protective mechanism elicited by the UPR [147, 148]. The use of chromatin immunoprecipitation led to the discovery that ATF4 regulates Parkin gene expression by binding to CREB/ATF sites in the *Parkin* promoter [148]. The resulting increase in Parkin protein protects against ER stress-induced cell death in neurons by preventing the toxic accumulation of Parkin substrates. Moreover, the protective function of Parkin could be partially explained with the discovery that Parkin promotes the production of sXBP-1, which upregulates the transcription of pro-survival genes [149]. Recent evidence indicates that Parkin controls the function of PS1 and PS2, suggesting a possible link between defective Parkin and the pathogenesis of both AD and PD [150]. LRRK2 also helps maintain neuronal integrity against induced Parkinsonism by alleviating the consequences of ER stress. Yuan et al. demonstrated that LRRK2 saves neuroblastoma cells and *C. elegans* dopaminergic neurons from 6-OHDA or α-synuclein toxicity [151]. They also demonstrated that loss of function mutations in LRRK2 compromises the expression of GRP78, resulting in the hyperactivation of p38 and elevated neuronal death. Collectively, impairment in these protective mechanisms in neurons provides an alternative disturbance that contributes to the progression of PD.

Amyotrophic lateral sclerosis

ALS is a progressive neurodegenerative disease characterized by the destruction of motor neurons, which leads to paralysis and poor patient prognosis [152]. Among cases of ALS, 10% are considered familial, while the remaining 90% of cases are sporadic [153]. A pathological hallmark of familial ALS is the formation of ubiquitinated cytoplasmic inclusions composed of misfolded superoxide dismutase-1 (SOD1) [154]. However, defects in the *SOD1* gene only account for 20% of familial ALS cases, and 2% of sporadic cases [155, 156]. An accrual of evidence now connects mutations in genes encoding chromosome 9 open reading frame 72 (C9orf72), transactive response DNA binding protein 43 (TDP43), and Fused in Sarcoma RNA-binding protein (FUS) (among others) to ALS pathology [155, 157–159]. In all, a large proportion of genetic alterations implicated in ALS promote disease onset and progression by either perturbing protein quality control mechanisms, RNA integrity or cytoskeletal dynamics [155]. As in other mutations associated with neurodegenerative diseases, ALS-associated mutations are expressed ubiquitously within the CNS (neurons and surrounding neuroglia), with strong evidence that both cell-autonomous and -nonautonomous mechanisms contribute to the progressive loss of motor neurons [155].

Mediators associated with the UPR are upregulated in the spinal cords of ALS patients and in mutant SOD1 transgenic mice [160–162]. For instance, CHOP is highly expressed in motor neurons, glial cells and spinal cords of mutant SOD1 transgenic mice [163]. A similar observation is seen in spinal cord samples of sporadic ALS patients [163]. ERAD impairment is considered a central mechanism by which mutant SOD1 induces ER stress in ALS. Here, mutant SOD1 protein has been shown to inhibit a specific component of the retro-translocation machinery involved in ERAD called Derlin-1 by directly interacting with its cytoplasmic C-terminus [164]. Failure to export misfolded substrates from the ER in NSC34 cells leads to their accumulation within the ER lumen, which promotes neuronal death by eliciting the IRE-1-TRAF2-ASK1 pathway [164].

Increased motor neuron loss and SOD1 aggregation is observed in SOD1^{G85R} PERK$^{+/-}$ mice compared to SOD1^{G85R} mice fully expressing PERK [165]. Interestingly, ATF4 deficiency in SOD1^{G85R} mice exacerbates SOD1 aggregation, but delays disease onset and reduces the expression of pro-apoptotic genes [166]. XBP1-null NSC34 motor neurons expressing mutant SOD1 are more apt to clear mutant SOD1 aggregates [167]. Moreover, silencing XBP1 in vivo provides protection against disease progression in mutant SOD1 mice [167]. Taken together, there is contradictory evidence regarding the protective effects of the UPR in experimental models of ALS, suggesting that the extent to which the UPR contributes to ALS is context-dependent.

PDI has been shown to be upregulated in SOD1^{G93A} ALS rats and mice [168]. Furthermore, post-mortem human brain samples exhibit greater PDI expression in comparison to controls, implying that PDI is induced in response to the abnormalities associated with ALS [169]. The protective role of PDI in ALS emanates from its ability to facilitate folding of misfolded assemblies, thereby reducing SOD1 aggregate-mediated toxicity [169]. As seen in PD, PDI expressed in spinal cords of ALS patients is highly S-nitrosylated [170]. Increased RNS production has been reported in ALS, and the resulting nitrosative stress may impair the function of PDI through this post-translational modification [171].

Aggregates composed of mutant TDP-43, FUS or C9orf72 also initiate the UPR program [172–174]. To this point, overexpressing ALS-associated mutant TDP-43 in Neuro2a neuroblastoma cells results in greater induction of CHOP, XBP1 and ATF6 [173]. Moreover, mutations in FUS contribute to the formation of cytoplasmic protein inclusions that trigger ER stress responses in NSC34 motor neurons, and are found to co-localize with PDI in post-mortem spinal cord samples from ALS patients [175, 176]. Lastly, a study expressing poly(GA) repeats in neuronal cultures, which model ALS-associated repeat expansions in the C9orf72 gene, contribute to neuronal death by inducing ER stress [172]. When treated with salubrinal or the chemical chaperone TUDCA, these neurons are rescued from ER stress-mediated cell death, indicating that mutations in the C9orf72 gene contribute to neurotoxicity by promoting ER dysfunction [172]. Overall, these findings highlight how pathological assemblies implicated in ALS contribute to motor neuron loss. Even with the present understanding that SOD1-linked mutations only account for a relatively small proportion of ALS cases, many studies investigating the relationship between ER stress and ALS largely utilize animal models expressing mutant SOD1. Therefore, it will be of importance to further elucidate the mechanisms by which ER stress is generated in other ALS models in order to fully grasp how ER stress aggravates ALS pathology.

Multiple sclerosis

MS is T lymphocyte-mediated autoimmune disease characterized by the spatiotemporal dissemination of white matter lesions within the CNS [177]. While the etiology of MS remains in question, it is thought to be initiated by autoreactive T lymphocytes that have breached the blood brain barrier (BBB) or the blood-cerebral spinal fluid-barrier and have mounted an autoimmune response directed toward self-CNS antigens [178]. Autoreactive B cells and innate immune cells, such as NK cells, have also been reported to localize to the CNS from the periphery during MS pathology [179]. In the early stages of MS, peripheral humoral and innate immune cells accumulate in the perivascular and ventricular spaces that separate the blood vessels from the adjacent brain tissue, reactivated by local antigen presenting cells and subsequently move into the brain parenchyma to promote severe neuroinflammation [180]. These reactive immune cells release a plethora of inflammatory mediators, including nitric oxide, ROS and inflammatory cytokines, which impair neuronal function and activates CNS-resident astrocytes and microglia. Together, the continuous secretion of soluble inflammatory mediators promotes the development of a neurotoxic microenvironment that facilitates demyelination, axonal degeneration and oligodendrocyte and neuronal death.

One explanation for the development of autoreactive T and B cells is that some viral antigens presented by major histocompatibility complex II in the periphery or the CNS share homology with that of myelin components. Effector lymphocytes that enter the perivascular space are reactivated by antigen presenting cells presenting myelin peptides that share sequence and structural similarities with foreign-peptides [181]. This phenomenon, molecular mimicry, is considered a potential mechanism by which pathogens break self-immunological tolerance and induce an autoimmune reaction. Pathogens sharing high degrees of peptide similarity with myelin-derived peptides include Human Herpes virus type 6 and Epstein Barr virus [182]. The inflammatory milieu brought about by infiltrating innate immune cells and reactive T lymphocytes in the initial stages of the disease promotes further T cell polarization to the T_H1 or T_H17 subsets to amplify neuronal damage. From a genetic standpoint, single polymorphisms within specific candidate genes increase the susceptibility of individuals to developing MS. Such candidate genes may include genes located within the human leukocyte antigen (HLA) locus and immunological non-HLA genes involved in central tolerance, cytokine production and homeostatic proliferation [177].

Real time qPCR analysis of CNS tissue from MS patients has revealed that the ER stress markers ATF4, GRP78 and CHOP are significantly upregulated in the white matter of MS patients relative to tissue from non-MS individuals [183]. In agreement with these findings, a study performing detailed semiquantitative immunohistochemical and molecular analysis on multiple CNS cell-types in active MS lesions found that GRP78 and CHOP were highly upregulated in astrocytes, microglia and oligodendrocytes [184]. The elevated expression of UPR markers in MS lesions points toward a possible link between impaired ER proteostasis and the development of active lesions.

There are multiple potential events hypothesized to induce ER stress during MS. Glutamate excitotoxicity is an important mechanism that contributes to autoimmune demyelination and lesion formation [185]. Glutamate induces the expression of GRP78, and GRP78 knockdown leads to a significant increase in excitotoxicity-induced apoptosis [186]. This suggests that glutamate excitotoxicity promotes neuronal death through an ER stress-dependent mechanism, and the upregulation of GRP78 helps neurons cope with the excessive amounts of glutamate. In accordance, GRP78 seems to be vital for maintaining cell survival during MS. Oligodendrocyte-selective heterozygous deletion of GRP78 in mice induced with experimental autoimmune encephalomyelitis (EAE), an experimental model used to mimic the symptoms of MS, aggravates disease severity and enhances oligodendrocyte death [187].

Hypoxia is another potential ER stress inducer that is characteristic in, though not restricted to, MS. Histological evidence points toward a similar hypoxic-type response in diseased tissue of MS patients, as the hypoxia-related antigen D-110 is strongly expressed in tissue also expressing high levels of CHOP [184]. Alternatively, expression of human endogenous retrovirus (HERV) envelop proteins may contribute to the pathology of MS by initiating neuroinflammatory and ER stress responses in the brain [12, 188]. For instance, the overexpression of the HERV envelope glycoprotein Syncytin-1 causes astrocytes to upregulate ER stress responses and the production of proinflammatory mediators that promote oligodendrocyte toxicity [12]. Finally, the inflammatory environment in the CNS could trigger ER stress in highly myelinating cells, such as oligodendrocytes. Due to their high demand for lipid synthesis, mature oligodendrocytes are more susceptible to ER stress when exposed to high levels of proinflammatory mediators. It was previously demonstrated that interferon (IFN)-γ drives ER stress and cell death in oligodendrocytes both in vitro and in vivo [189]. In this same study, mice that were haploinsufficient for PERK were more susceptible to forced expression of IFN-γ, leading to myelination defects and oligodendrocyte death. Therefore, excessive neuroinflammation may induce ER stress in myelinating cells which would not only disrupt their ability to myelinate neuronal axons, but can also lead to cell death.

ER stress-linked inflammation in neurodegenerative diseases

The development of ER stress is considered an underlying factor contributing to the clinical manifestations linked to many neurodegenerative disorders. In addition to the diseases previously described, pathological processes associated with other neuropathologies, such as prion diseases [190–193], human immunodeficiency virus associated-neurocognitive disorders (HAND) [193, 194] and a variety of lysosomal storage diseases [195], promote cellular and physiological challenges which perturb ER homeostasis. A unifying feature of all of these diseases is the presence of neuroinflammation [2, 196–198]. While few studies have directly examined the interactions between ER stress and inflammation in the CNS, there is evidence that these processes are intimately linked [24, 199, 200].

In brain tissue, microglia and astrocytes collaborate to mediate inflammation by integrating environmental information and carrying out an appropriate response. Microglia are CNS-resident phagocytic cells derived from the yolk sac. These sentinels of the CNS are the principal innate immune cell in the brain and have a key role in orchestrating inflammatory responses [201–203]. Astrocytes are also considered important regulators of the CNS, as they assist in neuronal metabolism, synaptic transmission, lay down the barriers isolating the neural tissue of the brain and coordinate the finely-tuned events of neuroinflammation along with microglia [3]. These glial cells possess a diverse repertoire of innate receptors, such as scavenger receptors and pattern recognition receptors, which allow them to augment the expression of inflammatory cytokines and chemokines under metabolic stress or interaction with PAMPs or DAMPs [204, 205].

Extracellular protein aggregates or oligomers underlie the pathology of various neurodegenerative disorders, and act as "danger signals" released from apoptotic or necrotic neurons [2]. These pathological assemblies can be recognized by innate immune receptors residing on neighboring glial cells [2, 206]. For example, Aβ oligomers are perceived to act as ligands for both the TNF-α receptor and toll-like receptor 4 [207]. Transient substrate-receptor interaction promotes an inflammatory response that initiates debris clearance via phagocytosis by microglia [2]. However, chronic exposure to these DAMPs or internalization of abnormal protein aggregates alters the functional properties of immunocompetent microglia and astrocytes to promote a reactive phenotype [2, 208]. In MS, autoreactive peripheral immune cells initiate an inflammatory response against myelin-derived antigen and promote neurotoxicity not only by compromising neuronal integrity directly, but causing astrocytes and microglia to secrete cytokines and other inflammatory mediators that contribute to demyelination [2, 209].

While chronic ER stress in neurons largely triggers signals to initiate apoptosis, extensive ER stress in glial cells has the potential to promote an inflammatory microenvironment characteristic in neurodegenerative diseases. Consistent with the role of astrocytes in mediating immunological homeostasis through its interactions with other cell types, the ER stress-induced upregulation in astrocytic inflammatory processes can encourage an inflammatory M1-like phenotype in microglia [92]. Similarly, neuronal ER stress has been shown to be positively correlated with microglial activation in a traumatic brain injury rat model [210]. ER stress not only influences pathways that result in the production of inflammatory mediators, but it also alters the responsiveness of cells to immunogenic stimuli. To this point, it has been documented that the administration of both prostaglandin E_2 and IFN-γ synergizes with ER stress to increase the production of IL-6 in glial cells [211]. Likewise, TNF-α autocrine signaling during ER stress significantly enhances the apoptotic signals of the UPR [80].

PERK knockdown experiments suggest that the association between ER stressed astrocytes and microglia activation is initially dependent on PERK signaling in astrocytes [92]. PERK haploinsufficiency and partial PERK inhibition using the small molecule PERK inhibitor GSK2606414 selectively attenuates the production of ER stress-induced inflammatory cytokines and chemokines, including IL-6, C-C Motif Chemokine Ligand (CCL)2 and CCL20 [212]. Interestingly, treating ER stressed astrocytes with ISRIB, a compound which reverses the translational block of phosphorylated eIF2α, attenuates ER stress-induced inflammatory gene expression [212]. We propose that the inflammatory signals induced during ER stress in astrocytes significantly relies on PERK-dependent eIF2α phosphorylation. These beneficial outcomes of PERK-eIF2α modulation fall in line with previous studies demonstrating that treating prion-diseased mice with GSK2606414 or ISRIB confers neuroprotection by partially recovering global translation rates [213, 214]. Conversely, preventing eIF2α dephosphorylation in response to tramatic brain injury using salubrinal is beneficial and attenuates neuroinflammation [11]. While it is becoming clear that PERK signaling has an important role in the regulation of neuroinflammation and neurodegeneration, a more complete understanding of the PERK-eIF2α pathway is needed to define the context and cell-specific roles. Therefore, manipulating the PERK-eIF2α axis without disturbing its homeostatic function could present an unappreciated way to alleviate aberrant neuroinflammation.

Conclusion

Many fundamental questions remain regarding the role of inflammation and ER stress in neurological diseases. Is inflammation beneficial or detrimental in neurodegenerative diseases? Most likely that it is important for tissue repair and neural regeneration, but detrimental when dysregulated. To complicate matters, the UPR system may be helpful or harmful depending on the level and spatial-temporal occurrence of ER stress. Cross-talk between the two programs may have beneficial functions through reciprocal regulation that promotes protective immunity. However, ER stress-induced amplification of inflammation may worsen chronic diseases [215].

Our understanding on if and how ER stress directly provokes an inflammatory reaction in neurodegenerative diseases remains to be clarified. Studies from our laboratory demonstrate that ER stress generated in murine astrocytes encourages PERK-dependent inflammatory signaling in vitro, suggesting that astrocytes themselves are potential contributors to neurotoxic inflammation in the face of ER dysfunction [92, 212]. Nevertheless, the relevance of these findings as it pertains to animal models and patients remains to be determined. Further, whether microglia respond to ER stress in the same vain has yet to be explored. Investigators must be cognizant of how agents used to manipulate the UPR will impinge on its homeostatic roles when devising pharmacological approaches to treat neurodegenerative diseases. Moreover, since both defective and chronic UPR signaling contribute to neuronal death in disease, developing agents which strictly attenuate pathways elicited by the ER stress response are insufficient. It is likely that targeting specific signaling components of the UPR that are predicted to enhance the pro-survival signals of the UPR or attenuate its inflammatory/apoptotic responses will possess more favorable outcomes.

In summary, ER stress and neuroinflammation are common pathological features of neurodegenerative diseases, and the mechanisms by which they interact during neurodegeneration remain to be elucidated. Further knowledge of this cross-talk will help us understand whether targeting cell stress pathways, such as ER stress in neurodegeneration, can control aberrant neuroinflammation and treat neurological disorders. To date, many studies have demonstrated beneficial effects of modulating ER stress pathways either genetically or pharmacologically in model organisms. However, the looming question remains: will targeting the UPR pathways be safe and beneficial in patients?

Abbreviations

AD: Alzheimer's disease; ALS: Amyotrophic Lateral Sclerosis; AP-1: Activator protein 1; APP: Aβ precursor protien; ASK1: Apoptosis signal-regulating kinase 1; ATF: Activating transcription factor; Aβ: Amyloid-β; BBB: Blood brain barrier; BiP: binding immunoglobulin protein; bZIP: basic leucine zipper; CHOP: CCAAT-enhancer-binding protein homologous protein; CNS: Central nervous system; DAMP: danger-associated molecular patterns; eIF2α: eukaryotic translation initiation factor 2α; ER: Endoplasmic reticulum; ERAD: ER-associated degradation; Ero1α: ER oxidoreductase α; FAD: Familial Alzheimer's disease; GADD34: Growth arrest and DNA damage-inducible protein 34; GCN2: General control non-derepressible 2; GRP: Glucose-regulated protein; GSK-3: Glycogen synthase kinase 3; HERV: human endogenous retrovirus; HLA: Human leukocyte antigen; IFN-γ: Interferon-γ; IKK: IκB kinase; IL: Interleukin; IRE-1α: Inositol-requiring 1α; IκB: inhibitors of κB;; JAK1: Januse kinase 1; JNK: c-Jun N-terminal kinase; Keap1: Kelch-like ECH-associated protein 1; LRRK2: Leucine-rich repeat kinase 2; MAPK: Mitogen activated protein kinase; MEF: Mouse embryonic fibroblasts; MS: Multiple Sclerosis; NFT: Neurofibrillary tangle; NF-κB: Nuclear factor kappa-light-chain-enhancer of activated B cells; NOD1/2: Nucleotide-binding oligomerization domain 1/2; Nrf-2: Nuclear factor-like 2, PAMP: pathogen associated molecular patterns; PD: Parkinson's disease; PDI: Protein disulphide isomerase; PERK: Double-stranded RNA dependent protein kinase-like ER kinase; PKR: Double stranded RNA-dependent kinase; PPI: Protein phosphatase 1; PS: Presenilin; RIDD: Regulated IRE1-dependent decay; RIPK2: Receptor-interacting serine/threonine-protein kinase 2; RNase: Endoribonuclease; RNS: Reactive nitrogen species; ROS: Reactive oxygen species; SRP: Signal-recognition particle; STAT: Signal transducers and activators of transcription; sXBP1: Spliced x-box-binding protein 1; TNF-α: Tumor-necrosis factor-α; TRAF2: TNF-α-receptor-associated factor 2; UPR: Unfolded protein response; WT: Wild-type; XBP1: X-box-binding protein 1

Acknowledgements

Not applicable.

Funding

The authors received funding from a Career Transition Award from the National Multiple Sclerosis Society (NMSS) (TA 3050-A-1), the West Virginia Clinical and Translational Science Institute (NIGMS U54GM104942) and the West Virginia Stoke CoBRE (NIGMS P20 GM109098).

Authors' contributions

NS performed the literature review and wrote the manuscript under the advisement of GM. NS, CS and SS graphed the illustrations and contributed to the content of the manuscript. GM edited the manuscript. All authors reviewed the manuscript before submission. All authors read and approved the final manuscript.

Authors' information

Not applicable.

Competing interests

The authors declare that they have no competing interests.

Consent for publication

Not applicable.

References

1. Heneka MT, Kummer MP, Latz E. Innate immune activation in neurodegenerative disease. Nat Rev Immunol. 2014;14(7):463–77.
2. Glass CK, Saijo K, Winner B, Marchetto MC, Gage FH. Mechanisms underlying inflammation in neurodegeneration. Cell. 2010;140(6):918–34.
3. Sofroniew MV. Astrocyte barriers to neurotoxic inflammation. Nat Rev Neurosci. 2015;16(5):249–63.
4. Prinz M, Priller J. Microglia and brain macrophages in the molecular age: from origin to neuropsychiatric disease. Nat Rev Neurosci. 2014;15(5):300–12.
5. Block ML, Hong JS. Microglia and inflammation-mediated neurodegeneration: multiple triggers with a common mechanism. Prog Neurobiol. 2005;76(2):77–98.
6. Perry VH, Nicoll JA, Holmes C. Microglia in neurodegenerative disease. Nat Rev Neurol. 2010;6(4):193–201.
7. DiSabato DJ, Quan N, Godbout JP. Neuroinflammation: the devil is in the details. J Neurochem. 2016;139(Suppl 2):136–53.
8. Lee KM, MacLean AG. New advances on glial activation in health and disease. World J Virol. 2015;4(2):42–55.
9. Hetz C, Mollereau B. Disturbance of endoplasmic reticulum proteostasis in neurodegenerative diseases. Nat Rev Neurosci. 2014;15(4):233–49.
10. Bellezza I, Grottelli S, Mierla AL, Cacciatore I, Fornasari E, Roscini L, et al. Neuroinflammation and endoplasmic reticulum stress are coregulated by cyclo(his-pro) to prevent LPS neurotoxicity. Int J Biochem Cell Biol. 2014;51:159–69.
11. Logsdon AF, Lucke-Wold BP, Nguyen L, Matsumoto RR, Turner RC, Rosen CL, et al. Salubrinal reduces oxidative stress, neuroinflammation and impulsive-like behavior in a rodent model of traumatic brain injury. Brain Res. 2016;1643:140–51.
12. Deslauriers AM, Afkhami-Goli A, Paul AM, Bhat RK, Acharjee S, Ellestad KK, et al. Neuroinflammation and endoplasmic reticulum stress are coregulated by crocin to prevent demyelination and neurodegeneration. J Immunol. 2011;187(9):4788–99.
13. Salminen A, Kauppinen A, Suuronen T, Kaarniranta K, Ojala J. ER stress in Alzheimer's disease: a novel neuronal trigger for inflammation and Alzheimer's pathology. J Neuroinflammation. 2009;6:41.
14. Drake TM. Unfolding the promise of translational targeting in neurodegenerative disease. NeuroMolecular Med. 2015;17(2):147–57.
15. Schechter I. Partial amino acid sequence of the precursor of immunoglobulin light chain programmed by messenger RNA in vitro. Science. 1975;188(4184):160_2.
16. Nyathi Y, Wilkinson BM, Pool MR. Co-translational targeting and translocation of proteins to the endoplasmic reticulum. Biochim Biophys Acta. 2013;1833(11):2392–402.
17. Siegel V, Walter P. Each of the activities of signal recognition particle (SRP) is contained within a distinct domain: analysis of biochemical mutants of SRP. Cell. 1988;52(1):39–49.
18. Walter P, Blobel G. Translocation of proteins across the endoplasmic reticulum. II. Signal recognition protein (SRP) mediates the selective binding to microsomal membranes of in-vitro-assembled polysomes synthesizing secretory protein. J Cell Biol. 1981;91(2 Pt 1):551–6.
19. Black BL, Jarett L, McDonald JM. The regulation of endoplasmic reticulum calcium uptake of adipocytes by cytoplasmic calcium. J Biol Chem. 1981;256(1):322–9.

20. Kim I, Xu W, Reed JC. Cell death and endoplasmic reticulum stress: disease relevance and therapeutic opportunities. Nat Rev Drug Discov. 2008;7(12):1013–30.
21. Tu BP, Weissman JS. Oxidative protein folding in eukaryotes: mechanisms and consequences. J Cell Biol. 2004;164(3):341–6.
22. Gomez-Navarro N, Miller EA. COP-coated vesicles. Curr Biol. 2016;26(2):R54–7.
23. Ellgaard L, McCaul N, Chatsisvili A, Braakman I. Co- and post-translational protein folding in the ER. Traffic. 2016;17(6):615–38.
24. Zhang K, Kaufman RJ. From endoplasmic-reticulum stress to the inflammatory response. Nature. 2008;454(7203):455–62.
25. Sun S, Shi G, Sha H, Ji Y, Han X, Shu X, et al. IRE1α is an endogenous substrate of endoplasmic-reticulum-associated degradation. Nat Cell Biol. 2015;17(12):1546–55.
26. Harding H, Zhang Y, Ron D. Protein translation and folding are coupled by an endoplasmic-reticulum-resident kinase. Nature. 1999;397(6716):271–4.
27. Shore GC, Papa FR, Oakes SA. Signaling cell death from the endoplasmic reticulum stress response. Curr Opin Cell Biol. 2011;23(2):143–9.
28. Hitomi J, Katayama T, Eguchi Y, Kudo T, Taniguchi M, Koyama Y, et al. Involvement of caspase-4 in endoplasmic reticulum stress-induced apoptosis and Abeta-induced cell death. J Cell Biol. 2004;165(3):347–56.
29. Egger L, Schneider J, Rheme C, Tapernoux M, Hacki J, Borner C. Serine proteases mediate apoptosis-like cell death and phagocytosis under caspase-inhibiting conditions. Cell Death Differ. 2003;10(10):1188–203.
30. Li J, Ni M, Lee B, Barron E, Hinton DR, Lee AS. The unfolded protein response regulator GRP78/BiP is required for endoplasmic reticulum integrity and stress-induced autophagy in mammalian cells. Cell Death Differ. 2008;15(9):1460–71.
31. Bertolotti A, Zhang Y, Hendershot LM, Harding HP, Ron D. Dynamic interaction of BiP and ER stress transducers in the unfolded-protein response. Nat Cell Biol. 2000;2(6):326–32.
32. Shen J, Chen X, Hendershot L, Prywes R. ER stress regulation of ATF6 localization by dissociation of BiP/GRP78 binding and unmasking of Golgi localization signals. Dev Cell. 2002;3(1):99–111.
33. Janssens S, Pulendran B, Lambrecht BN. Emerging functions of the unfolded protein response in immunity. Nat Immunol. 2014;15(10):910–9.
34. Credle JJ, Finer-Moore JS, Papa FR, Stroud RM, Walter P. On the mechanism of sensing unfolded protein in the endoplasmic reticulum. Proc Natl Acad Sci U S A. 2005;102(52):18773–84.
35. Ron D, Walter P. Signal integration in the endoplasmic reticulum unfolded protein response. Nat Rev Mol Cell Biol. 2007;8(7):519–29.
36. Haze K, Yoshida H, Yanagi H, Yura T, Mori K. Mammalian transcription factor ATF6 is synthesized as a transmembrane protein and activated by proteolysis in response to endoplasmic reticulum stress. Mol Biol Cell. 1999; 10(11):3787–99.
37. Schröder M, Kaufman R. The mammalian unfolded protein response. Annu Rev Biochem. 2005;74:739–89.
38. Ye J, Rawson R, Komuro R, Chen X, Davé U, Prywes R, et al. ER stress induces cleavage of membrane-bound ATF6 by the same proteases that process SREBPs. Mol Cell. 2000;6(6):1355–64.
39. Yamamoto K, Sato T, Matsui T, Sato M, Okada T, Yoshida H, et al. Transcriptional induction of mammalian ER quality control proteins is mediated by single or combined action of ATF6alpha and XBP1. Dev Cell. 2007;13(3):365–76.
40. Sidrauski C, Walter P. The transmembrane kinase Ire1p is a site-specific endonuclease that initiates mRNA splicing in the unfolded protein response. Cell. 1997;90(6):1031–9.
41. Lee KP, Dey M, Neculai D, Cao C, Dever TE, Sicheri F. Structure of the dual enzyme Ire1 reveals the basis for catalysis and regulation in nonconventional RNA splicing. Cell. 2008;132(1):89–100.
42. Tirasophon W, Lee K, Callaghan B, Welihinda A, Kaufman RJ. The endoribonuclease activity of mammalian IRE1 autoregulates its mRNA and is required for the unfolded protein response. Genes Dev. 2000;14(21):2725–36.
43. Lee K, Tirasophon W, Shen X, Michalak M, Prywes R, Okada T, et al. IRE1-mediated unconventional mRNA splicing and S2P-mediated ATF6 cleavage merge to regulate XBP1 in signaling the unfolded protein response. Genes Dev. 2002;16(4):452–66.
44. Yamamoto K, Yoshida H, Kokame K, Kaufman RJ, Mori K. Differential contributions of ATF6 and XBP1 to the activation of endoplasmic reticulum stress-responsive cis-acting elements ERSE, UPRE and ERSE-IIUPRE and ERSE-II. J Biochem. 2004;136(3):343–50.
45. Maurel M, Chevet E, Tavernier J, Gerlo S. Getting RIDD of RNA: IRE1 in cell fate regulation. Trends Biochem Sci. 2014;39(5):245–54.
46. Hollien J, Weissman JS. Decay of endoplasmic reticulum-localized mRNAs during the unfolded protein response. Science. 2006;313(5783):104–7.
47. Han D, Lerner AG, Vande Walle L, Upton JP, Xu W, Hagen A, et al. IRE1alpha kinase activation modes control alternate endoribonuclease outputs to determine divergent cell fates. Cell. 2009;138(3):562–75.
48. Upton JP, Wang L, Han D, Wang ES, Huskey NE, Lim L, et al. IRE1alpha cleaves select microRNAs during ER stress to derepress translation of proapoptotic Caspase-2. Science. 2012;338(6108):818–22.
49. Chen Y, Brandizzi F. IRE1: ER stress sensor and cell fate executor. Trends Cell Bio. 2013;23(11):547–55.
50. Starck SR, Tsai JC, Chen K, Shodiya M, Wang L, Yahiro K, Martins-Green M, Shastri N, Walter P: Translation from the 5′ untranslated region shapes the integrated stress response. Science 2016, 351(6272):aad3867.
51. Klann E, Dever TE. Biochemical mechanisms for translational regulation in synaptic plasticity. Nat Rev Neurosci. 2004;5(12):931–42.
52. Vattem KM, Wek RC. Reinitiation involving upstream ORFs regulates ATF4 mRNA translation in mammalian cells. Proc Natl Acad Sci U S A. 2004; 101(31):11269–74.
53. Wang M, Kaufman RJ. Protein misfolding in the endoplasmic reticulum as a conduit to human disease. Nature. 2016;529(7586):326–35.
54. Nishitoh H. CHOP is a multifunctional transcription factor in the ER stress response. J Biochem. 2012;151(3):217–9.
55. Oyadomari S, Mori M. Roles of CHOP/GADD153 in endoplasmic reticulum stress. Cell Death Differ. 2004;11(4):381–9.
56. Tabas I, Ron D. Integrating the mechanisms of apoptosis induced by endoplasmic reticulum stress. Nat Cell Biol. 2011;13(3):184–90.
57. Li G, Mongillo M, Chin K-T, Harding H, Ron D, Marks AR, et al. Role of ERO1-alpha-mediated stimulation of inositol 1,4,5-triphosphate receptor activity in endoplasmic reticulum stress-induced apoptosis. J Cell Biol. 2009;186(6): 783–92.
58. Görlach A, Klappa P, Kietzmann T. The endoplasmic reticulum: folding, calcium homeostasis, signaling, and redox control. Antioxid Redox Signal. 2006;8(9–10):1391–418.
59. Hansson MJ, Mansson R, Morota S, Uchino H, Kallur T, Sumi T, et al. Calcium-induced generation of reactive oxygen species in brain mitochondria is mediated by permeability transition. Free Radic Biol Med. 2008;45(3):284–94.
60. Gross E, Sevier CS, Heldman N, Vitu E, Bentzur M, Kaiser CA, et al. Generating disulfides enzymatically: reaction products and electron acceptors of the endoplasmic reticulum thiol oxidase Ero1p. Proc Natl Acad Sci U S A. 2006;103(2):299–304.
61. Brush MH, Weiser DC, Shenolikar S. Growth arrest and DNA damage-inducible protein GADD34 targets protein phosphatase 1 alpha to the endoplasmic reticulum and promotes dephosphorylation of the alpha subunit of eukaryotic translation initiation factor 2. Mol Cell Biol. 2003;23(4): 1292–303.
62. Marciniak S, Yun C, Oyadomari S, Novoa I, Zhang Y, Jungreis R, et al. CHOP induces death by promoting protein synthesis and oxidation in the stressed endoplasmic reticulum. Genes Dev. 2004;18(24):3066–77.
63. Urra H, Dufey E, Lisbona F, Rojas-Rivera D, Hetz C. When ER stress reaches a dead end. Biochim Biophys Acta. 2013;1833(12):3507–17.
64. Hollander MC, Zhan Q, Bae I, Fornace AJ. Mammalian GADD34, an apoptosis- and DNA damage-inducible gene. J Biol Chem. 1997;272(21): 13731–7.
65. Cullinan SB, Diehl JA. PERK-dependent activation of Nrf2 contributes to redox homeostasis and cell survival following endoplasmic reticulum stress. J Biol Chem. 2004,279(19):20108–17.
66. Cullinan SB, Zhang D, Hannink M, Arvisais E, Kaufman RJ, Diehl JA. Nrf2 is a direct PERK substrate and effector of PERK-dependent cell survival. Mol Cell Biol. 2003;23(20):7198–209.
67. Yoshida H, Matsui T, Yamamoto A, Okada T, Mori K. XBP1 mRNA is induced by ATF6 and spliced by IRE1 in response to ER stress to produce a highly active transcription factor. Cell. 2001;107(7):881–91.
68. Tsuru A, Imai Y, Saito M, Kohno K. Novel mechanism of enhancing IRE1alpha-XBP1 signalling via the PERK-ATF4 pathway. Sci Rep. 2016;6:24217.
69. Yoshida H, Okada T, Haze K, Yanagi H, Yura T, Negishi M, et al. ATF6 activated by proteolysis binds in the presence of NF-Y (CBF) directly to the cis-acting element responsible for the mammalian unfolded protein response. Mol Cell Biol. 2000;20(18):6755–67.
70. Cnop M, Foufelle F, Velloso LA. Endoplasmic reticulum stress, obesity and diabetes. Trends Mol Med. 2012;18(1):59–68.

71. Bommiasamy H, Back SH, Fagone P, Lee K, Meshinchi S, Vink E, et al. ATF6alpha induces XBP1-independent expansion of the endoplasmic reticulum. J Cell Sci. 2009;122(Pt 10):1626–36.
72. Trinh MA, Klann E. Translational control by eIF2α kinases in long-lasting synaptic plasticity and long-term memory. Neurobiol Learn Mem. 2013;105: 93–9.
73. Martínez G, Vidal RL, Mardones P, Serrano FG, Ardiles AO, Wirth C, et al. Regulation of memory formation by the transcription factor XBP1. Cell Rep. 2016;14(6):1382–94.
74. Tang G, Minemoto Y, Dibling B, Purcell NH, Li Z, Karin M, et al. Inhibition of JNK activation through NF-kappaB target genes. Nature. 2001;414(6861): 313–7.
75. Gilmore TD. Introduction to NF-kappaB: players, pathways, perspectives. Oncogene. 2006;25(51):6680–4.
76. Chen Z, Hagler J, Palombella VJ, Melandri F, Scherer D, Ballard D, et al. Signal-induced site-specific phosphorylation targets I kappa B alpha to the ubiquitin-proteasome pathway. Genes Dev. 1995;9(13):1586–97.
77. Tabary O, Boncoeur E, de Martin R, Pepperkok R, Clement A, Schultz C, et al. Calcium-dependent regulation of NF-(kappa)B activation in cystic fibrosis airway epithelial cells. Cell Signal. 2006;18(5):652–60.
78. van den Berg R, Haenen GR, van den Berg H, Bast A. Transcription factor NF-kappaB as a potential biomarker for oxidative stress. Br J Nutr. 2001; 86(Suppl 1):S121–7.
79. Deng J, Lu PD, Zhang Y, Scheuner D, Kaufman RJ, Sonenberg N, et al. Translational repression mediates activation of nuclear factor kappa B by phosphorylated translation initiation factor 2. Mol Cell Biol. 2004;24(23):10161–8.
80. Hu P, Han Z, Couvillon AD, Kaufman RJ, Exton JH. Autocrine tumor necrosis factor alpha links endoplasmic reticulum stress to the membrane death receptor pathway through IRE1alpha-mediated NF-kappaB activation and down-regulation of TRAF2 expression. Mol Cell Biol. 2006;26(8):3071–84.
81. Urano F, Wang X, Bertolotti A, Zhang Y, Chung P, Harding H, et al. Coupling of stress in the ER to activation of JNK protein kinases by transmembrane protein kinase IRE1. Science. 2000;287(5453):664–6.
82. Shaulian E, Karin M. AP-1 as a regulator of cell life and death. Nat Cell Biol. 2002;4(5):E131–6.
83. Keestra-Gounder AM, Byndloss MX, Seyffert N, Young BM, Chávez-Arroyo A, Tsai AY, et al. NOD1 and NOD2 signalling links ER stress with inflammation. Nature. 2016;532(7599):394–7.
84. Hetz C, Bernasconi P, Fisher J, Lee A-H, Bassik MC, Antonsson B, et al. Proapoptotic BAX and BAK modulate the unfolded protein response by a direct interaction with IRE1alpha. Science. 2006;312(5773):572–6.
85. Lamkanfi M, Kalai M, Vandenabeele P. Caspase-12: an overview. Cell Death Differ. 2004;11(4):365–8.
86. Yang C, Diiorio P, Jurczyk A, O'Sullivan-Murphy B, Urano F, Bortell R. Pathological endoplasmic reticulum stress mediated by the IRE1 pathway contributes to pre-insulitic beta cell apoptosis in a virus-induced rat model of type 1 diabetes. Diabetologia. 2013;56(12):2638–46.
87. Fischer H, Koenig U, Eckhart L, Tschachler E. Human caspase 12 has acquired deleterious mutations. Biochem Biophys Res Commun. 2002; 293(2):722–6.
88. Wang XZ, Ron D. Stress-induced phosphorylation and activation of the transcription factor CHOP (GADD153) by p38 MAP Kinase. Science. 1996; 272(5266):1347–9.
89. Lei K, Davis RJ. JNK phosphorylation of Bim-related members of the Bcl2 family induces Bax-dependent apoptosis. Proc Natl Acad Sci U S A. 2003; 100(5):2432–7.
90. Hosoi T, Sasaki M, Miyahara T, Hashimoto C, Matsuo S, Yoshii M, et al. Endoplasmic reticulum stress induces leptin resistance. Mol Pharmacol. 2008;74(6):1610–9.
91. Flores-Morales A, Fernandez L, Rico-Bautista E, Umana A, Negrin C, Zhang JG, et al. Endoplasmic reticulum stress prolongs GH-induced Janus kinase (JAK2)/signal transducer and activator of transcription (STAT5) signaling pathway. Mol Endocrinol. 2001;15(9):1471–83.
92. Meares GP, Liu Y, Rajbhandari R, Qin H, Nozell SE, Mobley JA, et al. PERK-dependent activation of JAK1 and STAT3 contributes to endoplasmic reticulum stress-induced inflammation. Mol Cell Biol. 2014;34(20):3911–25.
93. Lin JH, Li H, Yasumura D, Cohen HR, Zhang C, Panning B, et al. IRE1 signaling affects cell fate during the unfolded protein response. Science. 2007;318(5852):944–9.
94. Wang M, Kaufman RJ. The impact of the endoplasmic reticulum protein-folding environment on cancer development. Nat Rev Cancer. 2014;14(9):581–97.
95. Rutkowski DT, Arnold SM, Miller CN, Wu J, Li J, Gunnison KM, et al. Adaptation to ER stress is mediated by differential stabilities of pro-survival and pro-apoptotic mRNAs and proteins. PLoS Biol. 2006;4(11):e374.
96. Inagi R, Kumagai T, Nishi H, Kawakami T, Miyata T, Fujita T, et al. Preconditioning with endoplasmic reticulum stress ameliorates mesangioproliferative glomerulonephritis. J Am Soc Nephrol. 2008;19(5):915–22.
97. Mercado G, Valdes P, Hetz C. An ERcentric view of Parkinson's disease. Trends Mol Med. 2013;19(3):165–75.
98. Fouillet A, Levet C, Virgone A, Robin M, Dourlen P, Rieusset J, et al. ER stress inhibits neuronal death by promoting autophagy. Autophagy. 2012;8(6): 915–26.
99. Calabrese V, Cornelius C, Dinkova-Kostova AT, Calabrese EJ, Mattson MP. Cellular stress responses, the hormesis paradigm, and vitagenes: novel targets for therapeutic intervention in neurodegenerative disorders. Antioxid Redox Signal. 2010;13(11):1763–811.
100. Reitz C, Brayne C, Mayeux R. Epidemiology of Alzheimer disease. Nat Rev Neurol. 2011;7(3):137–52.
101. De Strooper B. Proteases and proteolysis in Alzheimer disease: a multifactorial view on the disease process. Physiol Rev. 2010;90(2):465–94.
102. Jucker M, Walker LC. Self-propagation of pathogenic protein aggregates in neurodegenerative diseases. Nature. 2013;501(7465):45–51.
103. Caceres A, Kosik KS. Inhibition of neurite polarity by tau antisense oligonucleotides in primary cerebellar neurons. Nature. 1990;343(6257):461–3.
104. Stoothoff WH, Johnson GV. Tau phosphorylation: physiological and pathological consequences. Biochim Biophys Acta. 2005;1739(2–3):280–97.
105. Gong CX, Iqbal K. Hyperphosphorylation of microtubule-associated protein tau: a promising therapeutic target for Alzheimer disease. Curr Med Chem. 2008;15(23):2321–8.
106. Veugelen S, Saito T, Saido TC, Chávez-Gutiérrez L, De Strooper B. Familial Alzheimer's disease mutations in Presenilin generate Amyloidogenic Aβ peptide seeds. Neuron. 2016;90(2):410–6.
107. Weggen S, Beher D. Molecular consequences of amyloid precursor protein and presenilin mutations causing autosomal-dominant Alzheimer's disease. Alzheimers Res Ther. 2012;4(2):9.
108. Mawuenyega KG, Sigurdson W, Ovod V, Munsell L, Kasten T, Morris JC, et al. Decreased clearance of CNS beta-amyloid in Alzheimer's disease. Science. 2010;330(6012):1774.
109. Duran-Aniotz C, Martinez G, Hetz C. Memory loss in Alzheimer's disease: are the alterations in the UPR network involved in the cognitive impairment? Front Aging Neurosci. 2014;6:8.
110. Lourenco MV, Clarke JR, Frozza RL, Bomfim TR, Forny-Germano L, Batista AF, et al. TNF-alpha mediates PKR-dependent memory impairment and brain IRS-1 inhibition induced by Alzheimer's beta-amyloid oligomers in mice and monkeys. Cell Metab. 2013;18(6):831–43.
111. Ma T, Trinh MA, Wexler AJ, Bourbon C, Gatti E, Pierre P, et al. Suppression of eIF2α kinases alleviates Alzheimer's disease-related plasticity and memory deficits. Nat Neurosci. 2013;16(9):1299–305.
112. Costa-Mattioli M, Sossin WS, Klann E, Sonenberg N. Translational control of long-lasting synaptic plasticity and memory. Neuron. 2009;61(1):10–26.
113. Cissé M, Duplan E, Lorivel T, Dunys J, Bauer C, Meckler X, et al. The transcription factor XBP1s restores hippocampal synaptic plasticity and memory by control of the Kalirin-7 pathway in Alzheimer model. Mol Psychiatry. 2016;
114. Segev Y, Barrera I, Ounallah-Saad H, Wibrand K, Sporild I, Livne A, et al. PKR inhibition rescues memory deficit and ATF4 Overexpression in ApoE epsilon4 human replacement mice. J Neurosci. 2015;35(38):12986–93.
115. Bomfim TR, Forny-Germano L, Sathler LB, Brito-Moreira J, Houzel JC, Decker H, et al. An anti-diabetes agent protects the mouse brain from defective insulin signaling caused by Alzheimer's disease- associated Abeta oligomers. J Clin Invest. 2012;122(4):1339–53.
116. Ferreiro E, Oliveira CR, Pereira C. Involvement of endoplasmic reticulum Ca2 + release through ryanodine and inositol 1,4,5-triphosphate receptors in the neurotoxic effects induced by the amyloid-beta peptide. J Neurosci Res. 2004;76(6):872–80.
117. Paula-Lima AC, Adasme T, SanMartín C, Sebollela A, Hetz C, Carrasco MA, et al. Amyloid β-peptide oligomers stimulate RyR-mediated Ca2+ release inducing mitochondrial fragmentation in hippocampal neurons and prevent RyR-mediated dendritic spine remodeling produced by BDNF. Antioxid Redox Signal. 2011;14(7):1209–23.
118. Demuro A, Parker I. Cytotoxicity of intracellular aβ42 amyloid oligomers involves Ca2+ release from the endoplasmic reticulum by stimulated production of inositol trisphosphate. J Neurosci. 2013;33(9):3824–33.

119. Abisambra JF, Jinwal UK, Blair LJ, O'Leary JC, Li Q, Brady S, et al. Tau accumulation activates the unfolded protein response by impairing endoplasmic reticulum-associated degradation. J Neurosci. 2013;33(22): 9498–507.
120. Nijholt DAT, Nölle A, van Haastert ES, Edelijn H, Toonen RF, Hoozemans JJM, et al. Unfolded protein response activates glycogen synthase kinase-3 via selective lysosomal degradation. Neurobiol Aging. 2013;34(7):1759–71.
121. Resende R, Ferreiro E, Pereira C, Oliveira C. ER stress is involved in Abeta-induced GSK-3beta activation and tau phosphorylation. J Neurosci Res. 2008;86(9):2091–9.
122. Ho Y-S, Yang X, Lau JC-F, Hung CH-L, Wuwongse S, Zhang Q, et al. Endoplasmic reticulum stress induces tau pathology and forms a vicious cycle: implication in Alzheimer's disease pathogenesis. J Alzheimers Dis. 2012;28(4):839–54.
123. Lasagna-Reeves CA, Castillo-Carranza DL, Guerrero-Muoz MJ, Jackson GR, Kayed R. Preparation and characterization of neurotoxic tau oligomers. Biochemistry. 2010;49(47):10039–41.
124. Katayama T, Imaizumi K, Sato N, Miyoshi K, Kudo T, Hitomi J, et al. Presenilin-1 mutations downregulate the signalling pathway of the unfolded-protein response. Nat Cell Biol. 1999;1(8):479–85.
125. Katayama T, Imaizumi K, Honda A, Yoneda T, Kudo T, Takeda M, et al. Disturbed activation of endoplasmic reticulum stress transducers by familial Alzheimer's disease-linked presenilin-1 mutations. J Biol Chem. 2001;276(46):43446–54.
126. Sato N, Imaizumi K, Manabe T, Taniguchi M, Hitomi J, Katayama T, et al. Increased production of beta-amyloid and vulnerability to endoplasmic reticulum stress by an aberrant spliced form of presenilin 2. J Biol Chem. 2001;276(3):2108–14.
127. Paschen W, Mengesdorf T. Endoplasmic reticulum stress response and neurodegeneration. Cell Calcium. 2005;38(3–4):409–15.
128. Mattson MP, Zhu H, Yu J, Kindy MS. Presenilin-1 mutation increases neuronal vulnerability to focal ischemia in vivo and to hypoxia and glucose deprivation in cell culture: involvement of perturbed calcium homeostasis. J Neurosci. 2000;20(4):1358–64.
129. Zatti G, Ghidoni R, Barbiero L, Binetti G, Pozzan T, Fasolato C, et al. The presenilin 2 M239I mutation associated with familial Alzheimer's disease reduces Ca2+ release from intracellular stores. Neurobiol Dis. 2004;15(2):269–78.
130. Sato N, Urano F, Yoon Leem J, Kim SH, Li M, Donoviel D, et al. Upregulation of BiP and CHOP by the unfolded-protein response is independent of presenilin expression. Nat Cell Biol. 2000;2(12):863–70.
131. Hartmann A, Hunot S, Michel PP, Muriel MP, Vyas S, Faucheux BA, et al. Caspase-3: a vulnerability factor and final effector in apoptotic death of dopaminergic neurons in Parkinson's disease. Proc Natl Acad Sci U S A. 2000;97(6):2875–80.
132. Schildknecht S, Gerding HR, Karreman C, Drescher M, Lashuel HA, Outeiro TF, et al. Oxidative and nitrative alpha-synuclein modifications and proteostatic stress: implications for disease mechanisms and interventions in synucleinopathies. J Neurochem. 2013;125(4):491–511.
133. Chartier-Harlin MC, Kachergus J, Roumier C, Mouroux V, Douay X, Lincoln S, et al. Alpha-synuclein locus duplication as a cause of familial Parkinson's disease. Lancet. 2004;364(9440):1167–9.
134. Michel PP, Hirsch EC, Hunot S. Understanding Dopaminergic cell death pathways in Parkinson disease. Neuron. 2016;90(4):675–91.
135. Scarffe LA, Stevens DA, Dawson VL, Dawson TM. Parkin and PINK1: much more than mitophagy. Trends Neurosci. 2014;37(6):315–24.
136. Corti O, Brice A. Mitochondrial quality control turns out to be the principal suspect in parkin and PINK1-related autosomal recessive Parkinson's disease. Curr Opin Neurobiol. 2013;23(1):100–8.
137. Pickrell AM, Youle RJ. The roles of PINK1, parkin, and mitochondrial fidelity in Parkinson's disease. Neuron. 2015;85(2):257–73.
138. Zimprich A, Biskup S, Leitner P, Lichtner P, Farrer M, Lincoln S, et al. Mutations in LRRK2 cause autosomal-dominant parkinsonism with pleomorphic pathology. Neuron. 2004;44(4):601–7.
139. Lee BD, Shin J-H, VanKampen J, Petrucelli L, West AB, Ko HS, et al. Inhibitors of leucine-rich repeat kinase-2 protect against models of Parkinson's disease. Nat Med. 2010;16(9):998–1000.
140. Ryu EJ, Harding HP, Angelastro JM, Vitolo OV, Ron D, Greene LA. Endoplasmic reticulum stress and the unfolded protein response in cellular models of Parkinson's disease. J Neurosci. 2002;22(24):10690–8.
141. Chung CY, Khurana V, Auluck PK, Tardiff DF, Mazzulli JR, Soldner F, et al. Identification and rescue of α-synuclein toxicity in Parkinson patient-derived neurons. Science. 2013;342(6161):983–7.
142. Uehara T, Nakamura T, Yao D, Shi Z-Q, Gu Z, Ma Y, et al. S-nitrosylated protein-disulphide isomerase links protein misfolding to neurodegeneration. Nature. 2006;441(7092):513–7.
143. Colla E, Jensen PH, Pletnikova O, Troncoso JC, Glabe C, Lee MK. Accumulation of toxic alpha-synuclein oligomer within endoplasmic reticulum occurs in alpha-synucleinopathy in vivo. J Neurosci. 2012;32(10):3301–5.
144. Cooper AA, Gitler AD, Cashikar A, Haynes CM, Hill KJ, Bhullar B, et al. Alpha-synuclein blocks ER-Golgi traffic and Rab1 rescues neuron loss in Parkinson's models. Science. 2006;313(5785):324–8.
145. Hoozemans JJM, van Haastert ES, Eikelenboom P, de Vos RAI, Rozemuller JM, Scheper W. Activation of the unfolded protein response in Parkinson's disease. Biochem Biophys Res Commun. 2007;354(3):707–11.
146. Smith WW, Jiang H, Pei Z, Tanaka Y, Morita H, Sawa A, et al. Endoplasmic reticulum stress and mitochondrial cell death pathways mediate A53T mutant alpha-synuclein-induced toxicity. Hum Mol Genet. 2005;14(24):3801–11.
147. Imai Y, Soda M, Takahashi R. Parkin suppresses unfolded protein stress-induced cell death through its E3 ubiquitin-protein ligase activity. J Biol Chem. 2000;275(46):35661–4.
148. Bouman L, Schlierf A, Lutz AK, Shan J, Deinlein A, Kast J, et al. Parkin is transcriptionally regulated by ATF4: evidence for an interconnection between mitochondrial stress and ER stress. Cell Death Differ. 2011;18(5): 769–82.
149. Duplan E, Giaime E, Viotti J, Sevalle J, Corti O, Brice A, et al. ER-stress-associated functional link between Parkin and DJ-1 via a transcriptional cascade involving the tumor suppressor p53 and the spliced X-box binding protein XBP-1. J Cell Sci. 2013;126(Pt 9):2124–33.
150. Duplan E, Sevalle J, Viotti J, Goiran T, Bauer C, Renbaum P, et al. Parkin differently regulates presenilin-1 and presenilin-2 functions by direct control of their promoter transcription. J Mol Cell Biol. 2013;5(2):132–42.
151. Yuan Y, Cao P, Smith MA, Kramp K, Huang Y, Hisamoto N, et al. Dysregulated LRRK2 signaling in response to endoplasmic reticulum stress leads to dopaminergic neuron degeneration in *C. elegans*. PLoS One. 2011; 6(8):e22354.
152. Matus S, Valenzuela V, Medinas DB, Hetz C. ER dysfunction and protein folding stress in ALS. Int J Cell Biol. 2013;2013:674751.
153. Zarei S, Carr K, Reiley L, Diaz K, Guerra O, Altamirano PF, et al. A comprehensive review of amyotrophic lateral sclerosis. Surg Neurol Int. 2015;6:171.
154. Deng HX, Hentati A, Tainer JA, Iqbal Z, Cayabyab A, Hung WY, et al. Amyotrophic lateral sclerosis and structural defects in cu,Zn superoxide dismutase. Science. 1993;261(5124):1047–51.
155. Taylor JP, Brown RH Jr, Cleveland DW. Decoding ALS: from genes to mechanism. Nature. 2016;539(7628):197–206.
156. Rosen DR, Siddique T, Patterson D, Figlewicz DA, Sapp P, Hentati A, et al. Mutations in cu/Zn superoxide dismutase gene are associated with familial amyotrophic lateral sclerosis. Nature. 1993;362(6415):59–62.
157. Rosen DR. Mutations in cu/Zn superoxide dismutase gene are associated with familial amyotrophic lateral sclerosis. Nature. 1993;364(6435):362.
158. Renton AE, Majounie E, Waite A, Simón-Sánchez J, Rollinson S, Gibbs JR, et al. A hexanucleotide repeat expansion in C9ORF72 is the cause of chromosome 9p21-linked ALS-FTD. Neuron. 2011;72(2):257–68.
159. Kwiatkowski TJ, Bosco DA, Leclerc AL, Tamrazian E, Vanderburg CR, Russ C, et al. Mutations in the FUS/TLS gene on chromosome 16 cause familial amyotrophic lateral sclerosis. Science. 2009;323(5918):1205–8.
160. Matus S, Glimcher LH, Hetz C. Protein folding stress in neurodegenerative diseases: a glimpse into the ER. Curr Opin Cell Biol. 2011;23(2):239–52.
161. Ilieva EV, Ayala V, Jové M, Dalfó E, Cacabelos D, Povedano M, et al. Oxidative and endoplasmic reticulum stress interplay in sporadic amyotrophic lateral sclerosis. Brain. 2007;130(Pt 12):3111–23.
162. Atkin JD, Farg MA, Walker AK, McLean C, Tomas D, Horne MK. Endoplasmic reticulum stress and induction of the unfolded protein response in human sporadic amyotrophic lateral sclerosis. Neurobiol Dis. 2008;30(3):400–7.
163. Ito Y, Yamada M, Tanaka H, Aida K, Tsuruma K, Shimazawa M, et al. Involvement of CHOP, an ER-stress apoptotic mediator, in both human sporadic ALS and ALS model mice. Neurobiol Dis. 2009;36(3):470–6.
164. Nishitoh H, Kadowaki H, Nagai A, Maruyama T, Yokota T, Fukutomi H, et al. ALS-linked mutant SOD1 induces ER stress- and ASK1-dependent motor neuron death by targeting Derlin-1. Genes Dev. 2008;22(11):1451–64.
165. Wang L, Popko B, Roos RP. The unfolded protein response in familial amyotrophic lateral sclerosis. Hum Mol Genet. 2011;20(5):1008–15.

166. Matus S, Lopez E, Valenzuela V, Nassif M, Hetz C. Functional contribution of the transcription factor ATF4 to the pathogenesis of amyotrophic lateral sclerosis. PLoS One. 2013;8(7):e66672.
167. Hetz C, Thielen P, Matus S, Nassif M, Court F, Kiffin R, et al. XBP-1 deficiency in the nervous system protects against amyotrophic lateral sclerosis by increasing autophagy. Genes Dev. 2009;23(19):2294–306.
168. Atkin JD, Farg MA, Turner BJ, Tomas D, Lysaght JA, Nunan J, et al. Induction of the unfolded protein response in familial amyotrophic lateral sclerosis and association of protein-disulfide isomerase with superoxide dismutase 1. J Biol Chem. 2006;281(40):30152–65.
169. Walker AK, Farg MA, Bye CR, McLean CA, Horne MK, Atkin JD. Protein disulphide isomerase protects against protein aggregation and is S-nitrosylated in amyotrophic lateral sclerosis. Brain. 2010;133(Pt 1):105–16.
170. Halloran M, Parakh S, Atkin JD. The role of s-nitrosylation and s-glutathionylation of protein disulphide isomerase in protein misfolding and neurodegeneration. Int J Cell Biol. 2013;2013:797914.
171. Parakh S, Atkin JD. Protein folding alterations in amyotrophic lateral sclerosis. Brain Res. 2016;1648(Pt B):633–49.
172. Zhang YJ, Jansen-West K, Xu YF, Gendron TF, Bieniek KF, Lin WL, et al. Aggregation-prone c9FTD/ALS poly(GA) RAN-translated proteins cause neurotoxicity by inducing ER stress. Acta Neuropathol. 2014;128(4):505–24.
173. Walker AK, Soo KY, Sundaramoorthy V, Parakh S, Ma Y, Farg MA, et al. ALS-associated TDP-43 induces endoplasmic reticulum stress, which drives cytoplasmic TDP-43 accumulation and stress granule formation. PLoS One. 2013;8(11):e81170.
174. Farg MA, Sundaramoorthy V, Sultana JM, Yang S, Atkinson RA, Levina V, et al. C9ORF72, implicated in amytrophic lateral sclerosis and frontotemporal dementia, regulates endosomal trafficking. Hum Mol Genet. 2014;23(13):3579–95.
175. Dormann D, Rodde R, Edbauer D, Bentmann E, Fischer I, Hruscha A, et al. ALS-associated fused in sarcoma (FUS) mutations disrupt Transportin-mediated nuclear import. EMBO J. 2010;29(16):2841–57.
176. Farg MA, Soo KY, Walker AK, Pham H, Orian J, Horne MK, et al. Mutant FUS induces endoplasmic reticulum stress in amyotrophic lateral sclerosis and interacts with protein disulfide-isomerase. Neurobiol Aging. 2012;33(12):2855–68.
177. Dendrou CA, Fugger L, Friese MA. Immunopathology of multiple sclerosis. Nat Rev Immunol. 2015;15(9):545–58.
178. Ransohoff RM, Kivisakk P, Kidd G. Three or more routes for leukocyte migration into the central nervous system. Nat Rev Immunol. 2003;3(7):569–81.
179. Hoglund RA, Maghazachi AA. Multiple sclerosis and the role of immune cells. World J Exp Med. 2014;4(3):27–37.
180. Goverman J. Autoimmune T cell responses in the central nervous system. Nat Rev Immunol. 2009;9(6):393–407.
181. Libbey JE, McCoy LL, Fujinami RS. Molecular mimicry in multiple sclerosis. Int Rev Neurobiol. 2007;79:127–47.
182. Virtanen JO, Jacobson S. Viruses and multiple sclerosis. CNS Neurol Disord Drug Targets. 2012;11(5):528–44.
183. Cunnea P, Mháille AN, McQuaid S, Farrell M, McMahon J, FitzGerald U. Expression profiles of endoplasmic reticulum stress-related molecules in demyelinating lesions and multiple sclerosis. Mult Scler. 2011;17(7):808–18.
184. Mháille AN, McQuaid S, Windebank A, Cunnea P, McMahon J, Samali A, et al. Increased expression of endoplasmic reticulum stress-related signaling pathway molecules in multiple sclerosis lesions. J Neuropathol Exp Neurol. 2008;67(3):200–11.
185. Werner P, Pitt D, Raine CS. Glutamate excitotoxicity–a mechanism for axonal damage and oligodendrocyte death in multiple sclerosis? J Neural Transm Suppl. 2000;60:375–85.
186. Yu Z, Luo H, Fu W, Mattson MP. The endoplasmic reticulum stress-responsive protein GRP78 protects neurons against excitotoxicity and apoptosis: suppression of oxidative stress and stabilization of calcium homeostasis. Exp Neurol. 1999;155(2):302–14.
187. Hussien Y, Podojil JR, Robinson AP, Lee AS, Miller SD, Popko B. ER chaperone BiP/GRP78 is required for Myelinating cell survival and provides protection during experimental autoimmune encephalomyelitis. J Neurosci. 2015;35(48):15921–33.
188. Dimcheff DE, Faasse MA, McAtee FJ, Portis JL. Endoplasmic reticulum (ER) stress induced by a neurovirulent mouse retrovirus is associated with prolonged BiP binding and retention of a viral protein in the ER. J Biol Chem. 2004;279(32):33782–90.
189. Lin W, Harding HP, Ron D, Popko B. Endoplasmic reticulum stress modulates the response of myelinating oligodendrocytes to the immune cytokine interferon-gamma. J Cell Biol. 2005;169(4):603–12.
190. Xu K, Zhu XP. Endoplasmic reticulum stress and prion diseases. Rev Neurosci. 2012;23(1):79–84.
191. Torres M, Castillo K, Armisen R, Stutzin A, Soto C, Hetz C. Prion protein misfolding affects calcium homeostasis and sensitizes cells to endoplasmic reticulum stress. PLoS One. 2010;5(12):e15658.
192. Torres M, Encina G, Soto C, Hetz C. Abnormal calcium homeostasis and protein folding stress at the ER: a common factor in familial and infectious prion disorders. Commun Integr Biol. 2011;4(3):258–61.
193. Cai Y, Arikkath J, Yang L, Guo ML, Periyasamy P, Buch S. Interplay of endoplasmic reticulum stress and autophagy in neurodegenerative disorders. Autophagy. 2016;12(2):225–44.
194. Akay C, Lindl KA, Shyam N, Nabet B, Goenaga-Vazquez Y, Ruzbarsky J, et al. Activation status of integrated stress response pathways in neurones and astrocytes of HIV-associated neurocognitive disorders (HAND) cortex. Neuropath Appl Neurobiol. 2012;38(2):175–200.
195. Wei H, Kim S-J, Zhang Z, Tsai P-C, Wisniewski KE, Mukherjee AB. ER and oxidative stresses are common mediators of apoptosis in both neurodegenerative and non-neurodegenerative lysosomal storage disorders and are alleviated by chemical chaperones. Human Mol Gen. 2008;17(4):469–77.
196. Bosch ME, Kielian T. Neuroinflammatory paradigms in lysosomal storage diseases. Front Neurosci. 2015;9:417.
197. Riemer C, Gültner S, Heise I, Holtkamp N, Baier M. Neuroinflammation in prion diseases: concepts and targets for therapeutic intervention. CNS Neurol Disord Drug Targets. 2009;8(5):329–41.
198. Gannon P, Khan MZ, Kolson DL. Current understanding of HIV-associated neurocognitive disorders pathogenesis. Curr Opin Neurol. 2011;24(3):275–83.
199. Martinon F, Glimcher LH. Regulation of innate immunity by signaling pathways emerging from the endoplasmic reticulum. Curr Opin Immunol. 2011;23(1):35–40.
200. Zanetti M, Rodvold JJ, Mahadevan NR. The evolving paradigm of cell-nonautonomous UPR-based regulation of immunity by cancer cells. Oncogene. 2016;35(3):269–78.
201. Alliot F, Godin I, Pessac B. Microglia derive from progenitors, originating from the yolk sac, and which proliferate in the brain. Brain Res Dev Brain Res. 1999;117(2):145–52.
202. Kawabori M, Yenari MA. The role of the microglia in acute CNS injury. Metab Brain Dis. 2015;30(2):381–92.
203. Katsumoto A, Lu H, Miranda AS, Ransohoff RM. Ontogeny and functions of central nervous system macrophages. J Immunol. 2014;193(6):2615–21.
204. Miranda-Hernandez S, Baxter AG. Role of toll-like receptors in multiple sclerosis. Am J Clin Exp Immunol. 2013;2(1):75–93.
205. Farina C, Aloisi F, Meinl E. Astrocytes are active players in cerebral innate immunity. Trends Immunol. 2007;28(3):138–45.
206. Bjorkqvist M, Wild EJ, Thiele J, Silvestroni A, Andre R, Lahiri N, et al. A novel pathogenic pathway of immune activation detectable before clinical onset in Huntington's disease. J Exp Med. 2008;205(8):1869–77.
207. Ledo JH, Azevedo EP, Beckman D, Ribeiro FC, Santos LE, Razolli DS, et al. Cross talk between brain innate immunity and serotonin signaling underlies depressive-like behavior induced by Alzheimer's Amyloid-beta Oligomers in mice. J Neurosci. 2016;36(48):12106–16.
208. Paresce DM, Ghosh RN, Maxfield FR. Microglial cells internalize aggregates of the Alzheimer's disease amyloid beta-protein via a scavenger receptor. Neuron. 1996;17(3):553–65.
209. Minagar A, Shapshak P, Fujimura R, Ownby R, Heyes M, Eisdorfer C. The role of macrophage/microglia and astrocytes in the pathogenesis of three neurologic disorders: HIV-associated dementia, Alzheimer disease, and multiple sclerosis. J Neurol Sci. 2002;202(1–2):13–23.
210. Harvey LD, Yin Y, Attarwala IY, Begum G, Deng J, Yan HQ, et al. Administration of DHA reduces endoplasmic reticulum stress-associated inflammation and alters Microglial or macrophage activation in traumatic brain injury. ASN Neuro. 2015;7(6):1–15.
211. Hosoi T, Honda M, Oba T, Ozawa K. ER stress upregulated PGE_2/IFNγ-induced IL-6 expression and down-regulated iNOS expression in glial cells. Sci Rep. 2013;3:3388.
212. Guthrie LN, Abiraman K, Plyler ES, Sprenkle NT, Gibson SA, McFarland BC, et al. Attenuation of PKR-like ER Kinase (PERK) signaling selectively controls endoplasmic reticulum stress-induced inflammation without compromising immunological responses. J Biol Chem. 2016;291(30):15830–40.
213. Halliday M, Radford H, Sekine Y, Moreno J, Verity N, le Quesne J, et al. Partial restoration of protein synthesis rates by the small molecule ISRIB prevents neurodegeneration without pancreatic toxicity. Cell Death Dis. 2015;6:e1672.

Blood cholesterol in late-life and cognitive decline: a longitudinal study of the Chinese elderly

Chaoran Ma[1], Zhaoxue Yin[2], Pengfei Zhu[3], Jiesi Luo[2], Xiaoming Shi[3*] and Xiang Gao[1*]

Abstract

Background: Previous studies regarding the lipid-cognition relation in older adults are limited and have generated mixed results. We thus examined whether higher blood cholesterol concentrations were associated with faster cognitive decline in a community-based longitudinal study of Chinese elderly.

Methods: The study included 1,159 Chinese adults aged over 60 years (women: 48.7%, mean age: 79.4 years), who were free of dementia, Parkinson disease and stroke at the baseline. Blood concentrations of total cholesterol (TC), high-density lipoprotein cholesterol (HDL-C), low-density lipoprotein cholesterol (LDL-C), and triglycerides (TG), were assessed at the baseline. Global cognitive functions were assessed using the Chinese Mini-Mental State Examination (MMSE) at in 2009, 2012 and 2014. Association between blood cholesterol and repeated cognitive function was analyzed with linear mixed models, adjusting for sociodemographic information, behavior and lifestyle, depression symptoms, physical examination, hypertension, and laboratory indexes.

Results: Higher baseline TC and LDL-C concentrations were significantly associated with greater cognitive decline. Adjusted mean difference in cognitive decline rate, comparing two extreme quartiles, was 0.28 points (MMSE score) per year (95% confident interval (CI): -0.54,–0.02; P-trend = 0.005) for TC and 0.42 points per year (95% CI: -0.69, -0.16; P-trend = 0.006) for LDL-C. In a subgroup analysis, the associations between all lipids and cognitive decline appeared to be more pronounced among individuals aged 100 years or older ($n = 90$), relative to others.

Conclusions: Higher blood concentrations of TC and LDL-C in late-life were associated with faster global cognitive decline.

Keywords: Lipid, Cognitive function, MMSE

Background

Cognitive impairment is one of the greatest causes of disability and becomes the primary public health issues globally. There are approximately 20–30% of Americans and 8% Chinese aged over 65 years with cognitive impairment, ranging from mild deficits to dementia [1–3]. Because of rapid world population ageing, the number of people living with cognitive impairment is expected to jump up dramatically. Currently, there have been no reversible treatments for cognitive impairment. Early intervention thus is significant for the prevention of cognitive impairment.

Previous studies indicated that high non-high density lipoprotein cholesterol (HDL-C) concentration in middle age was a potential risk factor for subsequent occurrence of cognitive impairment in later life [4–6]. However, the literature did not yield consistent results when it came to older adults [7–11]. In fact, the central nervous system has a separate supply and circulatory system of lipoproteins, with cholesterol solely through de novo synthesis and at a minimum from the periphery transfer [12]. On the one hand, high cholesterol is involved in synaptogenesis in the brain, facilitating compensatory repair of injured neuronal pathways in cognitive impairment [13, 14]. On the other hand, high cholesterol also

* Correspondence: shixm@chinacdc.cn; xxg14@psu.edu
[3]National Institute of Environmental Health, Chinese Center for Disease Control and Prevention, Beijing 100021, China
[1]Department of Nutritional Sciences, The Pennsylvania State University, University Park, PA 16802, USA
Full list of author information is available at the end of the article

plays a role in the accumulation of amyloid beta peptides, which accelerates the development of cognitive impairment [12]. However, those contradictory results in older adults may also lie in confounding factors when blood lipids and cognitive function were assessed. For example, individuals with high lipid concentrations were more likely to use of statins, which were suggested to be neuroprotective against cognitive dysfunction [15–18]. Previous studies were dominantly based on US or other high-income countries. According to the report from US Centers for Disease Control and Prevention, cholesterol-lowering medication (primarily statins) use increased with age, up to 48% of adults aged 75 and over [19]. Based on the new guidelines released by the American College of Cardiology (ACC) and the American Heart Association (AHA), a third of adults in the U.S. have been recommended to use statins, without lipid-cognition relation taken into account [20]. In this context it is of significance to understand the association between lipid profiles and cognitive function. Because only 0.4% of Chinese adults living in rural areas in China used statins, as suggested by a national survey between 2005 and 2009 [21, 22], Chinese rural areas would be an excellent setting for studying this important research question. In addition, although the risk of cognitive impairment increases with age, there has been only few studies concerning the oldest-old and there still have been no longitudinal data of a Chinese oldest old population.

In the current study, we examined whether higher blood cholesterol concentrations were associated with faster cognitive decline in a community-based longitudinal study of Chinese elderly living in rural areas.

Methods

Study population

This longitudinal study based on participants aged over 60 years in the Chinese Longitudinal Healthy Longevity Survey (CLHLS), an ongoing community-based study in seven longevity areas in China. CLHLS was established in half of the counties and cities in 22 of China's 31 provinces in 1998, and then was conducted in years of 2000, 2002, 2005, 2009, 2012 and 2014 [23]. Since the wave of 2009, in-depth study has been conducted in the eight longevity areas [24], which included cognitive function, laboratory assessment, the questionnaire assessment, physical examination and anthropometric measurement.

Of 3163 potential participants aged 60 years and over, we excluded 91 people with dementia, Parkinson disease and stroke based on questionnaire, and 127 people with unreliable body mass index (BMI) (BMI < 10 or BMI > 60). We also excluded 654 participants with a Mini-Mental State Examination (MMSE) score of less than or equal to 10 because cognitive function was too impaired to be able to complete the cognitive tests or questionnaires, leaving 2,291 eligible participants. There were 1,056 participants who died during the follow-up or loss of follow-up, and 76 people with incomplete covariate information, leaving 1,159 individuals with at least two cognitive tests during the follow-up for the current analysis. Specifically, 390 participants participated cognitive test in 2009, 1,116 participants participated cognitive test in 2012, and 1072 participants participated the test in 2014. Compared with those eligible participants, individuals who died or lost to follow up, had an older age, higher percentage of women, less years of education, lower BMI, blood total cholesterol (TC), low density lipoprotein cholesterol (LDL-C) and MMSE scores at the baseline ($P < 0.05$ for all). The study was approved by the Institutional Review Board of Peking University, China. Informed consent was obtained from the participants or their representatives.

Assessment of lipid profile

At the baseline, 12-h overnight fasting plasma TC, LDL-C, HDL-C, and triglyceride (TG) were measured by an Automatic Biochemistry Analyzer (Hitachi 7180, Japan), using commercially available diagnostic kits (Roche Diagnostic, Mannheim, Germany) in the central clinical lab at Capital Medical University in Beijing. TC and TG concentrations were both measured by standard enzymatic methods (CHOD-PAP and GPO-PAP; Roche Diagnostics). HDL-C was measured by a direct method, and LDL-C was determined by the Friedewald formula (LDL-C = TC - HDL-C - TG/2.17 (in mmol/L)). LDL-C plays a role in forming plaque, a thick, hard deposit that can clog arteries and make them less flexible, i.e., atherosclerosis. Less than 3.37 mmol/L of LDL-C concentration is considered normal. TG is used to store excess energy as another type of fate and high levels of TG are associated with atherosclerosis. The normal range of TG concentration is less than 1.70 mmol/L. HDL-C helps remove LDL-C from the arteries, and higher than 1.55 mmol/L of HDL-C concentration is the normal expected level. As a combination of LDL-C, TG and HDL-C, high concentrations of TC is also an atherogenic marker. The desirable concentration of TC is less than 5.18 mmol/L.

Assessment of cognitive function

Global cognitive functions were assessed at 2009, 2012 and 2014, using the validated Chinese version of MMSE, which was culturally translated into Chinese language on the basis of the international standard of MMSE questionnaire [25]. MMSE scores ranged from 0 to 30, with the indication that higher scores reflect better cognitive function.

Assessment of potential covariates

Potential covariates included sociodemographic information (age, sex, and education levels), behavior and lifestyle (smoking status, alcohol intake, and physical activity), depression symptoms, physical examination (BMI, and waist circumference), hypertension, and laboratory indexes (plasma glucose, C-reactive protein and uric acid). Among the above data, sociodemographic information, behavior and lifestyle and depression symptoms were collected at baseline via questionnaires, Weight and height were measured by trained medical personnel. BMI was calculated as body weight (kg) divided by the square of height (m^2). The waist circumference was measured to the nearest 0.1 cm at the midpoint between the bottom of the rib cage and the top of the iliac crest at the end of exhalation. Systolic and diastolic blood pressures were measured twice from the seated position using a mercury sphygmomanometer. The average of the two readings was used for analysis. Plasma glucose and uric acid were assessed together with the lipid profile by an Automatic Biochemistry Analyzer (Hitachi 7180, Japan), using commercially available diagnostic kits (Roche Diagnostic, Mannheim, Germany).

Statistical analyses

To evaluate the relation of blood lipid profile to cognition we examined mean performance at each assessment using linear mixed models (which permits examination of each time point, taking into account lipid profile status at baseline and an interaction between lipid profile status and time). We considered a number of potential confounders for inclusion in each model: model 1 was adjusted for sociodemographic information; model 2 was adjusted for sociodemographic information, behavior and lifestyle; model 3 was adjusted for all the covariates stated before. Education was categorized as illiteracy, 1–6 years or ≥6 years. Smoking status was categorized as non-smoker and smoker (0, 0.7–20.4, 20.5–44.4, or 44.5–220 pack-year). Alcohol intake was categorized as non-drinker and drinker (0, 0.4–2.11, 2.12–4.67, or 4.68–67.7 servings/d). BMI was categorized by 17.5, 17.5–23.0, 23.0–27.9, or ≥28.0 kg/m^2. Waist circumference was categorized by 50–73, 74–80, 81–88, or 89–155 cm. Plasma glucose was categorized by 0.15–3.93, 3.94–4.68, 4.69–5.41, or 5.42–36.04 mmol/L. C-reactive protein was categorized by <1, 1–2.9, or ≥3 mg/L. Uric acid was categorized by <240, 240–360, or ≥360 for women, and <240, 240–420, or ≥420 μmol/L for men. Physical activity, depression symptoms and hypertension were classified as yes or no. The estimate for the effect of "lipid profile status" reflected the cross-sectional impact of the lipid profile status on cognitive function at baseline and was presented as the "cross-sectional effect." The estimate for the effect of "time" reflected the annual change in cognitive function and was presented as "change over time." The estimate for "interaction" of the lipid profile status and time reflected the additional annual impact of the lipid profile status on cognitive function and was presented as "additional annual effect." We examined linear trends across quartiles of a given lipid using a continuous variable in which participants in a given category were assigned the median value.

Given the possibility that age (60–79 y, 80–99 y, and 100+ y) and sex at baseline could modify the association between lipid profile and cognitive decline, interaction terms for these variables and lipid profile were evaluated, and subgroup analyses by these variables were further conducted. All statistical analyses were conducted using SAS version 9.4 (SAS Institute, Inc, Cary, NC). Formal hypothesis testing will be 2-sided with a significant level of 0.05.

Results

Of 1,159 participants, 48.7% were women. The mean age was 79.4 years (ranged 60–112 y) and the mean education years was two years (ranged 0–19 years). Compared with those with a lower TC concentration, participants with a higher TC concentration had an older age, a higher percentage of women and hypertension, a higher BMI, blood uric acid and LDL-C concentration, and a larger waist circumference ($P < 0.05$) (Table 1). No differences were observed with other covariates.

Higher concentrations of TC and LDL-C were associated with faster decline in the MMSE score over time (Table 2). Adjusted mean difference in annual cognitive decline rate, comparing two extreme quartiles, was -0.28 points (95% confidence interval (CI): -0.54, -0.02; P trend = 0.005) for TC and -0.42 points (95% CI: -0.69, -0.16; P trend = 0.006) for LDL-C. The magnitudes were equivalent to 2.0- and 3.0-year ageing observed in the current study, respectively. In contrast, we did not observe significant relations between HDL-C/TG concentrations and cognitive decline (P trend > 0.05 for both).

We did not find any significant interaction between age, sex, and cognitive decline (P for interaction >0.05 for all; Figs. 1 and 2). However, in a subgroup analysis, the associations between all lipids and cognitive decline appeared to be more pronounced among individuals aged 100 years or older ($n = 90$), relative to others (Fig. 1 & Additional file 1).

Discussion

In this community-based longitudinal study of over 1,100 Chinese older adults living in rural area, we observed that higher blood concentrations of TC and LDL-C were associated with faster cognitive decline, independent of numerous potential co-determinants of

Table 1 Characteristics by quartile of baseline total cholesterol[a]

	Quartile 1	Quartile 2	Quartile 3	Quartile 4	P trend[b]
	0.35–3.46 mmol/L	3.47–4.14 mmol/L	4.15–4.84 mmol/L	4.85–8.79 mmol/L	
No.	290	287	293	289	
Age, y	78.4 (0.64)	79.0 (0.63)	80.4 (0.64)	80.0 (0.64)	0.03
Women, %	39.3	37.3	56.7	61.3	<0.001
Education, y	2.34 (0.18)	2.46 (0.18)	2.29 (0.18)	2.81 (0.19)	0.14
Smoking status, pack-year	8.59 (1.12)	8.87 (1.14)	7.59 (1.11)	10.98 (1.13)	0.25
Alcohol intake, servings/d	0.98 (0.47)	1.99 (0.48)	1.83 (0.47)	1.58 (0.48)	0.45
Physical activity, %	21.1	19.5	20.1	23.7	0.84
Depression symptoms, %	7.0	6.9	5.6	6.9	0.23
Body mass index, kg/m^2	21.0 (0.22)	21.6 (0.22)	21.6 (0.22)	22.5 (0.22)	<0.001
Waist circumference, cm	80.2 (0.63)	79.6 (0.64)	81.4 (0.63)	83.5 (0.63)	<0.001
Hypertension, %	49.7	55.4	61.4	59.2	0.02
LDL-C, mmol/L	1.66 (0.03)	2.11 (0.03)	2.59 (0.03)	3.45 (0.03)	<0.001
Glucose, mmol/L	5.10 (0.13)	4.71 (0.13)	4.99 (0.13)	4.88 (0.13)	0.51
Uric acids, μmol/L	272.5 (4.90)	278.2 (4.94)	284.1 (4.87)	299.9 (4.94)	<0.001

[a]Values are mean (standard error) adjusted for age and sex
[b]Adjusted for age and sex

decline, including diabetes, hypertension, and blood uric acids concentration.

Consistent with our findings, one 7-year longitudinal study with 6,855 French participants (mean age = 74 y) showed that higher TC and LDL-C concentrations in men were associated with a higher risk of cognitive decline over time [7]. Similar results were observed in another longitudinal study of 1037 US postmenopausal women with 4 years of follow-up (mean age = 71 y), reporting that individuals with decrement of TC over time was associated with lower odds of impairment [8]. In contrast, there have been a few US-based studies reporting that total serum cholesterol concentrations in subjects older than 65 years were not associated with the incidence of dementia during follow-up [10, 11]. Given that participants in those longitudinal studies were all Caucasians, racial and ethnic differences might account for the result discrepancies. Further, the cholesterol-lowering medication (primarily statins) use was up to 66.5% in high-income countries [22], while the using rate in China was only 1.7% throughout the country, much less in the rural areas (0.4%) [21, 22]. Consistently, in another national survey in China based on 23,129 Chinese adults aged 30-79 years with cardiovascular disease, only 1.4% of participants used statins during 2004–08; the prevalence of statin use was significantly lower among those with lower education and household income, relative to their counterparts [26]. In this context, we speculate that the different results observed in our studies and some previous studied conducted in high-income counties could be partially explained by statin use. However, there have been no longitudinal studies, to our knowledge, on the lipid-cognition relation in general population, stratified by statin use.

We also found that the lipid-cognition association was more pronounced in individuals aged 100 years or older, relative to others. This could be due to the faster cognitive decline rate in this age group, relative to their younger counterparts. However, significant association between lipid and cognitive function was not observed in a previous cross-sectional study conducted in centenarians [27]. One possible explanation for this discrepancy may be the current study's longer follow up period, which may have better captured cognitive trajectories. It is also possible that cardiovascular events due to the low prevalence of statin use could lead to cognitive decline. However, the interaction between age and cholesterol concentrations was not significant in the current study, which was probably due to the small number in centenarian group (n = 90). We cannot exclude the possibility of chance finding.

Some possible biological mechanisms may explain the observed association between high cholesterol concentrations and faster cognitive decline in the current study. Compared to cholesterol of the periphery with de novo synthesis and provided by diet half and half, brain cholesterol is stable, with the major input solely through de novo synthesis locally rather than transfer from the periphery. Therefore, the central nervous system contains its own supple of lipoproteins [12]. Brain cholesterol has been implicated to play a role in altering the degradation

Table 2 Mean difference and 95% confidence interval in annual cognitive decline according to quartile of lipid concentrations

	Quartile 1	Quartile 2	Quartile 3	Quartile 4	Cognitive decline for each mmol/L increment	P Trend
TC						
	0.35–3.46 mmol/L	3.47–4.14 mmol/L	4.15–4.84 mmol/_	4.85–8.79 mmol/L		
N	290	287	293	289		
Median (mmol/L)	2.88	3.83	4.45	5.38		
Model 1[a]	0 (ref.)	−0.10 (−0.33, 0.13)))	−0.25 (−0.49, −0.01)	−0.26 (−0.52, −0.003)	−0.09 (−0.16, −0.02)	0.009
Model 2[b]	0 (ref.)	−0.10 (−0.33, 0.13)	−0.26 (−0.50, −0.02)	−0.27 (−0.52, −0.01)	−0.09 (−0.16, −0.02)	0.008
Model 3[c]	0 (ref.)	−0.12 (−0.36, 0.12)	−0.28 (−0.52, −0.03)	−0.28 (−0.54, −0.02)	−0.10 (−0.17, −0.03)	0.005
LDL-C						
	0.20–1.85 mmol/L	1.86–2.39 mmol/L	2.40–2.97 mmol/L	2.98–5.69 mmol/L		
N	290	287	291	291		
Median (mmol/L)	1.51	2.14	2.66	3.44		
Model 1[a]	0 (ref.)	−0.24 (−0.47, −0.02)	−0.18 (−0.43, 0.06)	−0.38 (−0.64, −0.12)	−0.14 (−0.25, −0.03)	0.01
Model 2[b]	0 (ref.)	−0.25 (−0.47, −0.02)	−0.19 (−0.43, 0.06)	−0.40 (−0.66, −0.14)	−0.15 (−0.26, −0.04)	0.008
Model 3[c]	0 (ref.)	−0.26 (−0.48, −0.03)	−0.20 (−0.45, 0.04)	−0.42 (−0.69, −0.16)	−0.16 (−0.27, −0.04)	0.006
HDL-C						
	1.48–3.18 mmol/L	1.22–1.47 mmol/L	1.01–1.21 mmol/L	0.01–1.00 mmol/L		
N	293	286	289	291		
Median (mmol/L)	0.88	1.12	1.32	1.70		
Model 1[a]	0 (ref.)	0.12 (−0.11, 0.35)	−0.02 (−0.26, 0.22)	−0.04 (−0.30, 0.21)	0.01 (−0.24, 0.27)	0.91
Model 2[b]	0 (ref.)	0.12 (−0.12, 0.35) −0.03 (−0.27, 0.21)9-0.11, 0.36)	−0.03 (−0.29, 0.22) 9–0.27	−0.04 (−0.20, 0.22) 99((9–0.3	0.02 (−0.23, 0.28)	0.87
Model 3[c]	0 (ref.)	0.10 (−0.14, 0.34)	−0.04 (−0.29, 0.21)	−0.05 (−0.31, 0.21)	0.01 (−0.25, 0.27)	0.93
TG						
	0.13–0.67 mmol/L	0.68–0.92 mmol/L	0.93–1.32 mmol/L	1.33–8.05 mmol/L		
N	287	296	287	289		

Table 2 Mean difference and 95% confidence interval in annual cognitive decline according to quartile of lipid concentrations *(Continued)*

Median (mmol/L)	0.54	0.79	1.09	1.89		
Model 1[a]	0 (ref.)	0.17 (−0.13, 0.45)	0.14 (−0.15, 0.44)	0.16 (−0.13, 0.45)	0.06 (−0.02, 0.14)	0.13
Model 2[b]	0 (ref.)	0.17 (−0.12, 0.47)	0.14 (−0.15, 0.44)	0.16 (−0.12, 0.45)	0.06 (−0.02, 0.14)	0.13
Model 3[c]	0 (ref.)	0.17 (−0.13, 0.47)	0.14 (−0.16, 0.44)	0.18 (−0.11, 0.47)	0.06 (−0.02, 0.14)	0.12

Abbreviation: *TC* total cholesterol, *LDL-C* low density lipoprotein cholesterol, *HDL-C* high density lipoprotein cholesterol, *TG* triglyceride

[a]Adjusted for age, sex and education (illiteracy, 1–6 years, or ≥6 years)

[b]Adjusted for age, sex, education, smoking status (non-smoker and smoker (0.7–20.4, 20.5–44.4, or 44.5–220 pack-year)), alcohol intake (non-drinker and drinker (0.4–2.11, 2.12–4.67, or 4.68–67.7 servings/d)), physical activities (yes/no), depression symptoms (yes/no)

[c]Adjusted for age, sex, education, smoking status, alcohol intake, physical activity, depression, BMI (<17.5, 17.5–23.0, 23.0–27.9, or ≥28.0 kg/m^2), waist circumference (50–73, 74–80, 81–88, or 89–155 cm), hypertension (yes/no), plasma glucose (0.15–3.93, 3.94–4.68, 4.69–5.41, or 5.42–36.04 mmol/L), C-reactive protein (<1, 1–2.9, or ≥3 mg/L) and uric acid (women: <240, 240–360, or ≥360; men: <240, 240–420, or ≥420 μmol/L)

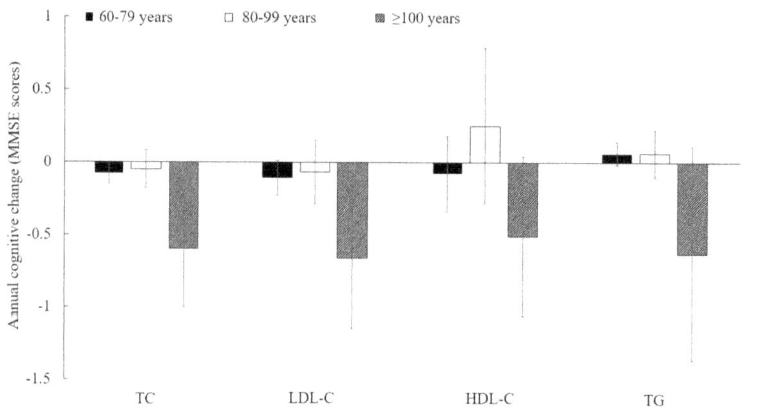

Fig. 1 Mean difference in annual cognitive change for each mmol/L increment of lipid concentrations, stratified by age [a]. Abbreviation: TC = total cholesterol; LDL-C = low density lipoprotein cholesterol; HDL-C = high density lipoprotein cholesterol; TG = triglyceride. P interaction > 0.50 for all, suggesting that the association between lipids and cognitive decline was not modified by age. [a]Adjusted for age, sex, education (illiteracy, 1–6 years, or ≥6 years), smoking status (non-smoker and smoker (0.7–20.4, 20.5–44.4, or 44.5–220 pack-year)), alcohol intake (non-drinker and drinker (0.4–2.11, 2.12–4.67, or 4.68–67.7 servings/d)), physical activities (yes/no), depression symptoms (yes/no), BMI (<17.5, 17.5–23.0, 23.0–27.9, or ≥28.0 kg/m^2), waist circumference (50–73, 74–80, 81–88, or 89–155 cm), hypertension (yes/no), plasma glucose (0.15–3.93, 3.94–4.68, 4.69–5.41, or 5.42–36.04 mmol/L), C-reactive protein (<1, 1–2.9, or ≥3 mg/L) and uric acid (women: <240, 240–360, or ≥360; men: <240, 240–420, or ≥420 μmol/L)

of the amyloid precursor protein, which could have impact on the accumulation of amyloid beta peptides, contributing to the pathogenesis of dementia [12]. In addition, hypercholesterolemia is involved in atherogenesis, which could result in macro- and micro- vascular diseases, deteriorating cognitive function both at subclinical [28, 29] and clinical levels [30].

Strengths of this study include its longitudinal design, inclusion of centenarians, and incorporation of time-dependent covariates. However, our study was limited by lack of a comprehensive neuropsychological battery to capture all detailed aspects of cognitive function. The MMSE is a relatively simple screening tool for dementia. Nevertheless, we measured the MMSE at three time points, which would allow us to capture the global pattern of cognitive change over time. Residual confounding is of concern because we did not collect information on ApoE genotype and dietary intake. Another limitation is high rate of loss to follow-up due to the old age and low education status of our participants. The diagnoses of dementia, Parkinson disease and stroke were not confirmed by review of medical records.

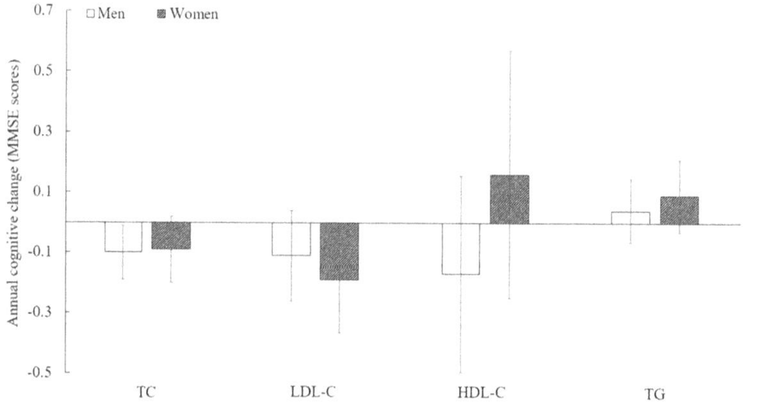

Fig. 2 Mean difference in annual cognitive change for each mmol/L increment of lipid concentrations, stratified by sex [a]. Abbreviation: TC = total cholesterol; LDL-C = low density lipoprotein cholesterol; HDL-C = high density lipoprotein cholesterol; TG = triglyceride.P interaction > 0.50 for all, suggesting that the association between lipids and cognitive decline was not modified by sex. [a] Adjusted for age, sex, education (illiteracy, 1–6 years, or ≥6 years), smoking status (non-smoker and smoker (0.7–20.4, 20.5–44.4, or 44.5–220 pack-year)), alcohol intake (non-drinker and drinker (0.4–2.11, 2.12–4.67, or 4.68–67.7 servings/d)), physical activities (yes/no), depression symptoms (yes/no), BMI (<17.5, 17.5–23.0, 23.0–27.9, or ≥28.0 kg/m^2), waist circumference (50–73, 74–80, 81–88, or 89–155 cm), hypertension (yes/no), plasma glucose (0.15–3.93, 3.94–4.68, 4.69–5.41, or 5.42–36.04 mmol/L), C-reactive protein (<1, 1–2.9, or ≥3 mg/L) and uric acid (women: <240, 240–360, or ≥360; men: <240, 240–420, or ≥420 μmol/L)

Conclusions

In conclusion, higher blood concentrations of TC and LDL-C in late-life were associated with faster global cognitive decline in this older Chinese rural population. The associations appeared to be stronger among those aged 100 years or older. Further studies with ApoE data available, larger sample size, and a comprehensive neuropsychological battery to capture specific cognitive effects are warranted to confirm our findings.

Abbreviations

ACC: American College of Cardiology; AHA: American heart association; BMI: Body mass index; CLHLS: Chinese longitudinal healthy longevity survey; HDL-C: High-density lipoprotein cholesterol; LDL-C: Low-density lipoprotein cholesterol; MMSE: Mini-mental state examination; TC: Total cholesterol; TG: Triglyceride.

Acknowledgements

Not applicable.

Funding

This work was supported by the National Natural Science Foundation of China (81273160 to X.M.S.); and the National Institute of Neurological Disorders And Stroke at the National Institutes of Health (NINDS 1R21NS087235-01A1 to X.G.).

Authors' contributions

CM analyzed and interpreted the data and was a major contributor in writing the manuscript. ZY participated in drafting/revising the manuscript. PZ participated in drafting/revising the manuscript. JL participated in drafting/revising the manuscript. XS acquired data and participated in drafting/revising the manuscript. XG conceptualized the research, participated in the analysis and interpretation of data and drafting the work, and gave final approval. All authors read and approved the final manuscript.

Competing interests

The authors declare that they have no competing interests.

Author details

[1]Department of Nutritional Sciences, The Pennsylvania State University, University Park, PA 16802, USA. [2]Division of Chronic Disease Control and Community Health, Chinese Center for Disease Control and Prevention, Beijing 102206, China. [3]National Institute of Environmental Health, Chinese Center for Disease Control and Prevention, Beijing 100021, China.

References

1. Association As. 2015 Alzheimer's disease facts and figures. Alzheimers Dement. 2015;11(3):332–84.
2. Roberts R, Knopman DS. Classification and epidemiology of MCI. Clin Geriatr Med. 2013;29(4):753–72.
3. Rodriguez JL, Ferri CP, Acosta D, Guerra M, Huang Y, Jacob KS, et al. Prevalence of dementia in Latin America, India, and China: a population-based cross-sectional survey. Lancet. 2008;372(9637):464–74.
4. Kaffashian S, Dugravot A, Nabi H, Batty GD, Brunner E, Kivimäki M, et al. Predictive utility of the Framingham general cardiovascular disease risk profile for cognitive function evidence from the Whitehall II study. Eur Heart J. 2011;32(18):2326–32.
5. Kivipelto M, Helkala EL, Hänninen T, Laakso MP, Hallikainen M, Alhainen K, et al. Midlife vascular risk factors and late-life mild cognitive impairment A population-based study. Neurology. 2001;56(12):1683–9.
6. Whitmer RA, Sidney S, Selby J, Johnston SC, Yaffe K. Midlife cardiovascular risk factors and risk of dementia in late life. Neurology. 2005;64(2):277–81.
7. Ancelin ML, Ripoche E, Dupuy AM, Samieri C, Rouaud O, Berr C, et al. Gender-specific associations between lipids and cognitive decline in the elderly. Eur Neuropsychopharmacol. 2014;24(7):1056–66.
8. Yaffe K, Barrett-Connor E, Lin F, Grady D. Serum Lipoprotein Levels, Statin Use, and Cognitive Function in Older Women. Arch Neurol. 2002;59:378–84.
9. Benito-Leon J, Vega-Quiroga S, Villarejo-Galende A, Bermejo-Pareja F. Hypercholesterolemia in elders is associated with slower cognitive decline: a prospective, population-based study (NEDICES). J Neurol Sci. 2015; 350(1-2):69–74.
10. Li G, Shofer JB, Kukull WA, Peskind ER, Tsuang DW, Breitner JC, et al. Serum cholesterol and risk of Alzheimer disease: a community-based cohort study. Neurology. 2005;65(7):1045–50.
11. Tan AS, Seshadri S, Beiser A, Wilson PWF, Kiel DP, Tocco M, et al. Plasma Total Cholesterol Level as a Risk Factor for Alzheimer Disease: The Framingham Study. Arch Intern Med. 2003;163(9):1053–7.
12. Bums M, Duff K. Cholesterol in Alzheimer's disease and tauopathy. Ann N Y Acad Sci. 2002;977:367–75.
13. Mauch DH, Nagler K, Schumacher S, Goritz C, Muller EC, Otto A, et al. CNS synaptogenesis promoted by glia-derived cholesterol. Science (New York, NY). 2001;294(5545):1354–7.
14. Goritz C, Mauch DH, Nagler K, Pfrieger FW. Role of glia-derived cholesterol in synaptogenesis: new revelations in the synapse-glia affair. J Physiol Paris. 2002;96(3-4):257–63.
15. Jick H, Zornberg GL, Jick SS, Seshadri S, Drachman DA. Statins and the risk of dementia. Lancet. 2000;356(9242):1627–31.
16. Wolozin B, Kellman W, Ruosseau P, Celesia GG, Siegel G. Decreased prevalence of Alzheimer disease associated with 3-hydroxy-3-methyglutaryl coenzyme A reductase inhibitors. Arch Neurol. 2000;57(10):1439–43.
17. Bettermann K, Arnold AM, Williamson J, Rapp S, Sink K, Toole JF, et al. Statins, risk of dementia, and cognitive function: secondary analysis of the ginkgo evaluation of memory study. J Stroke Cerebrovasc Dis. 2012;21(6):436–44.
18. Sparks DL, Kryscio RJ, Sabbagh MN, Connor DJ, Sparks LM, Liebsack C. Reduced risk of incident AD with elective statin use in a clinical trial cohort. Curr Alzheimer Res. 2008;5(4):416–21.
19. Gu QP, Paulose-Ram R, Burt VL, Kit BK. Prescription Cholesterol-lowering Medication Use in Adults Aged 40 and Over United States, 2003–2012. NCHS Data Brief. 2014;177:1–8.
20. Stone NJ, Robinson JG, Lichtenstein AH, Bairey Merz CN, Blum CB, Eckel RH, et al. 2013 ACC/AHA guideline on the treatment of blood cholesterol to reduce atherosclerotic cardiovascular risk in adults: a report of the American College of Cardiology/American Heart Association Task Force on Practice Guidelines. J Am Coll Cardiol. 2014;63(25 Pt B):2889–934.
21. Yang J, Chen T, Li W, Liu L, Teo K, Yusuf S, et al. Current Status of Medication Usage for Cardiovascular Disease and Hypertension in China (PURE-China Study). Circulation. 2012;126:A15144.
22. Salim Y, Shofiqul I, Chow CK, Rangarajan S, Dagenais G, Diaz R, et al. Use of secondary prevention drugs for cardiovascular disease in the community in high-income, middle-income, and low-income countries (the PURE Study): a prospective epidemiological survey. Lancet. 2011;378(9798):1231–43.
23. Yin Z, Shi X, Kraus VB, Brasher MS, Chen H, Liu Y, et al. Gender-dependent association of body mass index and waist circumference with disability in the Chinese oldest old. Obesity (Silver Spring, Md). 2014;22(8):1918–25.
24. Yin ZX, Shi XM, Kraus VB, Fitzgerald SM, Qian HZ, Xu JW, et al. High normal plasma triglycerides are associated with preserved cognitive function in Chinese oldest-old. Age Ageing. 2012;41(5):600–6.
25. Zeng Y, Vaupel JW. Functional capacity and self-evaluation of health and life of oldest old in China. J Soc ssues. 2002;58(4):733–48.
26. Chen Y, Li L, Zhang Q, Clarke R, Chen J, Guo Y, et al. Use of drug treatment for secondary prevention of cardiovascular disease in urban and rural communities of China: China Kadoorie Biobank Study of 0.5 million people. Int J Cardiol. 2014;172(1):88–95.

27. Huang CQ, Dong BR, Wu HM, Zhang YL, Wu JH, Lu ZC, et al. Association of cognitive impairment with serum lipid/lipoprotein among Chinese nonagenarians and centenarians. Dement Geriatr Cogn Disord. 2009; 27(2):111–6.
28. Wendell CR, Zonderman AB, Metter EJ, Najjar SS, Waldstein SR. Carotid intimal medial thickness predicts cognitive decline among adults without clinical vascular disease. Stroke. 2009;40(10):3180–5.
29. Wright CN, Festa JR, Paik MC, Schmiedigen A, Brown TR, Yoshita M, et al. White Matter Hyperintensities and Subclinical Infarction Associations with Psychomotor Speed and Cognitive Flexibility. Stroke. 2008;39(3):800–5.
30. de Haan EH, Nys GM, Van Zandvoort MJ. Cognitive function following stroke and vascular cognitive impairment. Curr Opin Neurol. 2006;19(6):559–64.

Intrastriatal injection of α-synuclein can lead to widespread synucleinopathy independent of neuroanatomic connectivity

Zachary A. Sorrentino[1,2], Mieu M.T. Brooks[1,2,4], Vincent Hudson III[1,2], Nicola J. Rutherford[1,2], Todd E. Golde[1,2,3], Benoit I. Giasson[1,2,3*] and Paramita Chakrabarty[1,2,3*]

Abstract

Background: Prionoid transmission of α-synuclein (αSyn) aggregates along neuroanatomically connected projections is posited to underlie disease progression in α-synucleinopathies. Here, we specifically wanted to study whether this prionoid progression occurs via direct inter-neuronal transfer and, if so, would intrastriatal injection of αSyn aggregates lead to nigral degeneration.

Methods: To test prionoid transmission of αSyn aggregates along the nigro-striatal pathway, we injected amyloidogenic αSyn aggregates into two different regions of the striatum of adult human wild type αSyn transgenic mice (Line M20) or non-transgenic (NTG) mice and aged for 4 months.

Results: M20 mice injected in internal capsule (IC) or caudate putamen (CPu) regions of the striatum showed florid αSyn inclusion pathology distributed throughout the neuraxis, irrespective of anatomic connectivity. These αSyn inclusions were found in different cell types including neurons, astrocytes and even ependymal cells. On the other hand, intra-striatal injection of αSyn fibrils into NTG mice resulted in sparse αSyn pathology, mostly localized in the striatum and entorhinal cortex. Interestingly, NTG mice injected with preformed human αSyn fibrils showed no induction of αSyn inclusion pathology, suggesting the presence of a species barrier for αSyn fibrillar seeds. Modest levels of nigral dopaminergic (DA) neuronal loss was observed exclusively in substantia nigra (SN) of M20 cohorts injected in the IC, even in the absence of frank αSyn inclusions in DA neurons. None of the NTG mice or CPu-injected M20 mice showed DA neurodegeneration. Interestingly, the pattern and distribution of induced αSyn pathology corresponded with neuroinflammation especially in the SN of M20 cohorts. Hypermorphic reactive astrocytes laden with αSyn inclusions were abundantly present in the brains of M20 mice.

Conclusions: Overall, our findings show that the pattern and extent of dissemination of αSyn pathology does not necessarily follow expected neuroanatomic connectivity. Further, the presence of intra-astrocytic αSyn pathology implies that glial cells participate in αSyn transmission and possibly have a role in non-cell autonomous disease modification.

Keywords: α-synuclein, Amyloid, Prion, Striatum, Dopaminergic Neurodegeneration, Astrocyte

* Correspondence: bgiasson@ufl.edu; pchakrabarty@ufl.edu
[1]Department of Neuroscience, University of Florida, 1275 Center Drive, PO Box 100159, Gainesville, FL 32610, USA
Full list of author information is available at the end of the article

Background

Intracellular accumulation of misfolded α-synuclein (αSyn) is a neuropathological hallmark of α-synucleinopathies [1–3]. Inclusions comprised of amyloidogenic αSyn aggregates, phosphorylated at Serine129 [4–6] are often found in neuronal cell bodies termed Lewy bodies (LB) or in neuronal projections, called Lewy neurites [1–3]. Nevertheless, how αSyn pathology initiates and spreads in the nervous system is still an area of intense research and debate.

In recent years, prion-like conformational templating has emerged as a plausible major mechanism that may explain the stereotypic progression of pathogenic αSyn into different brain regions [7–10]. Cell culture studies have shown that endogenous αSyn can be conformationally altered in the presence of exogenous pathologic αSyn to aggregate into inclusions [11–14], akin to classical prions [15, 16]. In vivo evidence for this prion-like characteristic of αSyn pathogenesis emerged from studies involving direct intracerebral injections of preformed αSyn amyloid fibrils in αSyn transgenic mice [17, 18]. More recently, studies have shown that peripheral (intramuscular, intraperitoneal or intravenous) injections of αSyn amyloid fibrils into rodents can induce progressive formation of αSyn pathology in the CNS [19–22]. However, the extent of induction and spread of seeded αSyn pathology in wild type nontransgenic (NTG) mice brains, on the other hand is more disparate; for example, while our group has observed that molecular templating and dissemination of pathogenic αSyn is an imprecise event in NTG mice [23], others have reported robust and widespread αSyn pathologies following exogenous αSyn challenge in NTG mice [14, 24–26]. Interestingly, injecting different molecular strains of αSyn can result in distinctive pathologies in rodents, possibly reflective of the spectrum of disease pathologies seen in different types of α-synucleinopathies [20, 27, 28]. Such dependence of seeded pathology on the presence of distinct conformer strains has been shown to exist in classical prion diseases [29]. Overall, these studies have established that αSyn can spread in the CNS by prion-like templating mechanisms [7–10].

Several recent publications have reported that following intracerebral injection of preformed αSyn fibrils, induction of intra-neuronal αSyn pathology leads to neurodegeneration, especially in the dopaminergic (DA) neurons of the nigrostriatal pathway [20, 24, 30]. This is reminiscent of selective neurodegeneration in α-synucleinopathies, such as Parkinson's disease [31]. Understanding how intercellular transmission of pathological αSyn along specific neuroanatomic projections leads to selective neurodegeneration in Parkinsonisms and related Lewy body dementias will allow us to design better therapeutics against these diseases. To test whether intrastriatal injection of pathological αSyn aggregates leads to selective nigral degeneration and further whether this is dependent on overexpression of human αSyn transgene, we administered preformed αSyn aggregates into the internal capsule (IC) or the caudate putamen (CPu) areas of either Line M20 (transgenic mice expressing human wild type (WT) αSyn [32]) or NTG mice. Our results indicate that while induction of αSyn pathology was sparse in NTG mice, M20 mice showed extensive Lewy-type inclusion pathology widely distributed throughout the brain, irrespective of anatomic connectivity. Surprisingly, we did not observe any αSyn inclusion pathology in DA neurons and only modest levels of DA neurodegeneration were noticed in M20 mice injected in the IC. We observed induction of gliosis that is associated with incipient αSyn pathology and interestingly, massive levels of pathological αSyn inclusions were detected within astrocytes in M20 mice. Overall, our results suggest that a combination of glial and neuronal inclusion pathology may result in distinctive αSyn strains that display widespread patterns of dissipation throughout the CNS without obvious direct neuroanatomic connectivity.

Methods

Expression and purification of recombinant αSyn protein

The bacterial expression plasmid pRK172 cDNA construct encoding full-length WT human or mouse αSyn was used to express these proteins in *E. coli* BL21 (DE3) and they were purified to homogeneity by size exclusion (Superdex 200 gel filtration) followed by ion exchange (Mono Q) chromatographies as previously described [33].

Fibril preparation of recombinant αSyn for mouse brain injection

Human αSyn recombinant protein or mouse αSyn recombinant protein was assembled into filaments by incubation at 37 °C at 5 mg/ml in sterile PBS (Invitrogen) with continuous shaking at 1050 rpm (Thermomixer R, Eppendorf, Westbury, NY). αSyn amyloid fibril assembly was monitored as previously described with K114 fluorometry [12]. αSyn fibrils were diluted to a concentration of 2 mg/mL in sterile PBS and gently sonicated at room temperature in a water bath sonicator for 1 h. This resulted in fragmentation of αSyn amyloid aggregates into shorter fibrils [17, 22]. These fibrils were imaged using transmission electron microscopy (EM) (Additional file 1: Figure S1), and were validated for induction of intracellular amyloid inclusion formation in cell culture as previously described [12]. For EM imaging, fibrils were adsorbed to 300-mesh carbon-coated copper grids, washed, stained with 1% uranyl acetate, and imaged at 100,000× magnification using a Hitachi H7600 transmission electron microscope (Hitachi).

Mouse husbandry and stereotactic injections

All procedures were performed according to the NIH Guide for the Care and Use of Experimental Animals and were approved by the University of Florida Institutional Animal Care and Use Committee. Line M20 mice express human WT αSyn and do not develop any intrinsic phenotype or αSyn pathology [32]. 2 months old M20 or NTG mice were bilaterally injected with 2 μl of 2 mg/ml human or mouse WT αSyn fibrils in the IC (coordinates from Bregma: A/P -0.5, L +/−1.5, D/V -3.0; Cohorts 1, 2, 4 and 5) or CPu (coordinates from Bregma: A/P + 0.5, L +/−2.0, D/V -3.5; Cohort 3 and Cohort 6). The inoculum was injected at a rate of 0.2 μl per min with the needle in place for 15 min at each site. Mice were analyzed 4–5 months following injection. Cohort sizes are described in Figs. 1 and 3.

Antibodies

The following antibodies were used to detect pathological αSyn phosphorylated at Ser129: 81A (B. Giasson; 1:10,000 for immunohistochemistry and 1:3000 for immunofluorescence; [5]) and EP1536Y (1:1000; AbCam, Cambridge, MA). The latter antibody specifically reacts with pSer129-αSyn and does not cross-react with phosphorylated low-molecular-mass neurofilament subunit [7]. Other antibodies used in this study are: Syn506, a conformation specific anti-αSyn antibody that preferentially detects αSyn in pathological inclusions (B. Giasson; 1:1000; [34]); anti-p62/sequestosome antibody (SQSTM1) (Proteintech, Chicago, IL); anti-glial fibrillary acidic protein (GFAP) (Dako, Carpentaria, CA); anti-Iba-1 antibody (1:1000; Wako, Richmond, VA) and anti-tyrosine hydroxylase (TH) antibody (Millipore, Billerica, MA).

Immunohistochemical and immunofluorescence analyses

Mouse brains and spinal cords were collected following intra-cardiac perfusion with PBS/heparin. Tissues were fixed with 70% ethanol/150 mM NaCl for 48 h followed by paraffin processing. Paraffin-embedded tissue sections were deparaffinized and hydrated through a series of graded ethanol solutions followed by washing with 0.1 M Tris, pH 7.6. The sections were blocked with 2% FBS in 0.1 M Tris, pH 7.6. Immunohistochemical detection was done using avidin-biotin complex (ABC) system (Vectastain ABC Elite Kit, Vector Laboratories, Burlingame, CA) and immunocomplexes were visualized with the chromogen 3,3′-diaminobenzidine (DAB). Sections were counterstained with hematoxylin. Slides were scanned using an Aperio ScanScope CS (Aperio Technologies Inc., Vista, CA) and images acquired using the ImageScopeTM software (Aperio Technologies Inc.). Quantification of immunostaining was done using the Pixel count Program (ImageScope, Aperio Technologies). For immunofluorescence detection, sections were incubated with secondary antibodies conjugated to Alexa fluor 594 or Alexa fluor 488 (Invitrogen, Eugene, OR) followed by Sudan Black treatment and staining with DAPI (Invitrogen, Eugene, OR). The sections were coverslipped with Fluoromount-G (Southern Biotech, Birmingham, AL) and visualized using an Olympus BX51 microscope mounted with a DP71 Olympus digital camera.

Stereological analysis of TH neurons in the substantia nigra

TH-positive neurons in the substantia nigra (SN) were counted by staining paraffin-embedded sections with an anti-TH polyclonal antibody (Millipore, Billerica, MA). Stereological counting of DA neurons was performed by counting and tallying TH-immunopositive neurons on every tenth section based on a previously published report [35].

Results

Induction and spread of pathological αSyn in M20 mice does not strictly follow neuroanatomic projections

To test the idea that induction of αSyn pathology follows pre-determined neuroanatomic pathways, we injected

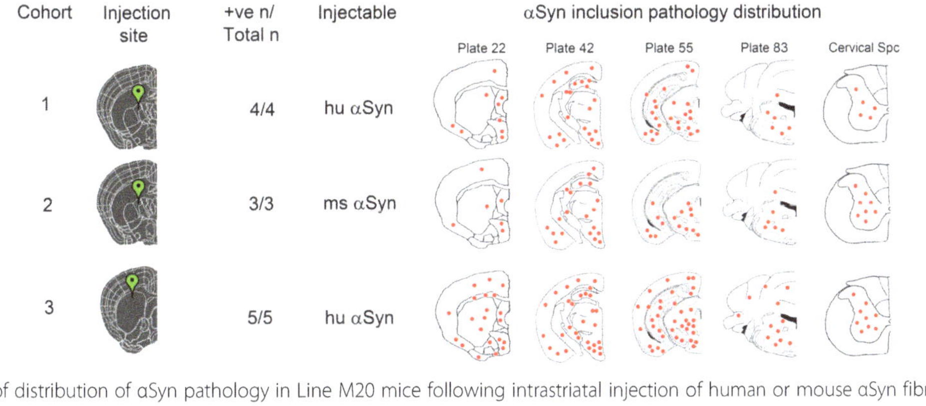

Fig. 1 Summary of distribution of αSyn pathology in Line M20 mice following intrastriatal injection of human or mouse αSyn fibrils. In Cohorts 1 and 2, mice were injected with human (hu) WT αSyn fibrils (Cohort 1) or mouse (ms) WT αSyn fibrils (Cohort 2) in the IC area whereas Cohort 3 mice were injected with human WT αSyn fibrils in the CPu. The total number of mice injected in each cohort as well as the number of mice actually displaying αSyn pathology is depicted (denoted as +ve n/Total n). Rostro-caudal distribution of αSyn inclusions is presented on a schematic brain and spinal cord map, with red dots depicting the relative abundance of αSyn inclusions in different brain and spinal cord locations. The numbers on top of the brain map schematics correspond to plates from the Paxinos Brain Atlas [57]

aggregated WT αSyn fibrils in two distinct regions of the striatum of 2 month old line M20 mice that overexpress human WT αSyn [32] as well as their NTG littermates. The M20 mice never intrinsically develop αSyn inclusion pathology or have overt phenotypes [32]. These injections were done to enable us to (1) study the efficiency of templated induction of WT αSyn pathology and (2) further conduct studies in NTG mice that are much less inherently susceptible to induction of αSyn inclusion pathology [23] so that we could better visualize and interpret frank transmission occurring via neuroanatomic connectivity. Cohorts 1 and 2 of M20 mice received bilateral injections into the IC while the Cohort 3 received bilateral injections in the CPu (Fig. 1). The IC, containing myelinated corticospinal tracts, intersects the caudate nucleus and putamen of the striatum. It serves as a conduit between motor areas, frontopontine, and thalamic peduncles to brain stem and cerebellar regions, and also between the thalamus and prefrontal cortex. Examination of Cohort 1 injected with human αSyn fibrils (Figs. 1 and 2a) or Cohort 2 injected with mouse αSyn fibrils (Figs. 1 and 2b) showed similar distribution of pSer129 αSyn/81A–immunopositive pathologies. αSyn pathology was further confirmed by staining sections with an additional antibody against pSer129-αSyn (EP1536Y) as well as an antibody raised against conformationally altered αSyn (Syn506). Immunostaining with p62/sequestosome confirmed that the intraneuronal and neuritic αSyn staining represented frank inclusion pathology (Fig. 2a-b). In both cohorts, robust αSyn inclusion pathology was found spread over multiple neuroanatomically connected areas as well as other areas of the brain that have no known direct connections to the IC. Overall, human αSyn fibril injected M20 mice (Cohort 1) showed profuse αSyn pathology in motor cortex, piriform cortex, somatosensory cortex, amygdala (basolateral and basomedial nuclei), ventral thalamus, IC, hypothalamus (ventromedial and dorsomedial), hippocampus, dentate gyrus, retrosplenial cortex, geniculate nucleus, SN region, retromammillary body, posterior commissure, cerebellar folia, vestibular nuclei and spinal cord (Figs. 1 and 2a, Additional file 2: Figure S2). Surprisingly, we observed very limited αSyn pathology in the CPu region. In M20 mice injected with mouse αSyn fibrils (Cohort 2), αSyn pathology was observed in all of these areas except there was sparse to no pathology in somatosensory cortex and retrosplenial cortex (Figs. 1 and 2b, Additional file 2: Figure S2). On the whole, this data shows that the induction and subsequent dissemination of the template αSyn pathology in M20 mice is widespread and not strictly restricted to areas that are neuroanatomically connected to the IC.

Since the IC provides connectivity between various brain areas supporting multiple, diverse, and dissociable functional regions, we next investigated whether injecting human αSyn fibrils directly into the CPu resulted in transmission of induced αSyn pathology into discrete areas linked by direct projections from this area (Cohort 3). The CPu area receives inputs from the cortex and sends projections directly into the globus pallidus, thalamus, and SN. Mice were examined for αSyn inclusion pathology following injection of human αSyn fibrils into the CPu. These M20 mice showed essentially a similar distribution of αSyn pathology as observed in Cohort 1 and Cohort 2 mice (Figs. 1 and 2c), indicating that templated induction of αSyn pathology follows similar patterns of distribution whether initiated in a white matter enriched area (IC) or a projection rich area (CPu). All M20 cohorts (Cohorts 1, 2 and 3) showed extensive perikaryal as well as axonal pathology; additionally, Cohort 3 mice showed pathology throughout the cortex especially in the visual and entorhinal cortex (Figs. 1 and 2c, Additional file 2: S2). On the whole, Cohort 3 of M20 mice showed relatively more robust and widespread distribution of αSyn inclusion pathology than mice injected with human αSyn fibrils or mouse αSyn fibrils in the IC (Cohorts 1, 2) (Fig. 2a-c). An important distinction between these cohorts is that the Cohort 3 mice seemed to develop relatively more robust αSyn pathology in and around the area of injection, i.e., striatum, than Cohort 1 and 2 mice, which had limited αSyn pathology proximal to the area of injection. We also observed robust induction of αSyn inclusion pathology in the ependymal cells abutting the lateral ventricles in the human αSyn fibril injected M20 mice in Cohorts 1 and 3 (Additional file 3: Figure S3).

Induction and spread of pathological αSyn in NTG mice is sparse and restricted

In our previous studies, we found that following intrahippocampal seeding, the templated induction of αSyn pathology in NTG mice is a relatively inefficient process compared to αSyn transgenic M20 mice [17, 23]. We reasoned that if there was any frank propagation of pathology along neuroanatomic connections, we would be able to clearly visualize this phenomenon in NTG mice that otherwise do not develop a surfeit of αSyn pathology outside of the area of injection. To characterize propagation of conformationally altered αSyn in NTG mice, we injected mouse αSyn fibrils (Cohort 4) or human αSyn fibrils (Cohort 5) into the IC (Figs. 3 and 4a) or mouse αSyn fibrils in the CPu (Cohort 6) (Figs. 3 and 4b). Cohort 5 had no detectable αSyn pathology and therefore no further analysis was done in these mice (data not shown). We noticed that in Cohorts 4 and 6, αSyn inclusion pathology was observed in dorsal striatum (CPu), thalamus, piriform cortex and entorhinal cortex (Figs. 3 and 4). Mice injected in the IC did not show appreciable αSyn pathology in the motor cortex, which is unexpected

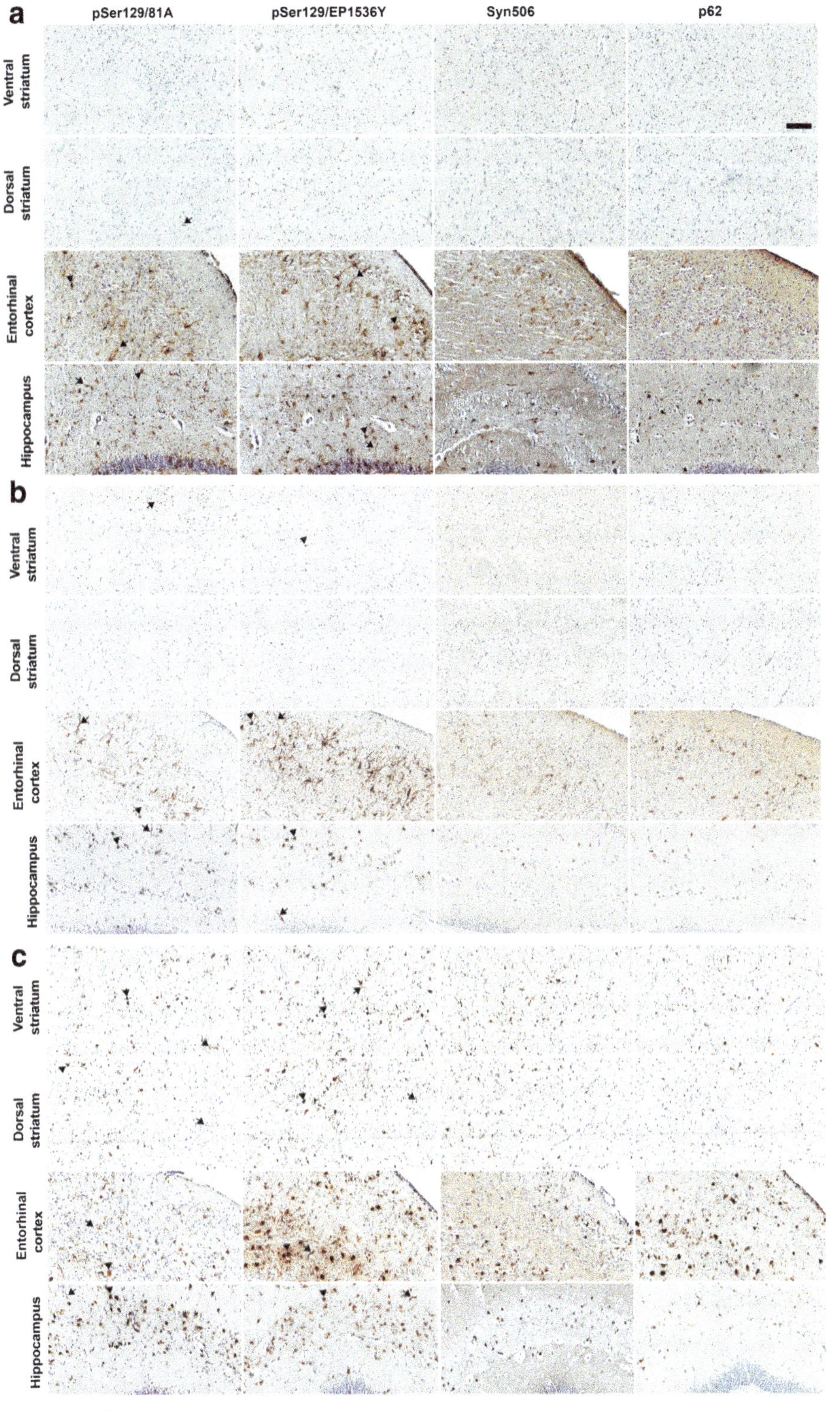

Fig. 2 (See legend on next page.)

(See figure on previous page.)

Fig. 2 Induction of αSyn pathology following injection of αSyn fibrils in the IC of line M20 mice. 2 month old Line M20 mice were injected with pre-formed human WT αSyn fibrils in IC (**a**, Cohort 1) or mouse WT αSyn fibrils in IC (**b**, Cohort 2) or human WT αSyn fibrils in the CPu (**c**, Cohort 3) and analyzed after 4 months. Abundant αSyn inclusion pathology, detected by pSer129-αSyn antibodies (81A and EP1536Y) was observed in most areas of the brain, even those that are not directly connected to the striatum, such as the hippocampus. Surprisingly, areas adjacent to the IC, such as the ventral and dorsal striatum had few pathological inclusions. Inclusion pathology was confirmed using a conformation-specific antibody against αSyn, Syn506, and p62/Sqstm1 antibody, which is a well-established marker of cytoplasmic LB inclusions. Both perikaryal (*arrowhead*) and neuritic (*arrow*) αSyn pathology were observed. The relative distribution and abundance of αSyn pathology in Cohort 3 was similar to Cohort 1, except that mice in Cohort 3 had relatively higher density of αSyn inclusion pathology in the striatum. Note that since 1 mouse in Cohort 2 died prematurely from hindlimb paralysis, neuropathological analysis could not be performed. Scale Bar, 100 μm; *n* = 3–5 mice

given that the IC is richly populated by corticospinal tracts (Figs. 3 and 4b). In both of these cohorts of NTG mice, the majority of the αSyn inclusions were perikaryal, with limited neuritic pathology (Fig. 4). Neither of these two cohorts showed any appreciable αSyn pathology in other areas that are neuroanatomically connected to the striatum, e.g., thalamus and SN region. Additionally, we did not observe any αSyn pathology in ependymal cells (Additional file 3: Figure S3), cerebellum or spinal cord (data not shown) of NTG mice.

Intra-striatal administration of αSyn aggregates does not necessarily induce degeneration of dopaminergic neurons in the substantia nigra

Tractographic studies have conclusively established that striatal neurons (both dorsal and ventral) project monosynaptically to DA neurons in the SN [36]. Especially, a majority of projections from the posterior aspect of the striatum has been shown to lead into the DA neurons of SN and retrorubral nucleus [37]. Therefore, we expected that direct injections of αSyn fibrils into the dorsal striatum (CPu) or IC (situated between caudate and putamen) should result in targeting DA neurons in the SN. Though we observed pSer129 αSyn immunopositive inclusions in the SN region and striatum of M20 transgenic mice, the αSyn inclusion pathology did not co-localize with the TH-immunopositive DA neuronal cell bodies (Additional file 4: Figure S4). We then conducted stereologic counting of TH-immunopositive DA neurons in M20 (Cohorts 1–3) or NTG mice (Cohorts 4–6) to explore whether seeded αSyn pathology affects survival of DA neurons in the SN. We observed a modest reduction in number of DA neurons in M20 transgenic mice injected in the IC with human αSyn fibrils (↓25.5%; Cohort 1) or mouse αSyn fibrils (↓20.6%; Cohort 2) (Fig. 5). Surprisingly, M20 transgenic mice injected with human αSyn fibrils in the CPu (Cohort 3) did not show any DA neuronal loss (Fig. 5). None of the NTG mice injected with either human αSyn fibrils (Cohort 5) or mouse αSyn fibrils (Cohorts 4 and 6) showed any nigral neuronal loss (Fig. 6).

Characterization of astrocytosis and microgliosis in αSyn seeded mice

To understand how gliosis is altered in αSyn seeded milieus, we conducted region-wise analysis of astrocytes and microglia in M20 and NTG mice. Overall, the induction of astrogliosis was much more consistently reproducible in M20 mice injected in the CPu (Cohort 3) compared to all other cohorts. In M20 mice, injection in CPu with human αSyn fibrils (Cohort 3) resulted in the most striking and consistent increases in astrocytosis

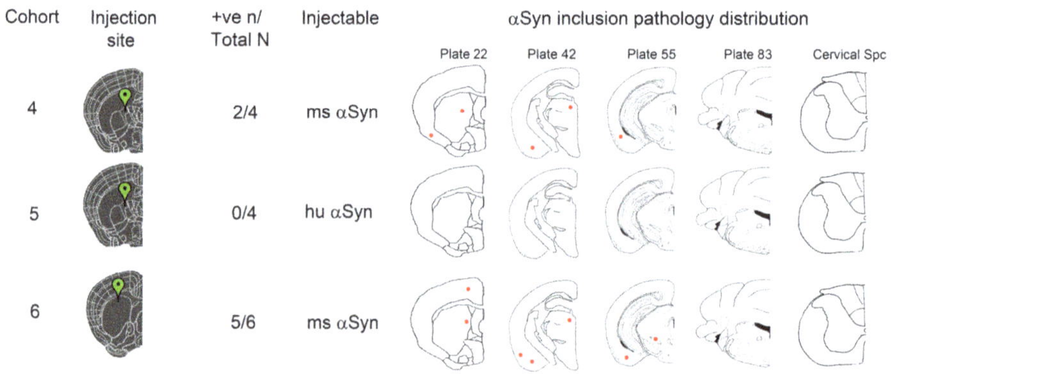

Fig. 3 Summary of distribution of αSyn pathology in NTG mice following intrastriatal injection of human or mouse αSyn fibrils. NTG mice were injected with mouse WT αSyn fibrils (Cohort 4) or human WT αSyn fibrils (Cohort 5) in the IC area whereas Cohort 6 mice were injected with mouse WT αSyn fibrils into the CPu. The total number of mice in each cohort as well as the number of mice displaying induced αSyn pathology is shown (denoted as +ve n/Total n). Rostro-caudal distribution of inclusions is presented on schematic brain maps, with red dots depicting the relative abundance of αSyn inclusions in different brain and spinal cord locations. The numbers on top of the brain schematic correspond to plates from the Paxinos Brain Atlas [57]

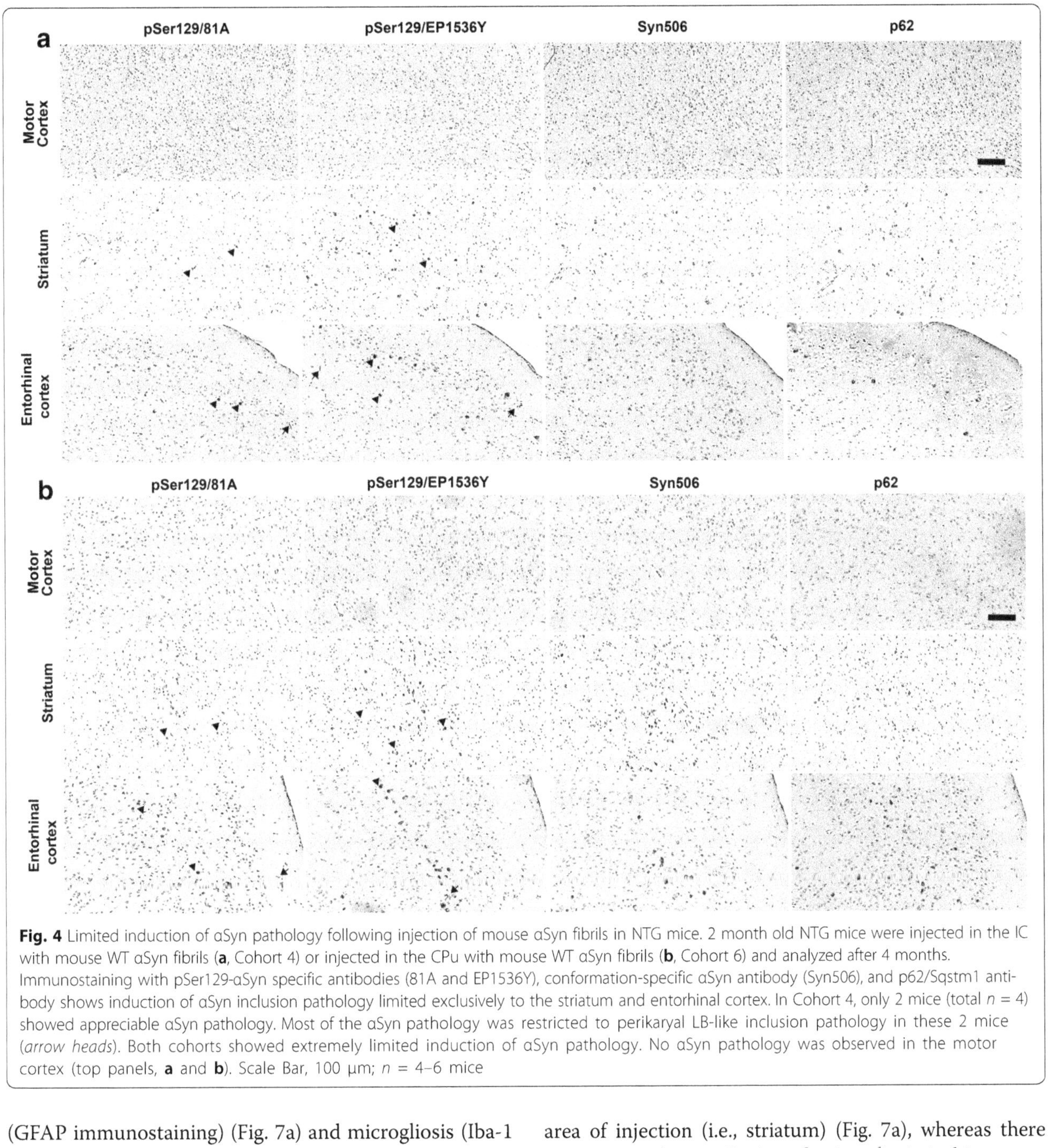

Fig. 4 Limited induction of αSyn pathology following injection of mouse αSyn fibrils in NTG mice. 2 month old NTG mice were injected in the IC with mouse WT αSyn fibrils (**a**, Cohort 4) or injected in the CPu with mouse WT αSyn fibrils (**b**, Cohort 6) and analyzed after 4 months. Immunostaining with pSer129-αSyn specific antibodies (81A and EP1536Y), conformation-specific αSyn antibody (Syn506), and p62/Sqstm1 antibody shows induction of αSyn inclusion pathology limited exclusively to the striatum and entorhinal cortex. In Cohort 4, only 2 mice (total $n = 4$) showed appreciable αSyn pathology. Most of the αSyn pathology was restricted to perikaryal LB-like inclusion pathology in these 2 mice (*arrow heads*). Both cohorts showed extremely limited induction of αSyn pathology. No αSyn pathology was observed in the motor cortex (top panels, **a** and **b**). Scale Bar, 100 μm; n = 4–6 mice

(GFAP immunostaining) (Fig. 7a) and microgliosis (Iba-1 immunostaining) (Fig. 7c) in the striatum. Other areas distal to the injection sites that displayed robust αSyn deposits in these mice, such as the hippocampus and entorhinal cortex, also showed increased GFAP and Iba-1 staining, albeit with more individual variability compared to striatum (Additional file 5: Figure S5, Fig. 7a and c).

Line M20 mice injected in IC (Cohorts 1 and 2) showed much more variability in astrogliosis across individual mice, in spite of consistently uniform distribution of αSyn pathology in these mice. In particular, Cohort 1 mice showed no induction of gliosis in and around the area of injection (i.e., striatum) (Fig. 7a), whereas there was increased astrogliosis and microgliosis in hippocampus and entorhinal cortex, albeit with more mouse-to-mouse variability; therefore, in a facile sense, induction of astrogliosis cannot be directly explained by the accretion of induced αSyn pathology (Additional file 5: Figure S5). Interestingly, there is also discordance between GFAP and Iba-1 immunostaining that is strikingly evident in the M20 mice injected in the IC (Cohorts 1 and 2) – for example, there was generally higher levels of astrogliosis in Cohort 2 compared to limited alterations in microgliosis (Fig. 7a and c; Additional file 5: Figure S5).

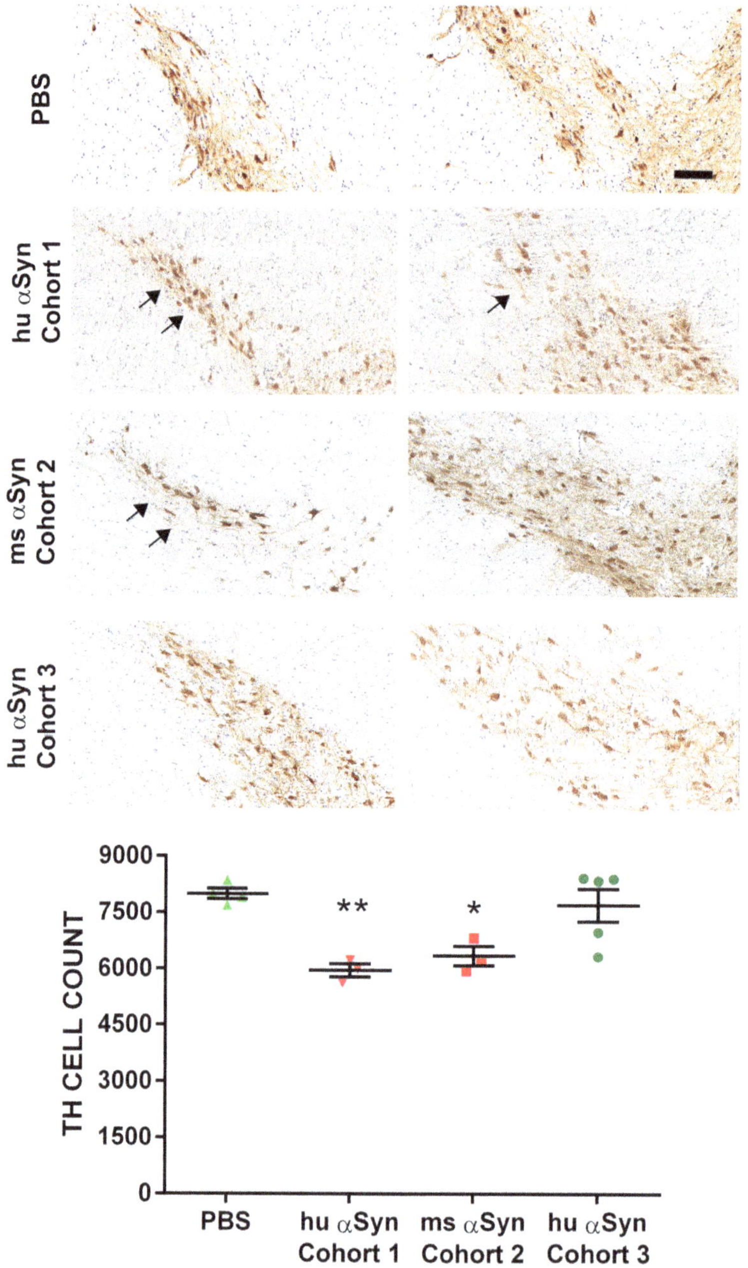

Fig. 5 Modest levels of nigral DA neuronal loss in line M20 mice injected in IC with αSyn fibrils. Line M20 mice were injected in the IC (Cohorts 1 and 2) or CPu (Cohort 3) with WT αSyn fibrils. Representative TH staining depicting SN-resident DA neurons in the dorsal (left panel) and ventral aspects (right panel) are shown. Mice that were injected with either human αSyn fibrils (Cohort 1) or mouse αSyn fibrils (Cohort 2) showed modest levels of DA degeneration as determined by counting TH-immunostained neurons in the SN (~20–25% compared to PBS injected control mice). The thinning of the nigral TH neuron layer is indicated by *arrows*. Cohort 3 mice injected with human αSyn fibrils did not display any nigral degeneration. PBS injected Line M20 mice were considered as control group for all cohorts. Scale Bar, 100 μm; $n = 3$–5/cohort. One way Anova, $^{**}p < 0.01$, $^{*}p < 0.5$

The extent of astrogliosis and microgliosis in NTG mice was variable throughout brain regions in the αSyn injected cohorts. Overall, in NTG mice injected in the IC (Cohorts 4 and 5) or CPu (Cohort 6), we observed sparse astrogliosis (Fig. 7b and d, Additional file 6: Figure S6). For example, Cohort 5 of NTG mice with no induction of αSyn inclusion pathology (i.e., injected in IC with human αSyn fibrils) expectedly does not show increased astrogliosis. Interestingly, with respect to mouse αSyn fibril injected cohorts, mice injected in the white matter rich IC area (Cohort 4) display higher (but variable) astrocytosis than in mice injected in the CPu (Cohort 6) (Fig. 7b, Additional file 6: Figure S6). Surprisingly, in spite of the presence of αSyn pathology, microgliosis was significantly downregulated in

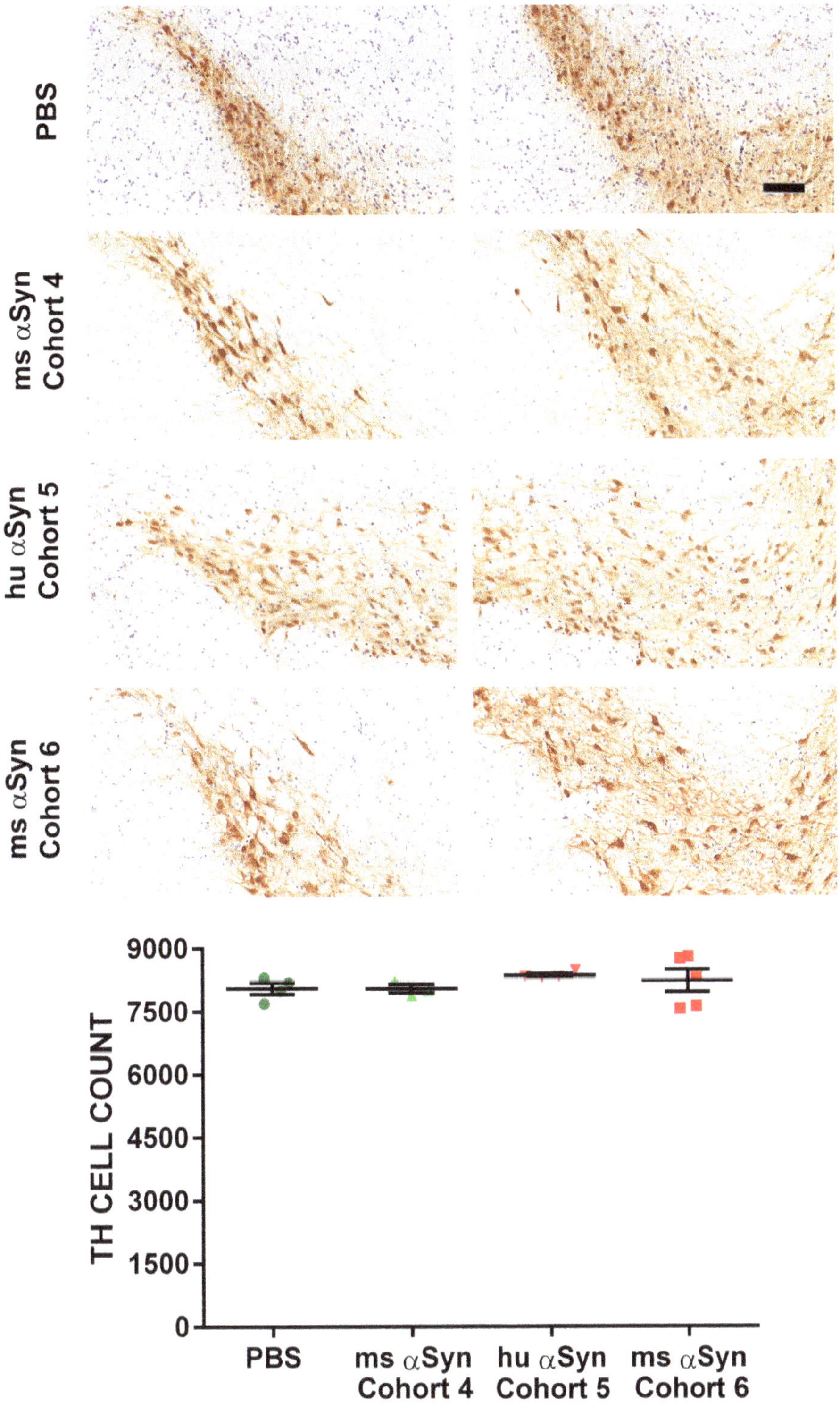

Fig. 6 Intrastriatal injection of αSyn fibrils in NTG mice does not result in nigral DA neurodegeneration. NTG mice were injected in the IC (Cohort 4, injected with mouse αSyn fibrils and Cohort 5, injected with human αSyn fibrils) or CPu (Cohort 6; injected with mouse αSyn fibrils). Representative TH staining depicting DA neurons in the dorsal and ventral aspects of SN are shown (left and right panels respectively). The total number of TH-immunostained neurons were unaltered in all cohorts compared to PBS injected mice. Scale Bar, 100 μm; *n* = 3–5/cohort

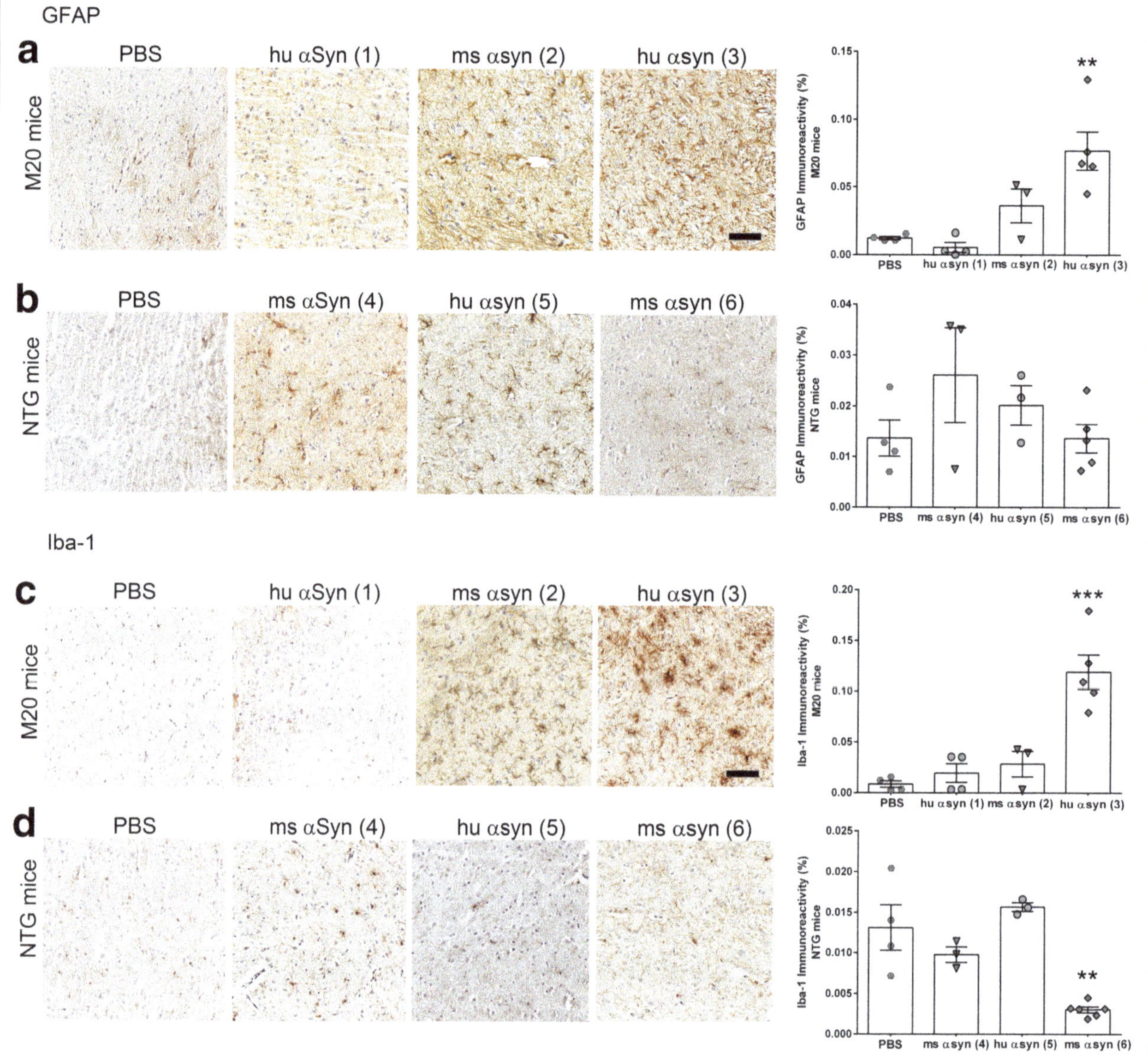

Fig. 7 Increased astrogliosis in line M20 mice injected with αSyn fibrils. Representative images of astrocytosis (GFAP immunostaining, **a-b**) and microgliosis (Iba-1 immunostaining, **c-d**) in the striatum region of line M20 (**a**, **c**) or NTG (**b**, **d**) mice injected with αSyn fibrils. Astrocytic and microglial activation was significantly upregulated in line M20 mice injected in the CPu with human αSyn fibrils (Cohort 3). Astrogliosis was variable in Cohort 1 of line M20 mice whereas in Cohort 2 of M20 mice, injection of mouse αSyn fibrils in the IC resulted in an insignificant trend towards increased GFAP and Iba-1 reactive astroglia. In all cohorts of NTG mice, the extent of astrogliosis was more variable (Cohorts 4, 5 and 6) and in Cohort 6, mice showed significantly lower microgliosis compared to control group. In all cases, genotype-matched PBS injected mice served as controls. Different cohorts are identified by numbers in parenthesis as described in Figs. 1 and 3. Scale Bar, 100 μm; n = 3–5/cohort; 1 way Anova, $^{***}p < 0.005$, $^{**}p < 0.01$

the striatum, hippocampus and entorhinal cortex of NTG mice injected with ms αSyn fibrils in the CPu (Cohort 6; Fig. 7d, Additional file 6: Figure S6).

Induction of robust αSyn pathology within nigral astrocytes but not TH neurons in M20 mice

In α-synucleinopathies, glial αSyn pathology is posited to contribute to progression of the disease and may be directly associated with DA neurodegeneration [38]. Therefore, we next investigated the localization of pSer129-αSyn pathology in glial cells and TH-immunopositive nigral DA neurons in M20 mice that showed frank nigral neurodegeneration (Cohort 1) (Fig. 8a) compared to M20 mice with no DA degeneration (Cohort 3) (Fig. 8b). In both these cohorts, which had widespread αSyn pathology and astrocytosis but differential DA neurodegeneration in the SN, we rarely observed any TH-resident pathological αSyn inclusions (Fig. 8a-b, Additional file 4: Figure S4B-C).

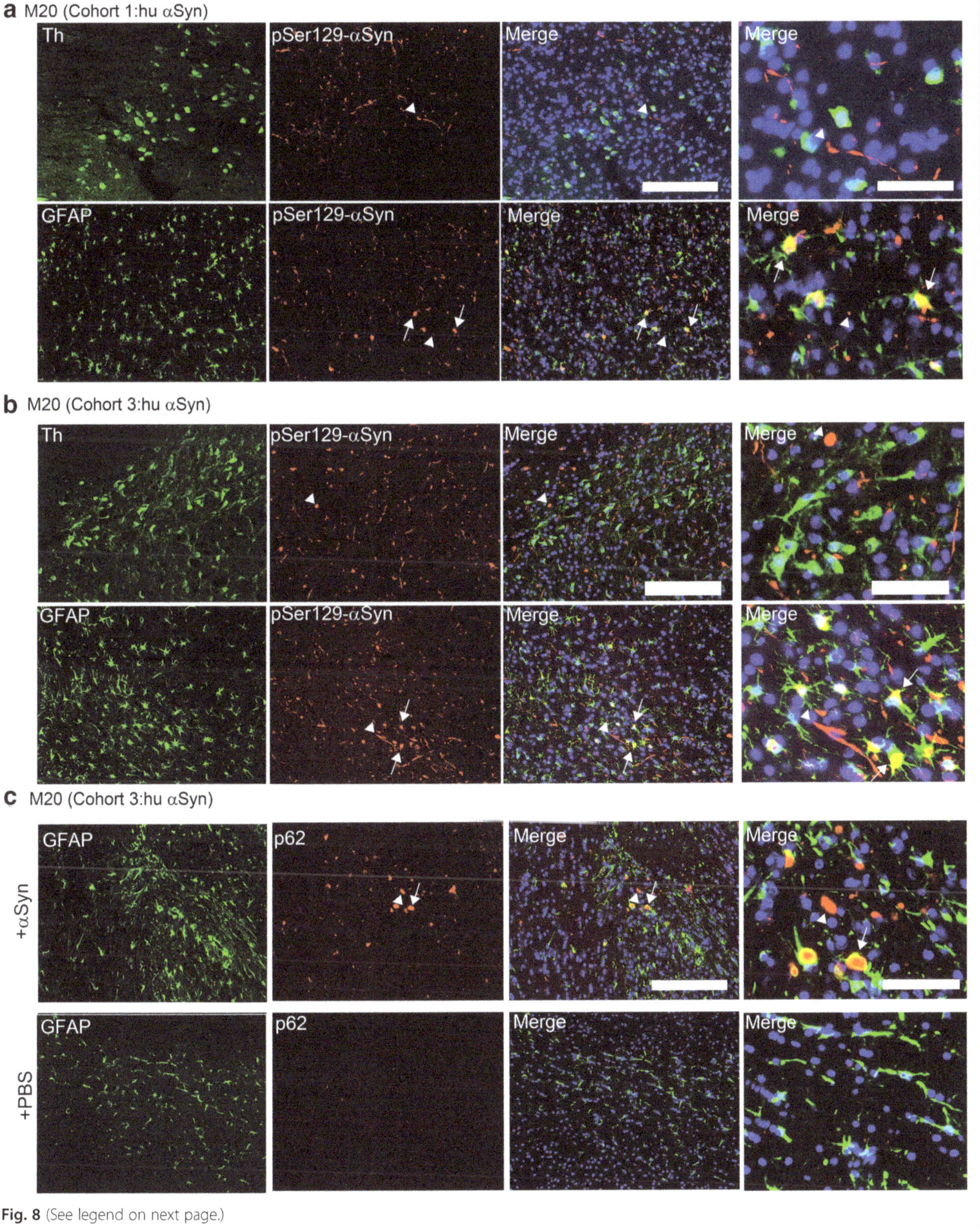

Fig. 8 (See legend on next page.)

(See figure on previous page.)

Fig. 8 αSyn aggregates preferentially co-localized within astrocytes but not in SN-resident DA neurons in line M20 mice injected with human WT αSyn fibrils. Representative immunofluorescence staining showing co-localization of pSer129 immunoreactive αSyn pathology (*red*) in the TH immunopositive DA neurons (*green*) or GFAP (*green*) immunopositive astrocytes in the SN region of human αSyn fibril injected M20 mice. In both cohorts of M20 mice injected in the IC or the CPu (**a-b**: Cohorts 1 and 3 respectively), astrocytes laden with pSer129-αSyn were present in abundance (*arrows*) while none of these LB type inclusions were identified within the TH-immunopositive DA neurons. Additionally, many cell body inclusions or neurites were present in populations that were not immunopositive for TH (*arrowheads*). Of note, the astrocytes with resident αSyn pathology resemble hypermorphic reactive state and co-localized with p62, an indicator of decreased autophagic flux (**c**). PBS injected mice represents the control mice (**c**). Cell nuclei were stained with DAPI (*blue*). The 3-color merged panel has been magnified (right panel) to visualize the localization of astrocytic pSer129 αSyn pathology in the SN. n = 3–5/cohort; Scale bar, 500 μm (all panels except right panel); 200 μm (merged panel, right)

Interestingly, a copious amount of pSer129-αSyn pathology was resident within the GFAP-immunopositive astrocytes in the SN in both these cohorts (Fig. 8a-b). We next tested whether astrocytic inclusion pathology was associated with autophagic alterations. Since p62 accumulates when autophagy is inhibited, and decreased levels can be observed when autophagy is induced, p62 may be used as a marker to study autophagic flux [39]. We noticed that these astrocytic inclusions were indeed immunopositive for p62, a cellular marker indicating inhibition of autophagy (Fig. 8c).

In Cohort 3, astrocyte resident pSer129-αSyn pathology was also observed in several other brain areas that had induced αSyn pathology, such as ventral midbrain, hippocampus and cortex in these mice (Additional file 7: Figure S7b). We also observed a similar distribution of astrocytic pSer129-αSyn pathology in Cohort 1 of M20 mice injected with human αSyn fibrils, though individual mice in this cohort showed variable induction of astrogliosis (Additional file 7: Figure S7A). In the NTG cohorts displaying induced αSyn pathology (Cohorts 4 and 6), we did not observe any astrocytic αSyn pathology in the ventral midbrain, entorhinal cortex or hippocampus (Additional file 8: Figure S8A–B).

Discussion

Templated conformational alterations in αSyn has been shown to induce LB-like pathology in mice, suggesting that this maybe a significant disease mechanism in human α-synucleinopathies [7–10]. While some reports have indicated that induced αSyn pathology spreads along neuroanatomic connections in a prionoid fashion [18, 20, 24–26, 40], we and others have previously reported that propagation of seeded αSyn pathology in mice can follow atypical or non-prionoid characteristics [17, 21, 41, 42]. Here, using human WT αSyn transgenic mice (M20) and NTG mice, we show that 1) injection of αSyn aggregates into two different areas of striatum results in widespread αSyn inclusion pathology in M20 mice, irrespective of neuroanatomic connectivity; 2) templated αSyn pathology following intra-striatal injection is not transmitted to DA neurons and causes moderate to no degeneration in DA neurons; 3) induction of αSyn pathology can be an inefficient process and spares the SN-resident TH-immunopositive neurons in NTG mice; and 4) αSyn laden astrocytes were readily observed in brain regions of M20 mice with robust αSyn pathology, suggesting that non-neuronal cells can also contribute to the dissemination of αSyn pathology. Overall, our observations indicate that, in addition to inter-neuronal transfer of seeded αSyn pathology along anatomic connections, simple diffusion or glia-mediated regional transfer may also affect the extent and distribution of pathologies in mouse models of α-synucleinopathies. In our study, a significant proportion of αSyn pathological inclusions induced by the administration of exogenous αSyn fibrils were localized within astrocytes throughout the CNS, in stark comparison to other published studies that have shown minimal glial involvement [18, 26]. It is possible that this unique property of our αSyn preparations along with potential maturation of αSyn pathology within the astroglia may generate unique αSyn conformers with distinctive strain-like properties that are preferentially transmitted via glial cells relative to direct inter-neuronal transfer. Induction of α-synucleinopathy by such astrocyte-discriminative αSyn conformers could be used to mechanistically understand the disease etiology in α-synucleinopathies with massive glial involvement, such as in multiple system atrophy [43, 44]. Whether the αSyn fibrils used in our studies indeed possess a preference for enhanced glial transmission relevant to disease pathogenesis in distinct spectra of α-synucleinopathies and how this impacts the progression and outcome of different subtypes of α-synucleinopathies will be examined in future studies.

Critical parameters that govern dissemination of αSyn seeds: concept of endogenous barriers

In the prion field, permissive transmission depends on overcoming the species barrier, which is determined by a range of possible conformers of a particular prion, its sequence, as well as its interaction with cellular co-factors such as chaperones [45–47]. One such endogenous 'barrier' relevant to α-synucleinopathies may be the subtle differences in the sequence of mouse and human αSyn (7/140 amino acids difference) [48] or their differential interactions with cellular co-factors. Based on this premise, mouse and human αSyn may have differential abilities in recruiting endogenous αSyn into pathological aggregates [26]. In support of this theory, we observed that in NTG mice, while mouse αSyn aggregates resulted in induction of αSyn pathology, human αSyn fibrils were ineffective. Therefore, it is likely that a 'species barrier' may determine the structural templating of αSyn and its dissemination in the brain. However, this notion is inconsistent with previous observations in NTG C57BL/6 J mice that intra-nigral injections of human or mouse αSyn aggregates result in identical patterns of pSer129-αSyn pathology [25]. Additionally, we found that the templated induction of pathological αSyn by mouse αSyn fibrils is an inefficient process in NTG mice compared to M20 mice. Since exogenous mouse αSyn aggregates do not necessarily recruit endogenous αSyn readily into pathological aggregates, this data suggests that the induction of αSyn pathology is a non-stochastic process dependent on the overall threshold barrier of αSyn protein. Therefore, it is possible that endogenous barriers such as a thresholding effect may regulate the induction and prionoid dissemination of αSyn pathology.

The 'species barrier' concept that can help explain why human WT αSyn fibrils are inefficient in seeding NTG mice is supported by the fact that there are sequence differences between human and mouse αSyn, albeit only 7 amino acids [48]. Interestingly, one of these alterations is an Ala in human αSyn compared to a Thr in mouse αSyn at residue 53, thus, mouse αSyn intrinsically has the Ala53Thr substitution that cause disease in human. In vitro mouse αSyn has a greater propensity to fibrilize into amyloid than human αSyn, akin to AlaThr53 human αSyn [49]. Although both mouse and human αSyn fibrils can cross-seed monomers of each other to polymerize into fibrils, homotypic seeding is usually more efficient in vitro [14]. Similarly, they both can initiate the aggregation of each other in vivo, but again homotypic seeding is more efficient [14]. However, as shown in extensive studies comparing the influences of amino acid alterations in mouse and human αSyn on the seeded-induction of aggregation, differences observed by in vitro cross-seeding do not always directly correlate with in vivo seeding efficiency [14]. The seeded induction of αSyn aggregation in vivo can be influenced by many differential factors unique to the αSyn seeds including cellular uptake, aggregate stability and cellular binding partners (eg. other proteins and lipids), in addition to subtle differences in the compatibility of unique conformers in initiating the recruitment and aggregation of intrinsic αSyn.

Mechanisms of de novo emergence of prions are still elusive. The aggregation of classical prions has been determined to be a non-stochastic process, whereby threshold of the prion protein determines the efficiency of prionoid transformation and propagation. Indeed, a criterion for prions is that these are formed more efficiently upon over-expression of the native protein. This was reported in the case of SUP35 and URE2 genes, where overproduction of each of these genes induce de novo formation of the respective prions [50, 51]. Indeed, in our present study as well as in previous studies, we have observed that templated induction of αSyn pathology is more efficient in mice overexpressing human αSyn than NTG mice [17, 23]. This suggests similarities between formation of classical prions and αSyn prionoid species. Overall, our study shows that the efficiency of induction of αSyn aggregation depends on the amount on available αSyn protein in the cell, suggesting that threshold of transgenic protein levels may be a determining factor for ensuring efficient prionoid induction of αSyn pathology.

In this present study and earlier studies [17], we have ascertained that M20 mice injected with αSyn aggregates show dramatic induction of astrogliosis and microgliosis. In sharp contrast to the observations by Rey et al. [26], we observed copious amounts of αSyn pathology co-localized with astrocytes, irrespective of the area of injection. This implies that, in addition to transneuronal transport, astrocytes and possibly other immune cells may also play key roles in the dissemination of pathological αSyn seeds. This has future therapeutic implications as glial cells can effectively act to reduce interneuronal transmission and more importantly clear extracellular αSyn seeds (reviewed in [52]). Indeed, it has been shown that both astrocytes and microglia can internalize and effectively degrade αSyn aggregates [53–56]. Collectively, these data suggest that glial cells that normally do not express or express very low levels of αSyn are not prone to seeding in some settings and this may play an important role in creating an endogenous barrier to the prionoid propagation of αSyn.

Does trans-neuronal propagation of templated αSyn pathology cause DA neurodegeneration?

The etiology of DA neurodegeneration in the SN of patients with LB diseases remain unknown. One theory is that trans-neuronal transmission of seeded αSyn pathology along the neuroanatomically connected nigro-striatal pathway causes significant DA neuronal death [18, 20, 24]. However, in our study, we observed only a 20–25% DA neurodegeneration in M20 mice following injection into the IC with either mouse or human αSyn fibrils. No DA neurodegeneration was noted in NTG mice or in M20 mice injected into the CPu, an area that is directly linked to the SN. Additionally, we were intrigued by our observations that DA neurons were impervious to seeded αSyn pathology in both NTG and M20 mice. We reasoned that this observation can be attributed to multiple complex scenarios such as (1) an initial wave of pathological αSyn inclusion pathology lead to DA neurodegeneration followed by astrocytic engulfment of released materials or (2) astrocytes are able to engulf extracellular αSyn directly during the templated induction and dissemination process [38]. In an effort to localize seeded αSyn pathology in the SN, we conducted immunofluorescent co-localization studies using antibodies against non-neuronal cells and found that a majority of these inclusions are present in astrocytes, but not in the nigral TH-immunopositive DA neurons. Since we did not observe any significant nigral DA neurodegeneration in some of these mice (Cohort 3 of M20 mice), our observations suggest that astrocytes likely engulf and scavenge pathological αSyn during the propagation process. Indeed, this is consistent with observations that even direct intra-nigral injection of αSyn aggregates does not necessarily cause nigral DA neurodegeneration [20, 25] but would be contrary to observations from other groups [18, 24]. Interestingly, whether glial cells, such as astrocytes, can have a disease modifying effect in α-synucleinopathies by acting as αSyn scavengers or as unwitting vehicles that aid in dissemination of αSyn, remains to be investigated.

Conclusions

Multiple independent reports, including this present study, show that αSyn aggregates display prionoid characteristics. Additionally, we show that contrary to expected routes of transmissibility exclusively following neuroanatomic connectivity, prionoid αSyn can be widely disseminated throughout the brain by various cellular networks - neurons as well as astrocytes. Therefore, our current findings, when aligned with the present literature, suggest that the mechanism influencing prionoid propagation of αSyn are complex and not always predictable by direct interneuronal connectivity. In fact, glial transmission of αSyn may also have a major impact on the pathological outcome in α-synucleinopathies. These findings are similar to disease pathogenesis by classical prion protein, where different strains of misfolded prions can have contextually-dependent transmission properties in the neuraxis [15, 16, 47]. Importantly, these properties open up potential therapeutic opportunities targeting such extracellular transfer of αSyn by utilizing endogenous immune and non-immune barriers.

Additional file

Additional file 1: Figure S1. Transmission EM images of αSyn fibrils. Recombinant WT αSyn fibrils (human or mouse) were sonicated and analyzed by EM following uranyl acetate staining. Scale bar, 100 nm.

Additional file 2: Figure S2. Robust αSyn inclusion pathology evident in the brains of M20 mice (Cohorts 1, 2 and 3). Robust αSyn inclusion pathology was observed in areas of the brain distal from the injection site such as motor cortex, brainstem, spinal cord and SN of M20 mice injected with αSyn fibrils (A, B, C: Cohorts 1, 2 and 3 respectively). αSyn pathology was identified using pSer129-αSyn antibodies (81A and EP1536Y), Syn506 antibody and p62/Sqstm1 antibody. Both perikaryal (arrowhead) and neuritic (arrow) αSyn pathology was observed. Scale Bar, 100 μm; $n = 3–5$ mice/group.

Additional file 3: Figure S3. Robust αSyn inclusion pathology evident in the ependymal cells lining the ventricles of M20 mice (Cohorts 1 and 3). M20 mice injected with human αSyn fibrils (Cohorts 1 and 3) show robust induction of αSyn pathology in the ependymal cells lining the lateral ventricles. αSyn pathology was identified using pSer129-αSyn antibodies (81A and EP1536Y), Syn506 antibody and p62/Sqstm1 antibody. The right panel shows a magnified image of p62-immunopositive ependymal cells. None of the NTG mice injected with αSyn fibrils showed any αSyn pathology in these cells; representative images from NTG Cohort 6 is shown as an example. Hu, human; ms, mouse. $n = 3–6$/cohort; scale bar, 100 μm (all panels except right panel); 50 μm (right panel).

Additional file 4: Figure S4. αSyn pathology was not detected in TH-immunopositive DA neurons in M20 or NTG mice injected with αSyn fibrils in the striatum. Representative images showing that pSer129-αSyn inclusion pathology (red, arrows) was not localized within nigral TH-immunopositive DA neurons (green) in any of the M20 (Cohorts 2 and 3, A and B respectively) or NTG (Cohorts 4 and 6, D and E respectively) mice injected with αSyn fibrils (A-B). Few αSyn inclusions were observed in the striatal neuronal cell bodies embedded within the TH-positive terminals of M20 mice injected with human αSyn fibrils in the CPu (C). Cell nuclei were stained with DAPI (blue). The 3-color merged panel has been magnified (right panel) to visualize the localization of pSer129 αSyn inclusions in the SN. NTG mice injected with human αSyn fibrils (Cohort 5) is not shown as this cohort had no αSyn inclusion pathology. Numbers in parenthesis denote cohort number as identified in Figs. 1 and 3. Hu, human; ms, mouse. $n = 3–6$/cohort; Scale bar, 500 μm (all panels except right panel); 200 μm (merged panel, right).

Additional file 5: Figure S5. Gliosis levels in forebrain areas of line M20 mice injected with human or mouse αSyn fibrils in the striatum. Representative images of astrocytosis (GFAP immunostaining) and microgliosis (Iba-1 immunostaining) in the hippocampus and entorhinal cortex (En. Cortex) of line M20 mice injected with αSyn fibrils in the IC (Cohorts 1 and 2) or CPu (Cohort 3). Though there was an overall trend towards higher astrocytic and microglial burden in M20 mice injected with αSyn fibrils which would be co-incident with αSyn inclusion pathology present in these brain areas, there seemed to be individual variability in astroglial numbers within each group. In all cases, PBS injected mice (genotype-matched) served as controls. Different cohorts are identified by numbers in parenthesis on top of corresponding panel. Hu, human; ms, mouse. Scale bar, 100 μm; $n = 3–5$/cohort; 1 way Anova.

Additional file 6: Figure S6. Gliosis levels in forebrains of NTG mice injected with αSyn fibrils in the striatum. Representative images of astrocytosis (GFAP immunostaining) and microgliosis (Iba-1 immunostaining) in the hippocampus and entorhinal cortex (En. Cortex) of NTG mice injected with WT αSyn fibrils in the IC (Cohorts 4 and 5) or CPu (Cohort 6). No significant alterations in GFAP staining was observed in any of the cohorts. Increased microgliosis was observed in the entorhinal cortex of NTG mice injected with mouse αSyn fibrils in the IC ($^*p < 0.05$) but not in the hippocampus of these mice. Strikingly, dampening of microgliosis was observed in forebrain areas of mice injected with human αSyn (Cohort 5; hippocampus, $^*p < 0.05$; entorhinal cortex, $p > 0.05$) as well as in the hippocampus and cortex of NTG mice injected with mouse αSyn fibrils (Cohort 6, $^{**}p < 0.01$). In all cases, PBS injected mice (genotype-matched) served as controls. Different cohorts are identified by numbers in parenthesis on top of panel. Hu, human; ms, mouse. Scale bar, 100 μm; $n = 3–6$/cohort; 1 way Anova, $^*p < 0.05$, $^{**}p < 0.01$.

Additional file 7: Figure S7. Astrocytic αSyn inclusions were abundant in midbrain and forebrain areas of line M20 mice injected with human αSyn fibrils (Cohorts 1 and 3). Representative immunofluorescence staining showing co-localization of pSer129 immunoreactive αSyn pathology (red) within the GFAP immunopositive astrocytes (green) in the ventral midbrain, hippocampus and motor cortex of human αSyn fibril injected M20 mice. In both cohorts (1 and 3) of these M20 mice, astrocytes laden with pSer129-αSyn were present in abundance (arrows). Additionally, several LB type inclusions or neurites (arrowheads) were also present in cells that were not immunopositive for GFAP. Cell nuclei were stained with DAPI (blue). The 3-color merged panel has been magnified (right panel) to visualize the localization of astrocytic pSer129 αSyn. Hu, human; ms, mouse. $n = 3–5$/cohort; Scale bar, 500 μm (all panels except right panel); 200 μm (merged panel, right).

Additional file 8: Figure S8. Astrocytic αSyn inclusions were absent in midbrain and forebrain areas of NTG mice injected with mouse αSyn fibrils (Cohorts 4 and 6). Representative immunofluorescence staining showing that pSer129 immunoreactive αSyn pathology (red; A-B) does not colocalize within the GFAP immunopositive astrocytes (green; A-B) in the ventral midbrain, hippocampus and motor cortex of mouse αSyn fibril injected NTG mice (Cohorts 4 and 6). Of note, most of these mice have low numbers of pSer129-αSyn pathology overall. Cell nuclei were stained with DAPI (blue). The 3-color merged panel has been magnified (right panel) to visualize the localization of pSer129 αSyn. Hu, human; ms, mouse. $n = 3$–6/cohort; Scale bar, 500 μm (all panels except right panel); 200 μm (merged panel, right).

Abbreviations
CPu: caudate putamen; DA: dopaminergic; EM: electron microscopy; GFAP: glial fibrillary acidic protein; Iba-1: ionized calcium-binding adapter molecule 1; IC: internal capsule; LB: Lewy body; NTG: nontransgenic; pSer129: αSyn phosphorylated on Serine 129; SN: substantia nigra; Sqstm1: Sequestosome1; TH: Tyrosine Hydroxylase; αSyn: α-synuclein

Acknowledgements
Not Applicable.

Funding
This work was supported by grants from the National Parkinson Foundation (NPF-UN203) and NIH/NINDS (NS089622). Publication of this article was funded in part by the University of Florida Open Access Publishing Fund. The authors declare no competing financial interests.

Authors' contributions
PC and BG conceived and coordinated the study, analyzed the data and wrote the manuscript; PC performed mouse injections; ZS performed immunostaining, drafted images for publication and participated in data analysis; MMB and VH performed tissue harvesting and immunostaining; NJR performed electron microscopy; TEG participated in data interpretation. All authors read and approved the final manuscript.

Competing interests
None of the authors have any competing interests in the manuscript.

Author details
[1]Department of Neuroscience, University of Florida, 1275 Center Drive, PO Box 100159, Gainesville, FL 32610, USA. [2]Center for Translational Research in Neurodegenerative Disease, University of Florida, Gainesville, FL 32610, USA. [3]McKnight Brain Institute, University of Florida, Gainesville, FL 32610, USA. [4]Current address: Department of Neuroscience, Mayo Clinic, Jacksonville, FL -32224, USA.

References
1. Waxman EA, Giasson BI. Molecular mechanisms of alpha-synuclein neurodegeneration. Biochim Biophys Acta. 2009;1792(7):616–24.
2. Goedert M, Spillantini MG, Del Tredici K, Braak H. 100 years of Lewy pathology. Nat Rev Neurol. 2013;9(1):13–24.
3. Cookson MR. The biochemistry of Parkinson's disease. Annu Rev Biochem. 2005;74:29–52.
4. Anderson JP, Walker DE, Goldstein JM, de Laat R, Banducci K, Caccavello RJ, Barbour R, Huang J, Kling K, Lee M, et al. Phosphorylation of ser-129 is the dominant pathological modification of alpha-synuclein in familial and sporadic Lewy body disease. J Biol Chem. 2006;281(40):29739–52.
5. Waxman EA, Giasson BI. Specificity and regulation of casein kinase-mediated phosphorylation of alpha-synuclein. J Neuropathol Exp Neurol. 2008;67(5):402–16.
6. Fujiwara H, Hasegawa M, Dohmae N, Kawashima A, Masliah E, Goldberg MS, Shen J, Takio K, Iwatsubo T. alpha-Synuclein is phosphorylated in synucleinopathy lesions. Nat Cell Biol. 2002;4(2):160–4.
7. Uchihara T, Giasson BI. Propagation of alpha-synuclein pathology: hypotheses, discoveries, and yet unresolved questions from experimental and human brain studies. Acta Neuropathol. 2016;131(1):49–73.
8. Guo JL, Lee VM. Cell-to-cell transmission of pathogenic proteins in neurodegenerative diseases. Nat Med. 2014;20(2):130–8.
9. Goedert M, Clavaguera F, Tolnay M. The propagation of prion-like protein inclusions in neurodegenerative diseases. Trends Neurosci. 2010;33(7):317–25.
10. Goedert M, Masuda-Suzukake M, Falcon B. Like prions: the propagation of aggregated tau and alpha-synuclein in neurodegeneration. Brain. 2016; 140(Pt 2):266–78.
11. Sacino AN, Thomas MA, Ceballos-Diaz C, Cruz PE, Rosario AM, Lewis J, Giasson BI, Golde TE. Conformational templating of alpha-synuclein aggregates in neuronal-glial cultures. Mol Neurodegener. 2013;8:17.
12. Waxman EA, Giasson BI. A novel, high-efficiency cellular model of fibrillar alpha-synuclein inclusions and the examination of mutations that inhibit amyloid formation. J Neurochem. 2010;113(2):374–88.
13. Luk KC, Song C, O'Brien P, Stieber A, Branch JR, Brunden KR, Trojanowski JQ, Lee VM. Exogenous alpha-synuclein fibrils seed the formation of Lewy body-like intracellular inclusions in cultured cells. Proc Natl Acad Sci U S A. 2009;106(47):20051–6.
14. Luk KC, Covell DJ, Kehm VM, Zhang B, Song IY, Byrne MD, Pitkin RM, Decker SC, Trojanowski JQ, Lee VM. Molecular and biological compatibility with host alpha-Synuclein influences fibril Pathogenicity. Cell Rep. 2016;16(12): 3373–87.
15. Eisenberg D, Jucker M. The amyloid state of proteins in human diseases. Cell. 2012;148(6):1188–203.
16. Aguzzi A, Heikenwalder M, Polymenidou M. Insights into prion strains and neurotoxicity. Nat Rev Mol Cell Biol. 2007;8(7):552–61.
17. Sacino AN, Brooks M, McKinney AB, Thomas MA, Shaw G, Golde TE, Giasson BI. Brain injection of alpha-Synuclein induces multiple Proteinopathies, Gliosis, and a neuronal injury marker. J Neurosci. 2014;34(37):12368–78.
18. Luk KC, Kehm VM, Zhang B, O'Brien P, Trojanowski JQ, Lee VM. Intracerebral inoculation of pathological alpha-synuclein initiates a rapidly progressive neurodegenerative alpha-synucleinopathy in mice. J Exp Med. 2012;209(5): 975–86.
19. Breid S, Bernis ME, Babila JT, Garza MC, Wille H, Tamguney G. Neuroinvasion of alpha-Synuclein Prionoids after Intraperitoneal and Intraglossal inoculation. J Virol. 2016;90(20):9182–93.
20. Peelaerts W, Bousset L, Van der Perren A, Moskalyuk A, Pulizzi R, Giugliano M, Van den Haute C, Melki R, Baekelandt V. alpha-Synuclein strains cause distinct synucleinopathies after local and systemic administration. Nature. 2015;522(7556):340–4.
21. Sacino AN, Brooks M, Thomas MA, McKinney AB, Lee S, Regenhardt RW, McGarvey NH, Ayers JI, Notterpek L, Borchelt DR, et al. Intramuscular injection of alpha-synuclein induces CNS alpha-synuclein pathology and a rapid-onset motor phenotype in transgenic mice. Proc Natl Acad Sci U S A. 2014;111(29):10732–7.
22. Ayers JI, Brooks MM, Rutherford NJ, Howard JK, Sorrentino ZA, Riffe CJ, Giasson BI. Robust central nervous system pathology in transgenic mice following peripheral injection of alpha-Synuclein fibrils. J Virol. 2017;91(2):pii: e02095-16.
23. Sacino AN, Brooks M, Thomas MA, McKinney AB, McGarvey NH, Rutherford NJ, Ceballos-Diaz C, Robertson J, Golde TE, Giasson BI. Amyloidogenic alpha-synuclein seeds do not invariably induce rapid, widespread pathology in mice. Acta Neuropathol. 2014;127(5):645–65.
24. Luk KC, Kehm V, Carroll J, Zhang B, O'Brien P, Trojanowski JQ, Lee VM. Pathological alpha-synuclein transmission initiates Parkinson-like neurodegeneration in nontransgenic mice. Science. 2012;338(6109):949–53.
25. Masuda-Suzukake M, Nonaka T, Hosokawa M, Oikawa T, Arai T, Akiyama H, Mann DM, Hasegawa M. Prion-like spreading of pathological alpha-synuclein in brain. Brain. 2013;136(Pt 4):1128–38.
26. Rey NL, Steiner JA, Maroof N, Luk KC, Madaj Z, Trojanowski JQ, Lee VM, Brundin P. Widespread transneuronal propagation of alpha-synucleinopathy triggered in olfactory bulb mimics prodromal Parkinson's disease. J Exp Med. 2016;213(9):1759–78.
27. Prusiner SB, Woerman AL, Mordes DA, Watts JC, Rampersaud R, Berry DB, Patel S, Oehler A, Lowe JK, Kravitz SN, et al. Evidence for alpha-synuclein prions causing multiple system atrophy in humans with parkinsonism. Proc Natl Acad Sci U S A. 2015;112(38):E5308–17.

28. Guo JL, Covell DJ, Daniels JP, Iba M, Stieber A, Zhang B, Riddle DM, Kwong LK, Xu Y, Trojanowski JQ, et al. Distinct alpha-synuclein strains differentially promote tau inclusions in neurons. Cell. 2013;154(1):103–17.
29. Mastrianni JA. The genetics of prion diseases. Genet Med. 2010;12(4):187–95.
30. Osterberg VR, Spinelli KJ, Weston LJ, Luk KC, Woltjer RL, Unni VK. Progressive aggregation of alpha-synuclein and selective degeneration of lewy inclusion-bearing neurons in a mouse model of parkinsonism. Cell Rep. 2015;10(8):1252–60.
31. Dawson TM, Dawson VL. Molecular pathways of neurodegeneration in Parkinson's disease. Science. 2003;302(5646):819–22.
32. Giasson BI, Duda JE, Quinn SM, Zhang B, Trojanowski JQ, Lee VM. Neuronal alpha-synucleinopathy with severe movement disorder in mice expressing A53T human alpha-synuclein. Neuron. 2002;34(4):521–33.
33. Giasson BI, Murray IV, Trojanowski JQ, Lee VM. A hydrophobic stretch of 12 amino acid residues in the middle of alpha-synuclein is essential for filament assembly. The J Biol Chem. 2001;276(4):2380–6.
34. Waxman EA, Duda JE, Giasson BI. Characterization of antibodies that selectively detect alpha-synuclein in pathological inclusions. Acta Neuropathol. 2008; 116(1):37–46.
35. Kitada T, Tong Y, Gautier CA, Shen J. Absence of nigral degeneration in aged parkin/DJ-1/PINK1 triple knockout mice. J Neurochem. 2009;111(3): 696–702.
36. Watabe-Uchida M, Zhu L, Ogawa SK, Vamanrao A, Uchida N. Whole-brain mapping of direct inputs to midbrain dopamine neurons. Neuron. 2012; 74(5):858–73.
37. Pan WX, Mao T, Dudman JT. Inputs to the dorsal striatum of the mouse reflect the parallel circuit architecture of the forebrain. Front Neuroanat. 2010;4:147.
38. Bruck D, Wenning GK, Stefanova N, Fellner L. Glia and alpha-synuclein in neurodegeneration: a complex interaction. Neurobiol Dis. 2016;85:262–74.
39. Bjorkoy G, Lamark T, Pankiv S, Overvatn A, Brech A, Johansen T. Monitoring autophagic degradation of p62/SQSTM1. Methods Enzymol. 2009;452:181–97.
40. Masuda-Suzukake M, Nonaka T, Hosokawa M, Kubo M, Shimozawa A, Akiyama H, Hasegawa M. Pathological alpha-synuclein propagates through neural networks. Acta Neuropathol Commun. 2014;2:88.
41. Sacino AN, Ayers JI, Brooks MM, Chakrabarty P, Hudson VJ 3rd, Howard JK, Golde TE, Giasson BI, Borchelt DR. Non-prion-type transmission in A53T alpha-synuclein transgenic mice: a normal component of spinal homogenates from naive non-transgenic mice induces robust alpha-synuclein pathology. Acta Neuropathol. 2016;131(1):151–4.
42. Mason DM, Nouraei N, Pant DB, Miner KM, Hutchison DF, Luk KC, Stolz JF, Leak RK. Transmission of alpha-synucleinopathy from olfactory structures deep into the temporal lobe. Mol Neurodegener. 2016;11(1):49.
43. Croisier E, Graeber MB. Glial degeneration and reactive gliosis in alpha-synucleinopathies: the emerging concept of primary gliodegeneration. Acta Neuropathol. 2006;112(5):517–30.
44. Fellner L, Jellinger KA, Wenning GK, Stefanova N. Glial dysfunction in the pathogenesis of alpha-synucleinopathies: emerging concepts. Acta Neuropathol. 2011;121(6):675–93.
45. Collinge J, Clarke AR. A general model of prion strains and their pathogenicity. Science. 2007;318(5852):930–6.
46. Kushnirov VV, Kryndushkin DS, Boguta M, Smirnov VN, Ter-Avanesyan MD. Chaperones that cure yeast artificial [PSI+] and their prion-specific effects. Curr Biol. 2000;10(22):1443–6.
47. Chien P, Weissman JS, DePace AH. Emerging principles of conformation-based prion inheritance. Annu Rev Biochem. 2004;73:617–56.
48. George JM. The synucleins. *Genome Biol.* 2002;3(1):REVIEWS3002.
49. Rochet JC, Conway KA, Lansbury PT Jr. Inhibition of fibrillization and accumulation of prefibrillar oligomers in mixtures of human and mouse alpha-synuclein. Biochemistry. 2000;39(35):10619–26.
50. Derkatch IL, Chernoff YO, Kushnirov VV, Inge-Vechtomov SG, Liebman SW. Genesis and variability of [PSI] prion factors in *Saccharomyces cerevisiae*. Genetics. 1996;144(4):1375–86.
51. Masison DC, Maddelein ML, Wickner RB. The prion model for [URE3] of yeast: spontaneous generation and requirements for propagation. Proc Natl Acad Sci U S A. 1997;94(23):12503–8.
52. Lee HJ, Bae EJ, Lee SJ. Extracellular alpha–synuclein-a novel and crucial factor in Lewy body diseases. Nat Rev Neurol. 2014;10(2):92–8.
53. Kim C, Ho DH, Suk JE, You S, Michael S, Kang J, Joong Lee S, Masliah E, Hwang D, Lee HJ, et al. Neuron-released oligomeric alpha-synuclein is an endogenous agonist of TLR2 for paracrine activation of microglia. Nat Commun. 2013;4:1562.
54. Lee HJ, Suk JE, Bae EJ, Lee JH, Paik SR, Lee SJ. Assembly-dependent endocytosis and clearance of extracellular alpha-synuclein. Int J Biochem Cell Biol. 2008;40(9):1835–49.
55. Lee HJ, Suk JE, Patrick C, Bae EJ, Cho JH, Rho S, Hwang D, Masliah E, Lee SJ. Direct transfer of alpha-synuclein from neuron to astroglia causes inflammatory responses in synucleinopathies. J Biol Chem. 2010;285(12):9262–72.
56. Stefanova N, Fellner L, Reindl M, Masliah E, Poewe W, Wenning GK. Toll-like receptor 4 promotes alpha-synuclein clearance and survival of nigral dopaminergic neurons. Am J Pathol. 2011;179(2):954–63.
57. Franklin KBJ, Paxinos G. Paxinos and Franklin's the mouse brain in stereotaxic coordinates. fourth ed. Amsterdam: Academic Press, an imprint of Elsevier; 2013.

Glycine-alanine dipeptide repeat protein contributes to toxicity in a zebrafish model of *C9orf72* associated neurodegeneration

Yu Ohki[1,2], Andrea Wenninger-Weinzierl[1], Alexander Hruscha[1], Kazuhide Asakawa[3], Koichi Kawakami[3], Christian Haass[1,2,4], Dieter Edbauer[1,4] and Bettina Schmid[1,4*]

Abstract

Background: The most frequent genetic cause of frontotemporal lobar degeneration (FTLD) and amyotrophic lateral sclerosis (ALS) is the expansion of a GGGGCC hexanucleotide repeat in a non-coding region of the chromosome 9 open reading frame 72 (*C9orf72*) locus. The pathological hallmarks observed in *C9orf72* repeat expansion carriers are the formation of RNA foci and deposition of dipeptide repeat (DPR) proteins derived from repeat associated non-ATG (RAN) translation. Currently, it is unclear whether formation of RNA foci, DPR translation products, or partial loss of C9orf72 predominantly drive neurotoxicity in vivo. By using a transgenic approach in zebrafish we address if the most frequently found DPR in human ALS/FTLD brain, the poly-Gly-Ala (poly-GA) protein, is toxic in vivo.

Method: We generated several transgenic UAS responder lines that express either 80 repeats of GGGGCC alone, or together with a translation initiation ATG codon forcing the translation of GA80-GFP protein upon crossing to a Gal4 driver. The GGGGCC repeat and GA80 were fused to green fluorescent protein (GFP) lacking a start codon to monitor protein translation by GFP fluorescence.

Results: Zebrafish transgenic for the GGGGCC repeat lacking an ATG codon showed very mild toxicity in the absence of poly-GA. However, strong toxicity was induced upon ATG initiated expression of poly-GA, which was rescued by injection of an antisense morpholino interfering with start codon dependent poly-GA translation. This morpholino only interferes with GA80-GFP translation without affecting repeat transcription, indicating that the toxicity is derived from GA80-GFP.

Conclusion: These novel transgenic *C9orf72* associated repeat zebrafish models demonstrate poly-GA toxicity in zebrafish. Reduction of poly-GA protein rescues toxicity validating this therapeutic approach to treat *C9orf72* repeat expansion carriers. These novel animal models provide a valuable tool for drug discovery to reduce DPR associated toxicity in ALS/FTLD patients with *C9orf72* repeat expansions.

Keywords: Zebrafish, *C9orf72*, poly-GA toxicity

Background

Expansion of the GGGGCC hexanucleotide repeat in the *C9orf72* intronic region was recently identified as a cause for amyotrophic lateral sclerosis (ALS) and frontotemporal lobar degeneration (FTLD) [1–3]. This repeat expansion is observed in around 40% of familial and 7% of sporadic cases of ALS and 25% of familial and 6% of sporadic cases of FTLD [4]. Affected patients have hundreds to several thousands of repeats, while healthy individuals generally have 2 to 23 repeats [1–3, 5]. The expanded repeat RNA is transcribed and accumulates in RNA foci, which have been detected in brain tissue, lymphoblasts, as well as fibroblasts derived from patients with the *C9orf72* associated repeat expansion [6]. This long repeat RNA transcript can sequester RNA binding proteins, including heterogeneous nuclear ribonucleoprotein A3 (hnRNPA3), hnRNPH, and nucleolin, and can lead to mis-regulation of RNA splicing [7–9]. Interestingly, despite the absence of an ATG start codon, the repeat

* Correspondence: bettina.schmid@dzne.de
[1]German Center for Neurodegenerative Diseases (DZNE), Feodor-Lynen-Str.17, 81377 Munich, Germany
[4]Munich Cluster for Systems Neurology (SyNergy), Feodor-Lynen-Str.17, 81377 Munich, Germany
Full list of author information is available at the end of the article

RNA is further subjected to unconventional **r**epeat **a**ssociated **n**on-ATG (RAN) translation [7, 9–11] resulting in dipeptide repeat proteins (DPRs) of Gly-Ala (poly-GA), Gly-Arg (poly-GR) and Gly-Pro (poly-GP) and additional Gly-Pro (poly-GP), Pro-Ala (poly-PA) and Pro-Arg (poly-PR) from the transcribed antisense strand. The DPRs form cytosolic coaggregates with p62 in the brains of patients with *C9orf72* repeat expansions [12–15] and have been shown to interfere with RNA metabolism and coaggregate with other proteins [16–20]. Additionally, interference of DPRs with nucleocytoplasmic transport has been identified independently in different model systems by unbiased genetic screens [21–25].

Three pathomechanisms have been postulated in *C9orf72* repeat expansion carriers, which are not mutually exclusive and most likely act in combination. First, haploinsufficiency due to reduced transcript levels of *C9orf72*. Second, toxicity of RNA foci by sequestration of important RNA binding proteins and disturbed RNA homeostasis. Third, toxicity of RAN translation products.

We set out to generate transgenic zebrafish lines with expanded GGGGCC repeats and poly-GA as a vertebrate animal model to address their contribution to toxicity. We generated two transgenic lines expressing 80 repeats of the GGGGCC sequence (ggggcc80) and two lines with the translation initiation codon ATG in front of the 80xGGGGCC repeat sequence driving expression of poly-GA protein fused to green fluorescent protein (GA80-GFP). We chose poly-GA since it is the most abundant DPR species found in patients with *C9orf72* repeat expansions [13, 26]. The transgenic zebrafish models with 80 repeats reproduced key pathological features, such as RNA foci, however RAN translation was not detectable. Transgenic zebrafish with 80 repeats of GGGGCC only showed minor toxicity (mild pericardial edema), which was greatly increased when we forced expression of poly-GA by 80 GGGGCC repeats with an ATG translational start codon in the GA frame (severe pericardial edema). By blocking poly-GA translation by an antisense approach, we show that the phenotypes can be partially rescued, demonstrating that poly-GA is toxic in vivo and that targeting poly-DPRs might be a useful therapeutic strategy for *C9orf72* repeat expansion carriers.

Results

Generation of a transgenic zebrafish model of *C9orf72* repeat expansion disease

We generated several transgenic zebrafish UAS-based responder lines expressing either 2 or 80 repeats with an ATG (Tg(UAS:ATG-2xGGGGCC-GFP) and Tg(UAS:ATG-80xGGGGCC-GFP)) in the GA reading frame as well as 80 GGGGGCC repeats without ATG (Tg(UAS:80xGGGGCC-GFP)) fused to GFP (Fig. 1a). We generated these lines by Tol2 mediated transposition into the zebrafish genome [27]. We confirmed successful germline transmission of the transgenes by PCR-based genotyping. The 80xGGGGCC repeat sequence was unstable and changes in repeat length were frequently observed in the F1 generation (data not shown). We selected stable transgenic lines with 80xGGGGCC repeats and confirmed the repeat length by PCR (Fig. 1b). To exclude potential toxicity mediated by the transgene integration site, we selected 2 independent lines (a and b) for Tg(UAS:ATG-2xGGGGCC-GFP) and Tg(UAS:ATG-80xGGGGCC-GFP), which we will refer to as GA2-GFPa/b and GA80-GFPa/b respectively. Comparable mRNA expression levels of the respective transgene were confirmed by semi-quantitative reverse transcription PCR (RT-PCR) upon crossing the responder lines to the gene trap Gal4 driver line SAGFF73A [28]. This line drives expression of high level of Gal4 ubiquitously at early embryonic stages and was used in all experiments to drive transgene expression of the respective UAS driver lines. All transgenic lines showed comparable RNA expression levels at 4 days post fertilization (dpf) (Fig. 1c). Additionally, we confirmed the expression of GA80-GFP protein by immunoblotting at 4 dpf (Fig. 1d). The GA2-GFPa/b larvae showed 7.2 fold higher GFP protein expression levels compared to the GA80-GFPa/b larvae (mean of line a and b). This suggests that despite nearly equal mRNA levels, less poly-GA is translated in the GA80-GFP fish than the GA2-GFP fish. A poly-GA specific antibody also detected the GA80-GFP protein (Fig. 1d), but failed to detect GA2-GFP, most likely because two GA repeats are too short to be recognized by the antibody.

Tg(UAS:80xGGGGCC-GFP) fish expressing repeat RNA without a start codon were generated and fish with a stable length of 80 repeats were selected by PCR (Fig. 1c). This line will be referred to as ggggcc80-GFP. Although the expression level of mRNA is similar to those of GA2-GFP and GA80-GFP expressing fish, poly-GA peptides derived from RAN translation were not detectable by Western blotting in the ggggcc80-GFP fish at 4 dpf (Fig. 1d). We also failed to detect poly-GR and poly-GP (data not shown). Thus, if RAN translation occurs in the ggggcc80-GFP line, it is below the detection limit of our specific antibodies.

RNA derived from GA80-GFP and ggggcc80-GFP lead to RNA foci formation

To test if pathological hallmarks of *C9orf72* repeat expansion disease are found in transgenic zebrafish with an expanded GGGGCC repeat, we analyzed RNA foci formation at 28 h post fertilization (hpf). GA80-GFP as well as ggggcc80-GFP zebrafish showed RNA foci in spinal cord neurons by in situ hybridization, whereas wild-type and GA2-GFP zebrafish did not show RNA foci (Fig. 2a and Additional file 1: Figure S1). We further

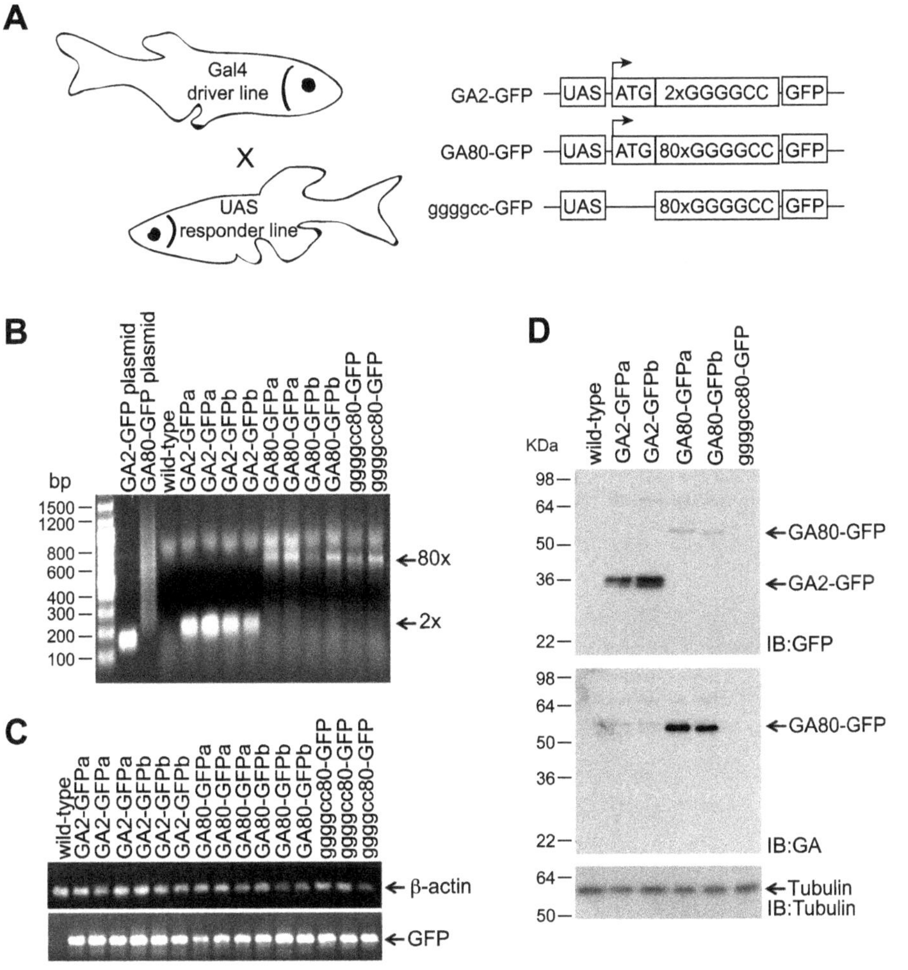

Fig. 1 Generation of transgenic zebrafish model of *C9ORF72* repeat expansion disease. **a** Schematic representation of Gal4 driver line zebrafish crossed to a UAS responder transgenic zebrafish to generate embryos that express a transgene under the control of the UAS. Schematic representation of the responder constructs used for the generation of transgenic zebrafish. **b** Genotyping by PCR of 1 dpf embryos. pCS2 + 2xGGGGCC and pCS2 + 80XGGGGCC constructs were used as standards for GA2-GFP and GA80-GFP in lane 2 and 3. Positions of 2xGGGGCC and 80xGGGGCC repeats are indicated by arrows. **c** Semi-quantitative RT-PCR analyses for the wild-type, GA2-GFPa/b, GA80-GFPa/b and ggggcc80-GFP zebrafish. Note that all transgenic lines showed similar expression level at 4 dpf embryos. **d** Immunoblotting of wild-type, GA2-GFPa/b, GA80-GFPa/b and ggggcc80-GFP with antibodies as indicated with embryonic lysates of 4 dpf old embryos

confirmed that the RNA foci are sensitive to RNaseA but not to DNase treatment, confirming the RNA nature of the foci (Fig. 2b and Additional file 1 Figure S1).

ggggcc80-GFP expression displays mild toxicity in zebrafish

We next analyzed ggggcc80-GFP transgenic fish for signs of toxicity. ggggcc80-GFP larvae showed a pericardial edema phenotype at 4 dpf. We categorized the phenotypes based on their severity in three groups: 1. wild-type, 2. mild edema and 3. severe pericardial edema as shown in Fig. 2c. Of the ggggcc80-GFP larvae 50.2 ± 13.7% (mean ± SD) were unaffected, 32.2 ± 8.2% had a mild pericardial edema and 17.2 ± 11.6% had a severe pericardial edema at 4 dpf (Fig. 2d). The edema phenotype precluded inflation of the swim bladder, inability to feed independently, and death during early larval stages. No abnormal phenotype was detectable in GA2-GFP larvae, suggesting that the expanded GGGGCC repeat causes the mild toxicity in the ggggcc80-GFP fish.

GA80-GFP protein expression is highly toxic in zebrafish

Poly-GA has previously been shown to be toxic in neurons and animal models [23, 29]. Expression of GA80-GFP protein was detected by diffuse green GFP expression and as GFP inclusions exclusively in the musculature by 2 and 4 dpf (Fig. 3a), whereas GA2-GFP fish showed only diffuse green fluorescence. Almost all GA80-GFPa expressing fish showed a severe pericardial edema (92.8 ± 2.8%) and only very few fish showed a mild pericardial edema (7.2 ± 2.8%) at 4 dpf. Similarly, the second transgenic line GA80-GFP-b had 97.5 ± 2.6%

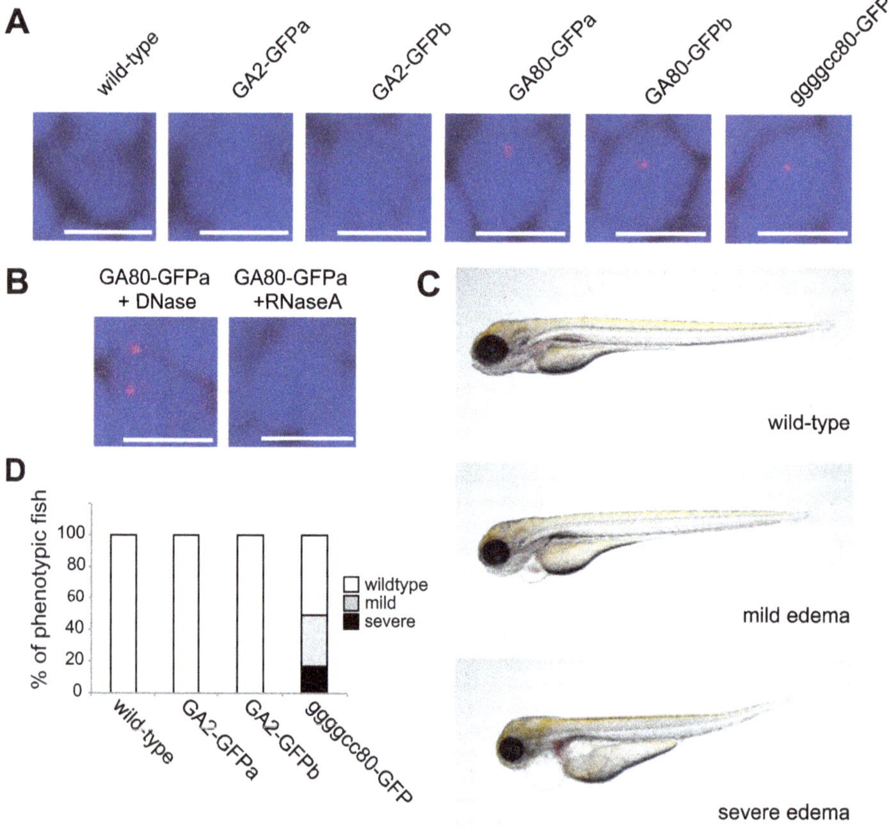

Fig. 2 RNA foci formation in transgenic zebrafish. **a**, **b** Cy3-labeled in situ probe detected dot-like structures in spinal cord in GA80-GFPa/b and ggggcc80-GFP zebrafish. **b** Foci were only detected in GA80-GFP and ggggcc-GFP fish whereas no foci were detected in wild-type and GA2-GFPa/b fish at 28 hpf. GA80-GFPa zebrafish were treated with RNaseA or DNase. Scale bar 10 µm. **c** Pericardial edema phenotype observed in ggggcc80-GFP zebrafish at 4 dpf. Phenotypic features are classified as wild-type, mild edema, and severe edema. **d** The average percentages of phenotypic fish of the three different phenotypic classes at 4 dpf are indicated in the bargraph (at least three independent clutches were analyzed with $n \geq 14$)

of the fish with an severe pericardial edema and 2.5 ± 2.6% with an mild pericardial edema at 4 dpf (Fig. 3b).

Additionally, GA80-GFPa/b fish also showed a strongly reduced circulation of red blood cells in 61.5 ± 9.0% (line a) and 21.6 ± 3.9% (line b) of the GFP positive embryos at 2 dpf, respectively. In contrast, wild-type, GA2-GFPa/b as well as ggggcc80-GFP fish did not show any circulation defect of red blood cells at 2 dpf (Fig. 3c,d), suggesting that poly-GA toxicity additionally impaired circulation. The circulation defect did not seem to be mediated by a heart defect since the GA80-GFPa fish had a normal heart beat at 2.5 dpf (data not shown). Phenotypic embryos with a strong edema and lack of circulation died around 5 dpf.

We further examined the length of the spinal motor neuron axons in GA80-GFPa zebrafish, since *C9orf72* repeat expansion carriers can suffer from motor neuron degeneration. No significant differences of the axonal length were observed at 28 hpf (Additional file 2: Figure S2A, B). In addition, there was no apparent difference in the overall neuronal outgrowth and branching at 2 dpf (Additional file 3: Figure S3A, B), indicating expression of neither an expanded GGGGCC repeat nor poly-GA protein affected neuronal outgrowth. Interestingly, aggregates of GA80-GFP were exclusively found in the musculature despite ubiquitous GA80-GFP protein expression in both transgenic GA80-GFP lines at 2 and 4 dpf. Larvae with a severe edema phenotype had more than twice as many inclusions compared to larvae with a mild phenotype at 4 dpf (Additional file 4: Figure S4A), suggesting that these embryos have higher expression levels, leading to higher toxicity and more inclusions. The overall structure of the muscle was not affected as determined by α-actinin staining at 2 dpf (Additional file 4: Figure S4B), suggesting that the GA80-GFP aggregates themselves are not toxic and that muscle defects are not the primary cause of toxicity in our zebrafish model.

Previously, we reported that knockout of the two orthologues of human TDP-43, a key protein in ALS/FTLD, in zebrafish (*tardbp−/−*, *tardbpl−/−*) showed a circulation phenotype accompanied with mispatterning

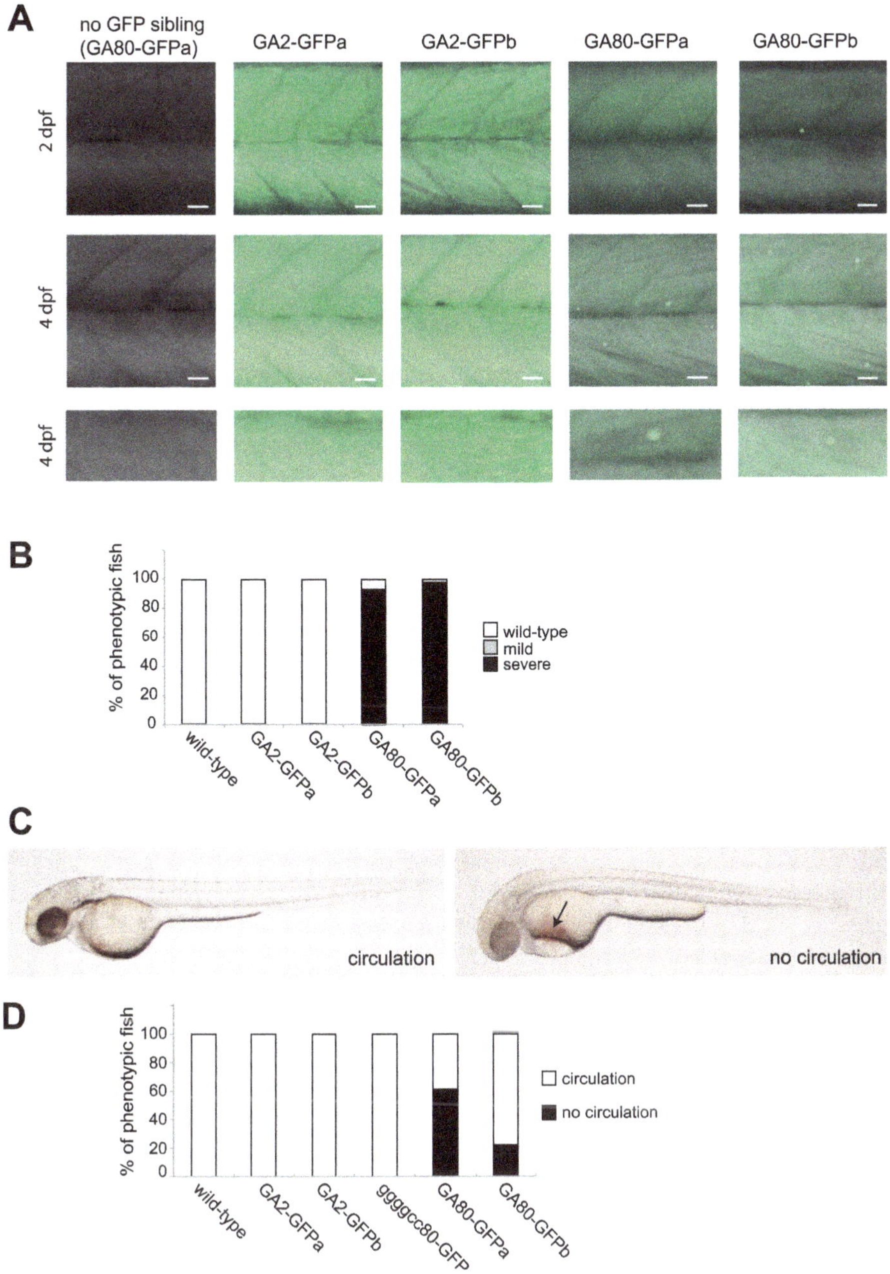

Fig. 3 Poly-GA protein elicits a toxic phenotype. **a** In vivo image of GA-GFP polypeptides at 2 and 4 dpf. Genotypes as indicated. No GFP sibling (GA80-GFP) refers to a sibling from a cross between a Gal4 driver and a UAS GA80-GFP responder fish that is GFP negative, and hence is either negative for the driver or the responder construct, or both constructs. GFP fluorescent images shown are merged with DIC pictures. Lowest panel is a magnification of the middle panel at 4 dpf. Lateral views of the trunk musculature. Scale bar 20 μm. **b** A strong pericardial edema phenotype was observed in GA80-GFPa/b zebrafish at 4 dpf. The average percentages of phenotypic fish of the three different classes are indicated in the bargraph. **c** GA80-GFPa/b zebrafish had mostly no circulation at 2 dpf. Red blood cells accumulate due to circulation defects (*arrow*). **d** The average percentages of fish with or without circulation are indicated in the bargraph (at least three independent clutches were analyzed with n ≥14)

and increased sprout formation of the vasculature [19]. Since *C9orf72* repeat expansion carriers show cytoplasmic TDP-43 mislocalization and presumably partial TDP-43 loss of function, we analyzed TDP-43 function in the repeat expressing fish. We examined vascular patterning in GA80-GFPa zebrafish by crossing them to Tg(kdrl:HsHRAS-mCherry)^{s896}, a reporter line expressing mCherry in all endothelial cells [20]. However, neither vascular mispatterning nor aberrant sprout formation as seen in *tardbp−/−*, *tardbpl−/−* fish were detected at 2.5 dpf (Additional file 5: Figure S5A, B), ruling out vascular patterning defects as the primary cause of the circulation phenotype. However, endothelial cells appeared thinner and less structured in GA80-GFPa larvae (Additional file 5: Figure S5), most likely due to the lack of perfusion. Reduction of zebrafish Tardbp function leads to an alternative splicing pattern of the second ortholgue Tardbpl, referred to as Tardbpl_tv1, which can fully replace Tardbp function. Impaired Tardbp function (for example by mislocalization) can therefore be monitored by upregulation of the compensatory Tardbpl_tv1 variant. We analyzed the expression levels of Tardbp as well as Tardbpl_tv1 by immunoblotting in GA80-GFPa zebrafish at 2 dpf. Increased levels of Tardbpl_tv1 would indicate partial loss of Tardbp. However, protein levels of Tardbp and Tardbpl_tv1 showed no differences in wild-type and GA80-GFP transgenic fish (Additional file 6: Figure S6), suggesting that the perfusion phenotype is mediated by a TDP-43 independent mechanism.

Antisense morpholino (AMO) rescues the edema phenotype in GA80-GFP zebrafish

Antisense morpholinos (AMO) are a useful tool to suppress the translation of genes of interest. Here, we designed AMOs targeting GAL4 as well as the ATG start codon of the GA80-GFP transgene (Fig. 4a) to further substantiate the correlation of GA80-GFP protein levels and toxicity. Injection of the AMO targeting GAL4 into the fertilized embryos in GA80-GFPa efficiently blocked translation of the transcriptional activator Gal4 and thereby efficiently reduced GA80-GFP protein expression at 2 dpf (Fig. 4b). Although control AMO injected transgenic zebrafish showed mostly the severe edema phenotype (95.8 ± 3.9%) and very few mild edema phenotypes (4.2 ± 3.9%), GAL4 AMO injected fish showed only few severe (4.8 ± 8.2%) and mild (8.6 ± 8.3%) and mostly unaffected zebrafish (86.7 ± 8.3%), indicating that AMO mediated GAL4 inhibition rescued the pericardial edema phenotype at 4 dpf (Fig. 4b).

To further address if toxicity is mediated by the expression of GA80-GFP protein we designed AMO targeting ATG start codon upstream of the GGGGCC repeat (ATG AMO) and aimed at reverting the phenotype by blocking translation of the poly-GA protein in the GA80-GFPa larvae. Upon injection of ATG AMO, GA80-GFP protein expression was severely reduced, as determined by immunoblot at 2 dpf (Fig. 4c). In addition, ATG targeting AMO reduced the severe pericardial edema phenotype in GA80-GFP expressing zebrafish demonstrating that poly-GA protein is a toxic species in vivo at 4 dpf (Fig. 4c.). We next examined the expression level of mRNA as well as RNA foci formation upon ATG targeting AMO injection, since they are blocking translation without changing the mRNA. mRNA expression levels analyzed at 2 dpf by semi-quantitative RT-PCR were unaffected in phenotypic fish upon ATG AMO injection and RNA foci were still detectable (Fig. 4d, e, Additional file 1 Figure S1) indicating that poly-GA was toxic in zebrafish and that the phenotypic rescue is mediated by reduction of GA80-GFP protein levels.

Discussion

Expansion of a GGGGCC repeat in a non-coding region of *C9orf72* is the most common cause of ALS/FTLD. Recently, RAN translation from the sense and antisense GGGGCC repeat transcript was observed in *C9orf72* repeat expansion carriers generating 5 different DPR species (poly-GA, -GR, -GP, -PA and -PR) [12–14, 30]. These DPRs coaggregate with p62 and form the characteristic star shaped inclusions in *C9orf72* repeat expansion carriers [13].

The relative contribution of RNA and DPR toxicity is still under debate since many conflicting results have been obtained in a variety of different model systems (reviewed in [31]). The GGGGCC repeat RNA forms foci in cells, animal models and patients and has been shown to be able to induce neuronal cell death and to sequester RNA binding proteins [8, 15, 20, 32]. However, there is only a weak correlation between RNA foci and neurodegeneration in patients [33–35]. In zebrafish RNA injection of 8x, 38x, and 72x GGGGCC repeats has been shown to cause RNA foci and cell death by apoptosis in a repeat length dependent manner [9]. This study did not report on RAN translation products upon repeat RNA injections in zebrafish. In line with these studies we observe RNA foci in two independent transgenic ggggcc80-GFP lines and RNA toxicity. In the ggggcc80-GFP fish we were not able to detect GA, GP, and GR species, most likely due to the relatively short repeat length or inefficient or even lack of RAN translation in early zebrafish that preclude detection of DPR species by Western blotting. This is in contrast to fly and mouse models in which repeat expression leads to DPR translation in the absence of a start codon [18, 20]. Whether the mild toxic effects seen in ggggcc80-GFP fish is due to RNA toxicity or low level DPRs remains to be determined. To further address DPR toxicity we focused on poly-GA since it is the most abundant species found in *C9orf72* repeat carriers and induced the neuronal cell death in primary cultured cell model as well as in animal models [16–18, 20]. We generated several transgenic zebrafish lines and demonstrated that poly-GA is toxic in zebrafish. In primary neurons poly-GA toxicity has been attributed to sequestration of Unc119 (a trafficking factor for myristylated proteins), interference with the ubiquitin proteasome system, and endoplasmic reticulum stress [16, 17]. Recently, poly-GR and poly-PR were shown to be the most toxic DPR species in *Drosophila* [18, 36]. Moreover, the arginine-rich DPR species are also toxic in primary neurons, potentially

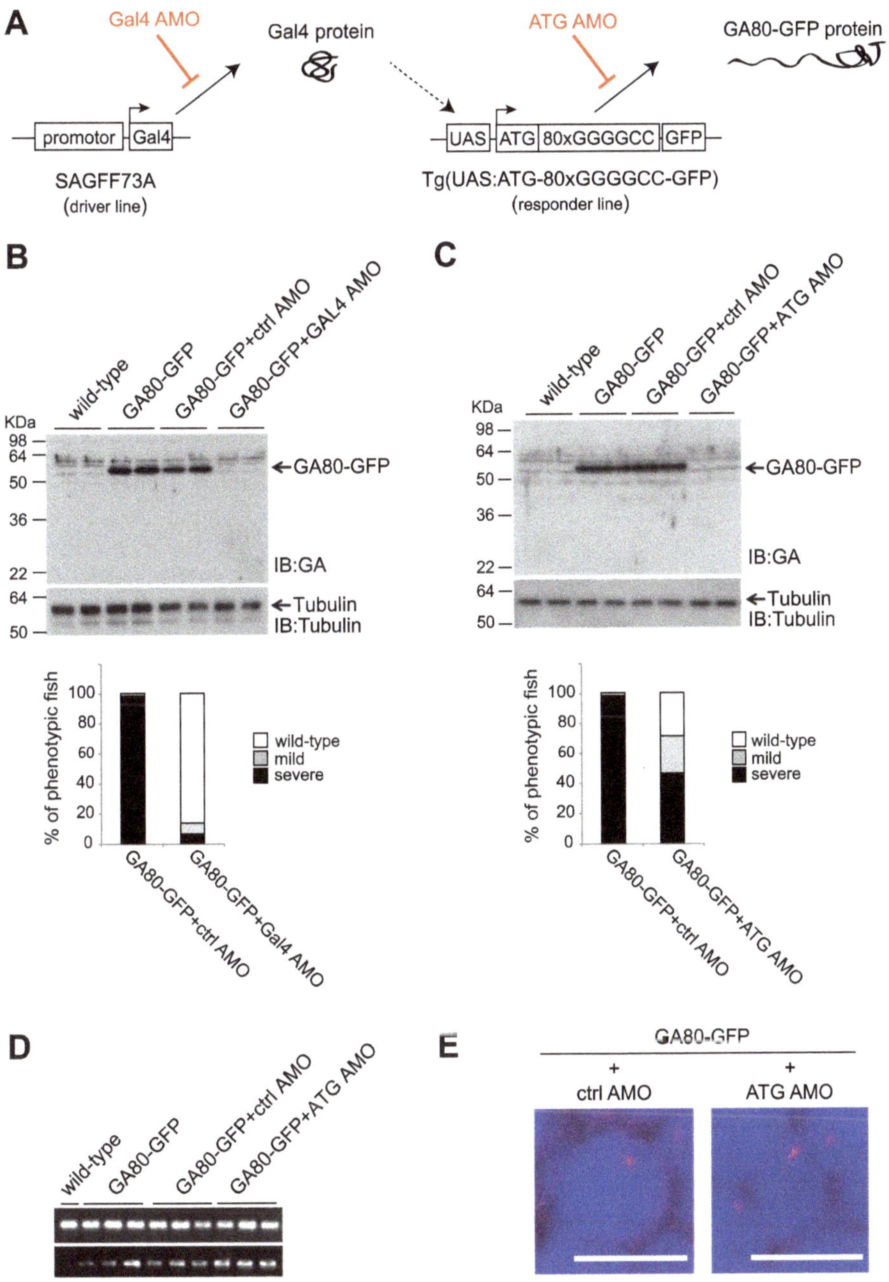

Fig. 4 Antisense morpholino rescued the toxic edema phenotype. **a** Representation of process of intervention for each morpholino during the generation of GA80-GFP protein in vivo. **b** GAL4 targeting AMO efficiently blocked Gal4 translation at 2 dpf shown by immunoblotting (*upper panel*). Quantification of the pericardial edema phenotype observed in GA80-GFP with injection of ctrl AMO or GAL4 targeting AMO at 4 dpf are shown as a bar graph (*lower panel*) ($p < 0{,}001$, 3 independent experiments with 3 clutches $n \geq 6$ are shown, unpaired t test). **c** ATG targeting morpholino efficiently inhibited the ATG dependent translation of poly-GA at 2 dpf (*upper panel*). Quantification of the pericardial edema phenotype observed in GA80-GFP upon injection of ctrl AMO or ATG targeting AMO at 4 dpf shown as a bar graph (*lower panel*) ($p < 0{,}005$, 3 independent experiments with 3 clutches $n \geq 19$ are shown, unpaired t test). **d** Semi-quantitative RT-PCR analyses of injected embryos at 2 dpf. **e** RNA foci formation was not affected upon injection with ctrl AMO or ATG AMO at 2 dpf. Scale bar 10 µm

affecting RNA synthesis [18, 19]. Interestingly, DPRs interfere with nucleocytoplasmic shuttling in *Drosophila*, cells, and yeast [21, 22, 24, 25]. Two independently generated BAC transgenic mouse models recapitulate *C9orf72* repeat associated pathology, however they lack neurodegeneration [34, 35]. In contrast, another BAC transgenic mouse model shows neurodegeneration and TDP-43 pathology [37]. Expression of high levels of *C9orf72* repeats by adeno associated virus in mouse brain also generate neurodegeneration and TDP-43 pathology [20]. These differences might reflect that sufficiently high expression levels are required to induce neurodegeneration. It remains unclear which DPR proteins contribute to ALS/FTLD pathogenesis in patients under physiological conditions. There is currently little evidence for a regional correlation of DPR aggregates in humans and neurodegeneration [38]. These animal models will be valuable tools to further dissect the relative contribution and synergistic effects of repeat RNA and DPRs to toxicity.

GA80-GFP fish showed a circulation defect at 2 dpf and a severe pericardial edema phenotype at 4 dpf. Interestingly, double knockout zebrafish (*tardbp−/−, tardbpl−/−*) also showed circulation defects at 2 dpf and vascular mispatterning, resulting in a pericardial edema phenotype reminiscent of the GGGGCC repeat induced phenotype [39]. Considering that partial loss of TDP-43 function could be linked to the pathogenesis of ALS/FTLD-TDP-43, including *C9orf72* repeat expansion carriers [40], we analyzed expression of Tardbp and Tardbpl_tv1 in GA80-GFP fish. However, no apparent changes in Tardbp and Tardbpl_tv1 protein level were observed upon transgene expression, indicating that neither RNA foci nor poly-GA lead to a loss of TDP-43 function in our zebrafish model. We speculate that potentially a common downstream pathway is affected in double knockout zebrafish (*tardbp−/−, tardbpl−/−*) and GA80-GFP zebrafish, resulting in a similar circulation defect. However, since pericardial edemas are a common phenotype, which can be caused by a variety of defects, we cannot exclude the possibility that these similar phenotypes have distinct causes. Unfortunately, the larval lethality precludes analysis of possible neurodegenerative phenotypes of the repeat expressing transgenic zebrafish during adulthood.

GA80-GFP leads to inclusion formation which was restricted to the musculature. Why the musculature was more prone to form inclusions in our model remains speculative. This might be due to higher expression levels of the GA80-GFP protein or driven by cell type specific other coaggregating proteins. There was no correlation of cell death and poly-GA aggregation in zebrafish, since we did not observe any degeneration of muscle cells. Interestingly, there is also no clear correlation between DPR aggregate formation and neuronal loss in *C9orf72* repeat expansion patients, raising the possibility that the aggregates themselves are not the toxic DPR species [26, 38, 41].

Conclusion

We developed a novel vertebrate animal model for *C9orf72* repeat expansion pathomechanisms and demonstrated that the DPR poly-GA is toxic in vivo. Selective inhibition of poly-GA production by antisense oligonucleotides decreased toxicity. These findings indicate that intervention with DPR expression might be an effective therapeutic strategy for patients with *C9orf72* repeat expansions.

Methods

Zebrafish

Zebrafish embryos were kept at 28.5 °C and staged as previously described [35]. AB and TLF were used as the wild-type strains. All experiments were performed in accordance with animal protection standard of Ludwig Maximilians University Munich and approved by the government of upper Bavaria (Regierung von Oberbayern, Munich, Germany).

Antibodies

Anti-tubulin (Sigma, T6199), anti-GFP (Clontech, 632377), anti-acetylated tubulin (Sigma, T6793), anti-Tardbp (clone 4A12 [19]), anti-Tardbpl_tv1 (clone 16C8 [19]), anti-znp-1 (DSHB), anti-α-actinin (Sigma, A7811), anti-GA (clone 5 F2 [16]), anti-GR (clone 5A2 [9]), anti-mouse IgG, HRP conj. (Promega, W4021), anti-rabbit IgG, HRP conj. (Promega, W4011), Alexa Fluor antibodies (Invitrogen).

Plasmid construction and generation of transgenic zebrafish

For the construction of the GA2-GFP and GA80-GFP plasmids, a Kozak sequence (GCCGCCACC) was inserted 3′ of the ATG.

For the generation of the GA80-GFP and ggggcc80-GFP plasmids were constructed as described in Additional file 7: Figure S7. pCS2 + eGFP plasmid [13] was PCR amplified by Phusion high fidelity polymerase (New England Biolabs) using the following primers:

GA80-GFP

A: pCS2-f1: 5′ -ggccgcaGGTGGCGGAGGTGGCGTGAGCAAGGGCGAGGAGC-3′
pCS2-r1: 5′ -gCATGGTGGCGGCCTTGGATCCGGAATTCGAATCGATGGGATCCTGCA-3′

B: pCS2-f2: 5′ - gcaGGTGGCGGAGGTGGCGTGAGCAAGGGCGAGGAGC-3′
pCS2-r2: 5′ - tagCATGGTGGCGGCCTTGGATCCGGAATTCGAATCGATGGGATCCTGCA-3′

ggggcc80xRNA

A′: pCS2-f1: 5′ - ggccgcaGGTGGCGGAGGTGGCGTGAGCAAGGGCGAGGAGC-3′
pCS2-r3: 5′ - gGGTGGCGGCCTTGGATCCGGAATTCGAATCGATGGGATCCTGCA-3′

B′ pCS2-f2: 5′ - gcaGGTGGCGGAGGTGGCGTGAGCAAGGGCGAGGAGC-3′
pCS2-r2: 5′ - tagCATGGTGGCGGCCTTGGATCCGGAATTCGAATCGATGGGATCCTGCA-3′

After purification of the PCR products generated by A/B or A'/B', the PCR products were co-incubated at following cycles (94 °C 2 min, 94 °C 30 s, 55 °C 30 s, 72 °C 2 min, 72 °C 10 min, 10 °C 10 min) to produce sticky end fragments digested by NotI/BfaI (New England Biolabs), like for circular plasmid generation. To prepare the ggggcc80-GFP plasmid for the generation of transgenic fish, the pEF-80xGGGGCC plasmid [9] was digested by BamHI and PmeI (New England Biolabs). Subsequently, the 80xGGGGCC fragment was purified and digested by BfaI and NotI. The fragment was then ligated to a PCR amplified pCS2+ plasmid vector backbone.

The pCS2 + ATG-80xGGGGCC-GFP and pCS2 + 80xGGGGCC plasmids were digested by StyI (New England Biolabs) and HpaI (New England Biolabs) and cloned into pT2KXIGdeltaIN plasmid (a gift from K. Kawakami, National Institute of Genetics, Shizuoka, Japan) to generate transgenic zebrafish by TOL2 mediated transposition. Our pT2KXIGdeltaIN plasmid harbored one point mutation in the UAS region that generated a novel StyI recognition site. We therefore had to reintroduce the StyI- StyI digested fragment that was previously lost during the cloning procedure into the pT2 + ATG-80xGGGGCC-GFP/+80xGGGGCC plasmids.

To generate the ATG-2xGGGGCC-GFP plasmid, the primer (ATG-short2:'- AAAAGATCCAAGGCCGCCA CCATGCTAGGGGCCGGGGCCGGGGCTCTCAAAC T-3'), which includes 2xGGGGCC and a T3 primer were used for amplification of the pCS2 + eGFP plasmid backbone [13]. Subsequently, the PCR product as well as pCS2 + ATG-80xGGGGCC-GFP were digested by StyI and HpaI and ligated to each other. The pT2 + ATG-2XGGGGCC-GFP plasmid was generated accordingly.

To generate the transgenic fish, 10 ng/μl of the corresponding plasmid and 100 ng/μl transposase mRNA were co-injected into 1 cell stage AB embryos.

GA2-GFP and GA80-GFP run at a higher molecular weight than the calculated 31,3 and 41,3 kDa (including the 33aa linker sequences) potentially due to posttranslational modifications. GFP coding sequence without a start codon was used.

Genotyping the repeat length by PCR

To extract genomic DNA from zebrafish embryos, Proteinase K (Roche) treatment (170 μg/ml, overnight) was performed at 65 °C. Subsequently, Proteinase K was inactivated at 95 °C for 10 min. To amplify the transgene, GFP specific primers were used for genotyping (GFP-3f: 5′- GTGGTGCCCATCCTGGTCGAGCT-3′ and GFP-3r: 5′- AGATCTGAGTCCGGACTTGTAC AG-3′).

To confirm the repeat length, Expand Long Template PCR System (Roche) was used with slight modifications: 98 °C 10 min, 97 °C 35 s, 55 °C 2min20s, 68 °C 2min20s, 68 °C 10 min, 55 °C 5 min, 50 °C 5 min, 10 °C. Steps from 2 to 4 were repeated in 49 cycles. [36]. 80rep-1f: 5′-CTAGAGGGTATATAATGGATC-3′ and 80rep-r2: 5′-CTGTGCTGGATATCTGCAGAATT-3′ were used for PCR.

Whole mount fluorescent in situ hybridization and motor axonal length measurement

Zebrafish embryos (28 hpf) were fixed in 4% paraformaldehyde (PFA) overnight. Protocol modified from Thisse et al. [42]. The embryo was gradually transferred into phosphate buffered saline Tween-20 (PBST), PBST with 30% methanol (MeOH), PBST with 60% MeOH and finally 100% MeOH and kept at −20 °C overnight. Before Proteinase K treatment, embryos were transferred into PBST with 60% MeOH, PBST with 30% MeOH and PBST. After Proteinase K digestion, re-fixation of embryos was performed by PFA for 15 min at room temperature. After washing with PBST for 5 × 10 min, embryos were preincubated with hybridization buffer (HYB+) for 1 h at 65 ° C. The Cy3(GGCCCC)$_4$ probe was synthesized by IDT (Integrated DNA Technologies) as previously described [2] and diluted into 10 ng/μl in HYB+ solution. Embryos were hybridized overnight at 65 °C. Afterwards, they were washed in HYB- for 3 × 30 min, 2 × saline sodium citrate with 0.1% Tween20 (SSCT) for 2 × 15 min, 0.2 × SSCT for 3 × 30 min, PBST 3 × 30 min at 65 °C. After 4,6-diamidin-2-phenylindol (DAPI) staining, embryos were mounted in 1.5% agarose.

DNaseI (Qiagen) or RNaseA (Thermo scientific) treatment of the embryos was performed after Proteinase K treatment, by incubation with the respective enzyme in PBST for 1.5 h at 37 °C prior in situ hybridization.

Measurement of axonal motor neuron axon length was previously described [19].

Semi-quantitative RT-PCR

The RNeasy kit (Qiagen) was used with on column DNaseI treatment for total RNA isolation. cDNA synthesis was performed with M-MLV reverse transcriptase (Invitrogen) and Random Primer Mix (NEB), followed by a RNaseH (Invitrogen) digest as previously described [16].

Antisense morpholino (AMO)

Sequences of AMO used in this study:

Control AMO (ctrl AMO) (CCTCTTACCTCAGTTA CAATTTATA), GAL4 targeting AMO (Gal4 AMO) (GTTCGATAGAAGACAGTAGCTTCAT) [37], and ATG targeting AMO (ATG AMO) (CCCCTAGCATGGTGG CGGCCTT) were all obtained from Genetools. AMOs were injected into fertilized embryos according to the manufacturer's instructions. The Gal4 AMO and the ATG AMO were used at 125 μM.

Western blotting and immunohistochemistry

A standard protocol was used as previously described [16]. To stain the anti-α-actinin or anti-acetylated tubulin, in vivo imaging for mCherry expression to analyze the vasculature, embryos at 2 dpf were fixed by 4% PFA.

Microscopy

Images were taken with a Cell Observer CSU-X1 (Yokogawa) Spinning Disk (Zeiss), AxioCam MRm (Zeiss) and Evolve 512 (Photometrics) or confocal microscope LSM710 (Zeiss). Brightness and contrast were adjusted using Zen blue or gray (Zeiss) and ImageJ. For in vivo imaging of GFP fluorescence, dechorionated zebrafish were incubated with Tricaine (3-amino benzoic acidethylester) (Sigma) for immobilization. Subsequently, zebrafish were mounted in the Metaphor (low melting temperature) agarose (LONZA).

Additional files

Additional file 1: Figure S1. RNA foci formation overview. Embryos of the indicated genotypes stained with a Cy3-labeled probe to visualize RNA foci formation by in situ hybridization. Between 13–33 cells per field of view showed RNA foci in the GA80-GFP larvae. All images were taken without DAPI fluorescence. Scale bar 10 μm.

Additional file 2: Figure S2. Spinal motor neuron axonal outgrowth is not affected. (A) Spinal motor neuron axon of GA80-GFP fish (Gal4 driver + UAS:ATG-80xGGGGCC-GFP responder) and the GFP negative siblings (Gal4 driver or UAS:ATG-80xGGGGCC-GFP alone, or wild-type) at 28 hpf. (B) Length of outgrowing spinal motor neuron axons measured from the exit point of the spinal cord to the tip of the growth cone in the 5 somites anterior of the end of the yolk expansion at 28 hpf (indicated by the numbers 1–5). Embryos are sorted by the genotypes wild-type, driver, responder, and driver + responder. Statistical analyses was performed in indicated genotypes. Scale bar 20 μm. Mean ± SD.

Additional file 3: Figure S3. Overall neuronal outgrowth is not affected. Overall neuronal outgrowth was analyzed in embryos stained with an antibody against acetylated tubulin at 2 dpf. Siblings of GA80-GFPa zebrafish expressing GFP (A) or not expressing GFP (B). Scale bar 100 μm.

Additional file 4: Figure S4. Muscle patterning is not affected. (A) Quantification of GFP inclusions in GA80-GFPa and GA80-GFPb larvae subdivided into mild and strong edema phenotypes at 4 dpf. (n = 4 per subgroup, mean ± SD). Amount of inclusions from GA80-GFP line a and b with mild and strong phenotypes were not significantly different (paired *t*-test). Inclusions were exclusively detected in the musculature in both lines. (B) The overall structure of the muscle was analyzed by α-actinin staining at 2 dpf in a GFP negative GA80-GFP embryo and (B) GFP positive sibling. Scale bar 20 μm.

Additional file 5: Figure S5. Vascular patterning is not affected. The vasculature was analyzed by incrossing with Tg(kdrl:HsHRAS-mCherry)^{s896} into the GA80-GFP expressing lines. mCherry expressed from the Tg(kdrl:HsHRAS-mCherry)^{s896} transgene is shown in Ga80-GFP-a transgenic zebrafish not expressing GFP (A) and siblings expressing GFP (B) at 2.5 dpf. Scale bar 20 μm.

Additional file 6: Figure S6. Tardbp function is not impaired in repeat expressing fish. (A) GA80-GFPa zebrafish expressing GFP and (B) siblings not expressing GFP. Western blot analysis of 2 dpf old embryos with antibodies as indicated. Tardbp/Tardbpl_tv1 bands indicated by arrow heads.

Additional file 7: Figure S7. Construction of repeat expressing plasmid in zebrafish. A representative scheme to generate the 80xggggcc repeat containing plasmid.

Acknowledgements
We thank B. Solchenberger, F. van Bebber, K. Strecker, L. Hasenkamp and S. Rothhaemel for the helpful discussion. K. Strecker for taking images by confocal microscopy. E. Kremmer for generating antibodies. W. Katharina, A. Rechenberg and M. Graf for technical assistance. S. Schlink and R. Rojas Rojas for taking care of zebrafish. This work was supported by the Helmholtz cross-program topic "Metabolic Dysfunction" to B. S., the Uehara Memorial Foundation and the National BioResource Project from the Ministry of Education, Culture, Sports, Science and Technology of Japan to K.K. and the European Research Council under the European Union's Seventh Framework Programme FP7/2014-2019 under grant agreement n° 617198 [DPR-MODELS] to D.E..

Authors' contributions
YO, AH, and BS designed the research. KA, KK, and DE shared materials. YO, AW-W, and AH performed the experiments. YO, KA, KK, CH, DE and BS wrote the paper. All authors read and approved the final manuscript.

Competing interests
The authors declare that they have no competing interests.

Author details
[1]German Center for Neurodegenerative Diseases (DZNE), Feodor-Lynen-Str.17, 81377 Munich, Germany. [2]Biomedical Center, Biochemistry, Ludwig-Maximilians University Munich, Feodor-Lynen-Str.17, 81377 Munich, Germany. [3]Division of Molecular and Developmental Biology, National Institute of Genetics, Mishima, Shizuoka 411-8540, Japan. [4]Munich Cluster for Systems Neurology (SyNergy), Feodor-Lynen-Str.17, 81377 Munich, Germany.

References

1. Gijselinck I, et al. A C9orf72 promoter repeat expansion in a Flanders-Belgian cohort with disorders of the frontotemporal lobar degeneration-amyotrophic lateral sclerosis spectrum: a gene identification study. Lancet Neurol. 2012;11(1):54–65.
2. Renton AE, et al. A hexanucleotide repeat expansion in C9ORF72 is the cause of chromosome 9p21-linked ALS-FTD. Neuron. 2011;72(2):257–68.
3. DeJesus-Hernandez M, et al. Expanded GGGGCC hexanucleotide repeat in noncoding region of C9ORF72 causes chromosome 9p-linked FTD and ALS. Neuron. 2011;72(2):245–56.
4. Majounie E, et al. Frequency of the C9orf72 hexanucleotide repeat expansion in patients with amyotrophic lateral sclerosis and frontotemporal dementia: a cross-sectional study. Lancet Neurol. 2012;11(4):323–30.
5. Renton AE, Chio A, Traynor BJ. State of play in amyotrophic lateral sclerosis genetics. Nat Neurosci. 2014;17(1):17–23.
6. Lagier-Tourenne C, et al. Targeted degradation of sense and antisense C9orf72 RNA foci as therapy for ALS and frontotemporal degeneration. Proc Natl Acad Sci U S A. 2013;110(47):E4530–9.
7. Haeusler AR, et al. C9orf72 nucleotide repeat structures initiate molecular cascades of disease. Nature. 2014;507(7491):195–200.
8. Mori K, et al. hnRNP A3 binds to GGGGCC repeats and is a constituent of p62-positive/TDP43-negative inclusions in the hippocampus of patients with C9orf72 mutations. Acta Neuropathol. 2013;125(3):413–23.
9. Lee YB, et al. Hexanucleotide repeats in ALS/FTD form length-dependent RNA foci, sequester RNA binding proteins, and are neurotoxic. Cell Rep. 2013;5(5):1178–86.
10. Todd PK, et al. CGG repeat-associated translation mediates neurodegeneration in fragile X tremor ataxia syndrome. Neuron. 2013;78(3):440–55.

11. Zu T, et al. Non-ATG-initiated translation directed by microsatellite expansions. Proc Natl Acad Sci U S A. 2011;108(1):260–5.
12. Ash PE, et al. Unconventional translation of C9ORF72 GGGGCC expansion generates insoluble polypeptides specific to c9FTD/ALS. Neuron. 2013;77(4):639–46.
13. Mori K, et al. The C9orf72 GGGGCC repeat is translated into aggregating dipeptide-repeat proteins in FTLD/ALS. Science. 2013;339(6125):1335–8.
14. Mori K, et al. Bidirectional transcripts of the expanded C9orf72 hexanucleotide repeat are translated into aggregating dipeptide repeat proteins. Acta Neuropathol. 2013;126(6):881–93.
15. Zu T, et al. RAN proteins and RNA foci from antisense transcripts in C9ORF72 ALS and frontotemporal dementia. Proc Natl Acad Sci U S A. 2013;110(51):E4968–77.
16. May S, et al. C9orf72 FTLD/ALS-associated Gly-Ala dipeptide repeat proteins cause neuronal toxicity and Unc119 sequestration. Acta Neuropathol. 2014;128(4):485–503.
17. Zhang YJ, et al. Aggregation-prone c9FTD/ALS poly (GA) RAN-translated proteins cause neurotoxicity by inducing ER stress. Acta Neuropathol. 2014;128(4):505–24.
18. Mizielinska S, et al. C9orf72 repeat expansions cause neurodegeneration in drosophila through arginine-rich proteins. Science. 2014;345(6201):1192–4.
19. Kwon I, et al. Poly-dipeptides encoded by the C9orf72 repeats bind nucleoli, impede RNA biogenesis, and kill cells. Science. 2014;345(6201):1139–45.
20. Chew J, et al. Neurodegeneration. C9ORF72 repeat expansions in mice cause TDP-43 pathology, neuronal loss, and behavioral deficits. Science. 2015;348(6239):1151–4.
21. Freibaum BD, et al. GGGGCC repeat expansion in C9orf72 compromises nucleocytoplasmic transport. Nature. 2015;525(7567):129–33.
22. Zhang K, et al. The C9orf72 repeat expansion disrupts nucleocytoplasmic transport. Nature. 2015;525(7567):56–61.
23. Zhang YJ, et al. C9ORF72 poly (GA) aggregates sequester and impair HR23 and nucleocytoplasmic transport proteins. Nat Neurosci. 2016;19(5):668–77.
24. Jovicic A, et al. Modifiers of C9orf72 dipeptide repeat toxicity connect nucleocytoplasmic transport defects to FTD/ALS. Nat Neurosci. 2015;18(9):1226–9.
25. Boeynaems S, et al. Drosophila screen connects nuclear transport genes to DPR pathology in c9ALS/FTD. Sci Rep. 2016;6:20877.
26. Schludi MH, et al. Distribution of dipeptide repeat proteins in cellular models and C9orf72 mutation cases suggests link to transcriptional silencing. Acta Neuropathol. 2015;130:537–55.
27. Kawakami K. Tol2: a versatile gene transfer vector in vertebrates. Genome Biol. 2007;8 Suppl 1:S7.
28. Asakawa K, Kawakami K. The Tol2-mediated Gal4-UAS method for gene and enhancer trapping in zebrafish. Methods. 2009;49(3):275–81.
29. Anonymous (!!! INVALID CITATION !!! {Zhang, 2014 #17;Mizielinska, 2014 #18; Kwon, 2014 #28;Chew, 2015 #44;Zhang, 2014 #17}).
30. Gendron TF, et al. Antisense transcripts of the expanded C9ORF72 hexanucleotide repeat form nuclear RNA foci and undergo repeat-associated non-ATG translation in c9FTD/ALS. Acta Neuropathol. 2013;126(6):829–44.
31. Haeusler AR, Donnelly CJ, Rothstein JD. The expanding biology of the C9orf72 nucleotide repeat expansion in neurodegenerative disease. Nat Rev Neurosci. 2016;17(6):383–95.
32. Mori K, et al. Reduced hnRNPA3 increases C9orf72 repeat RNA levels and dipeptide-repeat protein deposition. EMBO Rep. 2016;17(9):1314–25.
33. Hukema RK, et al. A new inducible transgenic mouse model for C9orf72-associated GGGGCC repeat expansion supports a gain-of-function mechanism in C9orf72-associated ALS and FTD. Acta Neuropathol Commun. 2014;2:166.
34. O'Rourke JG, et al. C9orf72 BAC transgenic mice display typical pathologic features of ALS/FTD. Neuron. 2015;88(5):892–901.
35. Peters OM, et al. Human C9ORF72 hexanucleotide expansion reproduces RNA foci and dipeptide repeat proteins but not neurodegeneration in BAC transgenic mice. Neuron. 2015;88(5):902–9.
36. Wen X, et al. Antisense proline-arginine RAN dipeptides linked to C9ORF72-ALS/FTD form toxic nuclear aggregates that initiate in vitro and in vivo neuronal death. Neuron. 2014;84(6):1213–25.
37. Liu Y, et al. C9orf72 BAC mouse model with motor deficits and neurodegenerative features of ALS/FTD. Neuron. 2016;90(3):521–34.
38. Mackenzie IR, et al. Dipeptide repeat protein pathology in C9ORF72 mutation cases: clinico-pathological correlations. Acta Neuropathol. 2013;126(6):859–79.
39. Schmid B, et al. Loss of ALS-associated TDP-43 in zebrafish causes muscle degeneration, vascular dysfunction, and reduced motor neuron axon outgrowth. Proc Natl Acad Sci U S A. 2013;110(13):4986–91.
40. Lee EB, Lee VM, Trojanowski JQ. Gains or losses: molecular mechanisms of TDP43-mediated neurodegeneration. Nat Rev Neurosci. 2012;13(1):38–50.
41. Gomez-Deza J, et al. Dipeptide repeat protein inclusions are rare in the spinal cord and almost absent from motor neurons in C9ORF72 mutant amyotrophic lateral sclerosis and are unlikely to cause their degeneration. Acta Neuropathol Commun. 2015;3(1):38.
42. Thisse C, Thisse B. High-resolution in situ hybridization to whole-mount zebrafish embryos. Nat Protoc. 2008;3(1):59–69.

Permissions

All chapters in this book were first published in MN, by BioMed Central; hereby published with permission under the Creative Commons Attribution License or equivalent. Every chapter published in this book has been scrutinized by our experts. Their significance has been extensively debated. The topics covered herein carry significant findings which will fuel the growth of the discipline. They may even be implemented as practical applications or may be referred to as a beginning point for another development.

The contributors of this book come from diverse backgrounds, making this book a truly international effort. This book will bring forth new frontiers with its revolutionizing research information and detailed analysis of the nascent developments around the world.

We would like to thank all the contributing authors for lending their expertise to make the book truly unique. They have played a crucial role in the development of this book. Without their invaluable contributions this book wouldn't have been possible. They have made vital efforts to compile up to date information on the varied aspects of this subject to make this book a valuable addition to the collection of many professionals and students.

This book was conceptualized with the vision of imparting up-to-date information and advanced data in this field. To ensure the same, a matchless editorial board was set up. Every individual on the board went through rigorous rounds of assessment to prove their worth. After which they invested a large part of their time researching and compiling the most relevant data for our readers.

The editorial board has been involved in producing this book since its inception. They have spent rigorous hours researching and exploring the diverse topics which have resulted in the successful publishing of this book. They have passed on their knowledge of decades through this book. To expedite this challenging task, the publisher supported the team at every step. A small team of assistant editors was also appointed to further simplify the editing procedure and attain best results for the readers.

Apart from the editorial board, the designing team has also invested a significant amount of their time in understanding the subject and creating the most relevant covers. They scrutinized every image to scout for the most suitable representation of the subject and create an appropriate cover for the book.

The publishing team has been an ardent support to the editorial, designing and production team. Their endless efforts to recruit the best for this project, has resulted in the accomplishment of this book. They are a veteran in the field of academics and their pool of knowledge is as vast as their experience in printing. Their expertise and guidance has proved useful at every step. Their uncompromising quality standards have made this book an exceptional effort. Their encouragement from time to time has been an inspiration for everyone.

The publisher and the editorial board hope that this book will prove to be a valuable piece of knowledge for researchers, students, practitioners and scholars across the globe.

List of Contributors

Peng Yin
State Key Laboratory of Molecular Developmental Biology, Institute of Genetics and Developmental Biology, Chinese Academy of Sciences, Beijing 100101, China

Guohao Wang
State Key Laboratory of Molecular Developmental Biology, Institute of Genetics and Developmental Biology, Chinese Academy of Sciences, Beijing 100101, China
Department of Human Genetics, Emory University School of Medicine, Atlanta, GA 30322, USA
University of Chinese Academy of Sciences, Beijing 100049, China

Sen Yan and Xiao-Jiang Li
State Key Laboratory of Molecular Developmental Biology, Institute of Genetics and Developmental Biology, Chinese Academy of Sciences, Beijing 100101, China
Department of Human Genetics, Emory University School of Medicine, Atlanta, GA 30322, USA

Huaqiang Yang, Bentian Zhao, Zhen Ouyang, Zhaoming Liu, Yu Zhao, Tao Liu, Nana Fan, Lin Guo and Liangxue Lai
Key Laboratory of Regenerative Biology, South China Institute for Stem Cell Biology and Regenerative Medicine, Guangzhou Institutes of Biomedicine and Health, Chinese Academy of Sciences, Guangzhou 510530, China

Chuan-En Wang and Shihua Li
Department of Human Genetics, Emory University School of Medicine, Atlanta, GA 30322, USA

Xudong Liu
State Key Laboratory of Molecular Developmental Biology, Institute of Genetics and Developmental Biology, Chinese Academy of Sciences, Beijing 100101, China
University of Chinese Academy of Sciences, Beijing 100049, China

Rebecca San Gil, Lezanne Ooi, Justin J. Yerbury and Heath Ecroyd
Illawarra Health and Medical Research Institute and School of Biological Sciences, University of Wollongong, Northfields Ave, Wollongong 2522, Australia

Honghuang Lin
National Heart Lung and Blood Institute's and Boston University's Framingham Heart Study, Framingham, MA, USA
Section of Computational Biomedicine, Department of Medicine, Boston University School of Medicine, 72 East Concord Street, B-616, Boston, MA 02118, USA

Alexa Beiser
National Heart Lung and Blood Institute's and Boston University's Framingham Heart Study, Framingham, MA, USA
Department of Neurology, Boston University School of Medicine, 72 East Concord Street, B-602, Boston, MA 02118, USA
Department of Biostatistics, Boston University School of Public Health, Boston, MA, USA

Claudia Satizabal and Sudha Seshadri
National Heart Lung and Blood Institute's and Boston University's Framingham Heart Study, Framingham, MA, USA
Department of Neurology, Boston University School of Medicine, 72 East Concord Street, B-602, Boston, MA 02118, USA

Zhijun Xie and Chengping Wen
College of Basic Medical Science, Zhejiang Chinese Medical University, Hangzhou, Zhejiang Province, China

Qiong Yang
Department of Biostatistics, Boston University School of Public Health, Boston, MA, USA

Daniel Levy and Tianxiao Huan
National Heart Lung and Blood Institute's and Boston University's Framingham Heart Study, Framingham, MA, USA
Population Sciences Branch, Division of Intramural Research, National Heart, Lung, and Blood Institute, Bethesda, MD, USA

Peter J. Munson
Mathematical and Statistical Computing Laboratory, Center for Information Technology, National Institute of Health, Bethesda, MD, USA

Roby Joehanes
Mathematical and Statistical Computing Laboratory, Center for Information Technology, National Institute of Health, Bethesda, MD, USA
Hebrew Senior Life, 1200 Centre Street Room #609, Boston, MA 02131, USA

Kimberly A. Fernandes and Michael P. Wilson
Department of Ophthalmology, Flaum Eye Institute, University of Rochester Medical Center, 601 Elmwood Ave, Rochester, NY 14642, USA

Stephanie B. Syc-Mazurek
Department of Ophthalmology, Flaum Eye Institute, University of Rochester Medical Center, 601 Elmwood Ave, Rochester, NY 14642, USA
Neuroscience Graduate Program, Rochester, USA

Peter Shrager
Department of Neuroscience, Rochester, USA

Richard T. Libby
Department of Ophthalmology, Flaum Eye Institute, University of Rochester Medical Center, 601 Elmwood Ave, Rochester, NY 14642, USA
Department of Biomedical Genetics, Rochester, USA
The Center for Visual Sciences, University of Rochester Medical Center, Rochester, NY 14642, USA

Daniela Diaz-Lucena
Network Center for Biomedical Research in Neurodegenerative Diseases (CIBERNED), Institute Carlos III, Ministry of Health, Feixa Llarga s/n, 08907 L'Hospitalet de Llobregat, Barcelona, Spain

Franc Llorens
Network Center for Biomedical Research in Neurodegenerative Diseases (CIBERNED), Institute Carlos III, Ministry of Health, Feixa Llarga s/n, 08907 L'Hospitalet de Llobregat, Barcelona, Spain
Department of Neurology, University Medical School, Göttingen, Germany

Matthias Schmitz and Inga Zerr
Department of Neurology, University Medical School, Göttingen, Germany
German Center for Neurodegenerative Diseases (DZNE), Göttingen, Germany

Waqas Tahir, Duru Ozbay, Susana Correia and Ângela Correia
Department of Neurology, University Medical School, Göttingen, Germany

Katrin Thüne
Network Center for Biomedical Research in Neurodegenerative Diseases (CIBERNED), Institute Carlos III, Ministry of Health, Feixa Llarga s/n, 08907 L'Hospitalet de Llobregat, Barcelona, Spain
German Center for Neurodegenerative Diseases (DZNE), Göttingen, Germany

Eirini Kanata, Eleni Kovatsi and Theodoros Sklaviadis
Laboratory of Pharmacology, School of Health Sciences, Department of Pharmacy, Aristotle University of Thessaloniki, Thessaloniki, Greece

Catharina Pleschka and Ina M. Vorberg
German Center for Neurodegenerative Diseases (DZNE), Bonn, Germany

Paula Garcia-Esparcia and Isidro Ferrer
Network Center for Biomedical Research in Neurodegenerative Diseases (CIBERNED), Institute Carlos III, Ministry of Health, Feixa Llarga s/n, 08907 L'Hospitalet de Llobregat, Barcelona, Spain
Bellvitge University Hospital-IDIBELL, Department of Pathology and Experimental Therapeutics, University of Barcelona, Hospitalet de Llobregat, Spain

Ira Milosevic
European Neuroscience Institute, Göttingen, Germany

Olivier Andréoletti
Institut National de la Recherche Agronomique/ Ecole Nationale Vétérinaire, Toulouse, France

Natalia Fernández-Borges and Juan Maria Torres
Centro de Investigación en Sanidad Animal (CISA-INIA), Madrid, Spain

Markus Glatzel and Susanne Krasemann
Institute of Neuropathology, University Medical Center Hamburg-Eppendorf, Hamburg, Germany

Raquel Sánchez-Valle
Alzheimer's Disease and Other Cognitive Disorders Unit, Neurology Department, Hospital Clínic, Institut d'Investigacions Biomediques August Pi i Sunyer (IDIBAPS), Barcelona, Spain

Konstantinos Xanthopoulos
Laboratory of Pharmacology, School of Health Sciences, Department of Pharmacy, Aristotle University of Thessaloniki, Thessaloniki, Greece
Unit of Lymphoid Malignancies, Division of Experimental Oncology, San Raffaele Scientific Institute, Milan, Italy

Shi Chen
Brain center, Zhongnan Hospital, Wuhan University, Wuhan, Hubei 430071, China
Taihe Hospital, Hubei University of Medicine, Shiyan, Hubei 442000, China

Zhiqiang Deng
Brain center, Zhongnan Hospital, Wuhan University, Wuhan, Hubei 430071, China
Taihe Hospital, Hubei University of Medicine, Shiyan, Hubei 442000, China
Department of Neurology, The Friedman Brain Institute, Icahn School of Medicine at Mount Sinai, New York 10029, USA

Zhenyu Yue and Patricia Sheehan
Department of Neurology, The Friedman Brain Institute, Icahn School of Medicine at Mount Sinai, New York 10029, USA

Jia Yu
Institute for Geriatrics and Rehabilitation, Beijing Geriatric Hospital, Beijing University of Chinese Medicine, Beijing 100095, People's Republic of China
Transgenic Section, Laboratory of Neurogenetics, National Institute on Aging, National Institutes of Health, Building 35, Room 1A112, MSC 3707, 35 Convent Drive, Bethesda, MD 20892-3707, USA

Chengsong Xie, Lixin Sun and Huaibin Cai
Transgenic Section, Laboratory of Neurogenetics, National Institute on Aging, National Institutes of Health, Building 35, Room 1A112, MSC 3707, 35 Convent Drive, Bethesda, MD 20892-3707, USA

Jinhui Ding
Computational Biology Core, Laboratory of Neurogenetics, National Institute on Aging, National Institutes of Health, Bethesda, MD 20892, USA

Yan Li
NINDS Protein/PeptideSequencing Facility, National Institute of Neurological Disorders and Stroke, National Institutes of Health, Bethesda, MD 20892, USA

Chen La
Transgenic Section, Laboratory of Neurogenetics, National Institute on Aging, National Institutes of Health, Building 35, Room 1A112, MSC 3707, 35 Convent Drive, Bethesda, MD 20892-3707, USA
Symptom Management Branch, National Institute of Nursing Research,
National Institutes of Health, Bethesda, MD 20892, USA

Hoon Shim
Transgenic Section, Laboratory of Neurogenetics, National Institute on Aging, National Institutes of Health, Building 35, Room 1A112, MSC 3707, 35 Convent Drive, Bethesda, MD 20892-3707, USA
Department of Anesthesiology, Albert Einstein College of Medicine, Bronx, New York 10467, USA

Cai-Xia Long
Transgenic Section, Laboratory of Neurogenetics, National Institute on Aging, National Institutes of Health, Building 35, Room 1A112, MSC 3707, 35 Convent Drive, Bethesda, MD 20892-3707, USA
Dendrite Morphogenesis and Plasticity Unit, National Institute of Neurological Disorders and Stroke, National Institutes of Health, Bethesda, MD 20892, USA

Li Zhong, Zongqi Wang, Daxin Wang, Zhe Wang, Linbei Wu, Ying Xu, Kai Wang, Jianguo Li, Ruizhi Huang and Dan Can
Fujian Provincial Key Laboratory of Neurodegenerative Disease and Aging Research, Institute of Neuroscience, Medical College, Xiamen University, Xiamen 361102, China

Guojun Bu
Fujian Provincial Key Laboratory of Neurodegenerative Disease and Aging Research, Institute of Neuroscience, Medical College, Xiamen University, Xiamen 361102, China
Department of Neuroscience, Mayo Clinic, Jacksonville, FL 32224, USA

Yuka A. Martens
Department of Neuroscience, Mayo Clinic, Jacksonville, FL 32224, USA

Olga C. Rodriguez
Lombardi Comprehensive Cancer Center, Department of Oncology, Georgetown University Medical Center, Washington, DC 20057, USA

Huaxi Xu
Fujian Provincial Key Laboratory of Neurodegenerative Disease and Aging Research, Institute of Neuroscience, Medical College, Xiamen University, Xiamen 361102, China
Neuroscience Initiative, Sanford Burnham Prebys Medical Discovery Institute, La Jolla, CA 92037, USA

Xiao-Fen Chen
Fujian Provincial Key Laboratory of Neurodegenerative Disease and Aging Research, Institute of Neuroscience, Medical College, Xiamen University, Xiamen 361102, China
Shenzhen Research Institute of Xiamen University, Shenzhen 518063, China

Bevan S. Main, Sonia Villapol, Stephanie S. Sloley, David J. Barton, Maia Parsadanian, Chinyere Agbaegbu, Kathryn Stefos, Mondona S. McCann and Patricia M. Washington
Laboratory for Brain Injury and Dementia, Department of Neuroscience, Georgetown University Medical Center, Washington, DC 20057, USA

Mark P. Burns
Laboratory for Brain Injury and Dementia, Department of Neuroscience, Georgetown University Medical Center, Washington, DC 20057, USA
Department of Neuroscience, Georgetown University Medical Center, New Research Building-EG11, 3970 Reservoir Rd, NW, Washington, D.C 20057, USA

Yingxue Ren, Joseph S. Reddy, Xue Wang and Yan W. Asmann
Department of Health Sciences Research, Mayo Clinic, Jacksonville, FL, USA

Marka van Blitterswijk, Mariet Allen, Minerva M. Carrasquillo, Dennis W. Dickson and Rosa Rademakers
Department of Neuroscience, Mayo Clinic, Jacksonville, FL, USA

Thomas G. Beach
Civin Laboratory for Neuropathology, Banner Sun Health Research Institute, Sun City, AZ, USA

Nilüfer Ertekin-Taner
Department of Neuroscience, Mayo Clinic, Jacksonville, FL, USA
Department of Neurology, Mayo Clinic, Jacksonville, FL, USA

Neil T. Sprenkle, Savannah G. Sims and Cristina L. Sánchez
Department of Microbiology, Immunology and Cell Biology, West Virginia University School of Medicine, One Medical Center Drive, BMRC, Morgantown, WV 311, USA

Gordon P. Meares
Department of Microbiology, Immunology and Cell Biology, West Virginia University School of Medicine, One Medical Center Drive, BMRC, Morgantown, WV 311, USA
Blanchette Rockefeller Neurosciences Institute, West Virginia University School of Medicine, Morgantown, WV, USA

Chaoran Ma and Xiang Gao
Department of Nutritional Sciences, The Pennsylvania State University, University Park, PA 16802, USA

Zhaoxue Yin and Jiesi Luo
Division of Chronic Disease Control and Community Health, Chinese Center for Disease Control and Prevention, Beijing 102206, China

Pengfei Zhu and Xiaoming Shi
National Institute of Environmental Health, Chinese Center for Disease Control and Prevention, Beijing 100021, China

Zachary A. Sorrentino, Vincent Hudson III and Nicola J. Rutherford
Department of Neuroscience, University of Florida, 1275 Center Drive, Gainesville, FL 32610, USA
Center for Translational Research in Neurodegenerative Disease, University of Florida, Gainesville, FL 32610, USA

Todd E. Golde, Benoit I. Giasson and Paramita Chakrabarty
Department of Neuroscience, University of Florida, 1275 Center Drive, Gainesville, FL 32610, USA
Center for Translational Research in Neurodegenerative Disease, University of Florida, Gainesville, FL 32610, USA
McKnight Brain Institute, University of Florida, Gainesville, FL 32610, USA

Mieu M. T. Brooks
Department of Neuroscience, University of Florida, 1275 Center Drive, Gainesville, FL 32610, USA
Center for Translational Research in Neurodegenerative Disease, University of Florida, Gainesville, FL 32610, USA
Department of Neuroscience, Mayo Clinic, Jacksonville, FL -32224, USA

Andrea Wenninger-Weinzierl and Alexander Hruscha
German Center for Neurodegenerative Diseases (DZNE), Feodor-Lynen-Str.17, 81377 Munich, Germany

Dieter Edbauer and Bettina Schmid
German Center for Neurodegenerative Diseases (DZNE), Feodor-Lynen-Str.17, 81377 Munich, Germany
Munich Cluster for Systems Neurology (SyNergy), Feodor-Lynen-Str.17, 81377 Munich, Germany

Yu Ohki
German Center for Neurodegenerative Diseases (DZNE), Feodor-Lynen-Str.17, 81377 Munich, Germany
Biomedical Center, Biochemistry, Ludwig-Maximilians University Munich, Feodor-Lynen-Str.17, 81377 Munich, Germany

Kazuhide Asakawa and Koichi Kawakami
Division of Molecular and Developmental Biology, National Institute of Genetics, Mishima, Shizuoka 411-8540, Japan

Christian Haass
German Center for Neurodegenerative Diseases (DZNE), Feodor-Lynen-Str.17, 81377 Munich, Germany
Biomedical Center, Biochemistry, Ludwig-Maximilians University Munich, Feodor-Lynen-Str.17, 81377 Munich, Germany
Munich Cluster for Systems Neurology (SyNergy), Feodor-Lynen-Str.17, 81377 Munich, Germany

Index

A

Amyotrophic Lateral Sclerosis, 1, 18-21, 28, 36-40, 65, 83, 85, 90, 92-95, 97, 111-112, 144, 152-153, 159, 161, 165, 168-169, 195, 204-205

Apolipoprotein-e, 125-126, 140

Astroglia, 21-22, 24, 26-36, 83, 188, 190, 194

Astroglial Cells, 24

Astrogliosis, 27, 72, 79-80, 103-104, 141, 184-186, 188, 190-191

Axonal Degeneration, 51, 57, 59-62, 93, 162

B

Bicinchoninic Acid, 101

Blood Brain Barrier, 125-126, 141, 162, 165

C

Casein Kinase 2, 88, 92

Cerebral Cortex, 1, 64, 67, 69-70, 72, 74-75, 102, 142, 149

Cerebrospinal Fluid, 53, 61, 64, 82-84, 126, 140-142

Chitinase 3-like 1, 64-65, 68, 82-83

Controlled Cortical Impact, 79, 83, 125-126, 140-142

Cyclophilin A, 125-126, 132, 140-141

Cytoplasmic Accumulation, 1-2, 16, 91, 106

D

Dementia, 38, 41, 43-44, 48-49, 64-66, 68, 74-76, 78, 80, 82-83, 85, 90, 92-95, 114, 125, 140-141, 143, 152, 159, 169-171, 173, 176-177, 204-205

Dual Leucine Kinase, 52, 55, 61-62

Dynein, 96-97, 101-102, 106-109, 111-112

E

Endoplasmic Reticulum Stress, 40, 51, 59, 62-63, 153, 165-169, 200

Entorhinal Cortex, 179, 182, 185, 188, 190, 192

Ependymal Cells, 179, 182, 184, 192

F

False Discovery Rate, 42, 44, 48, 50, 145, 152

Fibrillar Astrocytes, 64, 69, 74

Frontotemporal Dementia, 38, 65, 82-83, 85, 92-95, 143, 152, 169, 204-205

Frontotemporal Lobar Degeneration, 1, 18-19, 92-94, 143-144, 152, 195

G

Gene Expression, 1-2, 15-16, 27, 37, 41-46, 48-49, 56, 67, 93, 141, 143-145, 147, 149-152, 157, 161, 164

Glaucoma, 51-52, 55-57, 59-63

Glial Fibrillary Acidic Protein, 28, 36, 83, 99, 181, 193

Glutamate Receptor, 96, 108, 111

Granule Cell Layer, 103

Guanine Nucleotide Exchange Factor, 86, 90, 92, 95

H

Heat Shock Response, 21-22, 36-40

High-density Lipoprotein Cholesterol, 170

Huntington's Disease, 2, 19, 21, 24, 26, 36, 38, 40, 93, 97, 169

Hyperthermia, 23-24, 32, 37-39

L

Lewy Bodies, 64, 82-83, 160, 180

Low-density Lipoprotein, 114, 170, 177

M

Magnetic Resonance Imaging, 41, 49, 127, 140, 142

Matrix Metallopeptidase-9, 125-126

Microglia, 27, 31, 38-39, 79, 83-84, 105, 113-114, 116-118, 120-124, 141-142, 146-147, 152-154, 162-165, 169, 184, 191, 194

Mitogen-activated Protein Kinase, 51-52, 55, 61-62

Motor Neurons, 1, 3, 6, 9-10, 19, 21, 28-39, 85, 87, 91-92, 95-96, 102, 105, 107-108, 111, 161-162, 205

Multiple Sclerosis, 65, 82-83, 153, 159, 162, 165, 169

N

Neurodegenerative Diseases, 21, 36-39, 51-52, 57, 59, 62, 64, 78-79, 81-82, 91, 93-94, 109, 111, 113, 123, 144, 151-153, 158-159, 161, 163-165, 168, 193, 195, 204

Neuromuscular Junction, 96

Neuronal Cells, 1-2, 8, 14, 29, 87, 91, 99, 124, 190, 192

Neurovascular Unit, 60, 125-126, 140

O

Optic Nerve Crush, 51, 53, 61

Optineurin, 28, 36, 87, 89-90, 92-94

P

Paraformaldehyde, 18, 53, 61, 99, 115, 203

Parkinson's Disease, 64, 82, 97, 111, 141, 152-153, 159-160, 165, 167-168, 180, 193-194

Pericyte, 125, 132-133, 135-136, 138-142

Phosphate Buffered Saline, 53, 67, 99, 203

Postsynaptic Density, 100-101, 107-110

Prion Protein Gene, 68

Progranulin, 143-144, 152

Protein Homeostasis, 21, 36, 40, 85, 88, 92-93, 95, 159

R

Rapamycin Complex 1, 62, 86, 90, 92

Retinal Ganglion Cell, 51, 61-63

S

Sigma Receptor-1, 89-90, 92, 95

Single Nucleotide Polymorphisms, 143

Somatic Cell Nuclear Transfer, 2

Spinal Motor Neurons, 87, 95-96, 105, 107-108, 111

Splicing Factor Proline, 2-3

Sporadic Creutzfeldt-jakob Disease, 64, 82-83

Striatal Neurons, 21, 25-28, 36, 96, 99-100, 103, 184

Substantia Nigra Pars Compacta, 100, 103

Superoxide Dismutase 1, 18, 22, 36, 38-40, 89, 92, 95, 169

Surface Plasmon Resonance, 113, 116, 122-123

T

Thioflavin, 65

Total Intracranial Volume, 42, 48

Transmembrane Protein 106b, 143-144

Traumatic Brain Injury, 61, 63, 65, 78, 81, 83, 125-126, 140-142, 164-165, 169

Traumatic Optic Neuropathies, 51-52

Triglycerides, 44, 170, 177

U

Ubiquitin-proteasome System, 10, 38, 85, 94

Unfolded Protein Response, 29, 38-39, 60-63, 153, 165-169

V

Valosin-contain Protein, 90

Vascular Dementia, 64-65, 82-83

W

Western Blot, 3, 5, 7-8, 10-11, 13, 15, 17, 53-56, 61, 65, 67, 69, 72, 74-75, 80, 98, 100-101, 107-108, 110, 127, 132, 135, 204

White Matter Hyperintensities, 41, 48-50, 178

CPSIA information can be obtained
at www.ICGtesting.com
Printed in the USA
BVHW011050090222
628494BV00003B/173

9 781639 272778